Clinical Pharmacokinetics

Review Articles

Non-Opiate Abused Drugs

Therapeutic Monitoring of Cyclosporin

Saturable Kinetics in Renal Drug Excretion

Original Research Article

Nisoldipine Kinetics and Effects in Renal Failure

January 1989
Vol. 16, No. 1 (pp. 1-64)

CPKNDH (1) 1-64 (1989)
ISSN: 0312-5963

USA • JAPAN • UNITED KINGDOM • HONG KONG • AUSTRALIA • NEW ZEALAND

Clinical Pharmacokinetics

Contents Vol. 16, No. 1, 1989

Review Articles

Drug Disposition

1-26 Clinical Pharmacokinetics of Non-Opiate Abused Drugs
Busto, U.; Bendayan, R. and *Sellers, E.M.*

Drug Concentration Monitoring

27-37 Therapeutic Drug Monitoring of Cyclosporin: Practical Applications and Limitations
Rodighiero, V.

Clinical Pharmacokinetic Concepts

38-54 Saturable Pharmacokinetics in the Renal Excretion of Drugs
van Ginneken, C.A.M. and *Russel, F.G.M.*

Original Research Article

55-64 Influence of Renal Function on the Pharmacokinetics and Cardiovascular Effects of Nisoldipine After Single and Multiple Dosing
van Harten, J.; Burggraaf, J.; van Brummelen, P. and *Breimer, D.D.*

Clinical Pharmacokinetics is indexed in 'Current Contents', 'Index Medicus' and 'Excerpta Medica'.

Clinical Pharmacokinetics

Aim and Scope: The Journal aims to assist in the further development of clinical pharmacokinetics, to promote communication and increased awareness within this specialty area and to further postgraduate education in clinical pharmacology and therapeutics. The Journal places particular emphasis on review articles but also welcomes original research articles. Both types of article consider the pharmacokinetic properties of drugs as related to their actual clinical use. This definition includes bioavailability studies, drug pharmacokinetics, plasma concentration monitoring of pharmacodynamic response, the relationship of drug pharmacokinetics to the therapeutic efficacy or toxicity of drugs etc. – all studied within the context of disease, pregnancy, age or other clinical and pathophysiological determinants of drug response.

Submitted manuscripts of original research in clinical pharmacokinetics will be promptly considered for publication. Shorter communications (up to 2,000 words) will, because of their length, have priority for rapid publication. However, longer manuscripts will also be considered, particularly those which include a review of previous literature in the area of study; their publication will not necessarily be delayed. Priority will also be given to papers dealing with the relationship of pharmacokinetics to pharmacodynamic responses. Experimental data must be obtained from humans and relate to treatment of disease or to pathophysiological determinants of drug use. Animal or *in vitro* investigations and data from healthy human volunteers can be included only if they are relevant to the clinical pharmacokinetic problem under investigation. Studies conducted in healthy volunteers will only be considered if they offer major new findings or re-evaluate kinetics using improved methods of analysis.

Manuscripts: All enquiries relating to the editorial content of *Clinical Pharmacokinetics* should be directed to the Editor: George J. Mammen, ADIS Press Ltd, Private Bag, Mairangi Bay, Auckland 10, New Zealand. *Information for authors* appears on the back 2 pages of each issue.

Subscriptions: Two volumes are published annually with 6 issues per volume. The annual subscription price is North & South America $US420; Europe SwF650; rest of the world $US420. Subscriptions may be ordered from the office of ADIS Press most convenient to you, or through any bookseller or subscription agent. A subscription to *Clinical Pharmacokinetics* is accepted on the express condition that it will be used only internally, within an institution, company or national affiliate confined to one geographical location, and will not be copied and/or circulated outside these limits. An order for *Clinical Pharmacokinetics* constitutes an undertaking by the subscriber to comply with this condition.

Nth & Sth America	ADIS Press International Inc., Suite B-30, Oxford Court Business Center, 582 Middletown Boulevard, Langhorne, PA 19047, USA. Tel.: PA (215) 752-4500.
Europe	ADIS Press International Ltd (European Branch), Suite 15C, Manchester International Office Centre, Styal Rd, Wythenshawe, Manchester M22 5WL, England. Tel.: (61) 436-6428.
Japan (orders)	ADIS Press, c/- Maruzen Co., Ltd, 3-10 Nihonbashi 2-Chome, Chuo-ku, Tokyo 103, Japan. Tel.: Tokyo (3) 272-7211.
Japan (enquiries)	ADIS Press Limited (Representative Office), 4-38 Minamimori-machi 2-chome, Kita-ku, Osaka 530, Japan. Tel.: Osaka (6) 365-0709.
Australia	ADIS Press Australasia Pty Ltd, P.O. Box 132, Balgowlah, NSW 2093, Australia. Tel.: Sydney 949-2022.
New Zealand	ADIS Press Limited, Private Bag, Mairangi Bay, Auckland 10, New Zealand. Tel.: Auckland (09) 479-8100.
Rest of World	ADIS Press Publications Limited, 18/F Tung Sun Commercial Centre, 194-200 Lockhart Road, Wanchai, Hong Kong. Tel.: Hong Kong (5) 8920-633.

USA Postmasters: Send address changes to ADIS Press International Inc., Suite B-30, Oxford Court B-30, Oxford Court Business Center, 582 Middletown Blvd, Langhorne, PA 19047. Air freight and mailing in the USA by Publications Expediting Inc., 200 Meacham Avenue, Elmont, NY 11003.

Clinical Pharmacokinetics (ISSN 0312-5963) is published monthly by ADIS Press Limited, 41 Centorian Drive, Private Bag, Mairangi Bay, Auckland 10, New Zealand. Second class postage is paid at Jamaica, NY 11431. Printed in Hong Kong by Caritas Printing Training Centre.

Clinical Pharmacokinetics

Contents Vol. 16, No. 2, 1989

Leading Article

65-73 **Protein Binding Drug Displacement Interactions: Fact or Fiction?**
MacKichan, J.J.

Review Articles

Drug Disposition
74-85 Clinical Pharmacokinetics of Clofazimine: A Review
Holdiness, M.R.

Clinical Pharmacokinetics and Disease Processes
86-99 Clinical Pharmacokinetics and Therapeutic Use of Hydralazine in Congestive Heart Failure
Mulrow, J.P. and *Crawford, M.H.*

Pharmacokinetic-Pharmacodynamic Relationships
100-128 Pharmacokinetic-Pharmacodynamic Relationships of Oral Hypoglycaemic Agents: An Update
Marchetti, P. and *Navalesi, R.*

Clinical Pharmacokinetics is indexed in 'Current Contents', 'Index Medicus' and 'Excerpta Medica'.

Clinical Pharmacokinetics

Aim and Scope: The Journal aims to assist in the further development of clinical pharmacokinetics, to promote communication and increased awareness within this specialty area and to further postgraduate education in clinical pharmacology and therapeutics. The Journal places particular emphasis on review articles but also welcomes original research articles. Both types of article consider the pharmacokinetic properties of drugs as related to their actual clinical use. This definition includes bioavailability studies, drug pharmacokinetics, plasma concentration monitoring of pharmacodynamic response, the relationship of drug pharmacokinetics to the therapeutic efficacy or toxicity of drugs etc. – all studied within the context of disease, pregnancy, age or other clinical and pathophysiological determinants of drug response.

Submitted manuscripts of original research in clinical pharmacokinetics will be promptly considered for publication. Shorter communications (up to 2,000 words) will, because of their length, have priority for rapid publication. However, longer manuscripts will also be considered, particularly those which include a review of previous literature in the area of study; their publication will not necessarily be delayed. Priority will also be given to papers dealing with the relationship of pharmacokinetics to pharmacodynamic responses. Experimental data must be obtained from humans and relate to treatment of disease or to pathophysiological determinants of drug use. Animal or *in vitro* investigations and data from healthy human volunteers can be included only if they are relevant to the clinical pharmacokinetic problem under investigation. Studies conducted in healthy volunteers will only be considered if they offer major new findings or re-evaluate kinetics using improved methods of analysis.

Manuscripts: All enquiries relating to the editorial content of *Clinical Pharmacokinetics* should be directed to the Editor: George J. Mammen, ADIS Press Ltd, Private Bag, Mairangi Bay, Auckland 10, New Zealand. *Information for authors* appears on the back 2 pages of each issue.

Subscriptions: Two volumes are published annually with 6 issues per volume. The annual subscription price is North & South America $US420; Europe SwF650; rest of the world $US420. Subscriptions may be ordered from the office of ADIS Press most convenient to you, or through any bookseller or subscription agent. A subscription to *Clinical Pharmacokinetics* is accepted on the express condition that it will be used only internally, within an institution, company or national affiliate confined to one geographical location, and will not be copied and/or circulated outside these limits. An order for *Clinical Pharmacokinetics* constitutes an undertaking by the subscriber to comply with this condition.

Nth & Sth America	ADIS Press International Inc., Suite B-30, Oxford Court Business Center, 582 Middletown Boulevard, Langhorne, PA 19047, USA. Tel.: PA (215) 752-4500.
Europe	ADIS Press International Ltd (European Branch), Suite 15C, Manchester International Office Centre, Styal Rd, Wythenshawe, Manchester M22 5WL, England. Tel.: (61) 436-6428.
Japan (orders)	ADIS Press, c/- Maruzen Co., Ltd, 3-10 Nihonbashi 2-Chome, Chuo-ku, Tokyo 103, Japan. Tel.: Tokyo (3) 272-7211.
Japan (enquiries)	ADIS Press Limited (Representative Office), 4-38 Minamimori-machi 2-chome, Kita-ku, Osaka 530, Japan. Tel.: Osaka (6) 365-0709.
Australia	ADIS Press Australasia Pty Ltd, P.O. Box 132, Balgowlah, NSW 2093, Australia. Tel.: Sydney (02) 949-2022.
New Zealand	ADIS Press Limited, Private Bag, Mairangi Bay, Auckland 10, New Zealand. Tel.: Auckland (09) 479-8100.
Rest of World	ADIS Press Publications Limited, 18/F Tung Sun Commercial Centre, 194-200 Lockhart Road, Wanchai, Hong Kong. Tel.: Hong Kong (5) 8920-633.

USA Postmasters: Send address changes to ADIS Press International Inc., Suite B-30, Oxford Court B-30, Oxford Court Business Center, 582 Middletown Blvd, Langhorne, PA 19047. Air freight and mailing in the USA by Publications Expediting Inc., 200 Meacham Avenue, Elmont, NY 11003.

Clinical Pharmacokinetics (ISSN 0312-5963) is published monthly by ADIS Press Limited, 41 Centorian Drive, Private Bag, Mairangi Bay, Auckland 10, New Zealand. Second class postage is paid at Jamaica, NY 11431. Printed in Hong Kong by Caritas Printing Training Centre.

Clinical Pharmacokinetics

Contents Vol. 16, No. 3, 1989

Leading Article

129-133 Clinical Significance of Differences in Bioavailability of Medroxyprogesterone Acetate Preparations
Stockdale, A.D. and *Rostom, A.Y.*

Review Articles

Clinical Pharmacokinetics and Disease Processes

134-161 Clinical Pharmacokinetics in Organ Transplant Patients
Venkataramanan, R.; Habucky, K.; Burckart, G.J. and *Ptachcinski, R.J.*

Pharmacokinetic Drug Interactions

162-179 Food Interactions with Sustained-Release Theophylline Preparations: A Review
Jonkman, J.H.G.

Original Research Articles

180-185 Lack of Effect of Influenza Vaccine on the Pharmacokinetics of Antipyrine, Alprazolam, Paracetamol (Acetaminophen) and Lorazepam
Scavone, J.M.; Blyden, G.T. and *Greenblatt, D.J.*

186-191 Tianeptine and its Main Metabolite: Pharmacokinetics in Chronic Alcoholism and Cirrhosis
Royer, R.J.; Royer-Morrot, M.J.; Paille, F.; Barrucand, D.; Schmitt, J.; Defrance, R. and *Salvadori, C.*

Clinical Pharmacokinetics is indexed in 'Current Contents', 'Index Medicus' and 'Excerpta Medica'.

Clinical Pharmacokinetics

Aim and Scope: The Journal aims to assist in the further development of clinical pharmacokinetics, to promote communication and increased awareness within this specialty area and to further postgraduate education in clinical pharmacology and therapeutics. The Journal places particular emphasis on review articles but also welcomes original research articles. Both types of article consider the pharmacokinetic properties of drugs as related to their actual clinical use. This definition includes bioavailability studies, drug pharmacokinetics, plasma concentration monitoring of pharmacodynamic response, the relationship of drug pharmacokinetics to the therapeutic efficacy or toxicity of drugs etc. – all studied within the context of disease, pregnancy, age or other clinical and pathophysiological determinants of drug response.

Submitted manuscripts of original research in clinical pharmacokinetics will be promptly considered for publication. Shorter communications (up to 2,000 words) will, because of their length, have priority for rapid publication. However, longer manuscripts will also be considered, particularly those which include a review of previous literature in the area of study; their publication will not necessarily be delayed. Priority will also be given to papers dealing with the relationship of pharmacokinetics to pharmacodynamic responses. Experimental data must be obtained from humans and relate to treatment of disease or to pathophysiological determinants of drug use. Animal or *in vitro* investigations and data from healthy human volunteers can be included only if they are relevant to the clinical pharmacokinetic problem under investigation. Studies conducted in healthy volunteers will only be considered if they offer major new findings or re-evaluate kinetics using improved methods of analysis.

Manuscripts: All enquiries relating to the editorial content of *Clinical Pharmacokinetics* should be directed to the Editor: George J. Mammen, ADIS Press Ltd, Private Bag, Mairangi Bay, Auckland 10, New Zealand. *Information for authors* appears on the back 2 pages of each issue.

Subscriptions: Two volumes are published annually with 6 issues per volume. The annual subscription price is North & South America $US420; Europe SwF650; rest of the world $US420. Subscriptions may be ordered from the office of ADIS Press most convenient to you, or through any bookseller or subscription agent. A subscription to *Clinical Pharmacokinetics* is accepted on the express condition that it will be used only internally, within an institution, company or national affiliate confined to one geographical location, and will not be copied and/or circulated outside these limits. An order for *Clinical Pharmacokinetics* constitutes an undertaking by the subscriber to comply with this condition.

Nth & Sth America	ADIS Press International Inc., Suite B-30, Oxford Court Business Center, 582 Middletown Boulevard, Langhorne, PA 19047, USA. Tel.: PA (215) 752-4500.
Europe	ADIS Press International Ltd (European Branch), Suite 15C, Manchester International Office Centre, Styal Rd, Wythenshawe, Manchester M22 5WL, England. Tel.: (61) 436-6428.
Japan (orders)	ADIS Press, c/- Maruzen Co., Ltd, 3-10 Nihonbashi 2-Chome, Chuo-ku, Tokyo 103, Japan. Tel.: Tokyo (3) 272-7211.
Japan (enquiries)	ADIS Press Limited (Representative Office), 4-38 Minamimori-machi 2-chome, Kita-ku, Osaka 530, Japan. Tel.: Osaka (6) 365-0709.
Australia	ADIS Press Australasia Pty Ltd, P.O. Box 132, Balgowlah, NSW 2093, Australia. Tel.: Sydney (02) 949-2022.
New Zealand	ADIS Press Limited, Private Bag, Mairangi Bay, Auckland 10, New Zealand. Tel.: Auckland (09) 479-8100.
Rest of World	ADIS Press Publications Limited, 18/F Tung Sun Commercial Centre, 194-200 Lockhart Road, Wanchai, Hong Kong. Tel.: Hong Kong (5) 8920-633.

USA Postmasters: Send address changes to ADIS Press International Inc., Suite B-30, Oxford Court Business Center, 582 Middletown Blvd, Langhorne, PA 19047. Air freight and mailing in the USA by Publications Expediting Inc., 200 Meacham Avenue, Elmont, NY 11003.

Clinical Pharmacokinetics (ISSN 0312-5963) is published monthly by ADIS Press Limited, 41 Centorian Drive, Private Bag, Mairangi Bay, Auckland 10, New Zealand. Second class postage is paid at Jamaica, NY 11431. Printed in Hong Kong by Caritas Printing Training Centre.

Clinical Pharmacokinetics

Contents Vol. 16, No. 4, 1989

Review Articles

Drug Disposition

193-214 Clinical Pharmacokinetic Properties of the Macrolide Antibiotics: Effects of Age and Various Pathophysiological States (Part I)
Periti, P.; Mazzei, T.; Mini, E. and *Novelli, A.*

215-237 Clinical Pharmacology of 5-Fluorouracil
Diasio, R.B. and *Harris, B.E.*

Pharmacokinetic-Pharmacodynamic Relationships

238-253 Clinical Pharmacokinetic Considerations in the Control of Oral Anticoagulant Therapy
Shetty, H.G.M.; Fennerty, A.G. and *Routledge, P.A.*

Original Research Article

254-260 Phenytoin Dosage Predictions in Paediatric Patients
Yuen, G.J.; Latimer, P.T.; Littlefield, L.C. and *Mackey, R.W.*

Clinical Pharmacokinetics is indexed in 'Current Contents', 'Index Medicus' and 'Excerpta Medica'.

Clinical Pharmacokinetics

Aim and Scope: The Journal aims to assist in the further development of clinical pharmacokinetics, to promote communication and increased awareness within this specialty area and to further postgraduate education in clinical pharmacology and therapeutics. The Journal places particular emphasis on review articles but also welcomes original research articles. Both types of article consider the pharmacokinetic properties of drugs as related to their actual clinical use. This definition includes bioavailability studies, drug pharmacokinetics, plasma concentration monitoring of pharmacodynamic response, the relationship of drug pharmacokinetics to the therapeutic efficacy or toxicity of drugs etc. – all studied within the context of disease, pregnancy, age or other clinical and pathophysiological determinants of drug response.

Submitted manuscripts of original research in clinical pharmacokinetics will be promptly considered for publication. Shorter communications (up to 2,000 words) will, because of their length, have priority for rapid publication. However, longer manuscripts will also be considered, particularly those which include a review of previous literature in the area of study; their publication will not necessarily be delayed. Priority will also be given to papers dealing with the relationship of pharmacokinetics to pharmacodynamic responses. Experimental data must be obtained from humans and relate to treatment of disease or to pathophysiological determinants of drug use. Animal or *in vitro* investigations and data from healthy human volunteers can be included only if they are relevant to the clinical pharmacokinetic problem under investigation. Studies conducted in healthy volunteers will only be considered if they offer major new findings or re-evaluate kinetics using improved methods of analysis.

Manuscripts: All enquiries relating to the editorial content of *Clinical Pharmacokinetics* should be directed to the Editor: George J. Mammen, ADIS Press Ltd, Private Bag, Mairangi Bay, Auckland 10, New Zealand. *Information for authors* appears on the back 2 pages of each issue.

Subscriptions: Two volumes are published annually with 6 issues per volume. The annual subscription price is North & South America $US420; Europe SwF650; rest of the world $US420. Subscriptions may be ordered from the office of ADIS Press most convenient to you, or through any bookseller or subscription agent. A subscription to *Clinical Pharmacokinetics* is accepted on the express condition that it will be used only internally, within an institution, company or national affiliate confined to one geographical location, and will not be copied and/or circulated outside these limits. An order for *Clinical Pharmacokinetics* constitutes an undertaking by the subscriber to comply with this condition.

Nth & Sth America	ADIS Press International Inc., Suite B-30, Oxford Court Business Center, 582 Middletown Boulevard, Langhorne, PA 19047, USA. Tel.: PA (215) 752-4500.
Europe	ADIS Press International Ltd (European Branch), Suite 15C, Manchester International Office Centre, Styal Rd, Wythenshawe, Manchester M22 5WL, England. Tel.: (61) 436-6428.
Japan (orders)	ADIS Press, c/- Maruzen Co., Ltd, 3-10 Nihonbashi 2-Chome, Chuo-ku, Tokyo 103, Japan. Tel.: Tokyo (3) 272-7211.
Japan (enquiries)	ADIS Press Limited (Representative Office), 4-38 Minamimori-machi 2-chome, Kita-ku, Osaka 530, Japan. Tel.: Osaka (6) 365-0709.
Australia	ADIS Press Australasia Pty Ltd, P.O. Box 132, Balgowlah, NSW 2093, Australia. Tel.: Sydney (02) 949-2022.
New Zealand	ADIS Press Limited, Private Bag, Mairangi Bay, Auckland 10, New Zealand. Tel.: Auckland (09) 479-8100.
Rest of World	ADIS Press Publications Limited, 18/F Tung Sun Commercial Centre, 194-200 Lockhart Road, Wanchai, Hong Kong. Tel.: Hong Kong (5) 8920-633.

USA Postmasters: Send address changes to ADIS Press International Inc., Suite B-30, Oxford Court Business Center, 582 Middletown Blvd, Langhorne, PA 19047. Air freight and mailing in the USA by Publications Expediting Inc., 200 Meacham Avenue, Elmont, NY 11003.

Clinical Pharmacokinetics (ISSN 0312-5963) is published monthly by ADIS Press Limited, 41 Centorian Drive, Private Bag, Mairangi Bay, Auckland 10, New Zealand. Second class postage is paid at Jamaica, NY 11431. Printed in Hong Kong by Caritas Printing Training Centre.

Clinical Pharmacokinetics

Contents Vol. 16, No. 5, 1989

Review Articles

Drug Disposition

261-282 Clinical Pharmacokinetic Properties of the Macrolide Antibiotics: Effects of Age and Various Pathophysiological States (Part II)
Periti, P.; Mazzei, T.; Mini, E. and *Novelli, A.*

283-311 Clinical Pharmacokinetics of Epidural and Spinal Anaesthesia
Burm, A.G.L.

Original Research Articles

312-316 Clearance of the Antihistamine Doxylamine: Reduced in Elderly Men But Not in Elderly Women
Friedman, H.; Greenblatt, D.J.; Scavone, J.M.; Burstein, E.S.; Ochs, H.R.; Harmatz, J.S. and *Shader, R.I.*

317-325 Co-Trimoxazole (Sulphamethoxazole plus Trimethoprim): Peritoneal Barrier Transfer Pharmacokinetics
Svirbely, J.E.; Pesce, A.J.; Singh, S. and *O'Flaherty, E.J.*

Clinical Pharmacokinetics is indexed in 'Current Contents', 'Index Medicus' and 'Excerpta Medica'.

Clinical Pharmacokinetics

Aim and Scope: The Journal aims to assist in the further development of clinical pharmacokinetics, to promote communication and increased awareness within this specialty area and to further postgraduate education in clinical pharmacology and therapeutics. The Journal places particular emphasis on review articles but also welcomes original research articles. Both types of article consider the pharmacokinetic properties of drugs as related to their actual clinical use. This definition includes bioavailability studies, drug pharmacokinetics, plasma concentration monitoring of pharmacodynamic response, the relationship of drug pharmacokinetics to the therapeutic efficacy or toxicity of drugs etc. – all studied within the context of disease, pregnancy, age or other clinical and pathophysiological determinants of drug response.

Submitted manuscripts of original research in clinical pharmacokinetics will be promptly considered for publication. Shorter communications (up to 2,000 words) will, because of their length, have priority for rapid publication. However, longer manuscripts will also be considered, particularly those which include a review of previous literature in the area of study; their publication will not necessarily be delayed. Priority will also be given to papers dealing with the relationship of pharmacokinetics to pharmacodynamic responses. Experimental data must be obtained from humans and relate to treatment of disease or to pathophysiological determinants of drug use. Animal or *in vitro* investigations and data from healthy human volunteers can be included only if they are relevant to the clinical pharmacokinetic problem under investigation. Studies conducted in healthy volunteers will only be considered if they offer major new findings or re-evaluate kinetics using improved methods of analysis.

Manuscripts: All enquiries relating to the editorial content of *Clinical Pharmacokinetics* should be directed to the Editor: George J. Mammen, ADIS Press Ltd, Private Bag, Mairangi Bay, Auckland 10, New Zealand. *Information for authors* appears on the back 2 pages of each issue.

Subscriptions: Two volumes are published annually with 6 issues per volume. The annual subscription price is North & South America $US420; Europe SwF650; rest of the world $US420. Subscriptions may be ordered from the office of ADIS Press most convenient to you, or through any bookseller or subscription agent. A subscription to *Clinical Pharmacokinetics* is accepted on the express condition that it will be used only internally, within an institution, company or national affiliate confined to one geographical location, and will not be copied and/or circulated outside these limits. An order for *Clinical Pharmacokinetics* constitutes an undertaking by the subscriber to comply with this condition.

Nth & Sth America	ADIS Press International Inc., Suite B-30, Oxford Court Business Center, 582 Middletown Boulevard, Langhorne, PA 19047, USA. Tel.: PA (215) 752-4500.
Europe	ADIS Press International Ltd (European Branch), Suite 15C, Manchester International Office Centre, Styal Rd, Wythenshawe, Manchester M22 5WL, England. Tel.: (61) 436-6428.
Japan (orders)	ADIS Press, c/- Maruzen Co., Ltd, 3-10 Nihonbashi 2-Chome, Chuo-ku, Tokyo 103, Japan. Tel.: Tokyo (3) 272-7211.
Japan (enquiries)	ADIS Press Limited (Representative Office), 4-38 Minamimori-machi 2-chome, Kita-ku, Osaka 530, Japan. Tel.: Osaka (6) 365-0709.
Australia	ADIS Press Australasia Pty Ltd, P.O. Box 132, Balgowlah, NSW 2093, Australia. Tel.: Sydney (02) 949-2022.
New Zealand	ADIS Press Limited, Private Bag, Mairangi Bay, Auckland 10, New Zealand. Tel.: Auckland (09) 479-8100.
Rest of World	ADIS Press Publications Limited, 18/F Tung Sun Commercial Centre, 194-200 Lockhart Road, Wanchai, Hong Kong. Tel.: Hong Kong (5) 8920-633.

USA Postmasters: Send address changes to ADIS Press International Inc., Suite B-30, Oxford Court Business Center, 582 Middletown Blvd, Langhorne, PA 19047. Air freight and mailing in the USA by Publications Expediting Inc., 200 Meacham Avenue, Elmont, NY 11003.

Clinical Pharmacokinetics (ISSN 0312-5963) is published monthly by ADIS Press Limited, 41 Centorian Drive, Private Bag, Mairangi Bay, Auckland 10, New Zealand. Second class postage is paid at Jamaica, NY 11431. Printed in Hong Kong by Caritas Printing Training Centre.

# Clinical Pharmacokinetics

Contents Vol. 16, No. 6, 1989

Leading Article

327-336 Clinical Pharmacokinetics-Pharmacodynamics of Anticancer Drugs
Evans, W.E. and *Relling, M.V.*

Review Articles

Drug Disposition

337-364 Pharmacokinetics of the Newer Benzodiazepines
Garzone, P.D. and *Kroboth, P.D.*

Clinical Pharmacokinetics and Disease Processes

365-386 Clinical Pharmacokinetic Considerations in the Treatment of Patients with Leprosy
Venkatesan, K.

Original Research Article

387-391 Single-Dose and Steady-State Pharmacokinetics of Doxazosin Given in Combination with Chlorothiazide to Hypertensive Subjects
Conway, E.L.; McNeil, J.J.; Meng, L.; Drummer, O.H.; Howes, L.G.; Raymond, K. and *Louis, W.J.*

392-394 **Cumulated Contents**

Clinical Pharmacokinetics is indexed in 'Current Contents', 'Index Medicus' and 'Excerpta Medica'.

Clinical Pharmacokinetics

Aim and Scope: The Journal aims to assist in the further development of clinical pharmacokinetics, to promote communication and increased awareness within this specialty area and to further postgraduate education in clinical pharmacology and therapeutics. The Journal places particular emphasis on review articles but also welcomes original research articles. Both types of article consider the pharmacokinetic properties of drugs as related to their actual clinical use. This definition includes bioavailability studies, drug pharmacokinetics, plasma concentration monitoring of pharmacodynamic response, the relationship of drug pharmacokinetics to the therapeutic efficacy or toxicity of drugs etc. – all studied within the context of disease, pregnancy, age or other clinical and pathophysiological determinants of drug response.

Submitted manuscripts of original research in clinical pharmacokinetics will be promptly considered for publication. Shorter communications (up to 2,000 words) will, because of their length, have priority for rapid publication. However, longer manuscripts will also be considered, particularly those which include a review of previous literature in the area of study; their publication will not necessarily be delayed. Priority will also be given to papers dealing with the relationship of pharmacokinetics to pharmacodynamic responses. Experimental data must be obtained from humans and relate to treatment of disease or to pathophysiological determinants of drug use. Animal or *in vitro* investigations and data from healthy human volunteers can be included only if they are relevant to the clinical pharmacokinetic problem under investigation. Studies conducted in healthy volunteers will only be considered if they offer major new findings or re-evaluate kinetics using improved methods of analysis.

Manuscripts: All enquiries relating to the editorial content of *Clinical Pharmacokinetics* should be directed to the Editor: George J. Mammen, ADIS Press Ltd, Private Bag, Mairangi Bay, Auckland 10, New Zealand. *Information for authors* appears on the back 2 pages of each issue.

Subscriptions: Two volumes are published annually with 6 issues per volume. The annual subscription price is North & South America $US420; Europe SwF650; rest of the world $US420. Subscriptions may be ordered from the office of ADIS Press most convenient to you, or through any bookseller or subscription agent. A subscription to *Clinical Pharmacokinetics* is accepted on the express condition that it will be used only internally, within an institution, company or national affiliate confined to one geographical location, and will not be copied and/or circulated outside these limits. An order for *Clinical Pharmacokinetics* constitutes an undertaking by the subscriber to comply with this condition.

Nth & Sth America	ADIS Press International Inc., Suite B-30, Oxford Court Business Center, 582 Middletown Boulevard, Langhorne, PA 19047, USA. Tel.: PA (215) 752-4500.
Europe	ADIS Press International Ltd (European Branch), Suite 15C, Manchester International Office Centre, Styal Rd, Wythenshawe, Manchester M22 5WL, England. Tel.: (61) 436-6428.
Japan (orders)	ADIS Press, c/- Maruzen Co., Ltd, 3-10 Nihonbashi 2-Chome, Chuo-ku, Tokyo 103, Japan. Tel.: Tokyo (3) 272-7211.
Japan (enquiries)	ADIS Press Limited (Representative Office), 4-38 Minamimori-machi 2-chome, Kita-ku, Osaka 530, Japan. Tel.: Osaka (6) 365-0709.
Australia	ADIS Press Australasia Pty Ltd, P.O. Box 132, Balgowlah, NSW 2093, Australia. Tel.: Sydney (02) 949-2022.
New Zealand	ADIS Press Limited, Private Bag, Mairangi Bay, Auckland 10, New Zealand. Tel.: Auckland (09) 479-8100.
Rest of World	ADIS Press Publications Limited, 18/F Tung Sun Commercial Centre, 194-200 Lockhart Road, Wanchai, Hong Kong. Tel.: Hong Kong (5) 8920-633.

USA Postmasters: Send address changes to ADIS Press International Inc., Suite B-30, Oxford Court Business Center, 582 Middletown Blvd, Langhorne, PA 19047. Air freight and mailing in the USA by Publications Expediting Inc., 200 Meacham Avenue, Elmont, NY 11003.

Clinical Pharmacokinetics (ISSN 0312-5963) is published monthly by ADIS Press Limited, 41 Centorian Drive, Private Bag, Mairangi Bay, Auckland 10, New Zealand. Second class postage is paid at Jamaica, NY 11431. Printed in Hong Kong by Caritas Printing Training Centre.

Clinical Pharmacokinetics 16: 1-26 (1989)
0312-5963/89/00-1-0001/$13.00/0

Clinical Pharmacokinetics of Non-Opiate Abused Drugs

U. Busto, R. Bendayan, and *E.M. Sellers*

Clinical Psychopharmacology Program and Pharmacy Department, Addiction Research Foundation, Faculty of Pharmacy and Departments of Medicine and Pharmacology, University of Toronto, Toronto, Canada

Contents

Summary 1
1. Psychomotor Stimulants 2
1.1 Amphetamines 2
1.2 Caffeine 4
1.3 Cocaine 6
1.4 Nicotine 9
2. Hallucinogens 12
2.1 Cannabis 12
2.2 Phencyclidine (PCP) 14
3. Central Nervous System Depressants 16
3.1 Benzodiazepines 16

Summary

The present review discusses the available data on the kinetic properties of non-opiate abused drugs including psychomotor stimulants, hallucinogens and CNS-depressants. Some of the drugs of abuse reviewed here are illicit drugs (e.g. cannabis, cocaine), while others are effective pharmacological agents but have the potential to be abused (e.g. benzodiazepines).

Although some of the drugs mentioned in this review have been in use for centuries (e.g. caffeine, nicotine, cocaine, cannabis), knowledge of their kinetics and metabolism is very recent and in some cases still incomplete. This is partially due to the difficulties inherent in studying drugs of abuse in humans, and to the complex metabolism of some of these drugs (e.g. cannabis, caffeine) which has made it difficult to develop sensitive assays to determine biological pathways.

Although drugs of abuse may have entirely different intrinsic pharmacological effects, the kinetic properties of such drugs are factors contributing to abuse and dependence. The pharmacokinetic properties that presumably contribute to self-administration and drug abuse include rapid delivery of the drug into the central nervous system and high free drug clearance.

Kinetic characteristics also play an important role in the development of physical dependence and on the appearance of a withdrawal syndrome: the longer the half-life, the greater the likelihood of the development of physical dependence; the shorter the half-life, the earlier and more severe the withdrawal. The balance between these 2 factors, which has not yet been carefully studied, will also influence abuse patterns.

The clinical significance of kinetic characteristics with respect to abuse is discussed where possible.

Psychoactive drugs are among the most widely abused class of pharmacological agents. Although the proper clinical use of some of these drugs has represented an important step in the understanding and treatment of many psychiatric disorders, their inappropriate use can generate many medical, social and economic problems.

Research in the area of drugs of abuse has led to the development of methods to quantitate and predict abuse liability (Jasinski et al. 1984). Abused substances share at least 2 specific and measurable properties. Firstly, they are self-administered (as determined from animal and human studies) [Johanson & Schuster 1981], and, secondly, they produce behavioural, physiological and subjective effects that are associated with a sense of well-being or euphoria. The abuse potential of a drug is a function of the degree to which that drug produces pleasant subjective effects (i.e. 'reinforcing effects'), as well as the degree to which the same drug produces unpleasant effects (Griffiths et al. 1984a, 1985; Jasinski 1977). Highly abused drugs (e.g. cocaine) may be very powerful reinforcers despite producing significant adverse effects, or weak to moderate reinforcers with mild side effects (e.g. nicotine). Both the reinforcing properties (i.e. 'liking', 'euphoria') of a compound and the unpleasant side effects can be assessed in humans by using direct questioning, questionnaires or symptom checklists (Griffiths et al. 1984a; Jasinski 1977).

Another procedure frequently used to assess the abuse potential of a drug is to give the compound to experienced subjects who can compare the subjective effects of the drug with the effects of other drugs to which they have previously been exposed. It has been demonstrated that experienced subjects (i.e. those who have used enough drugs to be able to make an overall assessment) can clearly distinguish between drug effects induced by different pharmacological agents (e.g. narcotics, CNS stimulants, depressants) [Griffiths et al. 1984a,b; Jasinski 1977]. It is assumed that the abuse liability of a new drug will be similar to the abuse potential of the compound to which it has been related.

Another characteristic that may be a determinant of abuse liability is the development of physical dependence, which is the capacity of a drug to produce a withdrawal symptom(s) upon cessation after long term administration (Committee on Problems of Drug Dependence 1985). The methodology used to determine the dependence liability of drugs has been to detect the presence or absence of withdrawal symptoms and signs, by both rating scales and questionnaires (Dorian et al. 1983; Hill et al. 1963; Zilm & Sellers 1978).

Pharmacokinetics is an important field for the understanding of drug actions. The time course of the absorption, distribution, metabolism and excretion of drugs allows us to study how differences in kinetic properties may influence the use, misuse and abuse of psychoactive drugs (Boisse & Okamoto 1978; Kalant et al. 1971). Pharmacokinetic properties may also play an important role in predicting dependence and abuse potential of drugs. The pharmacokinetic properties of a drug liable to increased self-administration include rapid absorption, rapid entry into specific brain regions, high oral bioavailability, low protein binding, short half-life, small volume of distribution and high free drug clearance. In contrast, pharmacokinetic properties associated with drug dependence are long half-life and low free drug clearance. Therefore, the drug must be present in the body at high enough concentrations and for sufficient time to permit tolerance (tachyphylaxis) to develop (Busto & Sellers 1986).

This paper reviews the pharmacokinetics of non-opiate abused drugs including illicit drugs such as cocaine and cannabis, as well as those which have a legitimate role in therapeutics, but have the potential to be abused, such as benzodiazepines. The pharmacokinetics of the opiate drugs of abuse is the subject of a separate review, which will appear in a subsequent issue of the Journal. Where possible, the clinical significance that pharmacokinetic characteristics have with respect to the abuse of these types is discussed.

1. Psychomotor Stimulants

1.1 Amphetamines

The amphetamines (amphetamine, methamphetamine, methylphenidate and diethylpropion) are sympathomimetic agents that possess potent central nervous system stimulant effects. Moderate oral doses of these agents in normal subjects commonly produce elevation of mood, increased alertness, decreased appetite and an overall subjective feeling of well-being. The subjective effects are dependent on the user, the environment, the dose and the route of administration (Jaffe 1985).

Dissolved oral tablets of amphetamine or crystalline methamphetamine manufactured in illegal laboratories are commonly administered intravenously and are known as 'speed' (Gorrod 1973). The pharmacokinetic properties of amphetamine (2-amino-1-phenylpropane) are reviewed below.

1.1.1 Absorption

Limited data are available on the extent and rate of gastrointestinal absorption of amphetamine in humans. After a 15mg oral dose of *d*-amphetamine in 2 healthy subjects, peak serum concentrations were reached after 1.25 hours and serum concentrations were 48 and 40 μg/L under acidic urine conditions and 52 and 47 μg/L under uncontrolled urine pH conditions (urine pH is not changed by the administration of acid or alkaline fluids) [Beckett et al. 1969].

1.1.2 Distribution

Plasma protein binding of amphetamine in humans is low (20%) and is similar in drug-dependent and non-drug user subjects (Franksson & Anggard 1970) [table I]. The volume of distribution of amphetamine in drug non-users is smaller (3.5 to 4.6 L/kg) [Rowland 1969] than in drug dependent subjects (6.1 L/kg) [Anggard et al. 1970]. It has been suggested that the larger volume of distribution in drug-dependent subjects may be due to an increased affinity of the tissues for the drug. In amphetamine-dependent animals, higher tissue concentrations of the drug are found (Ellison et al. 1968). In animals, amphetamine distributes rapidly into tissues (i.e. kidneys, lungs, brain and liver); in rats, peak brain concentrations are reached 30 minutes after the intraperitoneal administration of amphetamine 1 mg/kg and are 5 to 8 times higher than in serum (Maickel et al. 1969). Cerebrospinal fluid amphetamine concentrations are 80% of the corresponding plasma concentrations, thus reflecting the extent of serum protein binding (Anggard et al. 1970).

1.1.3 Metabolism and Excretion

In humans, amphetamine appears to follow a linear pharmacokinetic 1-compartment open model over the dose range of 20 to 200mg (Gunne & Anggard 1973).

Amphetamine is a basic compound (pKa 9.9) and its renal excretion is significantly influenced by urinary pH and volume (Gunne & Anggard 1973). With uncontrolled urinary pH, it undergoes significant hepatic hydroxylation and deamination. Under these conditions, the excretion of unchanged amphetamine averages 14.5% while in the presence of urinary acidification excretion is increased to 55% (Beckett et al. 1965). In healthy men receiving 5mg ^{14}C-*d,l*-amphetamine orally, about 90% of the dose is excreted in the urine over 3 to 4 days. 70% of the dose is excreted in the urine within 1 day: 30% as unchanged drug, 21% as benzoic acid, 16% as hippuric acid and 3% as hydroxyamphetamine (Dring et al. 1970). The latter metabolite is pharmacologically active, but is unlikely to have a significant clinical effect. Under urinary acidification, total clearance of *d*-amphetamine is found to be significantly higher than under uncontrolled urine pH conditions; and the plasma elimination half-life is also significantly shorter (Anggard et al. 1970; Beckett et al. 1969; Davis et al. 1971).

Amphetamine plasma half-life is reported to be longer in drug-dependent subjects than in non-drug users (Anggard et al. 1970) [table I]. The longer plasma half-life observed in drug-dependent subjects may be due to an increased tissue affinity of the drug (increased volume of distribution) or to a decrease in systemic clearance, possibly due to an alteration of the drug metabolism.

The metabolism of *d,l*-amphetamine has been studied in subjects presenting with amphetamine psychosis. In the presence of acid urine, the renal elimination of unchanged amphetamine (67 to 73%) is more significant than in the presence of alkaline urine. Under these conditions a rapid improve-

Table I. Pharmacokinetic parameters of amphetamines (mean ± SD)

Drug	Reference	Subjects	Dosage/ Route (mg)	Protein binding (%)	$t_{1/2\beta}$ (min) [range]	Vd(L/kg) [range]	CL (L/min)
d-Amphetamine	Beckett et al. (1969)		15 PO				0.24-0.54[a] 0.016-0.12[b]
d,l-Amphetamine	Anggard et al. (1970)	Drug non-users	25 PO		3.5 ± 0.4[a] [2.2-4.4] 13.9 ± 3.4[c] [5.7-25.8]		
		Drug-dependent	25 PO		4.2 ± 0.6[a] [2.6-6.2] 21.8 ± 1.4[c] [17.9-26.0]		
		Drug-dependent	160-200 IV			6.11 ± 0.22 [4.8-7.6]	
	Franksson & Anggard (1970)	Drug non-users		23 ± 1.1			
		Drug-dependent		26 ± 1.0			

a Acidified urine.
b Urine pH not controlled.
c Alkaline urine.
Abbreviations: $t_{1/2\beta}$ = elimination half-life; Vd = volume of distribution; CL = total body clearance; PO = oral; IV = intravenous.

ment in psychotic symptoms is observed (Anggard et al. 1973). The intensity of the psychosis is found to correlate to the amount of basic polar metabolites of amphetamine excreted in urine, i.e. norephedrine, *p*-hydroxynorephedrine and hydroxyamphetamine, but not to the plasma amphetamine concentration. This suggests that amphetamine metabolites may play an important role in the development of paranoid psychosis in chronic amphetamine users (Anggard et al. 1973).

Understanding the pharmacokinetic properties of amphetamine allows the institution of a rational treatment for acute amphetamine overdose. Urine acidification and fluid administration can play a major role, as they enhance the renal elimination of the parent compound.

1.2 Caffeine

Caffeine (1,3,7-trimethylxanthine) is a xanthine alkaloid extensively consumed in tea, coffee, and many soft drinks, as well as in a variety of over-the-counter and prescription medications. It is the most widely and regularly consumed psychoactive substance in the world. It has been established that the average coffee drinker consumes between 100 and 200mg (2 to 4 cups) per day, with 20 to 30% of adult Americans consuming up to 600 mg/day and 10% consuming more than 1000 mg/day (Graham 1978; Greden 1979).

Caffeine has extensive pharmacological effects, is a central nervous system (CNS) stimulant, and increases blood pressure, catecholamines, renin and free fatty acids (Bellet et al. 1968; Robertson et al. 1978). After long term caffeine intake the pressor response disappears due to adaptation or tolerance to its circulatory effects (Ammon et al. 1983; Robertson et al. 1981).

If coffee is taken after a caffeine-free period, it produces alertness, excitation and an increase in blood pressure. Therefore, physicians should be aware of the patterns of caffeine use of patients, and the possible contribution of the use/abuse of the drug to the presenting signs and symptoms, especially in those individuals with disturbed sleep patterns, restlessness and tachycardia.

1.2.1 Absorption

Caffeine is usually ingested in an aqueous solution and is a lipophilic molecule which is rapidly and completely absorbed (Marks & Kelly 1973). Peak plasma concentrations of approximately 10 μg/L are reached at 30 to 60 minutes after the administration of 5 mg/kg (Blanchard & Sawers 1983a) or 50 to 750mg (Newton et al. 1981). More than 99% of the ingested dose is absorbed within 45 minutes (Bonati et al. 1982). Absorption in humans is more rapid following an oral dose than intramuscular injection (Sant'ambrogio et al. 1964). Animal studies indicate dose-dependent kinetics in rats at relatively low oral doses (10 mg/kg); however, human studies have not provided any evidence for dose-dependent bioavailability at usual doses (Aldridge et al. 1977; Newton et al. 1981). The rapid absorption of caffeine is probably responsible for the quick onset of subjective effects of alertness experienced after drinking coffee.

1.2.2 Distribution

Caffeine is distributed into all body tissues, rapidly crosses the blood-brain barrier and the placenta, and is also found in breast milk. Caffeine is only 15 to 30% protein bound and the apparent volume of distribution described for healthy subjects ranges between 0.54 and 0.70 L/kg (Axelrod & Reichenthal 1953; Blanchard & Sawers 1983a; Desmond et al. 1980; Parsons & Neims 1978; Patwardhan et al. 1980) [table II].

1.2.3 Metabolism and Excretion

Detailed studies of caffeine biotransformation pathways have been scarce until recently. The metabolism of caffeine in humans is complex, and the oxidative biotransformation occurs primarily in the liver via microsomal cytochrome P450. In humans, caffeine undergoes oxidative desmethylation and hydroxylation reactions and yields a number of products which are excreted in the urine (Burg 1975; Grant et al. 1983). The predominant pathways of formation of major metabolism of caffeine in humans indicate an initial 3-demethylation to paraxanthine, which is then converted to 1-methyluric acid, 1-methylxanthine and 1-7, methyluric acid with lesser amounts of other metabolites (Grant et al. 1983). The profile of metabolites, however, shows marked interindividual variability (Grant et al. 1983) and the metabolite ratio has been used as a marker of acetylator studies in humans (Grant et al. 1983). Some of the differences found in the metabolite ratio may be related to genetic differences or to different dosages used in the studies (Bergmann & Dikstein 1956). Only 0.5 to 1.5% of a caffeine dose is excreted as unchanged drug, indicating the almost complete biotransformation (Axelrod & Reichenthal 1953).

In healthy subjects, the elimination half-life of caffeine varies between 1.5 and 9.5 hours, the mean half-life being around 5 hours in most studies. The fairly wide range of elimination half-lives probably reflects interindividual variations in volume of distribution and clearance.

Total plasma clearance of caffeine has been calculated to be 0.078 L/h/kg (Patwardhan et al. 1980). However, the metabolic clearance of unbound drug is a better reflection of the metabolic capacity of the liver than total clearance. Although caffeine is only about 30% plasma protein bound, clearance and apparent volume of distribution may be influenced by differences between subjects in the unbound fraction. Free (unbound) clearance of caffeine has been shown to be 0.11 to 0.12 L/h/kg (Blanchard & Sawers 1983b), suggesting that plasma protein binding does not exert a substantial influence on the distribution pattern of caffeine.

The pharmacokinetics of caffeine are influenced by age, sex, smoking, concomitant diseases, and other drug use or abuse. The pharmacokinetics of caffeine in young and elderly males are similar. Although volume of distribution is significantly lower in elderly subjects (613 *vs* 524 ml/kg) [Blanchard 1982; Blanchard & Sawers 1983b], absorption and clearance are similar in elderly and young males, suggesting that the differences observed are not likely to exert clinically significant changes on caffeine kinetics. In contrast, newborn infants elimi-

Table II. Pharmacokinetic parameters of caffeine

Reference	Subjects (n)	Dosage/route (mg/kg)	Protein binding (%)	$t_{½β}$ (h)	Vd (L/kg)	CL (L/kg/h)	CL_R (ml/kg/h)
Blanchard & Sawers (1983b)	8 young	4.86 ± 0.3 IV	35.7	4.94[a]	0.61 ± 0.02	0.08 ± 0.03	0.93 ± 0.2
	8 elderly	4.99 ± 0.3 IV	35.0	3.70	0.42 ± 0.02	0.1 ± 0.03	1.06 ± 0.5
Bonati et al. (1982)	4 young	0.22 PO (in soft drink)		3.40[a]	0.03 ± 0.004	0.1 ± 0.03	
	4 young	1.0 PO (in mocha coffee)		4.20	0.05 ± 0.003	0.13 ± 0.014	
	4 young	1.54 PO (in aqueous sol.)		5.00	0.05 ± 0.006	0.12 ± 0.014	
	4 young	5.00 PO (in aqueous sol.)		6.30	0.04 ± 0.002	0.07 ± 0.009	
Desmond et al. (1980)	15[b]	250mg PO	31.3 ± 1.8	5.2	0.54 ± 0.02	0.12 ± 0.04	
Newton et al. (1981)	5 young	300mg PO		5.22	0.555-0.558	0.094-0.097	42.6-130.2
Parsons & Neims (1978)	13 smokers	5 PO (in aqueous sol.)		3.5	0.72 ± 0.07		
	13 non-smokers			6.0	0.61 ± 0.08	0.09 ± 0.02	

a Calculated as the harmonic mean.
b Age range 18-71.
Abbreviations: CL_R = renal clearance; for other abbreviations, see table I.

nate caffeine very slowly. In non-smoking adults, the plasma half-life of caffeine is 6 hours and clearance is 0.095 L/h/kg, while in preterm infants with apnoea these values are 103 hours and 0.09 L/h/kg, respectively (Aranda et al. 1979; Gorodischer et al. 1977; Parsons et al. 1976), probably due to decreased activity of the hepatic cytochrome P450 mono-oxygenase in neonates.

Smoking induces the activity of hepatic cytochrome P450 enzymes; therefore, the caffeine clearance in smokers is greater than in non-smokers (0.155 and 0.095 L/h/kg, respectively), and half-life is significantly shorter (3.5 *vs* 6 hours) due to increased metabolism. Increased clearance of caffeine has been postulated as a contributory factor to higher consumption of caffeine among cigarette smokers (Parsons & Neims 1978). Since induction of hepatic enzymes and liver function play such an important role in caffeine metabolism, it is predicted that use or abuse of drugs that are enzyme inducers (e.g. barbiturates) may alter caffeine kinetics. Impaired liver function, such as that occurring in alcoholic liver disease, slows caffeine elimination and prolongs caffeine half-life (Statland et al. 1976; Statland & Demas 1980).

1.3 Cocaine

Cocaine, a lipophilic weak base (pKa 8.6), is an alkaloid that exists in 2 chemical forms: cocaine hydrochloride ('snow', 'coke') and cocaine free-base ('crack', 'rocks'). Cocaine remains a very popular drug of abuse, especially in South and North America and also in Europe. In the past decade important information on the pharmacokinetic properties of various cocaine preparations has been released.

1.3.1 Absorption

Cocaine abuse occurs through various routes of administration: oral, intranasal, intravenous and smoking. In North America and Europe the intranasal and smoking routes of administration remain the most common.

Oral Route

For many years it was believed that cocaine was hydrolysed in the gastrointestinal tract and not absorbed into the systemic circulation (Ritchie & Cohen 1975). However, it is well known that native people of South America (more particularly Peru, Bolivia and northern Argentina) have chewed coca leaves for more than 3000 years with the production of marked pharmacological effects.

Significant concentrations of cocaine are present in the plasma of coca leaf chewers from South America (Paly et al. 1980). The method and pattern of chewing markedly affects the amount of cocaine present in blood. For example, after the administration of coca leaves (12g) containing 0.5% of cocaine, peak plasma concentrations are higher in experienced chewers (95 μg/L) than in those who are much less experienced and who do not swallow the leaves (38 μg/L). This also suggests that cocaine absorption occurs not only from the oral mucosa, but also from the gastrointestinal tract. When larger doses are administered (50g of coca containing 0.65% cocaine), mean peak plasma concentrations are 249 μg/L (range 130 to 859 μg/L).

In another study, healthy male subjects with a history of previous cocaine usage were administered cocaine hydrochloride (2 mg/kg) in gelatin capsules (to eliminate possible buccal absorption). Peak plasma cocaine concentrations occurred 50 to 90 minutes after oral administration, and ranged from 104 to 424 μg/L. Plasma concentrations decreased gradually over the next 2 to 3 hours (Van Dyke et al. 1978). Using similar oral cocaine doses, Wilkinson et al. (1980) found a mean peak plasma cocaine concentration of 242 μg/L, and an average time to reach the peak concentration (t_{max}) of 65 minutes. As in the previous study, cocaine was not detected in plasma until 30 minutes after administration. The delay observed for the rise in plasma drug concentration may be explained by the ionisation of cocaine in the acid medium of the stomach and a delay in reaching the alkaline environment of the small intestine where the non-ionised form is favoured and absorption occurs (Van Dyke et al. 1978; Wilkinson et al. 1980). As highly sensitive chromatographic assay techniques were used in the recent studies, it seems reasonable to exclude low assay sensitivity as a factor in the observed delay.

Intranasal Route

One of the most common routes of cocaine administration in North America is the intranasal route ('snorting'). Cocaine hydrochloride powder (20 to 30mg) is laid out and inhaled (absorption occurs through the nasal mucous membranes). The user generally experiences about 20 to 40 minutes of stimulation.

The pharmacokinetic properties of cocaine through the intranasal route have been studied and compared with those of the oral form (Van Dyke et al. 1978; Wilkinson et al. 1980), and of the intravenous form (Javaid et al. 1983).

After intranasal administration, rate and extent of absorption are highly variable (Wilkinson et al. 1980). Peak plasma concentrations of cocaine after intranasal administration occurred after 35 to 90 minutes in one study (Wilkinson et al. 1980), while t_{max} varied between 120 and 160 minutes after the administration of comparable cocaine doses (2 mg/kg) in another study (Van Dyke et al. 1978). Bioavailability appears to be dose-dependent after intranasal administration; the bioavailability of 64mg inhaled cocaine was only 28%, while after inhalation of 96mg it was 57% (Javaid et al. 1983). This high variability may be due to several factors, including variable nasal vasoconstriction induced by cocaine, previous metabolism in the nasal mucosa, significant plasma hydrolysis of cocaine by serum cholinesterase or a poor administration technique leading to a partial swallowing of the dose.

No major differences in kinetics are observed between the intranasally administered cocaine solution and cocaine powder (crystalline form) [Wilkinson et al. 1980].

Smoking of Cocaine

Recently, widespread smoking of cocaine has occurred in North America. Since 1983, the 'street' selling of cocaine powder (cocaine hydrochloride) has been almost exclusively replaced by that of cocaine free-base ('rocks') [Jekel et al. 1986]. Smoking free-base cocaine induces a rapid, temporary euphoric state of great intensity. In order to maintain this euphoric state, the drug is smoked at frequent intervals. This pattern of use is similar to the intravenous administration of cocaine or heroin and is associated with a high potential for dependency and overdose (Siegel 1979). Using a specially designed glass pipe, under a strictly controlled smoking protocol, Perez-Reyes et al. (1982b) have shown that around 32% of cocaine free-base originally placed in the pipe is inhaled. The inhaled cocaine free-base induced psychological and cardiovascular effects similar to those of 20mg of intravenous cocaine hydrochloride.

Smoking of cocaine paste is widespread among the young population of Peru, Bolivia, Colombia and Ecuador (Jeri et al. 1980). The paste is a crude extract of coca leaves that contains from 40 to 70% cocaine base along with cocaine salts, coca alkaloids and minimal amounts of residual organic solvents. The paste is mixed with tobacco or marijuana and then smoked (Paly et al. 1982).

Cocaine paste (75% cocaine) mixed with tobacco and administered to experienced volunteer smokers resulted in peak plasma cocaine concentrations of 462 μg/L after 3 minutes of smoking. This rapid rise in plasma cocaine concentration explains the dramatic pharmacological effects observed after smoking cocaine. Comparison of AUC data, corrected for dosage with those previously reported for oral and intranasal administration, indicated that the relative bioavailability of cocaine by smoking is about 70% (39 to 94%) [Paly et al. 1982].

1.3.2 Distribution

Tissue distribution and extent of plasma protein binding of cocaine have been determined in male rats (Nayak et al. 1976). 15 minutes after a single radiolabelled intravenous dose of cocaine, the highest concentrations of the drug are found in the brain, spleen, kidney and lung while the lowest concentrations are present in the muscle, heart and plasma. Cocaine concentrations in plasma decline very rapidly and are absent 4 hours after administration. The drug completely disappears from the brain, heart muscle and fat 6 hours after administration. In rats receiving multiple doses, brain to plasma ratios of cocaine are higher than in rats receiving a single dose of the drug.

Plasma protein binding of cocaine (0.1 to 1 mg/L) in rats is low (35%), and similar in the single- and multiple-dose-treated groups (Nayak et al. 1976). However, in humans, at lower concentrations (25 μg/L), plasma protein binding of cocaine is significant (91%). The drug appears to be not only bound to albumin, but possibly to α_1-acid glycoprotein (Edwards & Bowles 1987).

The steady-state volume of distribution of cocaine in human subjects with a history of drug abuse is large (1.96 L/kg), showing, as in animals, extensive extravascular distribution (Barnett et al. 1981; Chow et al. 1985) [table III].

After intravenous administration, cocaine has been reported to follow a linear pharmacokinetic 2-compartment open model in human subjects (Chow et al. 1985). The distribution phase is very rapid and the elimination half-life has been reported to range from 31 to 82 minutes (Barnett et al. 1981; Chow et al. 1985; Javaid et al. 1983) [table III]. After intranasal and oral cocaine administration, the elimination half-life of the drug is within the same range as after intravenous administration (Javaid et al. 1983; Wilkinson et al. 1980) [table III]. The mean half-life of cocaine paste (when smoked) has been reported to be 38 minutes (Paly et al. 1982).

1.3.3 Metabolism and Excretion

The excretion and metabolism of cocaine have been studied in male Wistar rats after short and long term treatment. Unchanged cocaine recovered in urine and faeces after 24 hours is very small (1.2 and 1.5%) and similar in both groups of rats. The percentage of the total dose recovered in urine is also the same in short (49.3%) and long term treated rats (51.6%). Urinary metabolites of [^{3}H]-cocaine, such as benzoylecgonine, benzoylnorecgonine, ecgonine and ecgonine methyl ester, as well as small amounts of unmetabolised cocaine, are identified

Table III. Pharmacokinetic parameters of cocaine

Reference	Dosage/route (mg)	$t_{½β}$ (min) [range]	Vd (L/kg) [range]	CL (L/min) [range]	CL_R (L/min) [range]
Barnett et al. (1981)	100 IV	[40.3-51.5]	[1.5-1.9]	[1.3-3.1]	
	200 IV	[32.3-78.9]	[1.2-1.6]	[0.7-1.2]	
Chow et al. (1985)	32 IV	48 ± 13	1.96 ± 0.2	2.1 ± 0.32	0.03 ± 0.013
		[31-63]	[1.77-2.29]	[1.8-2.1]	[0.01-0.043]
Javaid et al. (1983)	32 IV	42.6 ± 7.8	2.1 ± 0.6		
		[19.2-64.2]	[0.7-3.9]		
	64 IN	[29.1-101.4]			
	96 IN	[74.3-101.4]			
Wilkinson et al. (1980)	0.19-2.0 mg/kg IN	75 ± 5			
	(20% solution)	[57.2 - 93.5]			
	0.38 mg/kg IN	73 ± 10			
	(crystalline form)				
	2.0-3.0 mg/kg PO	57 ± 3			
	(crystalline form/capsule)				

Abbreviations: IN = intranasally; CL_R = renal clearance; for other abbreviations, see table I.

in urine. Norcocaine, the pharmacologically active metabolite, is not excreted, possibly due to its further biotransformation to benzoylnorecgonine (Nayak et al. 1976).

In humans, after oral ingestion of radiolabelled cocaine the major metabolite formed is an ecgonine methyl ester. This is a product of cocaine hydrolysis by plasma cholinesterase and liver esterase; it accounts for 32 to 49% of the urinary cocaine metabolites (Inaba et al. 1978; Stewart et al. 1977). Benzoylecgonine, a major metabolite of cocaine formed through hydrolysis, is not produced enzymatically in either plasma or liver but results from spontaneous formation at physiological pH (Stewart et al. 1979).

N-Demethylation of cocaine is also observed in humans; only a small fraction of cocaine is converted to norcocaine (2.6 to 6.2%) [Inaba et al. 1978]. Norcocaine produces some pharmacological effects in animals (Hawks et al. 1974), but the significance of this finding has not been evaluated in humans.

1.4 Nicotine

Cigarette smoking has been called 'the most addictive and dependence-producing form of object-specific self-administered gratification known to man' (Russell 1974). Estimates in 1984 suggest that 60 million Americans are addicted to tobacco, resulting annually in 400,000 premature deaths (Read 1984).

The potential role of nicotine in tobacco dependence has been identified in numerous studies (Griffiths & Henningfield 1982; Henningfield et al. 1985; Johnston 1931). As a consequence, marked interest in the pharmacokinetic properties of nicotine has emerged. Studying nicotine pharmacokinetics entails consideration of a multitude of factors including nicotine content in cigarette smoke, smoke and nicotine inhalation, physiological factors that alter the absorption, metabolism and elimination of the drug, and laboratory facilities for nicotine analysis (Darby et al. 1984).

1.4.1 Absorption

Cigarette smoke is a concentrated aerosol of liquid particles suspended in an atmosphere consisting mainly of nitrogen, oxygen and carbon dioxide. Nicotine is a liquid alkaloid (pKa 7.9) distilled from burning tobacco. It is highly ionised in cigarette smoke which has an acidic pH (5.5). Many factors, such as the tobacco blend, additives, wrapping paper, length of the tobacco rod and the filter design considerably modify the content of smoke (Darby et al. 1984). Smoking machines measure the yield of cigarettes, which is defined as being the yield of nicotine, tar and carbon monoxide obtained from a 35ml puff volume of 2 seconds' duration taken every minute during the burning time of a cigarette. Over the last 3 decades the yield of cigarettes sold in North America has decreased. Commercial low tar cigarettes contain 0.6 to 0.8mg nicotine, 6 to 14mg tar, and 7 to 15mg carbon monoxide (Guerin 1980).

Absorption of nicotine through cigarette smoking is affected by various factors, such as particle size, smoking pattern, smoke pH, and oral/buccal pH (for review see Svensson 1987). Minimal amounts of nicotine are absorbed from the buccal mucosa or the gastrointestinal tract, as nicotine is highly ionised in smoke. Absorption of nicotine through the oral mucosa has been demonstrated to be a linear function of oral pH; at pH 5 around 3% of a nicotine dose is absorbed, at pH 8 absorption rises to 20%. As alkalinity increases, cigarette taste is perceived as being stronger, bitter and unpleasant. Oral irritation from nicotine is known to be a direct function of the amount of nicotine present in un-ionised form (Kozlowski & Kleiman 1978). It is only when nicotine reaches the alveoli in the lungs that significant absorption occurs. At this site the factors which affect distribution and deposition include tidal volume, inspiratory and expiratory flow rates, vital capacity, lung morphology, particle size and density. The number of puffs taken, the puff volume and depth of inhalation are also important. Due to the significant complexity of the smoking process, the dose of nicotine consumed by the smoker cannot be predicted from the nicotine content of tobacco or its absorption characteristics. Most of the nicotine is lost into the surrounding air as sidestream smoke, or is retained in the cigarette butt; only 25% of the total nicotine content of a cigarette is present in the mainstream smoke. Habitual smokers may absorb up to 90% of the nicotine in the mainstream smoke; however, nonsmokers who do not inhale absorb much less nicotine. Peak serum concentrations in subjects who retain most of the mainstream smoke range from 31.3 to 40.1 μg/L (Armitage et al. 1975).

After oral ingestion of tobacco, nicotine is poorly absorbed from the stomach due to the acidity of the gastric fluid (Travell 1960). However, when it reaches the small intestine it is well absorbed, as the small intestine presents a more alkaline pH and a larger surface area than the stomach. Nevertheless, despite good absorption through the small intestine, the bioavailability of oral nicotine is very low due to extensive first-pass metabolism (F = 30%). Nicotine can also be absorbed after topical administration from contact with tobacco leaves (Benowitz et al. 1987; Gehlbach et al. 1974).

1.4.2 Distribution

Nicotine, being a weak lipophilic base, is rapidly and widely distributed to tissue compartments. The volume of distribution at steady-state is relatively large and highly variable in humans (Benowitz et al. 1982; Feyerabend et al. 1985; Rosenberg et al. 1980) [table IV]. The extent of nicotine protein binding in human plasma is very small (4.9 to 20%) [Benowitz et al. 1982; Svensson 1987].

Nicotine freely crosses the placenta and is found in amniotic fluid and in the umbilical cord blood of neonates (Hibberd et al. 1978; Luck & Nau 1984). Nicotine is also found in breast milk and the breast fluid of non-lactating females (Petrakis et al. 1978). The daily dose of nicotine received by a breast-feeding infant has been calculated to be between 5.9 and 9.3 μg/kg (Atkinson et al. 1988). This dosage may be clinically important (Luck and Nau 1985).

1.4.3 Metabolism and Excretion

After intravenous administration, nicotine pharmacokinetics follow a first-order 2-compartment model. Pharmacokinetic parameters evaluated in various studies reveal significant interindividual variability (table IV). This variability is mainly due to changes in the extent of hepatic drug metabolism and renal excretion. Nicotine is primarily metabolised in the liver, and to a small extent in the lungs and kidneys (Gorrod & Jenner

Table IV. Pharmacokinetic parameters of nicotine

Reference	Dosage (μg/kg/min)	Urine pH	Protein binding (%)	$t_{1/2\beta}$ (min) [range]	Vd (L/kg) [range]	CL (L/min) [range]	CL_R (L/min) [range]
Benowitz et al. (1982)	1.0 IV × 30 min	Acid	4.9 ± 2.9	98 ± 33 [66-128]	176 ± 72[b] [96-249]	1.28 ± 0.44 [0.89-1.9]	0.19 ± 0.06 [0.14-0.27]
	1.5 IV × 30 min	Acid		142 ± 58 [94-239]	186 ± 41[b] [117-222]	1.3 ± 0.32 [0.76-1.5]	0.2 ± 0.06 [0.095-0.23]
	2.0 IV × 30 min	Acid		114 ± 33 [74-151]	185 ± 46[b] [145-241]	1.3 ± 0.18 [1.12-1.56]	0.2 ± 0.07 [0.12-0.29]
Feyerabend et al. (1985)	25 μg/kg IV	Acid[c]		2.21 ± 0.34 [1.77-2.56]		0.915±0.146 [0.78-1.15]	
Rosenberg et al. (1980)	2 IV × 10 min	Acid		39 ± 4	1.0 ± 0.1[a]	1.3 ± 0.17	
		Alkaline		52 ± 5	1.0 ± 0.1[a]	0.97 ± 0.09	
	2 IV × 10 min (6 doses)	Acid		86 ± 7	1.7 ± 0.10[a]	1.03 ± 0.10	0.25 ± 0.045
		Alkaline		110 ± 6	1.7 ± 0.03[a]	0.79 ± 0.05	0.017 ± 0.000

a Vd_{area} in L/kg.
b Vd_{ss} in L.
c Subjects received 2g NH_4Cl 4 times/day.

Abbreviations: CL_R = renal clearance; Vd_{ss} = volume of distribution at steady-state; Vd_{area} = volume of distribution calculated from the area under the curve; for other abbreviations, see table I.

1975; Turner et al. 1975). The major metabolites of nicotine are cotinine and nicotine-*N*-oxide. Cotinine results from nicotine hydroxylation and oxidation by the cytochrome P450 and the cytoplasmic enzyme aldehyde oxidase. Nicotine-*N*-oxide results from nicotine oxidation by a microsomal flavoprotein system (Gorrod & Jenner 1975). Under uncontrolled urinary pH conditions around 10% of an intravenous nicotine dose is excreted unchanged in the urine. Nicotine-*N*-oxide is excreted unchanged in urine; however, cotinine is mainly eliminated by the liver (Beckett et al. 1971).

Nicotine elimination by the kidney involves glomerular filtration and tubular secretion. Renal elimination is urinary pH-dependent: in acid urine, nicotine is mostly ionised and tubular reabsorption is minimal; however, under alkaline urine conditions, nicotine renal clearance decreases significantly. These changes in renal clearance are followed by changes in the plasma elimination half-life (Rosenberg et al. 1980) [table IV].

The disposition kinetics of cotinine have been extensively studied. Cotinine is mainly metabolised in the liver; renal clearance of the drug averages only 17% of total clearance under uncontrolled urinary pH. In the presence of urine acidification, cotinine renal clearance is increased by about 50%; however, clearance is not affected by urine alkalinisation. Terminal half-life of cotinine in regular smokers is much longer than that observed for nicotine (15.8 + 4.0 hours). As cotinine is a more polar compound than nicotine, its volume of distribution is much smaller. Cotinine does not exhibit a potent pharmacological effect in humans (Benowitz et al. 1983; Matsukura et al. 1979). Due to its slow metabolic clearance and long half-life, cotinine is present in the blood of tobacco smokers in higher concentrations and remains much longer after cessation of smoking than nicotine. Blood and urine concentrations of cotinine have been used as markers of tobacco consumption and abstinence (Hall et al. 1984; Matsukura et al. 1979). The average blood cotinine concentration in smokers is around 300 μg/L, while non-smokers have concentrations below 10 μg/L (Benowitz et al. 1983).

2. Hallucinogens

2.1 Cannabis

Knowledge of the psychotropic effects of various preparations of *Cannabis sativa*, the plant from which marijuana and hashish are derived, dates from as early as 2700 BC. *Cannabis sativa* contains 61 known cannabinoids, of which at least 2, Δ^9-tetrahydrocannabinol (Δ^9-THC) and its 11-hydroxylated metabolite, are responsible for the observed psychopharmacological effects and its non-medical use (Turner et al. 1980; Wall 1971).

2.1.1 Absorption

Cannabis is usually smoked in cigarettes containing 5 to 30mg of Δ^9-THC. Rapid absorption occurs following 1 marijuana cigarette, with peak plasma concentrations of Δ^9-THC of 100 to 200 μg/L occurring after 3 to 8 minutes (Hollister et al. 1981; Lindgren et al. 1981; Ohlsson et al. 1980). Psychotropic effects are noted within minutes, with a duration of 2 to 3 hours (Lemberger et al. 1971). After oral ingestion, Δ^9-THC is well absorbed but produces lower peak plasma concentrations (6 μg/L) after 1 hour (Perez-Reyes et al. 1982a). The means by which Δ^9-THC is orally administered has importance since it may influence the subjective effects obtained (Lemberger 1976; Perez-Reyes et al. 1972, 1973b).

The bioavailability of Δ^9-THC after smoking has been suggested to be 10 times greater than after oral ingestion (Agurell et al. 1979). Recently, however, the systemic availability of Δ^9-THC after 3 different routes of administration was studied by Ohlsson et al. (1980). 11 healthy subjects were administered the drug intravenously (5mg), by smoking (19mg) and by mouth (20mg). The plasma concentrations 3 minutes after intravenous infusion ranged from 161 to 316 μg/L and fell rapidly afterwards. Similarly, after marijuana smoking, peak plasma concentrations occurred after 3 minutes, ranging from 33 to 118 μg/L, and the plasma profile after smoking was very similar to the intravenous curve, but at about half the concentrations. Interindividual differences in the 2 profiles were small. In contrast, plasma concentrations after oral doses were low and varied from subject to subject. Based on $AUC_{0\text{-}6h}$, systemic availability of Δ^9-THC after smoking varied between 8 and 24%, while oral administration resulted in a systemic availability ranging from 4 to 12% (Ohlsson et al. 1980).

As in the case of nicotine or other drugs taken by inhalation, the systemic availability of Δ^9-THC may be greatly influenced by the smoking patterns of subjects. Significant differences in the systemic availability have been reported (Lindgren et al. 1981). Heavy and habitual users were found to have a systemic availability of 23% compared with 10% in light and infrequent users, suggesting that heavy users smoke cigarettes more efficiently. This may be done by inhaling longer (length and hold of puff), by diminishing the interval between puffs, or by increasing the number of puffs.

2.1.2 Distribution

Δ^9-THC is rapidly transferred from blood to various tissues such as heart, salivary glands, fat, brain, liver and kidney (King & Forney 1967) and has also been found in breast milk. Lung contains the highest concentrations and brain the lowest (Agurell et al. 1970; Klausner & Dingell 1971). This rapid distribution results in a marked and rapid drop in the plasma concentrations after intravenous and inhaled administration of cannabis and accounts for the relatively short (2 to 3 hours) subjective effects of marijuana smoking compared with its long elimination half-life. When Δ^9-THC is administered orally, the plasma concentrations reach a peak and then decline rapidly. Δ^9-THC plasma levels become low while the concentrations of its metabolites increase, probably due to marked first-pass metabolism. Δ^9-THC is highly lipid soluble and has high tissue concentrations, with an apparent volume of distribution of 500L (table V). Only 5% of THC is free for pharmacological activity; the rest binds readily to plasma lipoproteins (Maykut 1985; Wahlqvist et al. 1970).

2.1.3 Metabolism and Excretion

Initial studies in humans were conducted by Lemberger et al. (1971). More recently the metabolism of Δ^9-THC has been studied in detail with improved analytical methodologies using intravenous, oral, and smoking routes of administration. Metabolism occurs in the liver by microsomal hydroxylation and non-microsomal oxidation (Wall & Perez-Reyes 1981). An active, equipotent, 11-hydroxy metabolite is rapidly formed within 10 minutes (Lemberger et al. 1970; Perez-Reyes et al. 1972) which is then oxidised to carboxylic and polar acids (Wall et al. 1976). 20 to 30% of a Δ^9-THC dose appears in the urine in the form of metabolites (Lemberger et al. 1970).

Peak concentrations of 11-OH-THC are higher than those of the parent compound after oral ingestion of marijuana but are very low (almost undetectable) after marijuana inhalation (Ohlsson et al. 1980; Perez-Reyes et al. 1973a). No differences have been reported in metabolic pattern between women and men; however, different patterns have been observed depending on the administration route: after intravenous doses, the ratio of Δ^9-THC to its active metabolite, 11-OH-THC, varies from 1 : 10 to 1 : 20, whereas after oral doses the ratio is 1 : 2. This is consistent with a first-pass effect (Wall et al. 1983).

Approximately equal proportions of Δ^9-THC and its 11-hydroxy metabolite are found in plasma at all times after oral Δ^9-THC administration. Maximum concentrations of the 11-hydroxy metabolite (6 to 8 μg/L) are found 2 or 3 hours after administration and remain at those levels for 6 hours after administration (Wall & Perez-Reyes 1981). The polar non-active metabolites were found at high concentrations (65 to 70 μg/L) for more than 24 hours. In contrast, after smoking or intravenous administration of Δ^9-THC, the active 11-hydroxy metabolite was a minor metabolic component, with plasma concentrations of only one-tenth of Δ^9-THC. The major metabolites found in plasma were the 11-nor-acid and the polar acids, which are, in turn, metabolites produced from 11-hydroxy-Δ^9-THC (Wall & Perez-Reyes 1981).

The faeces are the major excretion route of Δ^9-THC, irrespective of route of administration. The 11-hydroxy metabolite is a major component found in faeces. As much as 35% of total cannabinoids is excreted over a 72-hour period. In contrast, 10 to 15% of the dose is excreted in the urine over the same period as free and conjugated acid metabolites. The finding that Δ^9-THC is completely metabolised in humans has an implication for the testing of this drug, as the best strategy to determine whether a subject has smoked the drug would

Table V. Pharmacokinetic parameters of cannabis (Δ^9-tetrahydrocannabinol)

Reference	Subjects	Dosage (mg)	Vd_{ss} (L)	$t_{1/2\alpha}$ (min)	$t_{1/2\beta}$ (h)	CL (L/min)
Intravenous						
Hunt & Jones (1980)	6 males	–[a] 2	626 ± 296 (L/70kg)	2.78 ± 1.84	19.6 ± 4.1	0.6 ± 0.15
Lemberger et al. (1971)	4 non-users	0.5	658 ± 174		57 ± 4	
	5 chronic users	0.5	597 ± 76		27 ± 1	
Wall et al. (1983)	6 males	2.2-4	734 ± 444		36	0.25 ± 0.06
	6 females	2.2-4	523 ± 217		29	0.2 ± 0.05
Oral						
Hunt & Jones (1980)	6 males	30	742 ± 331	4.41 ± 0.94	18.7 ± 0.2	0.97 ± 0.3
Wall et al. (1983)	6 males	20			25	
	6 females	15			25	

a Dose not stated, but subjects were smoking 11-40 cannabis cigarettes/week.

Abbreviations: Vd_{ss} = volume of distribution at steady-state; $t_{1/2\alpha}$ = distribution half-life; for other abbreviations, see table I.

be to test not only for the parent drug, but for its metabolites which can be detected for prolonged periods (Lemberger et al. 1971).

A biphasic decay of plasma concentrations of Δ^9-THC is seen in healthy volunteers as well as in chronic smokers. Δ^9-THC elimination from the blood occurs rapidly during the first few hours (with a $t_{1/2}$ of 15 to 40 minutes). This phase corresponds with a distribution into tissues, and drug metabolism. The pharmacological effects described after marijuana smoking parallel the plasma concentration of the drug during this phase of rapid decline. The slower phase of decline differs significantly between first-time users ($t_{1/2}$ = 57 hours) and long term users ($t_{1/2}$ = 28 hours). The more rapid metabolism of Δ^9-THC in long term marijuana users may be the result of enzyme induction by Δ^9-THC or other constituents of marijuana cigarettes (Lemberger et al. 1971) [table V]. The apparent volume of distribution is high, of the order of 600L, and does not differ between non-users and long term users, suggesting that the difference in half-lives of the 2 groups is not due to different distribution but rather to an increased rate of metabolism in the latter group.

2.2 Phencyclidine (PCP)

Phencyclidine (PCP) is a popular drug of abuse. It is a lipophilic weak base (pKa 8.5) with pharmacological effects that appear to vary greatly with dosage, the user's previous experience, and the route of administration (Aronow et al. 1980; Perry 1976).

2.2.1 Absorption

PCP abuse occurs through either intravenous, oral or intranasal administration. After oral administration of small doses of PCP to healthy human volunteers, the bioavailability of the drug is highly variable (50 to 90%). This, together with the lack of purity of 'street' drugs, may contribute considerably to the potential for overdose among abusers (Cook et al. 1982a). The average time to reach peak plasma concentrations is 1.5 hours, which appears to coincide with the production of maximal pharmacological effects, although no definite correlation has been established between plasma PCP concentrations and effects (Beech et al. 1961; Cook et al. 1982a). Maximum serum PCP concentrations of 2.7 to 2.9 μg/L are achieved after oral and intravenous 1mg doses, respectively (Cook et al. 1982a).

The increase in popularity of PCP has been attributed to an increase in its use by smoking (Perry 1976). The pharmacokinetic properties of inhaled PCP have been studied in healthy human volunteers (Cook et al. 1982b). PCP and *l*-phenylcyclohexene (PC), a product of PCP pyrolysis, are found in smoke condensate from parsley cigarettes (70mm cigarette containing 650 to 720mg of parsley flakes) containing radiolabelled PCP. PCP and PC are absorbed from smoke; an average of 69 ± 5% of the total amount of PCP present in a cigarette is inhaled, 39% as PCP and 30% as PC. The pharmacological properties of PC are not well established; however, it appears to induce much less toxicity than PCP (Cook et al. 1982b). Following PCP inhalation, peak plasma concentrations (0.62 ± 0.09 nmol/L) occur within 5 to 20 minutes. In some subjects a second peak in the plasma concentration/time profile (0.57 ± 0.6 nmol/L) is observed, occurring between 1 and 3 hours. The presence of a second PCP peak may be due to the trapping of the drug in the membranes of the mouth, from where it could be released and absorbed from the gut or, alternatively, it could be due to absorption by the lung and bronchial tissue with an associated slower release into the systemic circulation. Accumulation of PCP in the lung tissue is possible, as a number of lipophilic amines are known to cumulate and persist in animal lung slices (Brown 1974; Wilson et al. 1979). Long term users report that they feel the first effects from smoking PCP within 2 to 5 minutes, the peak effect within 15 to 30 minutes, while the 'high' effects continue for 4 to 6 hours (Perry 1976).

2.2.2 Distribution

The extent of *in vitro* plasma protein binding of PCP in blood obtained from healthy men is reported to remain relatively constant (61.8 ± 6.2% to 68.9 ± 4.2%) over a concentration range of 0.007

to 5000 μg/L (Cook et al. 1982a). Male patients with mild to moderate alcoholic liver disease have a similar extent of PCP binding to healthy subjects, although age, and concentrations of albumin, bilirubin and high density lipoproteins, may differ (Giles et al. 1982). PCP binding to fatty acid free human serum albumin is only 23.8%, suggesting the presence of another major ligand for the binding of PCP in plasma. α_1-Acid glycoprotein is found to bind PCP significantly; changes in plasma concentrations of this protein are expected to induce major changes in the plasma free drug concentration (Giles et al. 1982).

The volume of distribution of PCP is large (6.2 ± 0.3 L/kg) [table VI], suggesting considerable distribution to extravascular tissues. The plasma elimination half-life is highly variable (7 to 51 hours) among subjects, irrespective of the route of administration (Cook et al. 1982a). Longer half-lives (over 3 days) have been reported in patients with PCP overdose (Done et al. 1978).

2.2.3 Metabolism and Excretion

The metabolic disposition of PCP is similar after intravenous, oral and intranasal administration (Cook et al. 1983). Within 10 days of intravenous PCP administration, 72.8% of a dose is recovered in the urine and 4.7% in the faeces. Faecal excretion of PCP after oral and intravenous doses is very small, suggesting low biliary secretion of the parent drug and metabolites. Around 1% of PCP dose is excreted in sweat (Cook et al. 1982a).

PCP is mainly eliminated by the liver through oxidative hydroxylation (Cook et al. 1982a; Wall et al. 1981; Wong & Biemann 1976). Following intravenous PCP administration under uncontrolled urinary pH, 19.4% of the excreted fraction in urine is composed of non-polar compounds (mainly unchanged drug), while 80.6% of the excreted fraction contains polar metabolites [mainly 4-phenyl-4-(1-piperidinyl) cyclohexanol]. The latter has been shown to have some pharmacological activity (Carroll et al. 1981).

PCP is a weakly basic lipophilic drug, and therefore urinary pH is an important determinant of its renal elimination. Under uncontrolled urinary pH conditions (pH 6.0 to 7.5), the average total clearance of PCP after intravenous administration is 22.8 ± 4.8 L/h and renal clearance is 1.98 ± 0.48 L/h (Cook et al. 1982a) [table VI], suggesting that under these urinary pH conditions PCP is mainly eliminated by metabolic processes. However, under urine alkalinisation (pH 7.4), renal clearance of PCP drops to 0.3 ± 0.18 L/h, while in the same subjects under urine acidification (pH 6.1), renal clearance is increased to 2.4 ± 0.78 L/h (Perez-Reyes et al. 1982c). At a lower urine pH (< 5.0)

Table VI. Pharmacokinetic parameters of phencyclidine

Reference	Dosage/Route	Protein binding (%)	$t_{1/2\beta}$ (h) [range]	Vd (L/kg) [range]	CL (L/min) [range]	CL_R (L/min) [range]
Cook et al. (1982a)	0.0012-0.012 mg/kg IV	64.5 ± 4.1 (at 100 μg/L)	16 ± 2 [7-23]	6.2 ± 0.3 [5.3-7.5]	0.38 ± 0.08 [0.26-0.77]	0.033 ± 0.008 [0.011-0.06]
	0.0125-0.0167 mg/kg PO		27 ± 5 [19-46]			0.037 ± 0.016
Cook et al. (1982b)	1.8 nmol/kg inhalation		24 ± 7 [10-51]		0.28 ± 0.05 [0.14-0.39]	0.033 ± 0.007 [0.015 - 0.043]
Perez-Reyes et al. (1982c)	0.5mg IV					Acid urine 0.040 ± 0.013 Alkaline urine 0.005 ± 0.003

Abbreviations: CL_R = renal clearance; for other abbreviations, see table I.

Aronow et al. (1978) reported a much higher PCP renal clearance of 8.04 ± 1.56 L/h.

PCP renal clearance is not only dependent on urine pH, but is also affected by urine flow rate. An increase in urine output through the administration of fluids and frusemide (furosemide) increases the renal elimination of PCP. These findings are extremely important for the treatment of acute PCP intoxication, where significant urine acidification and the maintenance of a high urine output dramatically enhance the elimination of the drug (Done et al. 1980).

3. Central Nervous System Depressants

3.1 Benzodiazepines

Benzodiazepine use is common. It has been shown that between 10 and 20% of the adult population of the western world has taken a sedative-hypnotic drug during the past year and 1 to 3% of the population remains on these drugs for longer than a year (Balter et al. 1984).

Problematical use of benzodiazepines may arise in at least 2 contexts that may be considered abusive: persistent therapeutic use, which is usually for a medical indication but for a longer duration than is generally recommended, and illicit use, in which the drug may be used outside medical indication and supervision (Cappell et al. 1987). The former type of usage seems to occur relatively frequently, and usually involves use of low (therapeutic) benzodiazepine doses (e.g. 5 to 40mg of diazepam per day). Dose increases or acute intoxication almost never occur, but a distinct risk of dependence exists. The latter usage of benzodiazepines is rare, but likely to involve high doses, multiple drug use, a pattern of pathological use, and clear impairment of normal functioning (Cappell et al. 1987).

3.1.1 Absorption

Benzodiazepines are lipophilic acids (diazepam pKa 3.4) with a high octanol/water partition coefficient (diazepam: 180).

The onset of action of the benzodiazepine depends on the absorption rate, and is the major determinant of the subjective effect after a single dose. Currently available data suggest that diazepam and midazolam are among the most rapidly absorbed benzodiazepines (table VII), while oxazepam, prazepam and halazepam are among the least rapidly absorbed. The differences between the absorption rates of the various drugs are of clinical significance. Diazepam, for example, produces quick effects and behavioural changes, whereas the effects of oxazepam appear slowly (Bliding 1974). Given that speed of onset of drug effect is a major determinant of the reinforcing effects, it follows that the relative potential for abuse of a benzodiazepine may be influenced by the rate of onset after oral administration. Recently available data support this hypothesis. A series of studies in patients with histories of drug abuse suggest that the abuse liability of diazepam is greater than that of oxazepam (Griffiths et al. 1984a,b) and subjects frequently cited the rapid onset of diazepam effects as a reason for preferring this drug over oxazepam. In addition, epidemiological studies show that while diazepam and oxazepam are used with the same frequency, illegal activities (such as prescription forgeries and theft reports) associated with diazepam are 2 to 2.5 times more frequent than those associated with oxazepam (Bergman & Griffiths 1986).

The pharmacokinetic profile of some benzodiazepines that are prodrugs has been used to take advantage of the slow transformation of the drug precursors into an active metabolite. For example, halazepam is rapidly converted into desmethyldiazepam, an active metabolite. In contrast to the rapid and marked effects of diazepam reported by drug abusers, very few subjective effects after halazepam administration are reported over the first hour after ingestion (Jaffe et al. 1983). Sedation and 'liking' effects are also delayed in the case of halazepam. To the extent that abuse liability is related to the onset and peak intensity of the reinforcing effects of drugs, these findings suggest that halazepam may have a lower potential for abuse than diazepam. No other prodrugs have been compared with diazepam in this respect. However, based on pharmacokinetic parameters, it has been suggested that prodrugs slowly converted to desmethyldiazepam (Greenblatt & Shader 1978) would also have

Table VII. Pharmacokinetic parameters of benzodiazepines

Drug	Dosage/Route (mg)	t_{max} (h) [range]	Bioavailability (F) [%]	Reference
Alprazolam	0.5-31 PO	0.7-1.6	Good (PO, liquid)	Abernethy et al. (1983); Evans (1981); Smith & Schoenfeld (1981)
Bromazepam	0.25-0.5 PO	1		Kaplan et al. (1976)
Chlordiazepoxide	20-50 PO, IM, IV	0.5-3.3	100 (PO) Poor (IM)	Greenblatt et al. (1978); Boxenbaum et al. (1977a,b); Shader et al. (1977); Greenblatt et al. (1974)
Clobazam	10-20 PO	1.3-1.7	Good (tablets, capsules, solutions)	Rupp et al. (1979); Vallner et al. (1978)
Clorazepate (see desmethyldiazepam)				
Desalkylflurazepam	PO	1		Greenblatt et al. (1975)
Desmethyldiazepam		1-1.8		Klotz et al. (1976)
Diazepam	1-40 PO, IM, IV	1.5-2	Good (tablets, suspension) Poor, irregular (50-60) (IM, suppositories)	Hillestad et al. (1974); Arnold (1975); Schwartz et al. (1965); Gamble et al. (1975); Baird & Hailey (1972)
Estazolam	2-16 PO	6		Allen et al. (1979)
Flunitrazepam	0.5-2 PO	1.5	Good (IM)	Cano et al. (1977)
Flurazepam (see desalkylflurazepam)	15-90 PO			Greenblatt et la. (1975); Kaplan et al. (1973b)
Halazepam (see desmethyldiazepam)				Greenblatt et al. (1983a); Chung et al. (1984)
Lorazepam	2-4 PO	1.5	90 (IM)	Greenblatt et al. (1979)
Lormetazepam			70-80	Humpel et al. (1979)
Medazepam (see desmethyldiazepam)				
Midazolam	5-15 PO, IV, IM	0.37-0.74	30-50 (PO)	Smith et al. (1981); Allonen et al. (1981); Greenblatt et al. (1981)
Nitrazepam	15-30 PO	2		Jochemsen & Breimer (1982); Kangas & Breimer (1981)
Oxazepam	15-45 PO	3 [0.5-8]		Alvan et al. (1977); MacLeod et al. (1978); Sellers et al. (1979); Greenblatt et al. (1980b)
Pinazepam (see desmethyldiazepam)				Pacifici et al. (1982)
Prazepam (see desmethyldiazepam)				Greenblatt & Shader (1978)
Temazepam	10-30 PO (soft and hard capsules)	0.75-1.0 (soft capsule) 1.4-4.7 (hard capsule)		Fuccella et al. (1977); Divoll & Greenblatt (1981); Bittencourt et al. (1979)
Triazolam	0.5-1.0 PO	1.6 [0.8-2.5]	Complete	Greenblatt et al. (1983b); Eberts et al. (1981); Adams et al. (1980); Metzler et al. (1977)

Abbreviations: t_{max} = time to reach peak plasma drug concentration; IM = intramuscular; IV = intravenous; PO = oral.

Table VIII. Pharmacokinetic parameters of benzodiazepines

Drug	Active metabolites	Protein binding (%) [range]	Vd (L/kg)	Mean $t_{½β}$ (h) [range]	CL (ml/min/kg)	Reference
Alprazolam	Hydroxyalprazolam	70 [65-80]	1-1.5	12 [6-18]	1.22	Moschitto & Greenblatt (1983); Bellantuono et al. (1980); Abernethy et al. (1983)
Bromazepam	3-Hydroxy-bromazepam	70		10-15		Kaplan et al. (1976); Garattini et al. (1977)
Chlordiazepoxide	Desmethyl-chlordiazepoxide, desmethyl-diazepam, oxazepam	95 [94-97]	0.26-0.58	10 [6-28]	0.21-0.54	Greenblatt et al. (1977, 1978); Boxenbaum et al. (1977a,b); MacLeod et al. (1977)
Clobazam	Demoxepam, desmethylclobazam	90 [85-92]	0.9-1.8	25 [16-49]	0.36-0.63	Greenblatt et al. (1983d); Tedeschi et al. (1981); Volz et al. (1979)
Desalkylflurazepam				80 [40-200]		Greenblatt et al. (1975); Greenblatt et al. (1983)
Desmethyldiazepam	Oxazepam	98	0.93-1.27	51 [51-120]		Mandelli et al. (1978); Klotz et al. (1976)
Diazepam	*N*-Desmethyl-diazepam, oxazepam, 3-hydroxydiazepam (temazepam)	[97-99]	0.95-20	31 [14-61]	0.39-0.51	van der Kleijn et al. (1971); Klotz et al. (1976); Thiessen et al. (1976); Andreasen et al. (1976); Kaplan et al. (1973a); Greenblatt et al. (1980a); Schwartz et al. (1965); Mandelli et al. (1978)
Estazolam	Hydroxyestazolam			17 [8-31]		Allen et al. (1979)
Flunitrazepam	Desmethyl-flunitrazepam, 7 amino derivative	85		25 [9-30]		Amrein (1978); Boxenbaum et al. (1978); Wickstrom et al. (1980)
Flurazepam	Hydroxyethyl-flurazepam, desalkylflurazepam flurazepam aldehyde					Greenblatt et al. (1975)
Halazepam (see desmethyldiazepam)						Greenblatt et al. (1983b)

Table VIII. Contd

Drug	Active metabolites	Protein binding (%) [range]	Vd (L/kg)	Mean $t_{1/2\beta}$ (h) [range]	CL (ml/min/kg)	Reference
Lorazepam	None	[90-93]	0.84-1.63	13 [8-25]	1 (0.8-1.3)	Greenblatt et al. (1979); Greenblatt & Shader (1978)
Lormetazepam				9-15	180-200	Humpel et al. (1979)
Medazepam (see desmethyldiazepam)						
Midazolam		[94-97]	0.8-1.72	2 [1.4-5]	6 (4-8)	Smith et al. (1981); Allonen et al. (1981); Greenblatt et al. (1981); Lauven et al. (1982)
Nitrazepam	None	[86-87]	1.50-2.76	[18-48]		Rieder & Wendt (1973); Kangas & Breimer (1981)
Oxazepam	None	97	0.52-2.0	7 [5.1-13]	0.6-2.85	Alvan et al. (1977); MacLeod et al. (1978); Sellers et al. (1979); Greenblatt et al. (1980b)
Pinazepam (see desmethyldiazepam)						Pacifici et al. (1982)
Prazepam (see desmethyldiazepam)						DiCarlo et al. (1971)
Temazepam	Oxazepam	97	1.3-1.5	12 [7.3-17.2]	0.97-1.36	Divoll & Greenblatt (1981)
Triazolam	None	90	NA	2.5 [2.1-4.6]	3.7-8.8	Eberts et al. (1981); Greenblatt et al. (1983c); Kroboth et al. (1984)

Abbreviations: see table I.

a slow onset of subjective effects, and therefore may have a lower potential for abuse than more rapidly absorbed benzodiazepines (diazepam) or other rapidly converted desmethyldiazepam precursors (e.g. clorazepate) [Busto & Sellers 1986]. This hypothesis has not yet been tested in rigorous experiments.

3.1.2 Distribution

Distribution of drugs into the brain is important for the reinforcement effect, since abused drugs must gain access to the site of action. Although other factors (e.g. blood flow, molecular size) play a role, high lipid solubility is associated with rapid access to the site of action into the brain. In the case of benzodiazepines the most lipid-soluble drugs (e.g. diazepam, midazolam) produce almost instantaneous effects if given intravenously. Half-life of the appearance of midazolam and diazepam in CSF is 0.28 and 0.44 minutes, respectively, which permits their use as pre-anaesthetic medication (Arendt et al. 1983; Smith et al. 1981).

The duration of action after a single benzodiazepine dose depends upon the rate and extent of drug distribution, as well as the rate of elimination once complete distribution has taken place. Lorazepam, for example, has a relatively short half-life (12 to 15 hours) but the effective duration of a single dose may be relatively long when compared with diazepam, which has a longer half-life (approximately 30 hours). This is due to the swift distribution of diazepam from blood to fatty tissues, causing a rapid termination of single-dose effect (George & Dundee 1977). Thus, it is important to note that a long elimination half-life does not necessarily imply long duration of action after single doses.

Benzodiazepines are highly bound to plasma proteins (table VII) and are readily distributed in the body. Due to their high lipid solubility, benzodiazepines are rapidly removed from plasma to brain and lungs, and also to adipose tissue. Volumes of distribution are typically 1 L/kg.

3.1.3 Metabolism and Elimination

The metabolic pathways of benzodiazepine include hydroxylation, desmethylation and glucuronidation. Several benzodiazepines are metabolised to 1 or more active metabolites, which are in many cases partially or totally responsible for the pharmacological effects. Others are metabolised to inactive metabolites through glucuronidation (e.g. oxazepam, lorazepam) [table VIII].

The average effect of drugs during long term use or multiple-dose therapy depends in part upon the rate and extent of drug accumulation. The steady-state concentration in turn is related to elimination half-life and free drug clearance. In addition, the clinical effect does not necessarily increase during multiple drug therapy, even when drug accumulation occurs (Hillestad et al. 1974); a consequence of tolerance or adaptation to the effect of the drug. Despite the fact that plasma diazepam and *N*-desmethyldiazepam concentrations in benzodiazepine abusers are 8 to 10 times greater than the therapeutic levels described in the literature (Harrison et al. 1984; Linnoila et al. 1980), patients do not appear intoxicated or impaired to trained observers. However, tolerance seems to develop differentially, and information processing and short term memory may not be impaired at high concentrations, while eye-hand coordination appears to deteriorate (Linnoila et al. 1980).

The elimination pharmacokinetics of benzodiazepines are closely related to the withdrawal reactions that these drugs produce. Drugs with a very short half-life, such as triazolam, will not sustain the high tissue concentrations required to produce physical dependence unless taken frequently and in high doses. On the other hand, drugs such as lorazepam, oxazepam and alprazolam will produce severe and rapid withdrawal symptoms when they are discontinued. This principle, which was postulated by Kalant for non-opiate drugs and by Hollister for benzodiazepines (Hollister 1980; Kalant et al. 1971), has recently been clinically confirmed in a placebo-controlled trial of benzodiazepine withdrawal after long term therapeutic use (Busto et al. 1986). The onset of withdrawal in patients taking benzodiazepines with short or intermediate half-life was 1 day after drug discontinuation, while for those using long acting benzodiazepines onset occurred 3 to 8 days after cessation of treatment. On an evaluation scale of 0 to 10, patients on rapidly eliminated benzodiazepines rated their symptoms as more severe than those on long acting benzodiazepines (9.7 *vs* 7.6). However, the difference was not clinically significant, probably due to the small number of subjects in which the analysis was possible. In addition, 7 of 8 patients refusing placebo treatment were taking rapidly eliminated benzodiazepines. The relationship between the appearance of a withdrawal reaction and drug self-administration has been further clarified in recent studies: patients undergoing withdrawal of benzodiazepines treat themselves by self-administering benzodiazepines from their own supply, thus establishing a clear relationship between withdrawal symptoms and persistent self-administration of drug (Cappell et al. 1987).

Slowly eliminated benzodiazepines are less liable to produce withdrawal reactions and, if they occur, they seem to be milder. The clearest therapeutic application of this pharmacokinetic principle is in the clinical management of benzodiazepine withdrawal. The understanding that

benzodiazepines with long half-lives produce a slow decrease of plasma concentrations, and therefore a milder withdrawal syndrome, has helped in the development of simplified detoxification treatment procedures. Patients who have been abusing high doses of benzodiazepines with short or intermediate half-lives are switched to equivalent doses of diazepam and gradually tapered off, capitalising on the long half-life of diazepam and its metabolite to minimise withdrawal symptomatology (Harrison et al. 1984).

References

Abernethy DR, Greenblatt DJ, Divoll M, Shader RI. Pharmacokinetics of alprazolam. Journal of Clinical Psychiatry 44: 45-47, 1983

Adams WJ, Rykert UM, Bombardt PA. High performance liquid chromatographic determination of triazolam in human serum. Analytical Letters 13: 149-161, 1980

Agurell S, Lindgren JE, Ohlsson H. Quantification of cannabinoids and their metabolites in biological fluids. In Nahas GG and Paton WD (Eds) Marihuana: biological effects, pp. 3-13, Pergamon Press, Oxford, 1979

Agurell S, Nilsson IM, Ohlsson A, Sandberg F. On the metabolism of tritium-labelled 1-tetrahydrocannabinol in the rabbit. Biochemical Pharmacology 19: 1333-1339, 1970

Aldridge A, Parsons WD, Neims AH. Stimulation of caffeine metabolism in the rat by 3-methylcholanthrene. Life Sciences 21: 967-974, 1977

Allen MD, Greenblatt DJ, Arnold DJ. Single- and multiple-dose kinetics of estazolam, a triazolobenzodiazepine. Psychopharmacology 66: 267-274, 1979

Allonen H, Ziegler G, Klotz U. Midazolam kinetics. Clinical Pharmacology and Therapeutics 30: 653-661, 1981

Alvan G, Siwers B, Vessman J. Pharmacokinetics of oxazepam in healthy volunteers. Acta Pharmacologica et Toxicologica 40 (Suppl. 1): 40-51, 1977

Ammon HPT, Bieck PR, Mandalaz D, Verspohl EJ. Adaptation of blood pressure to continuous heavy coffee drinking in young volunteers: a double-blind crossover study. British Journal of Clinical Pharmacology 15: 701-706, 1983

Amrein R. Zur Pharmacokinetic und zum Metabolismus von Flunitrazepam. In Ahnefeld et al. (Eds) Rohypnol (Flunitrazepam). Pharmakologische Grundlagen-Klinische Anwendung, pp. 8-24, Springer-Verlag, Berlin, 1978

Andreasen PB, Hendel J, Greisen G, Hvidger EF. Pharmacokinetics of diazepam in disordered liver function. European Journal of Clinical Pharmacology 10: 115-120, 1976

Anggard E, Gunne LM, Jonsson LE, Niklasson F. Pharmacokinetic and clinical studies on amphetamine dependent subjects. European Journal of Clinical Pharmacology 3: 3-11, 1970

Anggard E, Jonsson LE, Hogmark AL, et al. Amphetamine metabolism in amphetamine psychosis. Clinical Pharmacology and Therapeutics 14: 870-880, 1973

Aranda JV, Cook CE, Gorman W, Collinge JM, Loughnan PM, et al. Pharmacokinetic profile of caffeine in the premature newborn infant with apnea. Journal of Pediatrics 94: 663-668, 1979

Arendt RM, Greenblatt DJ, deJong RH, Bonin JD, Abernethy DR, et al. *In vitro* correlates of benzodiazepines cerebrospinal fluid uptake, pharmacodynamic action and peripheral distribution. Journal of Pharmacology and Experimental Therapeutics 227: 98-106, 1983

Armitage AK, Dollery CT, George CF, et al. Absorption and metabolism of nicotine from cigarettes. British Medical Journal 4: 313-316, 1975

Arnold E. A simple method for determining diazepam and its major metabolites in biological fluids: application in bioavailability studies. Acta Pharmacologica et Toxicologica 36: 335-352, 1975

Aronow R, Miceli JN, Done AK. Clinical observations during phencyclidine intoxication and treatment based on ion-trapping. National Institute of Drug Abuse Monograph Series 21: 218-228, 1978

Aronow R, Miceli JN, Done AK. A therapeutic approach to the acutely overdosed PCP patient. Journal of Psychedelic Drugs 12: 259-267, 1980

Atkinson HC, Begg EJ, Darlow BA. Drugs in human milk: clinical pharmacokinetic considerations. Clinical Pharmacokinetics 14: 217-240, 1988

Axelrod J, Reichenthal J. The fate of caffeine in man and a method for its estimation in biological material. Journal of Pharmacology and Experimental Therapeutics 107: 519-523, 1953

Baird ES, Hailey DM. Delayed recovery from a sedative: correlation of the plasma levels of diazepam with clinical effects after oral and intravenous administration. British Journal of Anaesthesia 44: 803-808, 1972

Balter MB, Manheimer DI, Mellinger GD, Uhlenhuth EH. A cross-national comparison of anti-anxiety/sedative drug use. Current Medical Research and Opinion 8 (Suppl. 4): 5-20, 1984

Barnett G, Hawks R, Resnick R. Cocaine pharmacokinetics in humans. Journal of Ethnopharmacology 3: 353-366, 1981

Beckett AH, Gorrod JW, Jenner P. The analysis of nicotine-1'-N-oxide in urine, in the presence of nicotine and cotinine, and its application to the study of *in vivo* nicotine metabolism in man. Journal of Pharmacy and Pharmacology 23: 55S-61S, 1971

Beckett AH, Rowland M, Turner P. Influence of urinary pH on excretion of amphetamine. Lancet 1: 303, 1965

Beckett AH, Salmon JA, Mitchard M. The relation between blood levels and urinary excretion of amphetamine under controlled acidic and under fluctuating urinary pH values using [^{14}C] amphetamine. Journal of Pharmacy and Pharmacology 21: 251-258, 1969

Beech HR, Davies BM, Morgenstern FS. Preliminary investigations of the effects of sernyl upon cognitive and sensory processes. Journal of Mental Sciences 109: 509-513, 1961

Bellantuono C, Reggi V, Tognoni G, Garattini S. Benzodiazepines: clinical pharmacology and therapeutic use. Drugs 19: 195-219, 1980

Bellet S, Kershbaum A, Finde EM. Response of free fatty acids to coffee and caffeine. Metabolism 17: 702-707, 1968

Benowitz NL, Jacob P, Jones RT, Rosenberg J. Interindividual variability in the metabolism and cardiovascular effects of nicotine in man. Journal of Pharmacology and Experimental Therapeutics 221: 368-372, 1982

Benowitz NL, Kuyt F, Jacob P, Jones RT, Osman AL. Cotinine disposition and effects. Clinical Pharmacology and Therapeutics 34: 604-610, 1983

Benowitz NL, Lake T, Keller KH, Lee LB. Prolonged absorption with development of tolerance to toxic effects after cutaneous exposure to nicotine. Clinical Pharmacology and Therapeutics 42: 119-120, 1987

Bergman U, Griffiths RR. Relative abuse of diazepam and oxazepam: prescription forgeries and theft/loss reports in Sweden. Drug and Alcohol Dependence 16: 293-301, 1986

Bergmann F, Dikstein S. Studies on uric acid and related compounds, III: observations on the specificity of mammalian xanthine oxidase. Journal of Biological Chemistry 223: 765-780, 1956

Bittencourt P, Richens A, Toseland PA, Wicks JFC, Latham AN.

Pharmacokinetics of the hypnotic benzodiazepine, temazepam. British Journal of Clinical Pharmacology 8: 31S-38S, 1979
Blanchard J. Protein binding of caffeine in young and elderly males. Journal of Pharmaceutical Sciences 71: 1415-1418, 1982
Blanchard J, Sawers SJA. The absolute bioavailability of caffeine in man. European Journal of Clinical Pharmacology 24: 93-98, 1983a
Blanchard J, Sawers SJA. Comparative pharmacokinetics of caffeine in young and elderly men. Journal of Pharmacokinetics and Biopharmaceutics 11: 109-126, 1983b
Bliding A. Effects of different rates of absorption of two benzodiazepines on subjective and objective parameters. European Journal of Clinical Pharmacology 7: 201-211, 1974
Boisse NR, Okamoto M. Physical dependence to barbital compared to pentobarbital, part IV: influence of elimination kinetics. Journal of Pharmacology and Experimental Therapeutics 204: 526-540, 1978
Bonati M, Latini R, Galletti F, Young JF, Tognoni G, et al. Caffeine disposition after oral doses. Clinical Pharmacology and Therapeutics 32: 98-106, 1982
Boxenbaum HG l, Geitner KA, Jack MK, Dixon WR, Kaplan SA. Pharmacokinetics and biopharmaceutical profile of chlordiazepoxide HCl in healthy subjects: single dose studies by intravenous, intramuscular and oral routes. Journal of Pharmacokinetics and Biopharmaceutics 5: 3-23, 1977a
Boxenbaum HG, Geitner KA, Jack ML, Dixon WR, Kaplan SA. Pharmacokinetic and bipharmaceutic profile of chlordiazepoxide HCl in healthy subjects: multiple-dose oral administration. Journal of Pharmacokinetics and Biopharmaceutics 5: 25-39, 1977b
Boxenbaum HG, Posmanter HN, Macasieb T, Geitner KA, Weinfeld RE, et al. Pharmacokinetics of flunitrazepam following single- and multiple-dose oral administration of healthy human subjects. Journal of Pharmacokinetics and Biopharmaceutics 6: 283, 1978
Brown EAB. The localization, metabolism and effects of drugs and toxicants in lung. Drug Metabolism Reviews 3: 33-87, 1974
Burg AW. Physiological disposition of caffeine. Drug Metabolism Reviews 4: 199-228, 1975
Busto U, Sellers EM. Pharmacokinetic determinants of drug abuse and dependence: a conceptual perspective. Clinical Pharmacokinetics 11: 144-153, 1986
Busto U, Sellers EM, Naranjo CA, Cappell H, Sanchez-Craig M, et al. Withdrawal reaction after long-term therapeutic use of benzodiazepines. New England Journal of Medicine 315: 854-859, 1986
Cano JP, Soliva M, Hartmann D, Ziegler WH, Amrein R. Bioavailability from various galenic formulations of flunitrazepam. Arzneimittel-Forschung 27: 2383-2388, 1977
Cappell H, Busto U, Kay G, Naranjo CA, Sellers EM, et al. Drug deprivation and reinforcement by diazepam in a dependent population. Psychopharmacology 91: 154-160, 1987
Carroll FI, Brine GA, Boldt KG, Cone EJ, Yousefnejad D, et al. Phencyclidine metabolism: resolution, structure, and biological activity of the isomers of the hydroxy metabolite, 4-phenyl-4-(1-piperidinyl) cyclohexanol. Journal of Medicinal Chemistry 24: 1047-1051, 1981
Chow MJ, Ambre JJ, Ruo TI, Atkinson AJ, Bowsher DJ, et al. Kinetics of cocaine distribution, elimination and chronotropic effects. Clinical Pharmacology and Therapeutics 38: 318-324, 1985
Chung M, Hilbert JM, Gural RP, Radwanski E, Symchowicz S, et al. Multiple-dose halazepam kinetics. Clinical Pharmacology and Therapeutics 35: 838-842, 1984
Committee on Problems of Drug Dependence. Report on the assessment of abuse liability and dependence potential. National Institute of Drug Abuse, United States Government Printing Office, Washington, D.C., 1985
Cook CE, Brine DR, Jeffcoat AR, Hill JM, Wall ME, et al. Phencyclidine disposition after intravenous and oral doses. Clinical Pharmacology and Therapeutics 31: 625-634, 1982a
Cook CE, Brine DR, Quin GD, Perez-Reyes M, DiGuiseppi SR. Phencyclidine and phenylcyclohexene disposition after smoking phencyclidine. Clinical Pharmacology and Therapeutics 31: 635-641, 1982b
Cook CE, Perez-Reyes M, Jeffcoat AR, Brine DR. Phencyclidine disposition in humans after small doses of radiolabeled drug. Federation Proceedings 42: 2566-2569, 1983
Darby TD, McNamee JE, Van Rossum JM. Cigarette smoking pharmacokinetics and its relationship to smoking behaviour. Clinical Pharmacokinetics 9: 435-449, 1984
Davis JM, Kopin IJ, Lemberger L, Axelrod J. Effects of urinary pH on amphetamine metabolism. Annals of New York Academy of Sciences 179: 493-501, 1971
Desmond PV, Patwardhan RV, Johnson RF, Schenker S. Impaired elimination of caffeine in cirrhosis. Digestive Diseases and Sciences 25: 193-197, 1980
DiCarlo FJ, Viau JP, Epps JE, Haynes LJ. Biotransformation of prazepam in man. Annals of the New York Academy of Sciences 179: 487, 1971
Divoll M, Greenblatt DJ. Plasma concentrations of temazepam, a 3-hydroxy benzodiazepine, determined by electron-capture gas-liquid chromatography. Journal of Chromatography 222: 125-128, 1981
Done AK, Aronow R, Miceli JN. The pharmacokinetics of phencyclidine in overdosage and its treatment. National Institute on Drug Abuse Research Monograph Series 21: 210-217, 1978
Done AK, Aronow R, Miceli JN. Pharmacokinetic bases for the diagnosis and treatment of acute PCP intoxication. Journal of Psychedelic Drugs 12: 253-258, 1980
Dorian P, Sellers EM, Kaplan H, Hamilton C. Evaluation of zopiclone physical dependence liability in normal volunteers. Pharmacology 27 (Suppl. 2): 228-234, 1983
Dring LG, Smith RL, Williams RT. The metabolic fate of amphetamine in man and other species. Biochemical Journal 116: 425-435, 1970
Eberts FS, Philopoulos Y, Reineke LM, Vliek RW. Triazolam disposition. Clinical Pharmacology and Therapeutics 29: 81-93, 1981
Edwards DJ, Bowles SK. Serum protein binding of cocaine. American Society for Clinical Pharmacology and Therapeutics. 88th Annual Meeting, Orlando, March 1987
Ellison T, Siegel M, Silverman AG, Okun R. Comparative metabolism of d,l H^3-amphetamine hydrochloride in tolerant and non tolerant cats. Proceedings of the Western Pharmacology Society 11: 75-77, 1968
Evans RL. Alprazolam. Drug Intelligence and Clinical Pharmacy 15: 633-638, 1981
Feyerabend C, Ings RMJ, Russell MAH. Nicotine pharmacokinetics and its application to intake from smoking. British Journal of Clinical Pharmacology 19: 239-247, 1985
Franksson G, Anggard E. The plasma protein binding of amphetamine, catecholamines and related compounds. Acta Pharmacologica et Toxicologica 28: 209-214, 1970
Fuccella LM, Bolcioni G, Tamassia V, Ferrario L, Tognoni G. Human pharmacokinetics and bioavailability of temazepam administered in soft gelatin capsules. European Journal of Clinical Pharmacology 12: 383-386, 1977
Gamble JAS, Dundee JW, Assaff RAE. Plasma diazepam levels after single dose oral and intramuscular administration. Anaesthesia 30: 164-169, 1975
Garattini S, Marcucci F, Mussini E. The metabolism and pharmacokinetics of selected benzodiazepines. In: Usdin & Forrest (Eds) Psychotherapeutic drugs part III: applications, pp. 1039-1087, M. Dekker, New York, 1977
Gehlbach SH, Williams WA, Perry LD, Woodall JS. Green-tobacco sickness: an illness of tobacco harvesters. Journal of the American Medical Association 229: 1880-1883, 1974

George KA, Dundee JW. Relative amnesic actions of diazepam, flunitrazepam and lorazepam in man. British Journal of Clinical Pharmacology 4: 45-50, 1977
Giles HG, Corrigall WA, Khouw V, Sellers EM. Plasma protein binding of phencyclidine. Clinical Pharmacology and Therapeutics 31: 77-82, 1982
Gorodischer R, Karplus M, Worszowski D, Bark H, Moses SW, et al. Caffeine pharmacokinetics in the neonate: humans and animal studies. Pediatric Research 11: 1013, 1977
Gorrod JW. The metabolism and excretion of amphetamines in man. In Frontiers in catecholamine research, pp. 945-950, 1973
Gorrod JW, Jenner P. The metabolism of tobacco alkaloids. In Essays in toxicology, pp. 35-78, Academic Press, New York, 1975
Graham DM. Caffeine: its identity, dietary sources, intake and biological effects. Nutrition Review 36: 97-102, 1978
Grant DM, Tang BK, Kalow W. Variability in caffeine metabolism. Clinical Pharmacology and Therapeutics 33: 591-602, 1983
Greden JF. Coffee, tea and you. The Sciences 19: 6-11, 1979
Greenblatt DJ, Abernethy DR, Divoll M, Harmatz JS, Shader RI. Pharmacokinetic properties of benzodiazepine hypnotics. Journal of Clinical Psychopharmacology 3: 129-132, 1983a
Greenblatt DJ, Allen MD, Harmatz S, Shader RI. Clinical pharmacokinetics of the newer benzodiazepines. Clinical Pharmacokinetics 8: 233-252, 1983b
Greenblatt DJ, Divoll M, Abernethy DR, Moschitto LJ, Smith RB, et al. Reduced clearance of triazolam in old age; relation to antipyrine oxidizing capacity. British Journal of Clinical Pharmacology 15: 303-309, 1983c
Greenblatt DJ, Divoll M, Abernethy DR, Ochs HR, Shader RI. Diazepam disposition determinants. Clinical Pharmacology and Therapeutics 27: 301-312, 1980a
Greenblatt DJ, Divoll M, Harmatz JS, Shader RI. Oxazepam kinetics: effects of age and sex. Journal of Pharmacology and Experimental Therapeutics 215: 86-91, 1980b
Greenblatt DJ, Divoll M, Puri SK, Ho I, Zinny MA, et al. Reduced single-dose clearance of clobazam in elderly men predicts increased multiple-dose accumulation. Clinical Pharmacokinetics 8: 83-94, 1983d
Greenblatt DJ, Locniskar A, Ochs HR, Lauven PM. Automated gas chromatography for studies of midazolam pharmacokinetics. Anesthesiology 55: 176-179, 1981
Greenblatt DJ, Shader RI. Prazepam and lorazepam, two new benzodiazepines. New England Journal of Medicine 299: 1342-1344, 1978
Greenblatt DJ, Shader RI, Franke K, MacLaughlin DS, Harmatz JS, et al. Pharmacokinetics and bioavailability of intravenous intramuscular and oral lorazepam in humans. Journal of Pharmaceutical Sciences 68: 57-63, 1979
Greenblatt DJ, Shader RI, Harmatz JS, Franke K, Koch-Weser J. Absorption rate, blood concentrations, and early response to oral chlordiazepoxide. American Journal of Psychiatry 134: 559-562, 1977
Greenblatt DJ, Shader RI, Koch-Weser J. Slow absorption of intramuscular chlordiazepoxide. New England Journal of Medicine 291: 1116-1118, 1974
Greenblatt DJ, Shader RI, Koch-Weser J. Flurazepam hydrochloride. Clinical Pharmacology and Therapeutics 17: 1-14, 1975
Greenblatt DJ, Shader RI, MacLeod SM, Sellers EM. Clinical pharmacokinetics of chlordiazepoxide. Clinical Pharmacokinetics 3: 381-394, 1978
Griffiths RR, Henningfield JE. Pharmacology of cigarette smoking behaviour. Trends in Pharmacological Sciences 3: 260-263, 1982
Griffiths RR, Lamb RJ, Ator NA, Roache JD, Brady JV. Relative abuse liability of triazolam: experimental assessment in animals and humans. Neuroscience and Behaviour Reviews 9: 133-151, 1985
Griffiths RR, McLeod DR, Bigelow GE, Liebson IA, Roache JD. Relative abuse liability of diazepam and oxazepam: behavioural and subjective dose effects. Psychopharmacology 84: 147-154, 1984a
Griffiths RR, McLeod DR, Bigelow GE, Liebson IA, Roache JD, et al. Comparison of diazepam and oxazepam: preference, liking and extent of abuse. Journal of Pharmacology and Experimental Therapeutics 229: 501-508, 1984b
Guerin MR. Chemical composition of cigarette smoke. In Gori and Bock (Eds) A safe cigarette?, pp. 191-203, Cold Spring Harbor Laboratory, Cold Spring Harbor, 1980
Gunne LM, Anggard E. Pharmacokinetic studies with amphetamines: relationships to neuropsychiatric disorders. Journal of Pharmacokinetics and Biopharmaceutics 1: 481-495, 1973
Hall SM, Henning RI, Jones RT, Benowitz NL, Jacob P. Blood cotinine levels as indicators of smoking treatment outcome. Clinical Pharmacology and Therapeutics 35: 810-814, 1984
Harrison M, Busto U, Naranjo CA, Kaplan HL, Sellers EM. Diazepam tapering in detoxification for high-dose benzodiazepine abuse. Clinical Pharmacology and Therapeutics 36: 527-533, 1984
Hawks RL, Kopin IJ, Colburn RW and Thoa NB. Norcocaine: a pharmacologically active metabolite of cocaine found in brain. Life Sciences 15: 2189-2195, 1974
Henningfield JE, Miyasato K, Jasinski DR. Abuse liability and pharmacodynamic characteristics of intravenous and inhaled nicotine. Journal of Pharmacology and Experimental Therapeutics 234: 1-12, 1985
Hibberd AR, O'Connor V, Gorrod JW. Detection of nicotine, nicotine-1-N-oxide and cotinine in maternal and fetal body fluids. In Gorrod JW (Ed.) Biological oxidation of nitrogen, pp. 353-361, Elsevier, Amsterdam, 1978
Hill HE, Haertzen CA, Wolbach AB, Miner EJ. The addiction research center inventory: standardization of scales which evaluate subjective effects of morphine, amphetamine, pentobarbital, alcohol, LSD-25, pyrahexyl and chlorpromazine. Psychopharmacologia 4: 167-183, 1963
Hillestad L, Hansen T, Melsom H. Diazepam metabolism in normal man. II. Serum concentration and clinical effect after oral administration and cumulation. Clinical Pharmacology and Therapeutics 16: 485-489, 1974
Hollister LE. Benzodiazepines: a look at the issues. Psychosomatics 21 (Suppl. 10): 4-8, 1980
Hollister LE, Gillespie HK, Ohlsson A, Lindgren JE, Wahlen A, et al. Do plasma concentrations of delta-9-tetrahydrocannabinol reflect the degree of intoxication? Journal of Clinical Pharmacology 21: 171S-177S, 1981
Humpel M, Illi V, Milius W, Wendt H, Kurowski M. The pharmacokinetics and biotransformation of the new benzodiazepine (lormetazepam) in humans. European Journal of Drug Metabolism and Pharmacokinetics 4: 237-243, 1979
Hunt CA, Jones RT. Tolerance and disposition of tetrahydrocannabinol in man. Journal of Pharmacology and Experimental Therapeutics 215: 35-44, 1980
Inaba T, Stewart DJ, Kalow W. Metabolism of cocaine in man. Clinical Pharmacology and Therapeutics 23: 547-552, 1978
Jaffe JH. Drug addiction and drug abuse. In Goodman et al. (Eds) The pharmacological basis of therapeutics, 7th ed., pp. 532-581, Macmillan Publishing Co. Inc., New York, 1985
Jaffe JH, Ciraulo DA, Nies A, Dixon RB, Monroe LL. Abuse potential of halazepam and of diazepam in patients recently treated for acute alcohol withdrawal. Clinical Pharmacology and Therapeutics 34: 623-630, 1983
Jasinski DR. Assessment of the abuse potentiality of morphine-like drugs (methods used in man). In Martin WR (Ed.) Handbook of experimental pharmacology, Vol. 45, pp. 197-258, Springer-Verlag New York Inc., New York, 1977
Jasinski DR, Johnson RE, Henningfield JE. Abuse liability as-

sessment in human subjects. Trends in Pharmacological Sciences 5: 196-200, 1984
Javaid JI, Musa MN, Fischman M, Schuster CR, Davis JM. Kinetics of cocaine in humans after intravenous and intranasal administration. Biopharmaceutics and Drug Disposition 4: 9-18, 1983
Jekel JF, Allen DF, Podlewski H, Clarke N, Dean-Patterson S, et al. Epidemic free-base cocaine abuse (case study from the Bahamas). Lancet 1: 459, 1986
Jeri FR, Sanchez CC, del Pozo L, et al. Further experience with the syndrome produced by coca paste smoking. In Jeri FR (Ed.) Cocaine, pp. 76-85, Pacific Press, Lima, 1980
Jochemsen R, Breimer DD. Assay of flunitrazepam, temazepam and desalkylflurazepam in plasma by capillary gas chromatography with electron-capture detection. Journal of Chromotography 227: 199-206, 1982
Johanson CE, Schuster CR. Animal models of drug self-administration. In Mello NK (Ed.) Advances in substance abuse: behavioural and biological research, Jai Press, Greenwich, Connecticut, 1981
Johnston L. Tobacco smoking and nicotine. Lancet 2: 742, 1931
Kalant H, LeBlanc AE, Gibbins RJ. Tolerance to, and dependence on, some non-opiate psychotropic drugs. Pharmacology Review 23: 135-191, 1971
Kangas L, Breimer DD. Clinical pharmacokinetics of nitrazepam. Clinical Pharmacokinetics 6: 346-366, 1981
Kaplan SA, de Silva JAF, Jack ML, Alexander K, Stroyny K, et al. Blood level profile in man following chronic oral administration of flurazepam hydrochloride. Journal of Pharmaceutical Sciences 62: 1932-1935, 1973b
Kaplan SA, Jack ML, Alexander K, Weinfeld RE. Pharmacokinetic profile of diazepam in man following single intravenous and oral and chronic oral administrations. Journal of Pharmaceutical Sciences 62: 1789-1796, 1973a
Kaplan SA, Jack ML, Weinfeld RE, Glover W, Weissman L, et al. Biopharmaceutical and clinical pharmacokinetic profile of bromazepam. Journal of Pharmacokinetics and Biopharmaceutics 4: 1-16, 1976
King LJ, Forney RB. The absorption and excretion of marijuana constituents, cannabinol and tetrahydrocannabinol. Proceedings of the Federal American Society of Experimental Biology 26: 540, 1967
Klausner HA, Dingell JV. The metabolism and excretion of delta 9-tetrahydrocannabinol in the rat. Life Sciences 10: 49-59, 1971
Klotz U, Antonin KH, Bieck PR. Comparison of the pharmacokinetics of diazepam after single and subchronic doses. European Journal of Clinical Pharmacology 10: 121-126, 1976
Kozlowski LT, Kleiman RM. Effects of oral pH on cigarette smoking. Pharmacology, Biochemistry and Behaviour 9: 477-480, 1978
Kroboth PD, Smith RB, Sorkin MI, Silver MR, Rault R, et al. Triazolam protein binding and correlation with alpha-1 acid glycoprotein concentration. Clinical Pharmacology and Therapeutics 36: 379-383, 1984
Lauven PM, Stoeckel H, Schwilden H. A microprocessor controlled infusion scheme for midazolam to achieve constant plasma levels. Anaesthesist 31: 15-20, 1982
Lemberger L. Pharmacokinetics of delta-9-tetrahydrocannabinol and its metabolites: importance and relationship in developing methods for detecting cannabis in biologic fluids. In Nahas et al. (Eds) Marihuana: chemistry, biochemistry and cellular effects, pp. 169-178, Springer-Verlag, New York, 1976
Lemberger L, Silberstein SD, Axelrod J, Kopin IJ. Marihuana: studies on the disposition and metabolism of delta-9-tetrahydrocannabinol in man. Science 170: 1320-1322, 1970
Lemberger L, Tamarkin NR, Axelrod J, Kopin IJ. Delta-9-tetrahydrocannabinol: metabolism and disposition in long-term marihuana smokers. Science 173: 72-74, 1971
Lindgren JE, Ohlsson A, Agurell S, Hollister L, Gillespie H. Clinical effects and plasma levels of delta-9-tetrahydrocannabinol in heavy and light users of cannabis. Psychopharmacology 74: 208-212, 1981
Linnoila M, Erwin CW, Brendle A, Skinner T, Routledge PA. Pharmacodynamics and pharmacokinetics of diazepam in an abuser. Acta Pharmacologica et Toxicologica 47: 75-77, 1980
Luck W, Nau H. Exposure of the fetus, neonate and nursed infant to nicotine and cotinine from maternal smoking. New England Journal of Medicine 311: 672, 1984
Luck W, Nau H. Nicotine and cotinine concentrations in serum and urine of infants exposed via passive smoking or milk from smoking mother. Journal of Pediatrics 107: 816-820, 1985
MacLeod SM, Greenblatt DJ, Sellers EM. Determination of intravenous chlordiazepoxide pharmacokinetics: plasma versus blood. Clinical Research 25: 273A, 1977
MacLeod SM, Sellers EM, Giles HG, Billings BJ, Martin PR, et al. Interaction of disulfiram with benzodiazepines. Clinical Pharmacology and Therapeutics 24: 583-589, 1978
Maickel RP, Cox RH, Miller FP, Segal DS, Russell RW. Correlation of brain levels of drugs with their behavioral effects. Journal of Pharmacology and Experimental Therapeutics 165: 216-224, 1969
Mandelli M, Tognoni G, Garattini S. Clinical pharmacokinetics of diazepam. Clinical Pharmacokinetics 3: 72-91, 1978
Marks V, Kelly JF. Absorption of caffeine from tea, coffee and coca cola. Lancet 1: 827, 1973
Matsukura S, Sakamoto N, Seino Y, Tamada T, Matsuyama H, et al. Cotinine excretion and daily cigarette smoking in habituated smokers. Clinical Pharmacology and Therapeutics 25: 555-561, 1979
Maykut MO. Health consequences of acute and chronic marihuana use. Progress in Neuro-Psychopharmacology and Biological Chemistry 9: 209-238, 1985
Metzler CM, Ko H, Boyer ME, Veldkamp W, Linet OI. Bioavailability and pharmacokinetics of orally administered triazolam in normal subjects. Clinical Pharmacology and Therapeutics 21: 111-112, 1977
Moschitto LJ, Greenblatt DJ. Concentration-independent plasma protein binding of benzodiazepines. Journal of Pharmacy and Pharmacology 35: 179-180, 1983
Nayak PK, Misra AL, Mule SJ. Physiological disposition and biotransformation of (^{3}H) cocaine in acutely and chronically treated rats. Journal of Pharmacology and Experimental Therapeutics 196: 556-569, 1976
Newton R, Broughton LJ, Lind MJ, Morrison PJ, Rogers HJ, et al. Plasma and salivary pharmacokinetics of caffeine in man. European Journal of Clinical Pharmacology 21: 45-52, 1981
Ohlsson A, Lindgren JE, Wahlen A, Agurell S, Hollister LE, et al. Plasma delta-9 tetrahydrocannabinol concentrations and clinical effects after oral and intravenous administration and smoking. Clinical Pharmacology and Therapeutics 28: 409-416, 1980
Pacifici GM, Placidi GF, Fornaro P, Gomeni R. Pinazepam: a precursor of *N*-desmethyldiazepam. European Journal of Clinical Pharmacology 22: 225-228, 1982
Paly D, Jatlow P, VanDyke C, et al. Plasma levels of cocaine in native Peruvian coca chewers. In Jeri FR (Ed.) Cocaine 1980, pp. 86-89, Pacific Press, Lima, 1980
Paly D, Jatlow P, VanDyke C, Jeri FR, Byck R. Plasma cocaine concentrations during cocaine paste smoking. Life Science 30: 731-738, 1982
Parsons W, Aranda JV, Neims AH. Elimination of caffeine in the newborn. Pediatric Research 10: 333, 1976
Parsons WD, Neims AH. Effect of smoking on caffeine clearance. Clinical Pharmacology and Therapeutics 24: 40-45, 1978
Patwardhan RV, Desmond PV, Johnson RF, Schenker S. Impaired elimination of caffeine by oral contraceptive steroids. Journal of Laboratory and Clinical Medicine 95: 603-608, 1980
Perez-Reyes M, DiGuiseppi S, Brine DR, Smith H, Cook CE.

Urine pH and phencyclidine excretion. Clinical Pharmacology and Therapeutics 32: 635-641, 1982c

Perez-Reyes M, DiGuiseppi S, Davis KH, Schindler VH, Cook CE. Comparison of effects of marihuana cigarettes of three different potencies. Clinical Pharmacology and Therapeutics 31: 617-624, 1982a

Perez-Reyes M, DiGuiseppi S, Ondrusek G, Jeffcoat AR, Cook CE. Free-base cocaine smoking. Clinical Pharmacology and Therapeutics 32: 459-465, 1982b

Perez-Reyes M, Lipton MA, Timmons MC, et al. Pharmacology of orally administered delta-9-tetrahydrocannabinol. Clinical Pharmacology and Therapeutics 14: 48-55, 1973b

Perez-Reyes M, Timmons MC, Lipton MA, Christensen HD, Davis KH, et al. A comparison of the pharmacological activity of delta-9-THC and its monohydroxylated metabolites in man. Experientia 29: 1009-1010, 1973a

Perez-Reyes M, Timmons MC, Lipton MA, Davis KH, Wall ME. Intravenous injection in man of 9-tetrahydrocannabinol and 11-OH-delta 9-tetrahydrocannabinol. Science 177: 633-635, 1972

Perry DC. PCP revisited. Clinical Toxicology 9: 339-348, 1976

Petrakis NL, Gruenke LD, Beelen TC, Castagnoli N, Craig JC. Nicotine in breast fluid of nonlactating women. Science 199: 303-305, 1978

Read RC. Systemic effects of smoking. American Journal of Surgery 148: 706-711, 1984

Rieder J, Wendt G. Pharmacokinetics and metabolism of the hypnotic nitrazepam. In Garattini et al. (Eds) The benzodiazepines, pp. 99-127, Raven Press, New York, 1973

Ritchie JM, Cohen PJ. Cocaine: procaine and other synthetic local anesthetics. In Goodman & Gilman (Eds) The pharmacological basis of therapeutics, 5th ed., pp. 379-403, Macmillan Publishing Co. Inc., New York, 1975

Robertson D, Frolich JC, Carr RK, Watson JT, Hollifield JW, et al. Effects of caffeine on plasma renin activity, catecholamines and blood pressure. New England Journal of Medicine 298: 181-186, 1978

Robertson D, Wade D, Workman R, Woosley RL, Oates JA. Tolerance to the humoral and hemodynamic effects of caffeine in man. Journal of Clinical Investigation 67: 1111-1117, 1981

Rosenberg J, Benowitz NL, Jacob P, Wilson KM. Disposition of kinetics and effects of intravenous nicotine. Clinical Pharmacology and Therapeutics 28: 517-522, 1980

Rowland M. Amphetamine blood and urine levels in man. Journal of Pharmaceutical Sciences 58: 508-509, 1969

Rupp W, Badian M, Christ O, Hadju P, Kulkarn RD, et al. Pharmacokinetics of single and multiple doses of clobazam in humans. British Journal of Clinical Pharmacology 7: 51S-57S, 1979

Russell MAH. The smoking habit and its classification. Practitioner 212: 791-800, 1974

Sant'ambrogio G, Mognoni P, Ventrella L. Plasma levels of caffeine after oral, intramuscular and intravenous administration. Archives Internationales de Pharmacodynamie et de Therapie 150: 259-263, 1964

Schwartz MA, Koechlin BA, Postma E, Palmer S, Krol G. Metabolism of diazepam in cat, dog, and man. Journal of Pharmacology and Experimental Therapeutics 149: 423-435, 1965

Sellers EM, Greenblatt DJ, Giles HG, Naranjo CA, Kaplan H, et al. Chlordiazepoxide and oxazepam disposition in cirrhosis. Clinical Pharmacology and Therapeutics 26: 240-246, 1979

Shader RI, Greenblatt DJ, Harmatz JS, Franke K, Koch-Weser J. Absorption and disposition of chlordiazepoxide in young and elderly male volunteers. Journal of Clinical Pharmacology 17: 709-718, 1977

Siegel RK. Cocaine smoking. New England Journal of Medicine 300: 373, 1979

Smith MT, Eadie MJ, Brophy TO. The pharmacokinetics of midazolam in man. European Journal of Clinical Pharmacology 19: 271-278, 1981

Smith RB, Schoenfeld MJ. Effect of food on the bioavailability of Xanax (alprazolam) following a single oral 1.0mg dose. Technical Report 8113-81-9122-016, 1981

Statland BE, Demas TJ. Serum caffeine half-lives: healthy subjects *vs* patients having alcoholic hepatic disease. American Journal of Clinical Pathology 73: 390-393, 1980

Statland BE, Demas T, Danis M. Caffeine accumulation associated with alcoholic liver disease. New England Journal of Medicine 295: 110-111, 1976

Stewart DJ, Inaba T, Lucassen M, Kalow W. Cocaine metabolism: cocaine and norcocaine hydrolysis by liver and serum esterases. Clinical Pharmacology and Therapeutics 25: 464-468, 1979

Stewart DJ, Inaba T, Tang BK, Kalow W. Hydrolysis of cocaine in human plasma by cholinesterase. Life Sciences 20: 1557-1563, 1977

Svensson CK. Clinical pharmacokinetics of nicotine. Clinical Pharmacokinetics 12: 30-40, 1987

Tedeschi G, Riva R, Baruzzi A. Clobazam plasma concentrations: pharmacokinetic study in healthy volunteers and data in epileptic patients. British Journal of Clinical Pharmacology 11: 619-622, 1981

Thiessen JJ, Sellers EM, Denbeigh P, Dolman L. Plasma protein binding of diazepam and tolbutamide in chronic alcoholics. Journal of Clinical Pharmacology 16: 345-351, 1976

Travell J. Absorption of nicotine from various sites. Annals of the New York Academy of Sciences 90: 13-30, 1960

Turner CE, Elsohly MA, Boeren EG. Constituents of cannabis sativa. Journal of Natural Products 43: 169-234, 1980

Turner DM, Armitage AK, Briant RH, Dollery CT. Metabolism of nicotine by the isolated perfused dog lung. Xenobiotica 5: 539-551, 1975

Vallner JJ, Needham TE, Jun HW, et al. Plasma levels of clobazam after three oral dosage forms in healthy subjects. Journal of Clinical Pharmacology 18: 319-324, 1978

van der Kleijn E, Van Rossum JM, Muskens ETJ, Rijntjes NVM. Pharmacokinetics of diazepam in dogs, mice, and humans. Acta Pharmacologica et Toxicologica 29: 109-129, 1971

Van Dyke C, Jatlow P, Ungerer J, Barash PG, Byck R. Oral cocaine: plasma concentrations and central effects. Science 200: 211-213, 1978

Volz M, Christ O, Kellner HM, Kuch H, Fehlhaber HW, et al. Kinetics and metabolism of clobazam in animals and man. British Journal of Clinical Pharmacology 7: 41S-50S, 1979

Wahlqvist M, Nilsson IM, Sandberg F, et al. Binding of delta-1-tetrahydrocannabinol to human plasma proteins. Biochemical Pharmacology 19: 2579, 1970

Wall ME. The *in vitro* and *in vivo* metabolism of tetrahydrocannabinol (THC). Annals of the New York Academy of Sciences 191: 23-29, 1971

Wall ME, Brine DR, Jeffcoat RA, Cook CE. Phencyclidine metabolism and disposition in man following a 100μg intravenous dose. Research Communications in Substance Abuse 2: 161-172, 1981

Wall ME, Brine DR, Perez-Reyes M. Metabolism of cannabinoids in man. In MC Braude and S Szara (Eds) The pharmacology of marihuana, pp. 93-113, Raven Press, New York, 1976

Wall ME, Perez-Reyes M. The metabolism of delta-9-tetrahydrocannabinol and related cannabinoids in man. Journal of Clinical Pharmacology 21: 178S-189S, 1981

Wall ME, Sadler BM, Brine D, Taylor H, Perez-Reyes M. Metabolism disposition and kinetics of delta-9-tetrahydrocannabinol in men and women. Clinical Pharmacology and Therapeutics 34: 352-363, 1983

Wickstrom E, Amrein R, Haefelfinger P, Hartmann D. Pharmacokinetic and clinical observations on prolonged adminis-

tration of flunitrazepam. Journal of Clinical Pharmacology 17: 189-196, 1980
Wilkinson P, Van Dyke C, Jatlow P, Barash P, Byck R. Intranasal and oral cocaine kinetics. Clinical Pharmacology and Therapeutics 27: 386-394, 1980
Wilson AGE, Pickett RD, Eling TE, Anderson MW. Studies on the persistence of basic amines in the rabbit lung. Drug Metabolism Reviews 7: 420-424, 1979
Wong LK, Biemann K. Metabolites of phencyclidine. Clinical Toxicology 9: 583-591, 1976
Zilm DH, Sellers EM. The quantitative assessment of physical dependence on opiates. Drug and Alcohol Dependence 3: 419-428, 1978

Authors' address: Dr *U. Busto*, Head, Pharmacy Discipline, Addiction Research Foundation, 33 Russell Street, Toronto, Ontario M5S 2S1 (Canada).

Clinical Pharmacokinetics 16: 27-37 (1989)
0312-5963/89/0001-0027/$05.50/0

Therapeutic Drug Monitoring of Cyclosporin
Practical Applications and Limitations

Vanni Rodighiero
Department of Pharmacology, University of Padova, Padova, Italy

Contents

Summary ... 27
1. Analytical Methods ... 28
 1.1 Radioimmunoassay and HPLC ... 28
 1.2 Factors Influencing Measured Cyclosporin Concentrations ... 29
  1.2.1 Temperature ... 29
  1.2.2 Haematocrit ... 29
  1.2.3 Intraerythrocytic Protein ... 29
  1.2.4 Infection ... 29
  1.2.5 Diurnal Variation ... 29
  1.2.6 Other Factors ... 29
 1.3 Monoclonal Antibodies ... 30
2. Factors Affecting Cyclosporin Kinetics ... 30
 2.1 Bile Deficit ... 30
 2.2 Gastrointestinal Status ... 31
 2.3 Time ... 31
 2.4 Food and Vehicle ... 32
 2.5 Lipoproteins ... 32
 2.6 Liver Function ... 32
 2.7 Renal Function ... 33
 2.8 Effects of Age ... 33
 2.9 Circadian Variations in Cyclosporin Clearance ... 33
 2.10 Drug Interactions ... 33
3. Conclusions ... 34

Summary *Cyclosporin, a potent immunosuppressive agent used to prevent rejection of transplanted organs, has a narrow therapeutic range and various toxic effects, mostly concentration-dependent. The kinetics of this drug present a large intra- and interindividual variability due to many factors resulting in marked variations of blood cyclosporin concentrations, and in a poor correlation between administered dose and concentrations. The knowledge of cyclosporin peculiarities and of factors affecting blood concentrations can provide a rational basis for establishing an adequate therapy for the individual patient, in conjunction with other laboratory and clinical data. Cyclosporin monitoring is a method of evaluating whether the therapeutic choice is correct. Cyclosporin concentrations can be measured in blood, plasma and serum using radioimmunoassay or high performance liquid chromatography. Different results are obtained, depending on the technique and on biological fluids used. Cyclosporin measurement presents many problems and difficulties.*

There is a need for standardisation and for quality assessment programmes. The recent development of monoclonal antibodies may represent a significant advance for cyclosporin monitoring. The most important factors affecting blood concentrations are: type of transplant, bile deficit, gastrointestinal dysfunction, food, variations of lipoprotein concentrations, impairment of liver function, age, drug coadministration. Therapeutic drug monitoring should be undertaken on a regular basis after the initiation of therapy with cyclosporin. After discharge from the hospital the patient and the attending physician should be aware of the factors which may require changes in cyclosporin therapy.

Cyclosporin is a cyclic endecapeptide with potent immunosuppressive properties. It has a narrow therapeutic range and various toxic effects, which are mostly concentration dependent (Busuttil et al. 1986; Irschik et al. 1984; Kennedy et al. 1985; Moyer et al. 1986; Scott & Higenbottam 1988). A large intra- and interindividual variability in cyclosporin kinetics has been observed (Burckart et al. 1986b; Lindholm et al. 1988; Ptachcinski et al. 1985b).

The pronounced differences in pharmacokinetic parameters, such as bioavailability and clearance, result in marked variations in blood cyclosporin concentrations and contribute to the poor correlation observed between administered dose and blood concentrations. Thus, neither blood concentrations nor effects of the drug can be predicted on the basis of the administered dose. Cyclosporin kinetics are influenced by a number of factors, such as interindividual variability, type of transplant, age, disease states, concomitant drug administration, diurnal variations and food. Knowledge of the peculiarities of cyclosporin and of factors affecting blood concentrations can provide a rational basis for establishing an appropriate therapy. Cyclosporin monitoring is a means of evaluating whether the therapeutic choice is correct. The essential tool for therapeutic monitoring is a reliable method for measuring drug concentrations in biological fluids, but the methods of measurement of cyclosporin present many problems and difficulties, imposing limitations on the practice of monitoring.

1. Analytical Methods

1.1 Radioimmunoassay and HPLC

At present 2 techniques are available for measuring cyclosporin concentrations in biological fluids: radioimmunoassay (RIA) and high performance liquid chromatography (HPLC). HPLC specifically measures the parent compound. Since RIA employs a polyclonal nonspecific antibody raised in sheep, which cross-reacts with a number of cyclosporin metabolites, it tends to overestimate cyclosporin concentrations (about 1.5 to 3.5-fold higher than those obtained by HPLC) [Venkataramanan et al. 1985a]. The biological fluids used as a sample matrix for cyclosporin determination are blood, plasma and serum.

Most clinical centres use RIA for several reasons: the small sample volumes needed, simplicity, easy sample preparation and short analysis time. Moreover, the instrumentation for RIA is usually part of existing laboratory equipment (Holt et al. 1986). HPLC assay has several limitations. It requires more laborious sample preparation, complex instrumentation, demanding technical expertise and a somewhat lengthy analysis time per sample (Kahan 1985). The RIA : HPLC ratio of cyclosporin concentrations is highly variable, depending on the patient's liver function, the post-transplant period and concomitant administration of other drugs affecting the metabolism of cyclosporin (Shaw et al. 1987). RIA : HPLC ratios of up to 15 : 1 have been observed (Ptachcinski et al. 1986b), with the greatest variability occurring in the early post-transplant period. In liver transplant patients with poor hepatic function cyclosporin metabolites accumulate in blood at this time because the elimination is impaired (Keown et al. 1986; Venkataramanan et al. 1985a), which may explain the high RIA : HPLC ratio observed (15 : 1). When circumstances indicate ratio variability may be high, the use of RIA may be misleading and it is better to monitor cyclosporin by a specific method.

1.2 Factors Influencing Measured Cyclosporin Concentrations

Cyclosporin is distributed in blood in the following way: about 50% in erythrocytes, 10% in leucocytes and 40% in plasma (Calabresi & Parks 1985). In plasma approximately 98% is bound to plasma proteins, mostly lipoproteins (Niederberger et al. 1983). In healthy subjects the concentration of cyclosporin in blood is approximately twice that measured in plasma (Niederberger et al. 1983). A number of factors can influence the pattern of cyclosporin distribution, and consequently the measured plasma concentration.

1.2.1 Temperature

The distribution of the drug in blood is temperature-dependent: when temperature increases, cyclosporin diffuses from erythrocytes into plasma, with the result that at 37°C plasma concentrations are about 2-fold higher than at 20°C (Wenk & Follath 1983). Thus, the measured concentration of cyclosporin in plasma depends on the temperature used for the separation of plasma. If this separation is performed at temperatures lower than 37°C, measured plasma concentrations do not reflect true levels *in vivo*.

1.2.2 Haematocrit

Cyclosporin distribution in blood may depend on haematocrit. An inverse correlation between variations of haematocrit and plasma concentrations of cyclosporin has been found *in vitro* (Niederberger et al. 1983; Rosano 1985). However, this has not been confirmed clinically, probably because *in vivo* the blood does not behave as a static, closed system, as there is a dynamic interchange between erythrocytes, plasma and tissues. Indeed, Holt et al. (1986) and Johnston et al. (1988) failed to find a significant correlation between haematocrit variations and either blood or plasma cyclosporin concentrations.

1.2.3 Intraerythrocytic Protein

Cyclosporin binds to an intraerythrocytic protein (Agarwal et al. 1986). The binding is rapid and reversible (Lemaire et al. 1986). It has been reported that erythrocytes become saturated at drug concentrations above 5 mg/L. Consequently, above this threshold the increase in plasma concentrations becomes non-linear. However, this effect has been shown to be an artefact of the separation temperature and the binding is directly proportional to concentration when plasma is separated at 37°C (Vine & Bowers 1987).

1.2.4 Infection

Infections, which are a frequent complication of transplantation, lead to an increase in leucocyte number and, presumably, to an increased binding of cyclosporin to leucocytes with alterations of distribution of the drug in blood.

Between plasma drug concentrations of 0.02 and 20 mg/L, the binding of cyclosporin to plasma proteins is independent of concentration, but it varies with temperature: about 70% of the drug is bound at 4°C, 93% at 20°C and 98% at 37°C (Niederberger et al. 1983). There is also an exchange/transfer of cyclosporin among the different serum lipoprotein classes and a transfer from albumin to lipoproteins (Mraz et al. 1983).

1.2.5 Diurnal Variation

The concentrations and clearance of cyclosporin have diurnal variations (Bowers et al. 1986; Venkataramanan et al. 1986b) [see also section 2.9]. Thus, blood samples for cyclosporin measurement should be drawn at a fixed time of the day.

1.2.6 Other Factors

It is evident that, depending on the nature of the analytical method (RIA or HPLC) and biological fluids used (blood, plasma, serum), different values of cyclosporin concentrations will be obtained. The kinetic parameters derived from these measurements will reflect these differences (Yee et al. 1984b). The available data are therefore difficult to interpret for therapeutic decision-making because of lack of uniformity, and different reference scales must be used. This situation has created a great deal of confusion among transplant surgeons (Moyer 1985).

Clearly, cyclosporin measurement presents many

problems and difficulties due to the analytical technique and sample matrix used, and the clinical condition of the patient. Furthermore, there are discrepancies in the values of cyclosporin measurement obtained by different laboratories using the same assay method and sample matrix, thus making it difficult to compare the results of different centres. This has been evidenced by the Swiss interlaboratory quality control programme (Frey et al. 1987) and by the quality assessment programme involving 27 centres in the United Kingdom (Johnston et al. 1986b), now extended to other centres in Europe and North America (Shaw et al. 1987). Clearly, there is a need for standardisation and the necessity of reference to an intra- and intercentre quality assessment programme in order to achieve comparable results. These problems have been faced by the Task Force on Cyclosporine Monitoring (Shaw et al. 1987), which has proposed a number of recommendations in order to standardise and to provide guidelines for effective therapeutic cyclosporin monitoring.

1.3 Monoclonal Antibodies

Recently monoclonal antibodies for cyclosporin measurement have been developed. Two of them are of particular interest, MAb1 and MAb2 (Quesniaux 1986; Quesniaux et al. 1987). MAb2 measures the drug plus most of its metabolites, but with a higher affinity as compared with the currently used nonspecific polyclonal antibody. MAb1 measures specifically cyclosporin. In preliminary studies the drug concentrations determined by using this antibody were similar to those obtained with HPLC (Holt et al. 1986; Schinella et al. 1987), and could be used in preference to HPLC in the future. These antibodies are under evaluation in a multicentre trial (Shaw et al. 1987), but a considerable body of data is needed before this assay can be applied to therapeutic monitoring. The use of monoclonal antibodies may represent a significant improvement for the future clinical monitoring of cyclosporin.

The drug's metabolites must also be taken into consideration. Cyclosporin is extensively metabolised by the liver and the metabolites are excreted into the bile (Burckart et al. 1988). 11 metabolites have been identified (Wang et al. 1988). High concentrations of metabolites M17 and M1 are present in the blood of transplant recipients (Freed et al. 1987a; Wang et al. 1988). The levels of M17, the major metabolite, are equal to or greater than those of cyclosporin, while the concentrations of M18 and M21 are much lower. M17 has a half-life (17.2 hours) longer than the parent compound (Vine & Bowers 1987). M17 and M1 are also found in large amounts in the kidney (Rosano et al. 1986). The metabolites were considered inactive, but it has been demonstrated that some of them have immunosuppressive activity. M17 and M1 *in vitro* have an immunosuppressive activity similar to that of cyclosporin (Freed et al. 1987a; Rosano et al. 1987), and similar results have been obtained with M18 (Freed et al. 1987b). The toxicity of these metabolites is unknown. Further investigations *in vivo* are needed, and a specific assay for metabolite measurement could be useful.

2. Factors Affecting Cyclosporin Kinetics

After oral administration the absorption of cyclosporin is variable and incomplete, with an absolute bioavailability of approximately 20 to 50% in normal subjects (Calabresi & Parks 1985). An even more marked intra- and interindividual variability in the extent of absorption has been observed in patients after organ transplantation (Burckart et al. 1986b). This contributes to the poor correlation between administered dose and steady-state concentration. Absorption is influenced by a variety of factors, among which only the most clinically relevant will be considered here.

2.1 Bile Deficit

Bile is necessary for absorption of fat-soluble substances from the gut. Since cyclosporin is lipophilic, any factor determining bile deficit can impair its absorption. Liver transplant patients often have a T-tube inserted in the common bile duct for external bile drainage. The clamping of this T-tube greatly improves the absorption of cyclosporin in these patients, most probably due to increased bile flow into the gut. An increase of the area under the blood concentration/time curve (AUC) has been observed, from 0.31 mg/L • h before to 0.95 mg/L • h after T-tube clamping (Mehta et al. 1988). A 2- to 6-fold rise of cyclosporin concentrations after T-tube clamping was reported by Andrews et al. (1985), with toxic levels (2.25 mg/L) in one patient. Cyclosporin dosage adjustments are needed whenever external bile diversion is instituted or discontinued.

Liver transplant recipients can have complications of bile duct reconstruction with biliary obstruction (Busutti1 et al. 1986), leading to a decrease in absorption of cyclosporin.

Liver transplant patients with poor hepatic function have a low bile production: Venkataramanan et al. (1985c) reported an output of 7.6 ml/h, *versus* 24.1 ml/h in patients with normal liver function. In the immediate postoperative period the new liver produces about 100 to 300 ml/day of bile (Busuttil et al. 1986), and this deficit can result in poor absorption of cyclosporin.

Patients with liver disease and high serum bilirubin levels (> 100 mg/L) absorb less than 5% of an oral dose of cyclosporin (Burckart et al. 1986b). Bioavailability in paediatric liver transplant patients with a decreased clearance of the drug is less than 5% (Burckart et al. 1986a). It has also been reported that oral administration of bile salts may improve the absorption of cyclosporin, as evidenced in cirrhotic patients (Burckart et al. 1986b).

2.2 Gastrointestinal Status

The absorption of oral cyclosporin can be impaired to a great extent by gastrointestinal dysfunction. Bone marrow transplant recipients with diarrhoea due to enteritis secondary to pretransplant chemoradiation therapy, acute graft-*vs*-host disease (GVHD) of the gut or infectious enteritis, absorb cyclosporin poorly, shown by greatly decreased AUC and trough concentrations (AUC in patients with diarrhoea > 500 ml/72h of 1.76 *versus* 4.62 mg/L • h in patients with diarrhoea < 500 ml/72h; trough concentrations in patients without gut dysfunction 428 *versus* 102 and 165 μg/L, respectively, in acute GVHD and chemoradiation enteritis) [Atkinson et al. 1983, 1984]. In paediatric liver transplant patients the onset of diarrhoea a few days after transplant led to poor cyclosporin absorption and required prolonged intravenous administration of the drug (Andrews et al. 1987). Postoperative ileus can also decrease the absorption of cyclosporin.

Gastric emptying can affect the absorption of cyclosporin, which takes place in the intestine. In renal allograft recipients the coadministration of metoclopramide, known to enhance gastric emptying, increases the rate and extent of cyclosporin absorption without significantly changing its elimination (AUC 3.37 mg/L • h without *versus* 4.12 mg/L • h with metoclopramide, C_{max} 388 *versus* 567 μg/L, t_{max} 3.3 *versus* 2.9 hours, respectively) [Wadhwa et al. 1987a].

2.3 Time

The bioavailability of cyclosporin increases with time after transplantation. In renal allograft recipients a 5-fold increase in bioavailability has been observed about 3 months after transplantation (Kahan et al. 1983). Another study reported that bioavailability rose by 50% during the first 3 months after renal transplantation, clearance being unchanged (Odlind et al. 1986). Heart and kidney transplant patients require a lower dosage with long term therapy to maintain steady serum concentrations of 200 to 300 μg/L (initial oral dose 17.5 *versus* 9.0 mg/kg/day after 8 weeks of therapy) [Keown et al. 1983]. In a group of kidney transplant recipients the bioavailability increased from 24.2% during the first 2 weeks after transplantation to 50.2% at 6 to 12 months (Kahan et al. 1986a). Different results were obtained by Tufveson et al. (1986), who found a 40% increase in bioavailability 3 months after renal transplantation with a return to pretransplant values after 6 to 12 months. The mechanism underlying the improvement of bioavailability is not known, but it probably depends on increased gastrointestinal absorption of cyclosporin. This change in bioavailability results in increased blood concentrations with time if the dosage is maintained. Thus, it is possible to reduce the dose but maintain the same concentration.

2.4 Food and Vehicle

The effect of food on oral cyclosporin absorption is controversial. Keown et al. (1982) reported that the administration of cyclosporin together with a standard meal delays and decreases absorption of the drug, but in a subsequent study the same group found no significant effect of food on cyclosporin absorption (administration following a standard test breakfast) [Keown et al. 1983]. Other authors have demonstrated that the absorption of cyclosporin is not affected by the administration of the drug with a standard hospital breakfast (Keogh et al. 1988; Lemaire et al. 1986). In contrast, Ptachcinski et al. (1985a) observed that food (drug administered with a standard hospital breakfast) enhances cyclosporin absorption with a 60.6% increase in AUC. The findings of these studies are conflicting and not conclusive. It is probable that the effect of food on cyclosporin absorption depends on the composition of the diet.

Cyclosporin is administered orally as an olive oil preparation because it is highly lipophilic. For palatability the preparation is dispersed in different vehicles (milk, milk plus chocolate flavouring or orange juice). These vehicles do not affect the absorption of cyclosporin in normal volunteers (Johnston et al. 1986a). Moreover, the kinetics of cyclosporin are not affected by 'Intralipid', a fat emulsion used for intravenous feeding as a caloric source (Wassef et al. 1986).

2.5 Lipoproteins

Lipoprotein concentrations can undergo considerable variations in renal and liver transplant recipients (Ptachcinski et al. 1986b). Hyperlipidaemia frequently develops within 6 months following heart transplantation (Ballantyne et al. 1987). Changes in lipoprotein concentrations may result in inverse changes in free drug fraction in plasma. A negative linear relationship between cyclosporin clearance and lipoprotein concentrations and composition was found by Lithell et al. (1986), and the gradual increase of lipoprotein concentrations with age has been considered as a factor that could explain the modifications of cyclosporin clearance and volume of distribution (Vd) observed in children and older persons (Yee et al. 1986).

2.6 Liver Function

Impairment of cyclosporin elimination significantly alters the kinetics of the drug. Heart transplant patients have a lower clearance and Vd than kidney or liver transplant recipients, with an increased AUC (CL 0.64 L/h/kg, Vd 6.0 L/kg, AUC 5.43 mg/L • h in heart transplant *versus* 0.74 L/h/kg, 8.7 L/kg and 1.94 mg/L • h, respectively, in renal transplant) [Kahan et al. 1986b; Venkataramanan et al. 1986a]. A lower dose is suggested for these patients. Cyclosporin is a drug with a low to intermediate extraction ratio and the impairment of liver function decreases its clearance. In renal transplant patients with impaired hepatic function a reduced clearance (0.53 *versus* 0.79 L/h/kg in patients with normal liver function) and a 30 to 50% increase in AUC have been observed (Kahan et al. 1986a). Bone marrow transplant recipients frequently develop hepatic dysfunction in the post-grafting period due to liver venocclusive disease, GVHD and other causes (Jones et al. 1987; Shulman et al. 1980). Moderate hepatic dysfunction in these patients (serum bilirubin 20 to 50 mg/L) induces a decrease in cyclosporin clearance (1.78 *versus* 3.14 L/h/kg in patients with normal liver function), accounting for a prolonged half-life (8.7 *versus* 3.5 hours), and a higher peak serum concentration (776 *versus* 383 μg/L) [Yee et al. 1984a]. The impairment of liver function in patients with hepatic cirrhosis results in a decrease of cyclosporin clearance (0.15 L/h/kg) and a prolongation of half-life (32.1 hours), compared with renal or bone marrow transplant recipients (Venkataramanan et al. 1985b). A reduced clearance of cyclosporin has also been observed in paediatric liver transplant patients with diminished liver function (Burckart et al. 1985).

2.7 Renal Function

Renal failure does not affect the clearance of cyclosporin (Follath et al. 1983; Venkataramanan et al. 1985a), as normally less than 1% of an administered dose is excreted unchanged into the urine. Transplant patients may require haemodialysis to treat acute tubular necrosis, surgical complications or drug-induced toxicity (Venkataramanan et al. 1984). Little cyclosporin is removed from the body by dialysis (less than 1% of a dose in 4 hours) because the drug is liposoluble and highly bound to plasma proteins, has a high molecular weight (1202 daltons) and a large Vd. However, in renal transplant recipients with acute tubular necrosis or requiring dialysis, the absorption of oral cyclosporin is decreased compared with patients with normal renal function (AUC 562 *versus* 818 μg/L • h) and the time to reach peak concentrations is longer (5 *versus* 3.62 hours) [Kahan et al. 1986a].

2.8 Effects of Age

Age is another factor affecting the kinetics of cyclosporin. Bone marrow transplant recipients over 40 years have a lower clearance (about half) and volume of distribution at steady-state (Vd_{ss}) [about a quarter] than patients 11 to 40 years old (Yee et al. 1986). These alterations can lead to higher plasma cyclosporin concentrations when older patients are given the same doses as younger patients. In renal transplant patients over the age of 45 years clearance decreases by 30% and the Vd by approximately the same percentage, with a 50% increase in AUC compared with younger patients, while the half-life is unchanged (Kahan et al. 1986a). The mechanisms underlying these modifications are not known, but may depend on age-related decreases in organ function and on the gradual increase of lipoprotein levels with age, with a corresponding decrease in free fraction of the drug. Thus, older patients can require lower doses than younger persons.

Paediatric liver transplant patients have a higher clearance of cyclosporin than adults (0.56 *versus* 0.33 L/h/kg) [Burckart et al. 1986a]. In bone marrow transplant recipients 0 to 10 years old, clearance and Vd_{ss} are about twice those in patients 11 to 40 years old (Yee et al. 1986). Children with renal transplant show a higher clearance (0.71 *versus* 0.34 L/h/kg) and a shorter half-life (7.3 *versus* 10.7 hours) than adults (Ptachcinski et al. 1986a). The decrease in half-life was confirmed by Neiberger et al. (1987) [317 *versus* 576 minutes in adults]. A 3-fold increase in clearance with an almost 50% reduction in AUC compared with adults was found by Kahan et al. (1986b), in accordance with the previously observed low concentrations of cyclosporin (below 100 μg/L) in children with renal transplant requiring a dose of 6 to 9.5 mg/kg of the drug (Klare et al. 1984). Because of the observed kinetic behaviour, children may require larger doses and at more frequent intervals than adults in order to achieve comparable cyclosporin concentrations.

2.9 Circadian Variations in Cyclosporin Clearance

The kinetics of cyclosporin seem to have circadian variations. In liver transplant patients clearance of the drug is higher during the night than during the day, with morning trough concentrations lower than evening levels (Venkataramanan et al. 1986b). Bowers et al. (1986) found that in 15 transplant recipients evening trough concentrations were 44.7% lower than those in the morning, but this was observed only for 18 of 24 concentration pairs (morning and evening) measured. Further studies are required to obtain more definitive results.

2.10 Drug Interactions

Cyclosporin is metabolised in the liver by the cytochrome P450 system (Kahan 1985), and any drug metabolised by this system may potentially interfere with cyclosporin metabolism. Drugs that

Table I. Drugs reported to interact pharmacokinetically with cyclosporin (after Ptachcinski et al. 1986; Scott & Higenbottam 1988; Wadhwa et al. 1987b)

Drug	Drug
Acyclovir	Nafcillin
Aminoglycosides	Nicardipine
Amphotericin B	Nifedipine
Carbamazepine	Non-steroidal anti-inflammatory drugs
Cephalosporins	Norethisterone
Cholestyramine	Oral contraceptives
Cimetidine	Phenobarbitone
Co-trimoxazole (sulphamethoxazole + trimethoprim)	Phenytoin
Danazol	Prazosin
Digoxin	Prednisolone
Diltiazem	Ranitidine
Enalapril	Rifampicin
Erythromycin	Spironolactone
Frusemide (furosemide)	Steroids (prednisone, prednisolone)
Imipenem/cilastatin	Sulphadimidine (sulfamethazine)
Indomethacin	Sulphadimidine + trimethoprim
Isoniazid	Sulphamethoxazole and/or trimethoprim
Josamycin	Thiazide diuretics
Ketoconazole	Trimethoprim
Mannitol	Verapamil
Melphalan	Warfarin
Methylprednisolone (high dose)	
Methyltestosterone	
Metoclopramide	

induce cytochrome P450 activity can increase the metabolism of cyclosporin, thus diminishing the blood drug concentrations, while drugs competing for cytochrome P450 can reduce cyclosporin metabolism, increasing blood drug concentrations. Several drugs enhance the nephrotoxicity of cyclosporin. The mechanisms of other interactions are poorly understood. This topic has been reviewed recently (Scott & Higenbottam 1988; Wadhwa et al. 1987b). The drugs known to interact with cyclosporin are listed in table I. Only some recently reported interactions will be considered here. Nafcillin decreases cyclosporin blood concentrations (trough level from 272 μg/L before to 42 μg/L after nafcillin), most probably due to induction of cytochrome P450 activity (Veremis et al. 1987). Josamycin increases plasma drug concentrations probably because of inhibition of cyclosporin metabolism (Kreft-Jais et al. 1987). Warfarin was found to decrease cyclosporin blood concentrations, but the patients were treated also with phenobarbitone (Snyder 1988) which itself increases cyclosporin metabolism. The administration of the antibiotic imipenem/cilastatin to rats results in reduced cyclosporin concentrations, probably because of increased hepatic cyclosporin metabolism (Mraz et al. 1987). Cholestyramine does not affect cyclosporin absorption, but variations in absorption were noted in some patients (Keogh et al. 1988). This suggests cyclosporin monitoring and the administration of oral cyclosporin 1 hour before or 4 hours after cholestyramine. Valproic acid and mevinolin (lovastatin) do not seem to affect the kinetics of cyclosporin (Ballantyne et al. 1987; Hillebrand et al. 1987). In rats indomethacin enhances the renal and hepatic toxicity of cyclosporin, while dimethyl dinoprostone (prostaglandin E_2) diminishes cyclosporin nephrotoxicity (Whiting et al. 1987). Another drug enhancing cyclosporin nephrotoxicity in renal transplant patients is ciprofloxacin (Elston & Taylor 1988).

The changes in cyclosporin concentrations due to drug interactions can be dramatic, and can have a significant impact on toxicity or immunosuppressive efficacy, with the risk of rejection. Cyclosporin is a drug with a low therapeutic index. If possible, it is better to avoid the concomitant administration of drugs affecting the kinetics of cyclosporin. If coadministration is unavoidable, careful monitoring of cyclosporin blood concentrations and appropriate modification of cyclosporin dosage are essential.

3. Conclusions

Cyclosporin cannot be administered on a fixed dosage schedule. Many factors can affect its kinetics, especially in the early post-transplant period, indicated by the marked variability observed in blood concentrations. These factors should be taken into consideration in order to establish the appropriate therapeutic regimen for the individual patient. Monitoring should be used in conjunction with other laboratory and clinical data to guide dosage adjustments for optimal efficacy with minimal toxicity. There are significant differences in the immunosuppressive protocols used by different centres (Shaw et al. 1987). The values of measured cyclosporin concentrations clearly depend on the biological fluid and the analytical technique used, but the optimal range of cyclosporin concentrations has not been defined as yet. The risks of rejection and toxicity vary inversely with increases or decreases in cyclosporin concentrations. For instance, in allograft recipients (kidney, pancreas, heart) having blood drug concentrations (RIA) below 200 μg/L the incidence of rejection was 21% with no nephrotoxicity or hepatotoxicity, while with levels above 800 μg/L the incidence of rejection and of toxicity was 3% and 23%, respectively (Irschik et al. 1984). In bone marrow transplant patients having serum trough concentrations (RIA) of < 150, 150 to 250 and > 250 μg/L the incidence of renal dysfunction was 73%, 95% and 100%, respectively (Kennedy et al. 1985). After the introduction of cyclosporin into clinical therapy there was initial use, perhaps overenthusiastic, of high doses, such as 18 mg/kg/day or even higher, with a notable incidence of toxic effects. As a result, and with the acquisition of experience in the use of cyclosporin, the doses were lowered. Now the trend is towards the use of cyclosporin in combination with other immunosuppressive agents (triple or quadruple therapy) [Cabrol et al. 1986; Kalayoglu et al. 1988; Sheil 1987; Sutherland et al. 1986]. Combined immunosuppressive therapy has a synergistic effect and allows the use of lower doses with less incidence of toxicity and rejection.

Therapeutic drug monitoring should be undertaken on a regular basis after the initiation of therapy with cyclosporin. Cyclosporin concentrations should be determined every 2 days, or even more frequently in the immediate postoperative period if needed, until the patient's clinical condition and cyclosporin levels are stable. The risk of rejection is greatest in the early post-transplant period and pathophysiological changes can occur rapidly: thereafter cyclosporin monitoring can be gradually reduced to every 1 to 2 months. Monitoring is required 2 to 3 days after any dosing change in patients with normal liver function because that is the period necessary to achieve a new steady-state concentration, due to the long half-life of cyclosporin. A longer monitoring period is necessary when liver function is impaired, because of the prolongation in cyclosporin half-life. Periodic monitoring should continue indefinitely while a patient is on cyclosporin therapy according to an individual schedule and, possibly, coincident with the clinical follow-up as an outpatient. After discharge from hospital the patient and the attending physician should be aware of the factors which may require changes in cyclosporin therapy, such as the onset of infections, concomitant administration of other drugs or impairment of liver function. Liver and kidney function should be routinely monitored.

References

Agarwal RP, McPherson RA, Threatte GA. Evidence of a cyclosporine-binding protein in human erythrocytes. Transplantation 42: 627-632, 1986

Andrews W, Fyock B, Gray S, Coln D, Hendrickse W, et al. Pediatric liver transplantation: the Dallas experience. Transplantation Proceedings 19: 3267-3276, 1987

Andrews W, Iwatsuki S, Shaw BW, Starzl TE. Letter. Transplantation 39: 338, 1985

Atkinson K, Biggs JC, Britton K, Short R, Mrongovius R, et al. Oral administration of cyclosporin A for recipients of allogeneic marrow transplants: implications of clinical gut dysfunction. British Journal of Haematology 56: 223-231, 1984

Atkinson K, Britton K, Paull P, Farrell C, Concannon A, et al. Detrimental effect of intestinal disease on absorption of orally administered cyclosporine. Transplantation Proceedings 15 (Suppl. 1): 2446-2449, 1983

Ballantyne CM, Jones PH, Payton-Ross C, Patsch W, Short HD, et al. Hyperlipidemia following heart transplantation: natural history and intervention with mevinolin (Lovastatin). Transplantation Proceedings 19 (Suppl. 5): 60-62, 1987

Bowers LD, Canafax DM, Singh J, Seifedlin R, Simmons RL, et al. Studies of cyclosporine blood levels: analysis, clinical utility, pharmacokinetics, metabolites and chronopharmacology. Transplantation Proceedings 18 (Suppl. 5): 137-143, 1986

Burckart G, Starzl T, Williams L, Sanghvi A, Gartner C, et al. Cyclosporine monitoring in pediatric liver transplant patients. Transplantation Proceedings 17: 1172-1175, 1985

Burckart GJ, Venkataramanan R, Ptachcinski RJ, Starzl TE, Gartner C, et al. Cyclosporine absorption following orthotopic liver transplantation. Journal of Clinical Pharmacology 26: 647-651, 1986a

Burckart GJ, Venkataramanan R, Ptachcinski RJ, Starzl TE, Griffith BP, et al. Cyclosporine pharmacokinetic profiles in liver, heart and kidney transplant patients as determined by high-performance liquid chromatography. Transplantation Proceedings 18 (Suppl. 5): 129-136, 1986b

Burckart GJ, Wang CP, Zeevi A, Venkataramanan R, Ptachcinski

RJ, et al. Cyclosporine metabolites in human bile: recovery and immunologic activity. Transplantation Proceedings 20 (Suppl. 1): 190-192, 1988
Busuttil RW, Goldstein LI, Danovitch M, Ament ME, Memsic LDF. Liver transplantation today. Annals of Internal Medicine 104: 377-389, 1986
Cabrol C, Gandjbakhch I, Pavie A, Cabrol A, Corcos T, et al. Indications and contraindications for cardiac transplantation: new trends in immunosuppressive therapy and results. Transplantation Proceedings 4 (Suppl. 3): 35-38, 1986
Calabresi P, Parks RE. Chemotherapy of neoplastic diseases. In Goodman & Gilman (Eds) The pharmacological basis of therapeutics, pp. 1240-1306, MacMillan Company, New York, 1985
Elston RA, Taylor J. Possible interaction of ciprofloxacin with cyclosporin A. Journal of Antimicrobial Chemotherapy 21: 679-680, 1988
Follath F, Wenk M. Vožeh S, Thiel G, Brunner F, et al. Intravenous cyclosporine kinetics in renal failure. Clinical Pharmacology and Therapeutics 34: 638-643, 1983
Freed BM, Rosano TG, Lempert N. *In vitro* immunosuppressive properties of cyclosporine metabolites. Transplantation 43: 123-127, 1987a
Freed BM, Rosano TG, Quick C, Lempert N. Effect of cyclosporine metabolites M17 and M18 on proliferation and IL-2 production in the mixed lymphocyte culture. Transplantation Proceedings 19: 1223-1226, 1987b
Frey BM, Appenzeller M, Gautschi K, Keller B, Vadas L, et al. Measurement of cyclosporine A by RIA in different centers are not comparable. Transplantation Proceedings 19: 1713-1714, 1987
Hillebrand G, Castro LA, Van Scheidt W, Beukelmann D, Land W, et al. Valproate for epilepsy in renal transplant recipients receiving cyclosporine. Transplantation 43: 915-916, 1987
Holt DW, Marsden JT, Johnston A. Measurement of cyclosporine: methodological problems. Transplantation Proceedings 18 (Suppl. 5): 101-110, 1986
Irschik E, Tilg H, Niederwieser D, Gastl G, Huber Ch, et al. Cyclosporin blood levels do correlate with clinical complications. Lancet 2: 692-693, 1984
Johnston A, Marsden JT, Hla KK, Henry A, Holt DW. The effect of vehicle on the oral absorption of cyclosporin. British Journal of Clinical Pharmacology 21: 331-333, 1986a
Johnston A, Marsden JT, Holt DW. The United Kingdom cyclosporin quality assessment scheme. Therapeutic Drug Monitoring 8: 200-204, 1986b
Johnston A, Marsden JT, Holt DW. The influence of haematocrit on blood cyclosporin measurements *in vivo*. British Journal of Clinical Pharmacology 25: 509-513, 1988
Jones RJ, Lee SK, Beschorner WE, Vogel VG, Grochow LB, et al. Venocclusive disease of the liver following bone marrow transplantation. Transplantation 44: 778-783, 1987
Kahan BD. Individualization of cyclosporine therapy using pharmacokinetic and pharmacodynamic parameters. Transplantation 40: 457-476, 1985
Kahan BD, Kramer WG, Wideman C, Flechner SM, Lorber MI, et al. Demographic factors affecting the pharmacokinetics of cyclosporine estimated by radioimmunoassay. Transplantation 41: 459-464, 1986a
Kahan BD, Kramer WG, Wideman CA, Frazier OH, Lorber MI, et al. Analysis of pharmacokinetic profiles in 232 renal and 87 cardiac allograft recipients treated with cyclosporine. Transplantation Proceedings 18 (Suppl. 5): 115-119, 1986b
Kahan BD, Ried M, Newburger J. Pharmacokinetics of cyclosporine in human renal transplantation. Transplantation Proceedings 15: 446-453, 1983
Kalayoglu M, Stratta RJ, Hoffmann RM, Sollinger HW, Belzer FO. Quadruple immunosuppressive therapy for liver transplantation. Transplantation Proceedings 20 (Suppl. 1): 524-529, 1988
Kennedy MS, Yee GC, McGuire TR, Leonard TM, Crowley JJ, et al. Correlation of serum cyclosporine concentration with renal dysfunction in marrow transplant recipients. Transplantation 40: 249-253, 1985
Keogh A, Day R, Critchley L, Duggin G, Baron D. The effect of food and cholestyramine on the absorption of cyclosporine in cardiac transplant recipients. Transplantation Proceedings 20: 27-30, 1988
Keown PA, Stiller CR, Laupacis AL, Howson W, Coles R, et al. The effects and side effects of cyclosporine: relationship to drug pharmacokinetics. Transplantation Proceedings 14: 659-661, 1982
Keown PA, Stiller CR, Sinclair NR, Carruthers G, Howson W, et al. The clinical relevance of cyclosporine blood levels as measured by radioimmunoassay. Transplantation Proceedings 15 (Suppl. 1): 2438-2441, 1983
Keown PA, Stiller CR, Stawecki M, Freeman D. Pharmacokinetics of cyclosporine in solid organ transplantation. Transplantation Proceedings 18 (Suppl. 5): 160-164, 1986
Klare B, Walter JV, Hahn H, Emmrich P, Land W. Cyclosporin in renal transplantation in children. Lancet 2: 692, 1984
Kreft-Jais C, Billaud EM, Gaudry C, Bedrossian J. Effect of josamycin on plasma cyclosporine levels. European Journal of Clinical Pharmacology 32: 327-328, 1987
Lemaire M, Maurer G, Wood AJ. Pharmacokinetics and metabolism. Progress in Allergy 38: 93-107, 1986
Lindholm A, Henricsson S, Lind M. Dahlqvist R. Intraindividual variability in the relative systemic availability of cyclosporin after oral dosing. European Journal of Clinical Pharmacology 34: 461-464, 1988
Lithell H, Odlind B, Selinus I, Lindberg A, Lindström B, et al. Is the plasma lipoprotein pattern of importance for treatment with cyclosporine? Transplantation Proceedings 18: 50-51, 1986
Mehta MU, Venkataramanan R, Burckart GJ, Ptachcinski RJ, Delamos B, et al. Effect of bile on cyclosporin absorption in liver transplant patients. British Journal of Clinical Pharmacology 25: 579-584, 1988
Moyer TP. Measurement of cyclosporine: a challenge to the professional laboratory organizations. Therapeutic Drug Monitoring 7: 123-124, 1985
Moyer TP, Johnson P, Faynor SM, Sterioff S. Cyclosporine: a review of drug monitoring problems and presentation of a simple, accurate liquid chromatographic procedure that solves these problems. Clinical Biochemistry 19: 83-89, 1986
Mraz W, Sido B, Knedel M, Hammer C. Concomitant immunosuppressive and antibiotic therapy: reduction of cyclosporine A blood levels due to treatment with imipenem/cilastatin. Transplantation Proceedings 19: 4017-4020, 1987
Mraz W, Zink RA, Graft A, Preis D, Illner WD, et al. Distribution and transfer of cyclosporine among the various human lipoprotein classes. Transplantation Proceedings 15 (Suppl. 1): 2426-2429, 1983
Neiberger R, Weiss R, Gomez M, Greifer J, Tellis VA, et al. Elimination kinetics of cyclosporine following oral administration to children with renal transplants. Transplantation Proceedings 19: 1525, 1987
Niederberger W, Lemaire M, Maurer G, Nussbaumer K, Wagner O. Distribution and binding of cyclosporine in blood and tissues. Transplantation Proceedings 15 (Suppl. 1): 2419-2421, 1983
Odlind B, Lindberg A, Tufveson G, Lindström B, Frödin L, et al. Longitudinal study of the pharmacokinetics of cyclosporine before and after renal transplantation. Transplantation Proceedings 18: 47-49, 1986
Ptachcinski RJ, Burckart GJ, Rosenthal JT, Venkataramanan R, Howrie DL, et al. Cyclosporine pharmacokinetics in children following cadaveric renal transplantation. Transplantation Proceedings 18: 766-767, 1986a
Ptachcinski RJ, Venkataramanan R, Burckart GJ. Clinical phar-

macokinetics of cyclosporine. Clinical Pharmacokinetics 11: 107-132, 1986b.

Ptachcinski RJ, Venkataramanan R, Rosenthal JT, Burckart GJ, Taylor RJ, et al. The effect of food on cyclosporine absorption. Transplantation 40: 174-176, 1985a

Ptachcinski RJ, Venkataramanan R, Rosenthal JT, Burckart GJ, Taylor RJ, et al. Cyclosporine kinetics in renal transplantation. Clinical Pharmacology and Therapeutics 38: 296-300, 1985b

Quesniaux V. The use of monoclonal antibodies to probe the surface of cyclosporine. Transplantation Proceedings 18 (Suppl. 5): 111-114, 1986

Quesniaux V, Tees R, Schreler MH, Maurer G, van Regenmortel MHV. Potential of monoclonal antibodies to improve therapeutic monitoring of cyclosporine. Clinical Chemistry 33: 32-37, 1987

Rosano TG. Effect of hematocrit on cyclosporine (cyclosporin A) in whole blood and plasma of renal-transplant patients. Clinical Chemistry 31: 410-412, 1985

Rosano TG, Freed BM, Pell MA, Dybas MT, Lempert N. Involvement of cyclosporine metabolites in therapeutic monitoring and immunosuppression. Transplantation Proceedings 19: 1699-1703, 1987

Rosano TG, Freed BM, Pell MA, Lempert N. Cyclosporine metabolites in human blood and renal tissue. Transplantation Proceedings 18 (Suppl. 5): 35-40, 1986

Schinella M, Perobelli L, Mazzi G, Determinazioni di ciclosporina e suoi metaboliti con anticorpi policlonali, monoclonali aspecifici e specifici (RIA) e con HPLC. Ligand Quarterly 6: 365-367, 1987

Scott JP, Higenbottam TW. Adverse reactions and interactions of cyclosporin Medical Toxicology 3: 107-127, 1988

Shaw LM, Bowers L, Demers L, Freeman D, Moyer T, et al. Critical issues in cyclosporine monitoring: report of the task force on cyclosporine monitoring. Clinical Chemistry 33: 1269-1288, 1987

Sheil AGR. Clinical organ transplantation. Transplantation Proceedings 19: 2782-2786, 1987

Shulman HM, McDonald GB, Matthews D, Doney KC, Kopecky KJ, et al. An analysis of hepatic venocclusive disease and centrilobular hepatic degeneration following bone marrow transplantation. Gastroenterology 79: 1178-1191, 1980

Snyder DS. Interaction between cyclosporine and warfarin. Annals of Internal Medicine 108: 311, 1988

Sutherland DER, Goetz FC, Najarian JS. Improved pancreas graft survival by use of multiple drug combination immunotherapy. Transplantation Proceedings 18: 1770-1773, 1986

Tufveson G, Odlind B, Sjöberg O, Lindberg A, Gabrielsson J, et al. A longitudinal study of the pharmacokinetics of cyclosporine A and *in vitro* lymphocyte responses in renal transplant patients. Transplantation Proceedings 18 (Suppl. 5): 16-24, 1986

Venkataramanan R, Burckart GJ, Ptachcinski RJ. Pharmacokinetics and monitoring of cyclosporine following orthotopic liver transplantation. Seminars in Liver Disease 5: 357-368, 1985a

Venkataramanan R, Burckart GJ, Ptachcinski RJ, Lee A, Hardesty RL, et al. Cyclosporine pharmacokinetics in heart transplant patients. Transplantation Proceedings 18: 768-770, 1986a

Venkataramanan R, Gray J, Ptachcinski RJ, Van Thiel DH, Burckart GJ, et al. Cyclosporine kinetics in liver disease. Clinical Pharmacology and Therapeutics 37: 234, 1985b

Venkataramanan R, Ptachcinski RJ, Burckart GJ, Yang SL, Starzl TE, et al. The clearance of cyclosporine by hemodialysis. Journal of Clinical Pharmacology 24: 528-531, 1984

Venkataramanan R, Starzl TE, Yang S, Burckart GJ, Ptachcinski RJ, et al. Biliary excretion of cyclosporine in liver transplant patients. Transplantation Proceedings 17: 286-289, 1985c

Venkataramanan R, Yang S, Burckart GJ, Ptachcinski RJ, Van Thiel DH, et al. Diurnal variation in cyclosporine kinetics. Therapeutic Drug Monitoring 8: 380-381, 1986b

Veremis SA, Maddux MS, Pollak R, Mozes MF. Subtherapeutic cyclosporine concentrations during nafcillin therapy. Transplantation 43: 913-915, 1987

Vine W, Bowers LD. Cyclosporine: structure, pharmacokinetics, and therapeutic drug monitoring. Critical Reviews in Clinical Laboratory Sciences 25: 275-311, 1987

Wadhwa NK, Schroeder TJ, O'Flaherty E, Pesce AJ, Myre SA, et al. The effect of oral metoclopramide on the absorption of cyclosporine. Transplantation 43: 211-213, 1987a

Wadhwa NK, Schroeder TJ, Pesce AJ, Myre SA, Clardy CW, et al. Cyclosporine drug interactions: a review. Therapeutic Drug Monitoring 9: 399-406, 1987b

Wang CP, Burckart GJ, Venkataramanan R, Ptachcinski RJ, Cuellar RE, et al. Cyclosporine metabolite profiles in the blood of liver transplant patients. Transplantation Proceedings 20 (Suppl. 1): 173-175, 1988

Wassef R, Cohen Z, Langer B. *In vivo* interaction of cyclosporine and Intralipid. Transplantation 41: 266-278, 1986

Wenk M, Follath F. Temperature dependency of apparent cyclosporin A concentrations in plasma. Clinical Chemistry 29: 1865, 1983

Whiting PH, Barnard N, Neilsch A, Simpson JG, Burke MD. Interactions between cyclosporin A, indomethacin and 16,16-dimethyl prostaglandin E_2: effects on renal, hepatic and gastrointestinal toxicity in the rat. British Journal of Experimental Pathology 68: 777-786, 1987

Yee GC, Kennedy MS, Storb R, Thomas ED. Effect of hepatic dysfunction on oral cyclosporine pharmacokinetics in marrow transplant patients. Blood 64: 1277-1279, 1984a

Yee GC, Kennedy MS, Storb R, Thomas ED. Pharmacokinetics of intravenous cyclosporine in bone marrow transplant patients. Transplantation 38: 511-513, 1984b

Yee GC, Lennon TP, Gmur DJ, Kennedy MS, Deeg HJ. Age-dependent cyclosporine: pharmacokinetics in marrow transplant recipients. Clinical Pharmacology and Therapeutics 40: 438-443, 1986

Author's address: *Vanni Rodighiero*, Department of Pharmacology, University of Padova, Largo E. Meneghetti 2, 35131 Padova (Italy).

Clinical Pharmacokinetics 16: 38-54 (1989)
0312-5963/89/0001-0038/$08.50/0

Saturable Pharmacokinetics in the Renal Excretion of Drugs

C.A.M. van Ginneken and *F.G.M. Russel*

Department of Pharmacology, University of Nijmegen, Nijmegen, The Netherlands

Contents

Summary 38
1. Urinary Drug Excretion 39
1.1 Glomerular Filtration and Passive Back Diffusion 39
1.2 Tubular Secretion 41
1.3 Active Reabsorption 42
2. Pharmacokinetics of Renal Drug Excretion 43
2.1 Accumulation Behaviour 46
3. Kinetic Drug Interactions 46
4. Tubular Secretion 47
4.1 Specificity 47
4.2 Clinical Implications 49

Summary

The renal excretion of drugs is the result of different mechanisms: glomerular filtration, passive back diffusion, tubular secretion and tubular reabsorption. Of these mechanisms the last 2 are saturable, as they involve carrier transport. This also implies that both tubular secretion and tubular reabsorption are susceptible to competition between similar substrates for a common carrier site. Furthermore, transport via these mechanisms is energy-dependent, so-called active transport, able to concentrate a drug.

Tubular secretion takes place in the proximal tubule of the nephron. Many organic compounds are actively secreted, but there are separate carrier systems for anions and cations. Anions appear to be transported actively over the basolateral membrane and by a less efficient non-active carrier-mediated process (facilitated diffusion) over the brush border membrane. As a result of these mechanisms, anions tend to accumulate in proximal tubular cells. For cations, however, the active transport step operates over the brush border membrane, whereas the uptake of the cation in the cell occurs via facilitated diffusion over the basolateral membrane.

Active reabsorption is most prominent for many nutrients and endogenous substrates (amino acids, glucose, vitamins), but various exogenous compounds also have a certain affinity for the reabsorptive carrier systems. Uricosuric drugs, for instance, interfere with carrier-mediated reabsorption of urate.

The occurrence of saturable excretion routes causes dose-dependent, non-linear pharmacokinetics. In clinical pharmacokinetics, tubular secretion can adequately be described with the use of a Michaelis-Menten equation. This implies that a compound undergoing tubular secretion exhibits a concentration-dependent renal clearance. At low plasma concentrations the clearance will be maximal, and for several drugs may be as high as the effective renal plasma flow. Increasing concentrations cause decreasing renal clearance, until eventually the secretion mechanism becomes fully saturated. Then the excretion of the drug in urine will depend primarily on its net rate of filtration. It is important to realise that the non-linear kinetics will be evident from the plasma kinetics only when the saturable pathway contributes to at least some 20% of the total body clearance. Interactions with other substrates, however, are likely to occur even when only a very small amount of drug is transported by the carrier system. Non-linear kinetics inevitably lead to disproportionate accumulation. Therefore, for any drug that is actively secreted, careful consideration should be given to the possibilities of drug-drug interaction and of unwanted drug accumulation with increasing doses.

Several mechanisms contribute to the excretion of drugs and other substances via the kidney, and are closely related to its anatomy and physiology. The functional units of the kidney are the nephrons, each consisting of a glomerulus, surrounded by a Bowman's capsule, and a tubular system (fig. 1). The nephron is surrounded by arterial and venous capillaries which provide a close contact between the blood circulation and the cells forming the glomerular and tubular lumen.

The excretion of drugs in urine is governed by 4 different processes:

1. *Glomerular filtration:* part of the blood flowing through the kidneys is ultrafiltered in the glomeruli (producing about 125ml of filtrate per minute).

2. *Passive back diffusion:* nearly all the water in the glomerular filtrate is reabsorbed in the renal tubuli. As a result, the concentration of drugs in the tubular urine increases markedly and a drug concentration gradient is established between urine and plasma. This gradient provides the driving force for diffusion of drug from urine to plasma.

3. *Tubular secretion:* some drugs are excreted from the capillaries surrounding the renal tubuli into the primary urine by a carrier-mediated process (tubular secretion), analogous to some endogenous 'waste' substances. This process is limited by a certain fixed maximum transport value and susceptible to competition by various compounds secreted by the same mechanism.

4. *Active tubular reabsorption:* some drugs are actively reabsorbed from the primary urine into the capillaries around the renal tubuli; this process is also analogous to that for endogenous substances (e.g. glucose). Like tubular secretion, this active reabsorption is saturable and susceptible to competition phenomena.

1. Urinary Drug Excretion

1.1 Glomerular Filtration and Passive Back Diffusion

Plasma water and the drug molecules present in it are filtered in the glomerulus. Drug molecules bound to plasma protein, notably albumin, are virtually excluded from this filtration since for all practical purposes the size of the pores in the glomerulus can be regarded as insufficient for the permeation of macromolecules. Kinetically, this implies that the *effective* clearance of a drug by glomerular filtration is equal to the glomerular filtration rate of an unbound substance (e.g. inulin) multiplied by the fraction of drug not bound to plasma protein. The effective clearance is further decreased by back-diffusion of the drug from the tubular fluid to the bloodstream. Nearly all the water in the filtrate is reabsorbed so that the concentration of drug molecules in the filtrate increases markedly. As a result, a large concentration gradient of drug molecules between primary urine and plasma develops, which becomes a driving force for (passive) back diffusion. As usual where permeation of biological membranes by non-active mechanisms is concerned, back diffusion is only possible for drug molecules which are sufficiently lipophilic in nature. This means that the drug should be un-ionised in urine: the pKa of the drug and the pH of the urine are thus important factors. When, for instance, the urine is acidic (by chance or by administration of acidifying agents) acid drugs

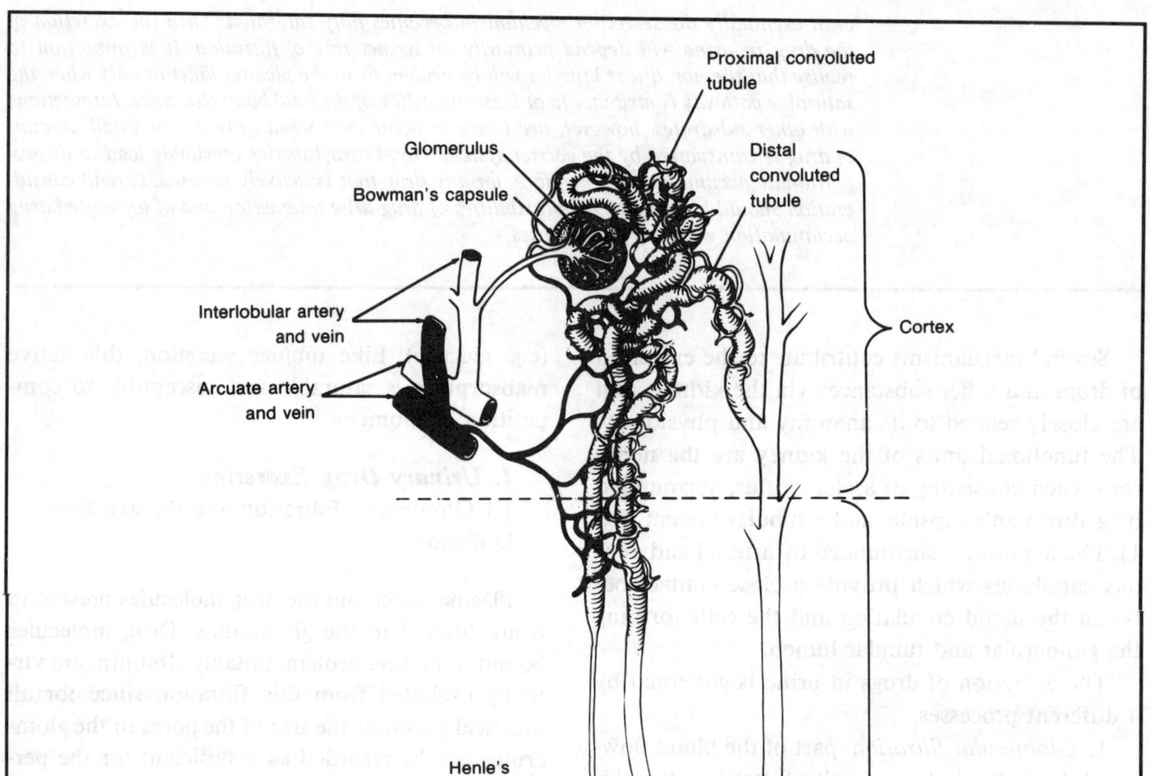

Fig. 1. The nephron with its arterial and venous supply. The components of the nephron are the glomerulus, surrounded by Bowman's capsule, the proximal tubule (part convoluted, part straight), the loop of Henle and the distal tubule flowing into the collecting tubule. A single layer of epithelial cells lines the lumen of the nephron throughout its length, and a close network of arterial and venous capillaries provides a close contact between the blood circulation and these cells. [From Junqueira et al. (1975), with permission.]

such as salicylic acid will tend to diffuse back into the peritubular capillaries. When the urine is alkaline, on the other hand, back diffusion will be negligible. For basic drugs the opposite holds true.

Another important factor for the degree of back diffusion is the relative amount of water reabsorption, which may also be considered as the urine flow. When less water is reabsorbed, more urine will be formed, and the concentration of drug in the tubular fluid will therefore be lower: this will result in a smaller concentration gradient and consequently less back diffusion. A clearcut relationship between the rate of drug excretion by the kidney and the urine flow may therefore be expected (and is indeed found), except for drugs with very low or very high lipophilicity, since the former will, and the latter will not, diffuse back in any case.

1.2 Tubular Secretion

A number of substances are excreted from the capillaries surrounding the renal tubules into the luminal fluid by a carrier-mediated process (tubular secretion). With several experimental techniques it has been shown independently that many organic compounds are actively secreted by the proximal tubular cells of the nephron. The pathways for organic anions and cations appear to be separate, but both transport systems are characterised by broad specificity. Tubular secretion is an active carrier-mediated process in that it is concentration-, temperature- and energy-dependent, and susceptible to competition by similar substrates (Grantham & Chonko 1986).

The characteristics of the renal organic anion transport system have been extensively studied with *p*-aminohippurate (PAH). Most of our knowledge about the exact anatomical location of PAH secretion derives from studies with isolated perfused rabbit tubules. The proximal tubule can be divided functionally into 3 segments, S_1, S_2 and S_3.

The highest rate of PAH secretion is seen in the S_2 segment of both the superficial and juxtamedullary nephrons of the rabbit kidney (Woodhall et al. 1978). Shimomura et al. (1981) showed that the affinity values in the 3 segments were the same, while the maximal transport rate in the S_2 segment was 5 to 6 times greater than in the other segments. They suggested that heterogeneity of PAH secretion along the proximal tubule is the result of an unequal distribution of transporters with common affinity. However, this pattern of heterogeneity is probably not representative for all mammalian species. For example, in the pig the S_1 segment is the predominant site of PAH secretion (Schäli & Roch-Ramel 1981).

Although protein binding always decreases the extent of glomerular filtration, the tubular secretion of most organic anions seems to be unaffected, presumably due to the high dissociation rate of the drug-protein complex relative to the duration of exposure to the secretory system. The affinity of the carrier system must also be high enough to compete effectively with the plasma-protein molecules for the available drug. These conditions do not appear to be universal, as there are examples of drugs for which protein binding impedes tubular secretion, e.g. frusemide (furosemide) [Bowman 1975; Hall & Rowland 1985]. In general, however, drug protein binding is easily reversible and dissociation rate constants higher than 10/second may be expected. The average life of a drug-protein complex would then be below 0.1 second, much shorter than the renal cortical transit time, which is in the order of seconds at least. These estimates suggest that the carrier molecule can compete effectively with the plasma protein molecule and that tubular secretion will proceed without much impediment by plasma protein binding.

A number of *in vivo* and *in vitro* techniques (Ullrich & Greger 1985) have been employed to study the sequence of movement of organic anions through the proximal tubular cells. In particular, the relatively new technique of isolated renal plasma membrane vesicles has proved to be of great value for the study of transport mechanisms at specific membrane sites. Most studies have been carried out with an archetype of secreted anions, i.e. PAH (Pritchard 1987).

The first step in tubular secretion involves the carrier-mediated uptake of PAH from the interstitial fluid across the peritubular (basolateral) membrane into the proximal tubular cell. This process is active since it has been shown that PAH is taken up against an electrochemical gradient, to achieve intracellular concentrations up to 30 times higher than those in the extracellular fluid. There is abundant evidence to indicate the PAH transport is coupled to the transmembrane sodium gradient. However, recent studies with basolateral membrane vesicles have shown that this sodium-coupled mechanism can also be stimulated by an opposing anion gradient, suggesting a sodium gradient-stimulated anion exchange mechanism (Russel et al. 1988a).

The movement of PAH out of the cell across the brush border membrane into the tubular lumen occurs by carrier-mediated (facilitated) diffusion, a process which can be considered as passive in the sense that the substance is transported down its electrochemical gradient. Recent studies strongly support the involvement of an anion exchange mechanism in the brush border membrane, but there are also indications for a (gated) channel that mediates the movement of PAH out the cell (Pritchard 1987). At present it is not clear whether both types of transport proceed via a single carrier, or whether different carriers are involved.

The PAH transport system in the brush border membrane has a lower affinity but higher capacity than the transport system in the basolateral membrane. Both transport systems are competitively inhibited by probenecid, but the basolateral membrane system is more susceptible to inhibition (Russel et al. 1988a).

It is to be expected that a similar situation will exist for other acidic drugs that are secreted in the tubule. When the facilitated diffusion in the brush border has a much lower capacity and operates at a lower rate than the active system in the basolateral membrane, the combination of mechanisms results in a potential accumulation of the drug in the tubular cell. A clinically important example is the cephalosporin antibiotics, which accumulate in the tubular cell and may exert a pronounced nephrotoxic action (Tune 1975).

With cationic drugs the situation is different. For the archetypal *N*-methylnicotinamide a two-carrier transport has also been postulated, but here the active stage occurs in the brush border membrane while transport in the basolateral membrane proceeds by facilitated diffusion (Kinsella et al. 1979; Rennick 1981a,b). Accumulation in the tubular cell from the combined action of these mechanisms is unlikely.

1.3 Active Reabsorption

Carrier-mediated reabsorption from the tubular fluid occurs for many endogenous compounds which are indispensable to the body, e.g. glucose, amino acids and some vitamins. The physicochemical properties of these nutrients preclude their effective return to the circulation by passive back diffusion. Glucose, for example, is not normally present in the voided urine because it is completely reabsorbed from the glomerular filtrate in the proximal tubules. Only when the amounts delivered to the kidney exceed the transport capacity of the carrier system does glucose appear in the urine. In fact, the presence of glucose in urine indicates an abnormally high glucose level in blood which, for instance, is a main feature of diabetes mellitus.

Renal excretion of most organic anions is dominated by tubular secretion. Reabsorption, if any, usually occurs by simple diffusion. However, some compounds are known to be transported by tubular secretion as well as active reabsorption. Urate is an interesting example of an endogenous anion that undergoes bidirectional active transport (Lang 1981). The combined action of opposing transport mechanisms explains the paradoxical effects of drugs like salicylate, probenecid and phenylbutazone on urate excretion. In low doses they act as hyperuricaemic drugs by inhibiting tubular urate secretion, but with high doses they exert a hypouricaemic effect by inhibiting tubular urate reabsorption (Gutman & Yü 1961; Yü & Gutman 1955, 1959).

Exogenous organic anions for which active bidirectional transport has been reported are *m*-hydroxybenzoate, nicotinate and pyrazinoate. The transport systems involved in the specific secretion and reabsorption of these compounds have still not been fully described, but there is evidence that they are, at least in part, different from the urate system (Weiner 1985).

Another mechanism capable of reabsorbing various substances from the tubular fluid is endocytosis. From a purely kinetic point of view endocytosis behaves similarly to carrier-mediated transport, but the mechanism is very different. In endocytosis, vesicles are formed from the brush border membrane, incorporating fluid and substances from the lumen of the tubule. The vesicles fuse with primary lysosomes and are subsequently transferred to secondary lysosomes, where the incorporated substances are metabolised or released in the cytoplasm. Endocytosis is the normal mechanism for protein reabsorption in the kidney, but drugs may also be reabsorbed by this route. It is known, for instance, that aminoglycoside antibiotics such as gentamicin enter the tubular fluid only by glomerular filtration but may be reabsorbed by an endocytosis-like mechanism. It appears that aminoglycosides bind to anionic binding sites on the brush border membrane, and that this provides a stimulus for endocytosis (Cojocel & Hook 1983). This process forms the first step in the mechanism of the well-known aminoglycoside nephrotoxicity. As can be seen from the discussion in section 1.2 there are significant differences in the mechanisms of toxicity of cephalosporins and aminoglycosides.

2. Pharmacokinetics of Renal Drug Excretion

The basic relationship governing the renal excretion of drugs is the following:

$$RER = CL_R \times C_p \quad \text{(Eq. 1)}$$

where RER = renal excretion rate (amount of drug excreted per unit of time); CL_R = renal plasma clearance (volume of plasma cleared of drug per unit of time); and C_p = plasma concentration (e.g. mg/L). When only glomerular filtration occurs, CL_R equals the glomerular filtration rate (GFR): about 7.5 L/h (inulin clearance) in humans for drugs not bound to plasma proteins. For a bound drug the clearance by glomerular filtration is equal to its free fraction multiplied by the inulin clearance. In many cases the net GFR is further reduced by passive back diffusion of the drug from the filtrate passing through the tubular system. Although the rate of back diffusion will depend upon the flow and the pH of the tubular urine, the renal clearance of a drug that undergoes filtration and back diffusion alone can be regarded as a constant, since variations in its value caused by flow and pH changes will average out when the duration of study is long enough. This means that the renal excretion rate as a function of time is a pure reflection of the plasma concentration curve; it is thus possible to obtain time constants for elimination from renal excretion data alone. When tubular secretion occurs in addition to filtration and back diffusion, clearance will become a concentration-dependent function. In most cases the clearance by tubular secretion can be adequately described with the use of the Michaelis-Menten equation:

$$CL_{TS} = \frac{T_m}{K_T + C_p} \quad \text{(Eq. 2)}$$

where CL_{TS} = that part of the renal clearance that proceeds by tubular secretion; T_m = the (apparent) transport maximum of the carrier system (maximum amount of drug that can be secreted per unit of time); and K_T = the apparent Michaelis-Menten constant for the drug with respect to its secretory carrier (the units of K_T are those of concentration).

It should be noted that to date it has not been established whether or not plasma protein binding restricts secretion of the drug for the general case. Drugs that are almost completely extracted in the kidney (PAH and similar compounds) are evidently not hindered by binding to plasma protein. Other compounds, however, exhibit features which indicate that tubular secretion is at least partly restricted by protein binding (Russel et al. 1988).

Tubular secretion is always accompanied by glomerular filtration. Therefore, equation 1 becomes:

$$RER = \left(CL_{GF} + \frac{T_m}{K_T + C_p}\right) \cdot C_p \quad \text{(Eq. 3)}$$

where CL_{GF} = net clearance resulting from glomerular filtration and passive back diffusion.

There are two extremes for this equation:

1. When $C_p \ll K_T$:

$$RER = \left(CL_{GF} + \frac{T_m}{K_T}\right) \cdot C_p \qquad \text{(Eq. 4)}$$

In this situation the excretion kinetics are linear, renal clearance is maximal, and its value may be as high as renal plasma flow. It should be noted that application of diagnostics for measuring the renal plasma flow requires the assumption that the plasma concentration of the diagnostic is negligible with respect to its K_T value, as otherwise the renal plasma flow will be underestimated.

2. When $C_p \gg K_T$:

$$RER = CL_{GF} \cdot C_p + T_m \qquad \text{(Eq. 5)}$$

The secretory mechanism is now fully saturated, and with increasing plasma concentrations the linear glomerular filtration process will become the dominant factor in renal excretion. Eventually the renal clearance will equal the GFR again.

In most cases, renal excretion is not the only pathway of drug elimination. The total rate of elimination, then, will be larger than the RER. Usually the clearance of glomerular filtration can be totalled with other linear clearances to a total linear clearance CL_{lin}, so that the decay of the amount (A) of drug in time is given by the following differential equation:

$$\frac{dA}{dt} = -\left(CL_{lin} + \frac{T_m}{K_T + C_p}\right) \cdot C_p \qquad \text{(Eq. 6)}$$

It is useful to rearrange this equation with the aid of the following expression for the maximum attainable clearance (CL_{max}):

$$CL_{max} = CL_{lin} + \frac{T_m}{K_T} \qquad \text{(Eq. 7)}$$

When f is the fraction of CL_{max} that proceeds via the capacity-limited pathway then:

$$\frac{T_m}{K_T} = f \cdot CL_{max} \qquad \text{(Eq. 8)}$$

or

$$T_m = f \cdot K_T \cdot CL_{max} \qquad \text{(Eq. 8a)}$$

Equation 6 can now be rewritten as:

$$\frac{dA}{dt} = -\left(1 - f + \frac{f \cdot K_T}{K_T + C_p}\right) \cdot CL_{max} \cdot C_p \qquad \text{(Eq. 9)}$$

This equation can be integrated analytically but the resulting equation is implicit in C_p (van Ginneken et al. 1974). The use of computer programs with integrating subroutines makes the analytical integration of differential equations superfluous, so that the various relevant parameters of this type of equation are readily accessible. The occurrence of a saturable mechanism of elimination in principle leads to a non-linear plasma curve when plotted on a semilogarithmic scale (fig. 2). Nevertheless, a non-linear plasma curve is not a prerequisite for partly non-linear elimination: a saturable mechanism of elimination will only be visible in the plasma curve when the plasma concentration is high enough with respect to the apparent Michaelis-Menten constant *and* when the non-linear mechanism contributes at least some 20% to the total elimination capacity. Therefore, in many cases tubular secretion will not be reflected in the plasma curve of a drug unless specific aspects such as unusual accumulation on repeated dosage or drug-drug interaction are taken into account. To date no comprehensive kinetic description of carrier-mediated reabsorption has been accomplished, although interesting efforts have been made (Garrett 1978). The main reason for this is the fact that it is extremely difficult to estimate the drug concentration at the luminal site of the reabsorptive carrier. The classical compartmental analysis is insufficient in this respect. More promising is the application of physiologically based kinetic kidney models.

In classical pharmacokinetics renal clearance is considered as a process operating directly from the central compartment. It is implicitly assumed that an equilibrium exists between the concentrations

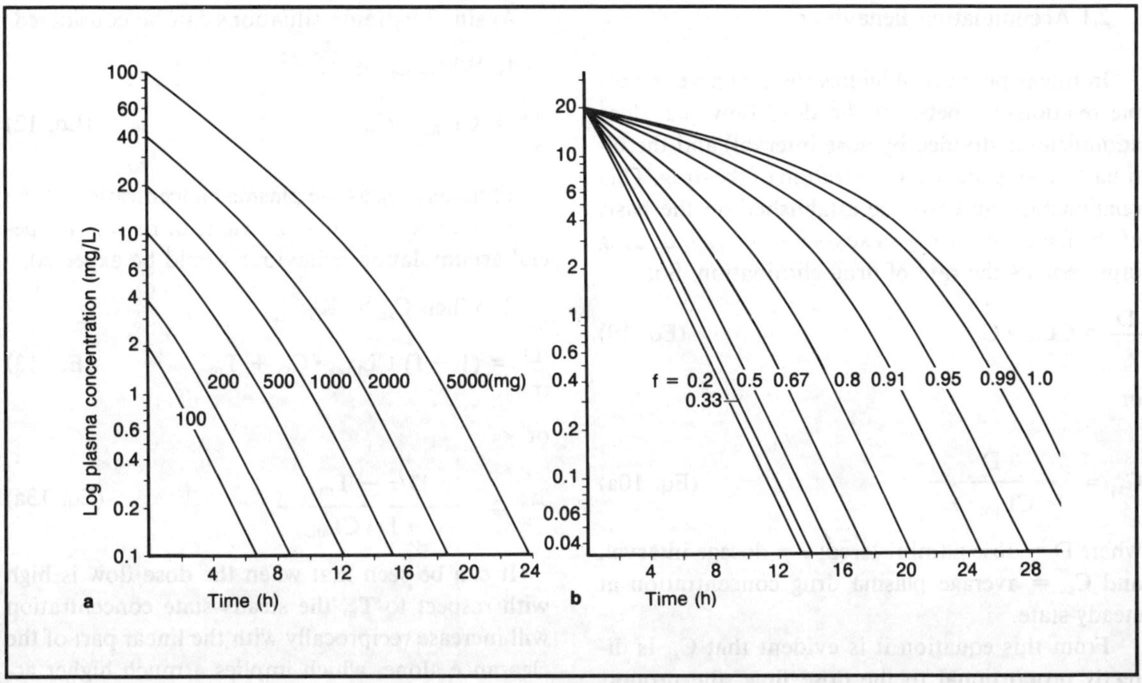

Fig. 2. Simulated plasma concentration curves for drugs eliminated from the body by active tubular secretion combined with one or more linear, non-saturable pathways. For all curves the volume of distribution (Vd) and the transport maximum (T_m) of the tubular secretion are kept constant: Vd = 50L and T_m = 50 mg/h. **(a)** Dose variation from 100 to 5000mg of a drug that is two-thirds eliminated by tubular secretion (f = 0.67). The apparent Michaelis-Menten constant (K_T) of the tubular secretion is 3 mg/L. At concentrations below 1 mg/L all curves run parallel. In **(b)** the fraction of the total body clearance that proceeds via tubular secretion is varied from 0.2 to 1. The maximum attainable total body clearance is kept constant at 25 L/h. Again, at low plasma concentrations all curves run parallel. It is also clear that the plasma curves show no sign of saturation when f ⩽ 0.2.

of drug in plasma and urine. However, this assumption is only valid in some special cases: particularly when carrier-mediated transcellular transport is involved, a simple equilibrium between plasma and urine is unlikely on theoretical grounds. For example, experiments on plasma kinetics and renal excretion of iodopyracet in dogs revealed that the classic Michaelis-Menten approach is unable to cover the pharmacokinetic profile of this compound (Hekman & van Ginneken 1982). The main reason is that the equilibrium assumption is not valid for iodopyracet and other drugs that are eliminated by tubular secretion so rapidly that at low plasma concentrations the rate of excretion becomes limited by the renal plasma flow.

The limitations of classical pharmacokinetics have led to the need for a more physiological approach. Recently, a prototype of a new generation of physiologically based pharmacokinetic models was proposed, in which the kidney is set apart as a subsystem containing several compartments, e.g. plasma, glomerular, tubular and luminal (Hekman & van Ginneken 1982, 1983). With such a model the transport systems can be accommodated at the exact site where they are operating. By using this type of kinetic modelling it appeared possible to describe the excretion kinetics of iodopyracet in a consistent way. It has been shown that the flow-dependent profile is no more than a limiting case of this general approach, whereas the Michaelis-Menten equilibrium state follows directly from the model. Furthermore, the models appeared to be useful in describing drug interactions at the level of tubular secretion (Russel et al. 1987a,b, 1988b).

2.1 Accumulation Behaviour

In linear pharmacokinetics there is a very simple relationship between the dose flow (i.e. dose administered divided by dose interval) and the ultimate mean plateau concentration of the drug. This relationship can easily be established on the basis of the fact that during steady-state the rate of drug input equals the rate of drug elimination. So:

$$\frac{D}{\tau} = CL_{tot} \cdot C_{ss} \quad \text{(Eq. 10)}$$

or

$$C_{ss} = \frac{D}{CL_{tot} \cdot \tau} \quad \text{(Eq. 10a)}$$

where D = dose administered; τ = dosage interval; and C_{ss} = average plasma drug concentration at steady-state.

From this equation it is evident that C_{ss} is directly proportional to the dose flow, the proportionality constant being the total body clearance (CL_{tot}). Changes in clearance by saturable elimination or protein binding will, of course, have a direct influence on the accumulation characteristics of the drug.

Since in the case of Michaelis-Menten kinetics the clearance decreases with increasing plasma concentration, we may anticipate at least one important implication: that in long term administration, accumulation will occur to higher levels than would be expected with linear kinetics. The average steady-state concentration may be mathematically formulated with the use of equations analogous to equation 10 (Gibaldi & Perrier 1982).

By substituting the clearance from equation 9 into equation 10 under steady-state conditions the following expression is obtained:

$$\frac{D}{\tau} = \left(1 - f + \frac{f \cdot K_T}{K_T + C_{ss}}\right) \cdot CL_{max} \cdot C_{ss} \quad \text{(Eq. 11)}$$

This equation can be rearranged into a quadratic formula for C_{ss} which always has two roots, the positive one of which is the actual value of the steady-state concentration (van Ginneken 1982).

Again, 2 extreme situations can be considered.

1. When $C_{ss} \ll K_T$:

$$\frac{D}{\tau} = CL_{max} \cdot C_{ss} \quad \text{(Eq. 12)}$$

Thus, as long as the plasma concentration of the drug remains far below the value of its K_T, no special accumulation behaviour would be expected.

2. When $C_{ss} \gg K_T$:

$$\frac{D}{\tau} = (1 - f)\, CL_{max} \cdot C_{ss} + T_m \quad \text{(Eq. 13)}$$

or

$$C_{ss} = \frac{D/\tau - T_m}{(1 - f) \cdot CL_{max}} \quad \text{(Eq. 13a)}$$

It can be seen that when the dose flow is high with respect to T_m the steady-state concentration will increase reciprocally with the linear part of the clearance alone, which implies a much higher accumulation than expected from low-dose kinetics. In a hypothetical situation, when all clearance mechanisms are saturable (f = 1) a steady-state will not be reached, but the plasma concentration will increase to infinity.

3. *Kinetic Drug Interactions*

In the case of elimination by tubular secretion in combination with linear pathways, there are 3 different ways in which a drug's clearance can be modified by simultaneous administration of another substance. This can best be shown by returning to the general expressions for the total body clearance:

$$CL_{tot} = CL_{lin} + \frac{T_m}{K_T + C_p}$$

$$= \left(1 - f + \frac{f \cdot K_T}{K_T + C_p}\right) \cdot CL_{max} \quad \text{(Eq. 14)}$$

Three possibilities of drug interactions exist:

1. A compound may cause a change of the ac-

tual value of CL_{lin}. Obvious examples are substances that influence the pH of the urine and thereby the degree of back diffusion of ionisable drugs. In this way both CL_{max} and f will change (in opposite directions).

2. A compound may cause a change of T_m. A decrease can be the result of non-competitive inhibition of the carrier transport system or of (increased) degradation of carriers. Only relatively toxic compounds may be expected to cause such changes. An increase may follow from induction of carrier sites. There is some evidence that during the development of the secretory system induction by substrate is possible (Hook & Hewitt 1977).

3. The most common type of interaction at the level of the transport system is a competitive interaction between substances with an affinity for the same carrier. When an interacting drug I with an apparent Michaelis-Menten constant K_I is introduced, the K_T of the first substrate will increase according to the well-known formula:

$$K_{T,I} = K_T\left(1 + \frac{I}{K_I}\right) \quad \text{(Eq. 15)}$$

where $K_{T,I}$ = the apparent Michaelis-Menten constant of the drug in the presence of a concentration I of a competing substance; and K_I = the apparent Michaelis-Menten constant of the inhibitor.

This implies that a competitive inhibitor will cause a concentration-dependent increase of K_T and consequently a decrease of CL_{TS}. It is interesting to note that a competitive inhibitor may mask the signs of saturation of tubular secretion by increasing K_M although the transport rate of the substrate is reduced.

As far as the quantitative aspects of kinetic drug interactions are concerned, the measurement of half-lives in the presence or absence of an inhibitor (e.g. probenecid in combination with anionic drugs) has only a limited value since the half-life is principally dependent on the concentration of both the drug and the inhibitor. The half-life is inversely proportional to the clearance and the clearance in the presence of the inhibitor is given by:

$$CL_{tot} = CL_{lin} + \frac{T_m}{K_T(1 + I/K_I) + C_p} \quad \text{(Eq. 16)}$$

When the concentration I is very high with respect to K_I and when the term $K_T(1 + I/K_I) \gg C_p$ it is possible for the carrier transport to be fully inhibited and for the clearance to be diminished to CL_{lin}. In most cases, however, the carrier system will be only partly blocked.

4. Tubular Secretion

4.1 Specificity

One of the remarkable characteristics of the renal organic anion system is that it accepts compounds with a tremendous diversity in chemical structure. A wide variety of drugs and their metabolites as well as numerous endogenous substrates are excreted by the kidney through tubular secretion. A list with a number of representative compounds is given in table I.

A considerable effort has been made, particularly by Despopoulos (1965) and Møller and Sheikh (1983), to elucidate the structural features necessary for transport. However, none of these attempts has led to a comprehensive model accounting for all the structures that are accepted by the anion system. Recently, Ullrich and co-workers (1987a,b) showed that an organic backbone and a negative charge are in fact sufficient for affinity to the PAH transport system in the basolateral membrane. It has been suggested that this apparent lack of substrate specificity, which is unusual for carrier-mediated processes, stems from multiple transport systems with overlapping structural specificities (Hewitt et al. 1977; Ullrich et al. 1985). However, at present the evidence for this hypothesis is not conclusive.

Until now, less attention has been paid to the organic cation secretory system. Nevertheless the list of cations known to be secreted in the proximal tubule is rapidly increasing (table II). Among those secreted are primary, secondary, tertiary and quaternary amines (Rennick 1981a). It appears that all of these substances show a mutually competitive inhibition in secretion, but no cross-inhibition by

Table I. Compounds known to be secreted by the renal organic anion transport system

	Reference		Reference
Endogenous compounds			
Aromatic amino acids	Williams & Huang (1981)	Hydroxyindoleacetate	Hakim et al. (1970)
Bile salts	Bárány (1975); Zins & Weiner (1968)	Oxalate	Greger et al. (1978); Weinman et al. (1978)
Bilirubin	Baines et al. (1968)	Prostaglandins	Bito & Barody (1978); Irish (1979); Rennick (1977)
cAMP	Blonde et al. (1974); Coulson (1976)	Urate	Lang (1981); Poulsen & Praetorius (1954); Praetorius & Kirk (1950)
cGMP	Blonde et al. (1974); Coulson (1976)		
Fatty acids	Barac-Nieto & Cohen (1968); Barac-Nieto (1971)		
Drug Metabolites			
Acetylated sulfonamides	Arita et al. (1972); Shimoda et al. (1986); Vree et al. (1983, 1986a)	Glycine conjugates	Knoefel & Huang (1959); Knoefel et al. (1962); Mudge et al. (1962); Smith et al. (1945); Wu & Elliott (1961)
N-Acetylcysteine conjugates	Inoue et al. (1981); Monks & Lau (1987); Newton et al. (1986); Scheffer & Stevens (1987); Smith & Francis (1983)	Pyrazinoate	Fanelli & Weiner (1973); Weiner & Tinker (1972)
Gentisate	Weiner et al. (1964)	Sulphate conjugates	Duggin & Mudge (1975); Watrous et al. (1970)
Glucuronide conjugates	Little et al. (1985); Meffin et al. (1983); Schachter & Manis (1958); Sperber (1948)		
Glutathione conjugates	Kramer et al. (1987); Lash & Jones (1985); Monks & Lau (1987); Newton et al. (1986)		
Drugs			
Acyclovir	deMiranda et al. (1981)	Iothalamate sodium	Odlind et al. (1985)
Acetazolamide	Weiner et al. (1959); Sweeney et al. (1986)	Methotrexate	Bourke et al. (1975); Lui et al. (1985); Aherne et al. (1978)
p-Aminohippurate	Häberle (1981); Pritchard (1987)	Nitrofurantoin	Paul et al. (1959); Watari et al. (1985)
p-Aminosalicylate	Huang et al. (1960)	Penicillins	Barza et al. (1975); Bergan (1984); Eagle & Newman (1947); Kamiya et al. (1983); Sjövall et al. (1985); Bins & Mattie (1988)
Benzoates	Weiner et al. (1964)	Pentopril	Rakhit et al. (1987)
Bumetanide	Rennick (1977); Smith & Lau (1983)	Phenosulfonphthalein	Goldring et al. (1936); Ochwadt & Pitts (1968)
Cephalosporins	Ings et al. (1985); Kamiya et al. (1983); Kirby & Regamey (1973); Tune (1975); Bins & Mattie (1988)	Phenylbutazone	Gutman et al. (1960); Weiner et al. (1964)
Captopril	Drummer et al. (1985); Drummer & Jarrott (1986); Singhvi et al. (1982)	Piretanide	Odlind et al. (1983)
Chlorthalidone	Fleuren et al. (1979)	Probenecid	Dayton et al. (1963); Weiner et al. (1960)
Cisplatin	Caterson et al. (1983); Jacobs et al. (1980)	Quinolones	Vree et al. (1986b)
Diatrizoate	Mudge et al. (1971)	Salicylates	Blonde et al. (1974); Gutman et al. (1955); Schachter & Manis (1958)
Diflunisal	Baer et al. (1978)	Saccharin	Goldstein et al. (1978)
Diodrast	Mudge et al. (1971)	Sulphinpyrazone	Lentjes et al. (1986); Perel et al. (1969)
Enoxacin	(Dobbs et al. (1987)	Sulphonamides	Hori et al. (1976); Kamiya et al. (1983); Owada et al. (1974)
Enprofylline	Borga et al. (1986)	Thiazides	Welling (1986)
Ethacrynic acid	Odlind (1979b)	Thymidine	Zaharko et al. (1979)
Frusemide (furosemide)	Bowman (1975); Odlind (1979a,b)	Tienilic acid	Kerremans et al. (1982)
Gossypol	Goldinger et al. (1985)	Zidovudine	Klecker et al. (1987)
Hippuran	Milton & Odlind (1985); Smith et al. (1938)		
Hydrochlorothiazide	Koopmans et al. (1985)		
Ibuprofen	van Ginneken (1976)		
Indomethacin	Baber et al. (1978); Skeith et al. (1978)		
Iodipamide	Berndt & Mudge (1968); Milton & Odlind (1985)		

Abbreviations: cAMP = cyclic adenosine monophosphate; cGMP = cyclic guanidine monophosphate.

anions. The assumption of a single cation carrier system is sufficient given the present level of knowledge (Somogyi 1987).

4.2 Clinical Implications

Tubular secretion is an important process in the renal handling of many drugs, and may therefore be the basis of a variety of clinical implications. The presence of tubular secretion is often a vital link in the disposition of and response to drugs with an intratubular site of action (e.g. diuretics, uricosurics and some antibiotics), especially when these drugs are highly bound to plasma proteins (Brater 1983).

The organic anion transport system may also play a role in the development of nephrotoxicity with compounds that are highly accumulated in the proximal tubular cells, thereby exerting a direct toxic effect. A clinically important example is cephaloridine (Tune et al. 1974), and it has been suggested that the acute renal failure sometimes seen with renal contrast agents is also a consequence of very high intracellular drug concentrations (Humes & Weinberg 1986).

Since carrier-mediated processes are involved in organic anion secretion, there will be potential problems of saturation and competition. Saturation of tubular secretion invariably leads to a decrease of the total body drug clearance, and consequently to a risk of unwanted drug accumulation in the body (Brater 1980). Drug interactions at the level of tubular secretion have been described many times. In principle, all compounds listed in table I and II have the potential to compete with each other's tubular secretion. For instance, it has been reported that several drugs are able to increase the half-life of penicillin in man (Kampmann et al. 1972). An interaction with life-threatening consequences has been described recently between methotrexate and non-steroidal anti-inflammatory drugs (King et al. 1987; Maiche 1986; Singh et al. 1986; Thyss et al. 1986). Interactions between drugs and endogenous substances may also have clinical consequences, e.g. the interaction with urate transport.

Table II. Compounds known to be secreted by or to have affinity for the renal organic cation transport system

	Reference		Reference
Endogenous compounds			
(Acetyl)choline	Rennick (1981a,b)	Various catecholamines	Rennick (1981a,b)
Creatinine	Shannon (1938)		
Drugs[a]			
Acecainide (*N*-acetylprocainamide)	Lai et al. (1985); Somogyi et al. (1983); Somogyi & Bochner (1984)	Procainamide	Christian et al. (1984); Lai et al. (1988); Somogyi et al. (1983); Somogyi & Bochner (1984)
Amiloride	Knauf et al. (1985)		
Atropine	Hinderling et al. (1985)	Pseudoephedrine	Till & Benet (1979)
Cimetidine	Christian et al. (1984); Drayer et al. (1982); Gersema et al. (1987); Muirhead et al. (1986); Somogyi & Gugler (1985); Somogyi et al. (1983)	Quinine	Notterman et al. (1986)
		Quinidine	Notterman et al. (1986)
		Ranitidine	Muirhead et al. (1988); Somogyi & Bochner (1984); Van Crugten et al. (1986)
Disopyramide	Braun et al. (1987); Lima et al. (1985)		
Emepronium bromide	Pilbrant & Norlén (1985)	Triamterene	Muirhead et al. (1986); Muirhead et al. (1988); Sörgel et al. (1985)
Famotidine	Lin et al. (1988); Takabatake et al. (1985)	Trimethoprim	Cacini (1987); Cacini & Myre (1985); Vlasses et al. (1986)
Metformin	Somogyi et al. (1987)		
Pindolol	Hsyu & Giacomini (1985)		
Various other *β*-blockers	Hinderling et al. (1984)		

a In animals various other cationic drugs are known to be secreted (Rennick 1981a,b).

It is clear that a proper understanding of the processes of tubular secretion, and the renal handling of drugs in general, is a prerequisite for careful drug prescribing.

References

Aherne GW, Piall E, Marks V, Mould G, White WF. Prolongation and enhancement of serum methotrexate concentrations by probenecid. British Medical Journal 1: 1097-1099, 1978

Arita T, Hori R, Takada M, Akuzu S, Misawa A. Transformation and excretion of drugs in biological systems. VII. Effect of biotransformation in renal excretion of sulfonamides. Chemical and Pharmaceutical Bulletin 20: 570-580, 1972

Baber N, Halliday L, Sibeon R, Littler T, Orme MLE. The interaction between indomethacin and probenecid. Clinical Pharmacology and Therapeutics 24: 298-307, 1978

Baer JE, Breault GO, Russo HF. Diflunisal renal clearance in anesthetized dogs. Effect of probenecid, urine flow and urine pH. Archives Internationales de Pharmacodynamie et de Thérapie 235: 204-210, 1978

Baines AD, Gottschalk CW, Lassier WE. Microinjection study of *p*-aminohippurate excretion in rat kidneys. American Journal of Physiology 214: 703-709, 1968

Barac-Nieto M. Renal uptake of *p*-aminohippuric acid *in vitro*. Effects of palmitate and *L*-carnitine. Biochimica et Biophysica Acta 233: 446-452, 1971

Barac-Nieto M, Cohen JJ. Non-esterified fatty acid uptake by dog kidney. Effects of probenecid and chlorothiazide. American Journal of Physiology 215: 98-107, 1968

Bárány EH. *In vitro* uptake of bile acids by choroid plexus, kidney cortex and anterior uvea. I. The iodipamide-sensitive transport systems in the rabbit. Acta Physiologica Scandinavica 93: 250-268, 1975

Barza M, Brusch J, Bergeron MG, Kemmotsu O, Weinstein L. Extraction of antibiotics from the circulation by liver and kidney: effect of probenecid. Journal of Infectious Diseases 131: 586-597, 1975

Bergan T. Pharmacokinetics of beta-lactam antibiotics. Scandinavian Journal of Infectious Diseases 42: 83-98, 1984

Berndt WO, Mudge GH. Renal excretion of iodipamide. Comparative study in the dog and rabbit. Investigative Radiology 3: 414-426, 1968

Bins JW, Mattie H. Saturation of the tubular excretion of β-lactam antibiotics. British Journal of Clinical Pharmacology 25: 41-50, 1988

Bito LZ, Barody RA. Comparison of renal prostaglandin and *p*-aminohippuric acid transport processes. American Journal of Physiology 234: F80-88, 1978

Blonde L, Wehmann RE, Steiner AL. Plasma clearance rates and renal clearance of ^{3}H-labeled cyclic AMP and ^{3}H-labeled cyclic GMP in the dog. Journal of Clinical Investigation 53: 163-172, 1974

Borgå O, Larsson R, Lunell E. Effects of probenecid on enprofylline kinetics in man. European Journal of Clinical Pharmacology 30: 221-223, 1986

Bourke RS, Cheda G, Bremer A, Watanabe O, Tower DB. Inhibition of renal tubular transport of methotrexate by probenecid. Cancer Research 35: 110-116, 1975

Bowman RH. Renal secretion of [^{35}S]furosemide and its depression by albumin binding. American Journal of Physiology 229: 93-98, 1975

Brater DC. The pharmacological role of the kidney. Drugs 19: 31-48, 1980

Brater DC. Pharmacodynamic considerations in the use of diuretics. Annual Review of Pharmacology and Toxicology 23 45-62, 1983

Braun J, Sörgel F, Gluth WP, Oie S. Bioavailability of disopyramide in normal volunteers using unbound concentration. European Journal of Clinical Pharmacology 32: 625-629, 1987

Cacini W. *In vivo* renal tubular secretion of trimethoprim without metabolism. Biochemical Pharmacology 36: 2693-2695, 1987

Cacini W, Myre SA. Uptake of trimethoprim by renal cortex. Biochemical Pharmacology 19: 3483-3488, 1985

Caterson R, Etheredge S, Snitch P, Duggin G. Mechanisms of renal excretion of cisdichlorodiamine platinum. Research Communications in Chemical Pathology and Pharmacology 41: 255-264, 1983

Christian Jr CD, Meredith CG, Speeg Jr KV. Cimetidine inhibits renal procainamide clearance. Clinical Pharmacology and Therapeutics 36: 221-227, 1984

Cojocel C, Hook JB. Aminoglycoside nephrotoxicity. Trends in Pharmacological Sciences 4: 174-179, 1983

Coulson R. Metabolism and excretion of exogenous adenosine 3′,5′-monophosphate and guanosine 3′,5′-monophosphate. Studies in the isolated perfused rat kidney and in the intact rat. Journal of Biological Chemistry 251: 4958-4967, 1976

Dayton PG, Yü TF, Chen W, Berger L, West LA, et al. The physiological disposition of probenecid, including renal clearance in man, studied by an improved method for its estimation in biological material. Journal of Pharmacology and Experimental Therapeutics 140: 278-286, 1963

deMiranda P, Good SS, Laskin OL, Krashny HC, Connor JD, et al. Disposition of intravenous radioactive acyclovir. Clinical Pharmacology and Therapeutics 30: 662-672, 1981

Despopoulos A. A definition of substrate specificity in renal transport of organic anions. Journal of Theoretical Biology 8: 163-192, 1965

Dobbs BR, Gazeley LR, Campbell AJ, Edwards IR. The effect of age on the pharmacokinetics of enoxacin. European Journal of Clinical Pharmacology 33: 101-104, 1987

Drayer DE, Romankiewicz J, Lorenzo B, Reidenberg MM. Age and renal clearance of cimetidine. Clinical Pharmacology and Therapeutics 31: 45-50, 1982

Drummer OH, Jarrott B. The disposition and metabolism of captopril. Medicinal Research Reviews 6: 75-97, 1986

Drummer OH, Thompson J, Hooper R, Jarrott B. Effect of probenecid on the disposition of captopril and captopril dimer in the rat. Biochemical Pharmacology 34: 3347-3351, 1985

Duggin GG, Mudge GH. Renal tubular transport of paracetamol and its conjugates in the dog. British Journal of Pharmacology 54: 359-366, 1975

Eagle H, Newman E. The renal clearance of penicillins F, G, K and X. Journal of Clinical Investigation 26: 903-918, 1947

Fanelli Jr GM, Weiner IM. Pyrazinoate excretion in the chimpanzee: Relation to urate disposition and the actions of uricosuric drugs. Journal of Clinical Investigation 52: 1946-1957, 1973

Fleuren HLJ, Verwey-van Wissen C, Van Rossum JM. Dose-dependent urinary excretion of chlorthalidone. Clinical Pharmacology and Therapeutics 25: 806-812, 1979

Garrett ER. Pharmacokinetics and clearances related to renal processes. International Journal of Clinical Pharmacology 16: 155-172, 1978

Gersema LM, Park GD, Kitt TM, Spector R. The effect of dietary protein-calorie restriction on the renal elimination of cimetidine. Clinical Pharmacology and Therapeutics 42: 471-475, 1987

Gibaldi M, Perrier D. Pharmacokinetics, pp. 271-290, Dekker, New York, 1982

Goldinger JM, Lee SH, Hong SK. Renal transport of gossypol in the rabbit. Proceedings of the Society for Experimental Biology and Medicine 179: 50-54, 1985

Goldring W, Clarke RW, Smith HW. The phenol red clearance

in normal man. Journal of Clinical Investigation 15: 221-228, 1936
Goldstein RS, Hook JB, Bond JT. Renal tubular transport of saccharin. Journal of Pharmacology and Experimental Therapeutics 204: 690-695, 1978
Grantham JJ, Chonko AM. Renal handling of organic anions and cations. In Brenner & Rector (Eds) The kidney, pp. 663-700, Saunders, Philadelphia, 1986
Greger L, Lang F, Oberleithner H, Deetjen P. Handling of oxalate by the rat kidney. Pflügers Archiv: European Journal of Physiology 374: 243-248, 1978
Gutman AB, Dayton PG, Yü TF, Berger L, Chen W, et al. A study of the inverse relationship between pK_a and rate of renal excretion of phenylbutazone analogs in man and dog. American Journal of Medicine 29: 1017-1033, 1960
Gutman AB, Yü TF. A three-component system for regulation of uric acid in man. Transactions of the Association of American Physicians 74: 353-365, 1961
Gutman AB, Yü TF, Sirota JH. A study by simultaneous clearance techniques of salicylate excretion in man. Effect of alkalinization of the urine by bicarbonate administration; effect of probenecid. Journal of Clinical Investigation 34: 711-721, 1955
Häberle DA. Characteristics of *p*-aminohippurate transport in the mammalian kidney. In Greger et al. (Eds) Renal transport of organic substances, pp. 188-209, Springer Verlag, Berlin, 1981
Hakim R, Watrous WM, Fujimoto JM. The renal tubular transport and metabolism of serotonin (5-HT) and 5-hydroxyindoleacetic acid (5-HIAA) in the chicken. Journal of Pharmacology and Experimental Therapeutics 175: 749-762, 1970
Hall S, Rowland M. Influence of fraction unbound upon the renal clearance of furosemide in the isolated perfused rat kidney. Journal of Pharmacology and Experimental Therapeutics 232: 263-268, 1985
Hekman P, van Ginneken CAM. Kinetic modeling of the renal excretion of iodopyracet in the dog. Journal of Pharmacokinetics and Biopharmaceutics 10: 77-92, 1982
Hekman P, van Ginneken CAM. Simultaneous kinetic modelling of plasma levels and urinary excretion of salicyluric acid and the influence of probenecid. European Journal of Drug Metabolism and Pharmacokinetics 3: 239-249, 1983
Hewitt WR, Wagner PA, Bostwick EF, Hook JB. Transport ontogeny and selective substrate stimulation as models for identification of multiple renal organic anion transport systems. Journal of Pharmacology and Experimental Therapeutics 202: 711-723, 1977
Hinderling PH, Gundert-Remy U, Schmidlin O. Integrated pharmacokinetics and pharmacodynamics of atropine in healthy humans I: pharmacokinetics. Journal of Pharmaceutical Sciences 74: 703-710, 1985
Hinderling PH, Schmidlin O, Seydel JK. Quantitative relationships between structure and pharmacokinetics of beta-adrenoceptor blocking agents in man. Journal of Pharmacokinetics and Biopharmaceutics 12: 263-287, 1984
Hook JB, Hewitt WR. Development of mechanisms for drug excretion. American Journal of Medicine 62: 497-506, 1977
Hori R, Sunayashiki K, Kamiya A. Pharmacokinetic analysis of renal handling of sulfamethizole. Journal of Pharmaceutical Sciences 65: 463-465, 1976
Hsyu PH, Giacomini KM. Steroselective renal clearance of pindolol in humans. Journal of Clinical Investigation 76: 1720-1726, 1985
Huang KC, Moore KB, Campbell Jr PJ. Renal excretion of para-aminosalicylic acid. A two-way transport system in the dog. American Journal of Physiology 199: 5-8, 1960
Humes HB, Weinberg JM. Toxic nephropathies. In Brenner & Rector (Eds) The kidney, pp. 1491-1532, Saunders, Philadelphia, 1986
Ings RMJ, Reeves DS, White LO, Bax RP, Bywater MJ, et al. The human pharmacokinetics of cefotaxime and its metabolites and the role of renal tubular secretion on their elimination. Journal of Pharmacokinetics and Biopharmaceutics 13: 121-142, 1985
Inoue M, Okajima K, Morino Y. Renal transtubular transport of mercapturic acid *in vivo*. Biochimica et Biophysica Acta 641: 122-128, 1981
Irish JM. Secretion of prostaglandin E_2 by rabbit proximal tubules. American Journal of Physiology 237: F268-273, 1979
Jacobs C, Kalman SM, Tretton M, Weiner MW. Renal handling of *cis*-diaminedichloroplatinum (II). Cancer Treatment Reports 64: 1223-1226, 1980
Junqueira LC, Carneiro J, Contopoulos AN. Basic histology, p. 356, Lange Medical Publications, Los Altos, 1975
Kamiya A, Okumura K, Hori R. Quantitative investigation on renal handling of drugs in rabbits, dogs, and humans. Journal of Pharmaceutical Sciences 72: 440-443, 1983
Kampmann J. Hansen JM, Siersbaek-Nielsen K, Laursen H. Effect of some drugs on penicillin half-life in blood. Clinical Pharmacology and Therapeutics 13: 516-519, 1972
Kerremans ALM, Gribnau FWJ, Tan Y, van Ginneken CAM. Pharmacokinetic and pharmacodynamic studies of tienilic acid in healthy volunteers. European Journal of Clinical Pharmacology 22: 515-521, 1982
King HW, Macfarlane AW, Graham RM, Verbov JL. Near fatal drug interactions with methotrexate given for psoriasis. British Medical Journal 295: 752-753, 1987
Kinsella JL, Holohan PD, Pessah NI, Ross CR. Transport of organic ions in renal cortical luminal and antiluminal membrane vesicles. Journal of Pharmacology and Experimental Therapeutics 209: 443-450, 1979
Kirby WMM, Regamey C. Pharmacokinetics of cefazolin compared with four other cephalosporins. Journal of Infectious Diseases 128: S341-346, 1973
Klecker RW, Collins JM, Yarchoan R, Thomas R, Jenkins JF, Broder S, Myers CE. Plasma and cerebrospinal fluid pharmacokinetics of 3′-azido-3′deoxythymidine: a novel pyrimidine analog with potential application for the treatment of patients with AIDS and related diseases. Clinical Pharmacology and Therapeutics 41: 407-412, 1987
Knauf H, Reuter K, Mutschler E. Limitation on the use of amiloride in early renal failure. European Journal of Clinical Pharmacology 28: 61-66, 1985
Knoefel PK, Huang KC. Biochemorphology of renal tubular transport: hippuric acid and related substances. Journal of Pharmacology and Experimental Therapeutics 126: 296-303, 1959
Knoefel PK, Huang KC, Jarboe CH. Renal disposal of salicyluric acid. American Journal of Physiology 203: 6-10, 1962
Koopmans PP, Kateman WGPM, Tan Y, van Ginneken CAM, Gribnau FWJ. Effects of indomethacin and sulindac on hydrochlorothiazide kinetics. Clinical Pharmacology and Therapeutics 37: 625-628, 1985
Kramer RA, Foureman G, Greene KE, Reed DJ. Nephrotoxicity of *S*-(2-chloroethyl)glutathione in the Fischer rat: evidence for γ-glutamyltranspeptidase-independent uptake by the kidney. Journal of Pharmacology and Experimental Therapeutics 242: 741-748, 1987
Lai MY, Jiang FM, Chung CH, Chen HC, Chao PDL. Dose dependent effect of cimetidine on procainamide disposition in man. International Journal of Clinical Pharmacology, Therapy and Toxicology 26: 118-121, 1988
Lang F. Renal handling of urate. In Greger et al. (Eds) Renal transport of organic substances, pp. 234-261, Springer Verlag, Berlin, 1981
Lash LH, Jones DP. Uptake of the glutathione conjugate *S*-(1,2-dichlorovinyl)glutathion by renal basal-lateral membrane vesicles and isolated kidney cells. Molecular Pharmacology 28: 278-282, 1985

Lentjes EWGM, Russel FGM, van Ginneken CAM. Renal clearance of sulphinpyrazone in man. European Journal of Clinical Pharmacology 31: 473-478, 1986
Lima JJ, Boudoulas H, Shields BJ. Stereoselective pharmacokinetics of disopyramide enantiomers in man. Drug Metabolism and Disposition 13: 572-577, 1985
Lin JH, Los LE, Ulm EH, Duggan DE. Kinetic studies on the competition between famotidine and cimetidine in rats. Evidence of multiple renal secretory systems for organic cations. Drug Metabolism and Disposition 16: 52-56, 1988
Little JM, Chari MV, Lester R. Excretion of cholate glucuronide. Journal of Lipid Research 26: 583-592, 1985
Lui CY, Lee MG, Chiou WL. Urinary pH and urine flow independent renal clearance of methotrexate in dogs. Journal of Pharmacokinetics and Biopharmaceutics 13: 159-171, 1985
Maiche AG. Acute renal failure due to concomitant action of methotrexate and indomethacin. Lancet 1: 1390, 1986
Meffin PJ, Zilm DM, Veenendaal JR. A renal mechanism for the clofibric acid-probenecid interaction. Journal of Pharmacology and Experimental Therapeutics 227: 739-742, 1983
Milton A, Odlind B. Renal tubular accumulation of organic substances: a new *in vivo* method which differentiates between luminal and peritubular uptake. Acta Physiologica Scandinavica 123: 237-248, 1985
Møller JV, Sheikh MI. Renal organic anion transport system: Pharmacological, physiological and biochemical aspects. Pharmacological Reviews 34; 315-358, 1983
Monks TJ, Lau SS. Renal transport processes and glutathione conjugate-mediated nephrotoxicity. Drug Metabolism and Disposition 15: 437-441, 1987
Mudge GH, Berndt WO, Saunders A, Beattie B. Renal transport of diatrizoate in the rabbit, dog, and rat. Nephron 8: 156-172, 1971
Mudge GH, Garlid K, Weiner IM. Renal tubular secretion of *o*-acetylaminohippurate. American Journal of Physiology 203: 881-885, 1962
Muirhead M, Bochner F, Somogyi A. Pharmacokinetic drug interactions between triamterene and ranitidine in humans: alterations in renal and hepatic clearances and gastrointestinal absorption. Journal of Pharmacology and Experimental Therapeutics 244: 734-739, 1988
Muirhead MR, Somogyi AA, Rolan PE, Bochner F. Effect of cimetidine on renal and hepatic drug elimination; studies with triamterene. Clinical Pharmacology and Therapeutics 40: 400-407, 1986
Newton JF, Hoefle D, Gemborys MW, Mudge GH, Hook JB. Metabolism and excretion of a glutathione conjugate of acetaminophen in the isolated perfused rat kidney. Journal of Pharmacology and Experimental Therapeutics 237: 519-524, 1986
Notterman DA, Drayer DE, Metakis L, Reidenberg MM. Stereoselective renal tubular secretion of quinidine and quinine. Clinical Pharmacology and Therapeutics 40: 511-517, 1986
Ochwadt BK, Pitts RF. Disparity between phenol red and diodrast clearance in the dog. American Journal of Physiology 187: 318-322, 1956
Odlind B, Relation between tubular secretion of furosemide and its saluretic effect. Journal of Pharmacology and Experimental Therapeutics 208: 515-521, 1979a
Odlind B. Relation between tubular secretion and effects of five loop diuretics. Journal of Pharmacology and Experimental Therapeutics 211: 238-244, 1979b
Odlind B, Beermann B, Selén G, Persson AEG. Renal tubular secretion of piretanide and its effects on electrolyte reabsorption and tubuloglomerular feedback mechanism. Journal of Pharmacology and Experimental Therapeutics 225: 742-746, 1983
Odlind B, Hällgren R, Sohtell M, Lindström B, Is ^{125}I iothalamate an ideal marker for glomerular filtration? Kidney International 27: 9-16, 1985
Owada E, Takahashi K, Hori R, Arita T. Transformation and excretion of drugs in biological systems. X. Renal excretion mechanisms of sulfonamides in rabbits. Chemical and Pharmaceutical Bulletin 22: 594-600, 1974
Paul MF, Bender RC, Nohle EG. Renal excretion and nitrofurantoin (Furadantin). American Journal of Physiology 197: 580-584, 1959
Perel JM, Dayton PG, Snell MM, Yü TF, Gutman AB. Studies of interactions among drugs in man at the renal level. Probenecid and sulfinpyrazone. Clinical Pharmacology and Therapeutics 10: 834-840, 1969
Pilbrant A, Norlén LJ. Pharmacokinetics and pharmacodynamics of emepronium bromide (Cetiprin®) after intravenous administration in man. Acta Pharmacologica et Toxicologica 56: 289-297, 1985
Poulsen H, Praetorius E. Tubular excretion of uric acid in rabbits. Acta Pharmacologica et Toxicologica 10: 371-378, 1954
Praetorius E, Kirk JE. Hypouricemia: with evidence for tubular elimination of uric acid. Journal of Laboratory and Clinical Medicine 35: 856-868, 1950
Pritchard JB. Luminal and peritubular steps in renal transport of *p*-aminohippurate. Biochimica et Biophysica Acta 906: 295-308, 1987
Rakhit A, Kochak GM, Tipnis V, Hurley ME. Inhibition of renal clearance of furosemide by pentopril, an angiotensin-converting enzyme inhibitor. Clinical Pharmacology and Therapeutics 41:580-586, 1987
Rennick BR. Renal tubular transport of prostaglandins: inhibition by probenecid and indomethacin. American Journal of Physiology 233: F133-137, 1977
Rennick BR. Renal tubule transport of organic cations. American Journal of Physiology 240: F83-89, 1981a
Rennick BR. Renal tubular transport of organic cations. In Greger et al. (Eds) Renal transport of organic substances, pp. 178-188, Springer Verlag, Berlin/Heidelberg/New York, 1981b
Russel FGM, Van der Linden PEM, Vermeulen WG, Heijn M, Van Os CH, et al. $Na^+$and H^+ gradient-dependent transport of *p*-aminohippurate in membrane vesicles from dog kidney cortex. Biochemical Pharmacology 37: 2639-2649, 1988a
Russel FGM, Wouterse AC, van Ginneken CAM. Physiologically based pharmacokinetic model for the renal clearance of salicyluric acid and the interaction with phenolsulfonphthalein in the dog. Drug Metabolism and Disposition 15: 695-701, 1987a
Russel FGM, Wouterse AC, van Ginneken CAM. Physiologically based pharmacokinetic model for the renal clearance of phenolsulfonphthalein and the interaction with probenecid and salicyluric acid in the dog. Journal of Pharmacokinetics and Biopharmaceutics 15: 349-368, 1987b
Russel FGM, Wouterse AC, van Ginneken CAM. Physiologically based kidney model for the renal clearance of iodopyracet and the interaction with probenecid in the dog. Biopharmaceutics and Drug Disposition, in press, 1988b
Schachter D, Manis JG. Salicylate and salicylate conjugates. Fluorimetric estimation, biosynthesis and renal excretion in man. Journal of Clinical Investigation 37: 800-807, 1958
Schäli C, Roch-Ramel F. Uptake of ^{3}H-PAH and ^{14}C-urate into isolated proximal segments of the pig kidney. American Journal of Physiology 241: F591-596, 1981
Scheffer VH, Stevens JL. Mechanism of transport for toxic cysteine conjugates in rat kidney cortex membrane vesicles. Molecular Pharmacology 32: 293-298, 1987
Shannon JA. The renal excretion of creatinine in man. Journal of Clinical Investigation 14: 403-410, 1938
Shimoda M, Kokue EI, Tanaka N, Hayama T. Contribution of renal active secretion in renal excretion of N^4-acetylsulfamonomethoxine in conscious pigs. Journal of Pharmacobio-Dynamics 9: 865-870, 1986

Shimomura A, Chonko AM, Grantham JJ. Basis for heterogeneity of para-aminohippurate secretion in rabbit proximal tubules. American Journal of Physiology 240: F430-436, 1981

Singh RR, Malaviya AN, Pandley JN, Guleria JS. Fatal interaction between methotrexate and naproxen. Lancet 1: 1390, 1986

Singhvi SM, Duchin KL, Willard DA, McKinstry DW, Migdalof BH. Renal handling of captopril: effect of probenecid. Clinical Pharmacology and Therapeutics 32: 182-189, 1982

Sjövall J, Westerlund D, Alván G. Renal excretion of intravenously infused amoxycillin and ampicillin. British Journal of Clinical Pharmacology 19: 191-201, 1985

Skeith MD, Sunkin PA, Healey LA. Renal excretion of indomethacin and its inhibition by probenecid. Clinical Pharmacology and Therapeutics 9: 89-93, 1978

Smith AG, Francis JE. Evidence for the active renal secretions of *S*-pentachlorophenyl-*N*-acetyl-*L*-cysteine by female rats. Biochemical Pharmacology 32: 3797-3801, 1983

Smith DE, Lau HSH. Determinants of bumethanide response in the dog: effect of probenecid. Journal of Pharmacokinetics and Biopharmaceutics 11: 31-46, 1983

Smith HW, Finkelstein N, Aliminosa L, Crawford B, Graber M. The renal clearances of substituted hippuric acid derivatives and other aromatic acids in dog and man. Journal of Clinical Investigation 24: 388-404, 1945

Smith HW, Goldring W, Chasis H. The measurement of the tubular excretory mass, effective bloodflow and filtration rate in the normal human kidney. Journal of Clinical Investigation 17: 263-278, 1938

Somogyi A. New insights into the renal secretion of drugs. Trends in Pharmacological Sciences 8: 354--357, 1987

Somogyi A, Bochner F. Dose and concentration dependent effect of ranitidine on procainamide disposition and renal clearance in man. British Journal of Clinical Pharmacology 18: 175-181, 1984

Somogyi A, Gugler R. Effect of variations in urine pH and flow rate on cimetidine renal disposition in man. Biopharmaceutics and Drug Disposition 6: 345-349, 1985

Somogyi A, McLean A, Heinzow B. Cimetidine-procainamide pharmacokinetic interaction in man: evidence for tubular secretion of basic drugs. European Journal of Clinical Pharmacology 25: 339-345, 1983

Somogyi A, Stockley C, Keal J, Rolan P, Bochner F. Reduction of metformin renal tubular secretion by cimetidine in man. British Journal of Clinical Pharmacology 23: 545-551, 1987

Sörgel F, Hasegawa J, Lin ET, Williams RL. Oral triamterene disposition. Clinical Pharmacology and Therapeutics 38: 306-312, 1985

Sperber I. The excretion of some glucuronic acid derivatives and phenol sulfuric esters in the chicken. Annals of the Royal Agricultural College of Sweden 15: 317-349, 1948

Sweeney KR, Chapron DJ, Brandt JL, Gomolin IH, Feig PU, et al. Toxic interaction between acetazolamide and salicylate: case reports and a pharmacokinetic explanation. Clinical Pharmacology and Therapeutics 40: 518-524, 1986

Takabatake T, Ohta H, Maekawa M, Yamamoto Y, Ishida Y, et al. Pharmacokinetics of famotidine, a new H_2-receptor antagonist, in relation to renal function. European Journal of Clihical Pharmacology 28: 327-331, 1985

Thyss A, Milano G, Kubar J, Namer M, Schneider M. Clinical and pharmacokinetic evidence of a life-threatening interaction between methotrexate and ketoprofen. Lancet 1: 256-258, 1986

Till AE, Benet LZ. Renal excretion of pseudoephedrine in the rat. Journal of Pharmacology and Experimental Therapeutics 211; 555-560, 1979

Tune BM. Relationship between the transport and toxicity of cephalosporins in the kidney. Journal of Infectious Diseases 132; 189-194, 1975

Tube BM, Fernholt M, Schwartz A. Mechanism of cephaloridine transport in the kidney. Journal of Pharmacology and Experimental Therapeutics 191: 311-317, 1974

Ullrich KJ, Greger R. Approaches to the study of tubule transport functions. In Seldin & Giebisch (Eds) The kidney: physiology and pathophysiology, pp. 427-469, Raven Press, New York, 1985

Ullrich KJ, Rumrich G, Fritsch G, Klöss S. Contraluminal para-aminohippurate (PAH) transport in the proximal tubule of the rat kidney. II., Specificity: aliphatic dicarboxylic acids. Pflügers Archiv: European Journal of Physiology 408: 38-45, 1987a

Ullrich KJ, Rumrich G, Klöss S. Contraluminal para-aminohippurate (PAH) transport in the proximal tubule of the rat kidney. III. Specificity: monocarboxylic acids. Pflügers Archiv: European Journal of Physiology 409: 547-554, 1987b

Ullrich KJ, Rumrich G, Klöss S, Lang HJ. Contraluminal sulfate transport in the proximal tubule of the rat kidney. V. Specificity: phenolphthaleins, sulfonphthaleins, and other sulfo dyes, sulfamoylcompounds and diphenyamine-2-carboxylates. Pflügers Archiv: European Journal of Physiology 404: 311-318, 1985

Van Crugten J, Bochner F, Keal J, Somogyi A. Selectivity of the cimetidine-induced alterations in the renal handling of organic substrates in humans. Studies with anionic, cationic and zwitterionic drugs. Journal of Pharmacology and Experimental Therapeutics 236: 481-487, 1986

van Ginneken CAM. Pharmacokinetics of antipyretic and anti-inflammatory analgesics, pp. 109-119, PhD Thesis, Nijmegen, 1976

van Ginneken CAM. Linear and nonlinear processes in pharmacokinetics. In Bozler & Van Rossum (Eds) Pharmacokinetics during drug development: data analysis and evaluation techniques, pp. 67-91, Gustav Fischer Verlag, Stuttgart-New York, 1982

van Ginneken CAM, Van Rossum JM, Fleuren HLJM. Linear and nonlinear kinetics of drug elimination. Journal of Pharmacokinetics and Biopharmaceutics 2: 395-415, 1974

Vlasses PH, Lottes SR, Chase SL, Greenspon AJ, Andress E, et al. Trimethoprim decreases the renal clearance of procainamide and *N*-acetylprocainamide. Clinical Pharmacology and Therapeutics 39: 233, 1986

Vree TB, Hekster CA, Braakman M, Janssen T, Oosterbaan M et al. Pharmacokinetics, acetylation-deacetylation, renal clearance, and protein binding of sulphamerazine, N_4-acetylsulphamerazine, and N_4-trideuteroacetylsulphamerazine in 'fast' and 'slow' acetylators. Biopharmaceutics and Drug Disposition 4: 271-291, 1983

Vree TB, Hekster YA, Tijhuis MW, Termond EFS, Nouws JFM. Pharmacokinetics, metabolism and renal excretion of sulfatroxazole and its 5-hydroxy- and N_4-acetyl-metabolites in man. Biopharmaceutics and Drug Disposition 7: 239-252, 1986a

Vree TB, Wijnands WJA, Guelen PJM, Baars AM, Hekster YA. Pharmacokinetics: metabolism and renal excretion of quinolones in man. Pharmaceutisch Weekblad – Scientific Edition 8: 29-34, 1986b

Watari N, Aizawa K, Kaneniwa N. Dose- and time-dependent kinetics of the renal excretion of nitrofurantoin in the rabbit. Journal of Pharmaceutical Sciences 74: 165-170, 1985

Watrous WM, May DG, Fujimoto JM. Mechanism of the renal tubular transport of morphine and MES in the chicken. Journal of Pharmacology and Experimental Therapeutics 172: 224-229, 1970

Weiner IM. Organic acids and bases and uric acid. In Seldin & Giebisch (Eds) The kidney: physiology and pathophysiology, pp. 1703-1724, Raven Press, New York, 1985

Weiner IM, Blanchard KC, Mudge GH. Factors influencing renal excretion of foreign acids. American Journal of Physiology 207: 953-963, 1964

Weiner IM, Tinker JP. Pharmacology of pyrazinamide: metabolic and renal function related to the mechanism of drug induced

urate retention. Journal of Pharmacology and Experimental Therapeutics 180: 411-434, 1972
Weiner IM, Washington II JA, Mudge GH. Studies on the renal excretion of salicylate in the dog. Bulletin of the Johns Hopkins Hospital 105: 284-297, 1959
Weiner IM, Washington II JA, Mudge GH. On the mechanism of action of probenecid on renal tubular secretion. Bulletin of the Johns Hopkins Hospital 106: 333-346, 1960
Weinman EJ, Frankfurt SJ, Ince A, Samsom S. Renal tubular transport of organic acids. Studies with oxalate and para-aminohippurate in the rat. Journal of Clinical Investigation 61: 801-806, 1978
Welling PG. Pharmacokinetics of the thiazide diuretics. Biopharmaceutics and Drug Disposition 7: 501-535, 1986
Williams WM, Huang KC. Structural specificity in the renal tubular transport of tyrosine. Journal of Pharmacology and Experimental Therapeutics 219: 69-74, 1981
Woo E, Greenblatt DJ. Pharmacokinetic and clinical implications of quinidine protein binding. Journal of Pharmaceutical Sciences 68 466-470, 1979
Woodhall PB, Tisher CC, Simonson CA, Robinson RK. Relationship between para-aminohippurate secretion and cellular morphology in rabbit proximal tubules. Journal of Clinical Investigation 61: 1320-1329, 1978
Wu H, Elliott HC. Urinary excretion of hippuric acid by man. Journal of Applied Physiology 16: 553-556, 1961
Yü TF, Gutman AB. Paradoxical retention of uric acid by uricosuric drugs in low dosage. Proceedings of the Society for Experimental Biology and Medicine 90: 542-547, 1955
Yü TF, Gutman AB. Study of the paradoxical effects of salicylate in low, intermediate and high dosage on the renal mechanisms for excretion of urate in man. Journal of Clinical Investigation 38: 1298-1315, 1959
Zaharko DS, Bolten BJ, Chinten D, Wiernik PH. Pharmacokinetic studies during phase I trials of high-dose thymidine infusions. Cancer Research 39: 4777-4781, 1979
Zins GR, Weiner IM. Bidirectional transport of taurocholate by the proximal tubule of the dog. American Journal of Physiology 215: 840-845, 1968

Authors' address: Professor *C.A.M. van Ginneken*, Department of Pharmacology, University of Nijmegen, P.O. Box 9101, 6500HB Nijmegen (The Netherlands).

Clinical Pharmacokinetics 16: 55-64 (1989)
0312-5963/89/0001-0055/$05.00/0

Influence of Renal Function on the Pharmacokinetics and Cardiovascular Effects of Nisoldipine After Single and Multiple Dosing

J. van Harten, J. Burggraaf, P. van Brummelen and *D.D. Breimer*

Center for Bio-Pharmaceutical Sciences, Division of Pharmacology, and Department of Nephrology, University Hospital, Leiden, The Netherlands, Duphar Research Laboratories, Weesp, The Netherlands, and Hoffman-LaRoche, Basle, Switzerland

Summary *The pharmacokinetics and cardiovascular effects of the calcium entry blocker nisoldipine (10mg twice daily) were studied in 6 patients with renal failure (creatinine clearance 23 ± 9 ml/min) and 6 healthy control subjects after a single dose and 1 week of oral administration. No significant differences in elimination half-life, area under the concentration/time curve, peak plasma drug concentration and time to reach that peak were observed between renal patients and control subjects, and between single-dose and short term administration. The decrease in systolic blood pressure and increase in heart rate were similar in both groups, but the decrease in diastolic blood pressure was more pronounced in the patients. This can be explained by increased haemodynamic sensitivity for nisoldipine. Adverse effects were mainly restricted to the first day of administration.*

The second-generation dihydropyridine calcium entry blocker nisoldipine (fig. 1) is currently being investigated for the treatment of hypertension (Deeg et al. 1987; Rosendorff & Goodman 1985) and angina pectoris (Lam et al. 1985; Lopez et al. 1985). The metabolism of nisoldipine takes place predominantly in the liver, and includes oxidation of the dihydropyridine nucleus, side-chain hydroxylation, and ester cleavage (Scherling et al. 1987). The metabolites are mainly excreted in urine, but a small fraction is excreted in faeces (Müller et al. 1986). The pharmacokinetics of nisoldipine in healthy subjects has recently been described: it is a high clearance substance with a mean systemic availability of approximately 4% and a systemic clearance that depends very much on liver blood flow (Ahr et al. 1987; van Harten et al. 1988a,b).

Pharmacokinetics may be changed in renal failure through impaired urinary excretion of drugs or metabolites, and also through diminished plasma

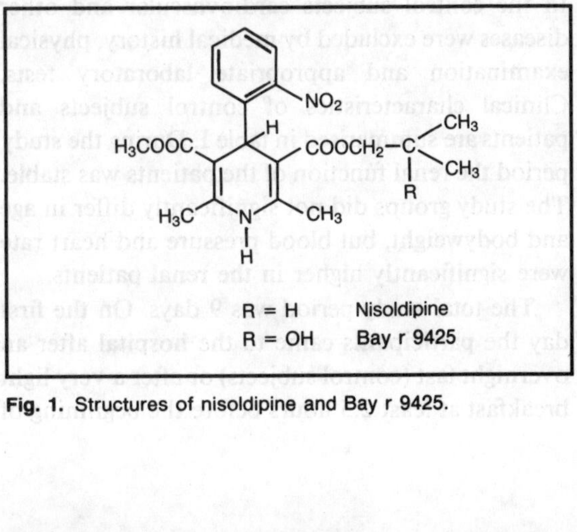

Fig. 1. Structures of nisoldipine and Bay r 9425.

protein binding. The latter results in an increased volume of distribution, and an increased plasma elimination half-life (Bennet et al. 1977; Dettli 1976; Gibson 1980; Keller et al. 1984; Neureth & Szelezhi 1981; Reidenberg 1977). Depending on the elimination characteristics of the substance, decreased plasma protein binding may result in increased free plasma concentrations and, therefore, possibly in enhanced pharmacological effects (Gibson 1980). In addition, pharmacological sensitivity to drugs may be different in renal failure (Danhof et al. 1984; Dundee & Richards 1954; Galeazzi et al. 1979). For the calcium entry blocker nifedipine it has been shown that patients with chronic renal failure are more sensitive to the blood-pressure-lowering effect than healthy control subjects (Kleinbloesem et al. 1985).

The aim of the present study was to investigate the influence of chronic renal failure on the pharmacokinetics and haemodynamic effects of nisoldipine after single-dose and short term oral administration. The study of the influence of renal function on the pharmacokinetics of nisoldipine and its effects on blood pressure and heart rate is particularly important, since nisoldipine has been postulated as delaying the progression of chronic renal failure in humans (Eliahou et al. 1987).

Subjects and Methods

Protocol

The study was carried out in 6 patients with chronic renal failure and 6 healthy control subjects. In the control subjects cardiovascular and other diseases were excluded by medical history, physical examination and appropriate laboratory tests. Clinical characteristics of control subjects and patients are summarised in table I. During the study period the renal function of the patients was stable. The study groups did not significantly differ in age and bodyweight, but blood pressure and heart rate were significantly higher in the renal patients.

The total study period was 9 days. On the first day the participants came to the hospital after an overnight fast (control subjects) or after a very light breakfast at least 2.5 hours before the beginning of the study. Beverages containing alcohol were not permitted during the study day, and caffeine was prohibited until dinner, which was supplied 8 hours after nisoldipine administration. A light lunch was supplied 6 hours after drug administration. The participants remained in a semirecumbent position until 4 hours after drug dosing. After this time they were allowed to sit and walk in the study room, but they resumed the semirecumbent position at least 15 minutes before measurement of blood pressure and heart rate. An indwelling cannula (Venflon®) with a heparin lock (20 U/ml) was inserted in a forearm vein for collection of blood samples up to 11 hours after dosing, when the participants left the hospital.

At 9.30 a.m. the participants received nisoldipine 10mg in tablet form. Blood samples for determination of plasma nisoldipine and one of its metabolites were drawn before dosing, and after 15, 30, 45, 60 and 90 minutes and 2, 3, 4, 5, 6, 8, 11, 24 and 32 hours. Simultaneously, blood pressure and heart rate were measured up to 8 hours. Blood samples were drawn before nisoldipine administration, after 1 hour and again after 6 hours, for determination of plasma noradrenaline (norepinephrine) and intact parathyroid hormone (PTH) [amino acids 1-84].

From the third to seventh days the subjects took nisoldipine orally in a dose of 10mg twice daily (approximately 9 a.m. and 9 p.m.). On the eighth day they returned to the hospital, and participated in an experiment identical to that on the first day. The purpose and nature of the experiments were explained at a pre-study visit, and all subjects gave their consent. The protocol was approved by the medical ethics committee of the Leiden University Hospital. The data of 5 of the control subjects were also used in another study, and as a part of that study liver blood flow was assessed by an intravenous injection of indocyanine green 0.5 mg/kg before and 45 minutes after oral administration of nisoldipine.

Methods

Plasma nisoldipine and one of its metabolites were measured by gas chromatography with electron capture detection (van Harten et al. 1987).

Table I. Clinical characteristics of healthy control subjects and patients, and concomitant medication

Subject	Age (y)	Weight (kg)	SBP/DBP (mm Hg)	HR (bpm)	CL_{cr}[a] (ml/min)	Diagnosis[b]	Previous medication[c]	Co-medication[c]
Controls								
1	23	63	118/64	56	110			
2	23	77	110/55	58	140			
3	37	80	119/73	52	126			
4	49	90	121/76	54	124			
5	55	84	128/76	52	107			
6	56	67	147/88	51	67			
Mean	41	77	124/72	54	112			
± SD	± 15	± 10	± 13/11	± 3	± 25			
Patients								
1	26	66	135/76	62	12	I	1,2,3	5,6,7
2	26	79	121/72	61	32	I		6,7,8
3	35	67	150/93	60	20	II		8,9,10
4	45	79	149/91	68	12	II		8,9,10,11
5	58	81	150/85	62	31	I		6,7,12
6	59	89	159/90	67	30	I	4	6,7,12
Mean	42	77	144[d]/85[d]	63[e]	23			
± SD	± 15	± 9	± 14/9	± 3	± 9			

a In the control subjects CL_{cr} was calculated using the formula of Cockroft & Gault (1976):

$$CL_{cr}\ (ml/min) = \frac{[140 - Age\ (y)]\ [Bodyweight\ (kg)]}{72 \times [Serum\ creatinine\ (mg/dl)]}$$

b I = chronic allograft rejection; II = polycystic renal disease.

c 1 = atenolol, 2 = ranitidine, 3 = calcium gluconate, 4 = nifedipine, 5 = frusemide (furosemide), 6 = prednisone, 7 = azathioprine, 8 = aluminium hydroxide, 9 = sodium bicarbonate, 10 = allopurinol, 11 = dihydrotachysterol, 12 = compound vitamin B.

d $p < 0.05$.

e $p < 0.001$.

Abbreviations: SBP = systolic blood pressure; DBP = diastolic blood pressure; HR = heart rate; CL_{cr} = creatinine clearance.

Plasma noradrenaline was determined in duplicate by a single isotope radioenzymatic assay (Peuler & Johnson 1977). PTH was measured radioimmunologically (Lindall et al. 1983). Blood pressure and heart rate were assessed using an automatic device (Dinamap®, Critikon Inc., Tampa, Florida, USA).

The elimination half-life ($t_{1/2}$) of nisoldipine was calculated from the terminal part of the concentration/time curve. Peak plasma concentrations (C_{max}) and time to reach C_{max} (t_{max}) were directly derived from the individual plasma concentration/time curves. Area under the curve (AUC) values of nisoldipine and its side-chain hydroxylated metabolite Bay r 9425 were estimated by lin-log trapezoidal rule and subsequent extrapolation to infinity (single-dose experiment on day 1) or up to 12 hours after nisoldipine administration (short term experiment on day 8). Statistical comparisons were made by use of Wilcoxon's signed rank test for paired data and Wilcoxon's rank sum test for differences of 2 independent groups.

Results

Individual plasma concentration/time curves of nisoldipine in renal patients and control subjects after single-dose and short term administration are given in figure 2. The profiles were similar in renal

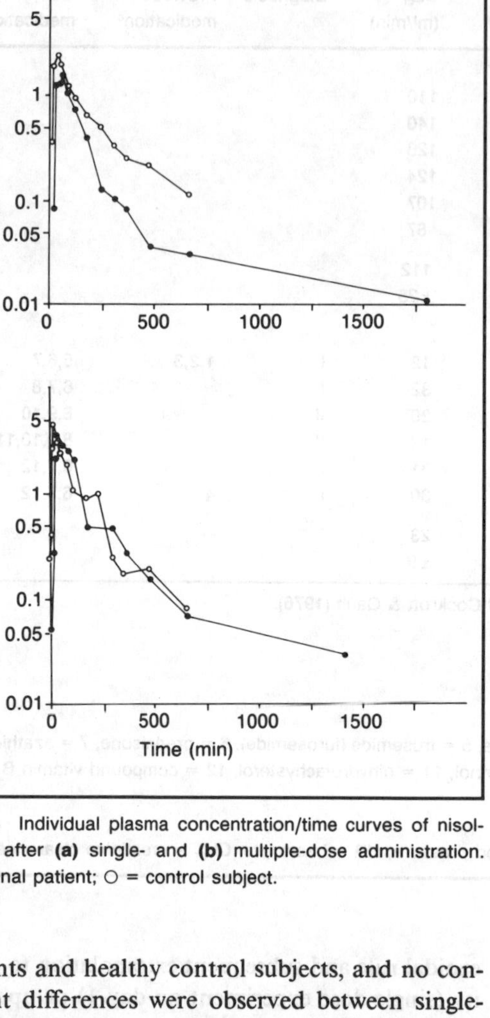

Fig. 2. Individual plasma concentration/time curves of nisoldipine after **(a)** single- and **(b)** multiple-dose administration. ● = renal patient; ○ = control subject.

patients and healthy control subjects, and no consistent differences were observed between single- and multiple-dose administration. Individual pharmacokinetic parameters are given in table II. Mean $t_{1/2}$ was approximately 8 hours, and C_{max} of approximately 2 μg/L was reached after 1 to 2 hours. The half-lives of nisoldipine were very variable, not only between subjects (compare patients 2 and 3 with patients 4, 5 and 6), but also within subjects (see patient 1). AUC values were low and variable and it was calculated that the apparent clearance (assuming complete absorption) after oral administration (hereafter called 'oral clearance') was very high, on average being 30 to 40 L/min. Plasma concentrations of the side-chain hydroxylated dihydropyridine metabolite of nisoldipine (Bay r 9425; fig. 1) were comparable with concentrations of nisoldipine, and no significant differences in AUC were found in either group, AUC values being 8.9 ± 4.4 and 9.2 ± 5.3 μg/L • h in renal patients, and 13.0 ± 8.9 and 12.0 ± 6.8 μg/L • h in the control subjects after single-dose and short term nisoldipine administration, respectively. Plasma concentrations of nisoldipine before drug administration at day 8 were 0.16 ± 0.10 μg/L in the control subjects and 0.09 ± 0.13 μg/L in the renal patients. These values did not differ from those obtained 12 hours after single-dose nisoldipine administration, indicating that no accumulation of nisoldipine occurred during 1 week of oral treatment.

In figure 3 the effects of single- and multiple-dose nisoldipine on blood pressure and heart rate are shown. Systolic blood pressure slightly decreased in both groups after single-dose and short term nisoldipine. Increases in heart rate were also comparable in the two groups. Diastolic blood pressure, however, decreased much more in the renal patients than in the healthy control subjects.

The relationship between plasma concentrations of nisoldipine and percentage changes in diastolic blood pressure for all individual data points up to 6 hours after nisoldipine administration is shown in figure 4. Plasma concentrations of nisoldipine were in the same range in patients and control subjects for both single-dose and short term administration. In the control group a poor relationship between plasma concentrations of nisoldipine and decreases in diastolic blood pressure was found, whereas in the patient group a much better correlation was observed, decrease in diastolic pressure being highly dependent on plasma nisoldipine. Regression data for both blood pressure and heart rate are given in table III. The relationship between plasma concentration of nisoldipine and decrease in blood pressure, as reflected by the correlation coefficient, is more pronounced in renal patients than in control subjects. Unlike that for diastolic blood pressure, the slope of the regression equation for systolic blood pressure was the same

Table II. Pharmacokinetic parameters after single and multiple doses of nisoldipine

Subject	Single dose					Multiple dosing				
	$t_{1/2}$ (h)	AUC (μg/L • h)	C_{max} (μ/L)	t_{max} (h)	t_{last} (h)	$t_{1/2}$ (h)	AUC (μg/L • h)	$C_{max)}$ (μg/L)	t_{max} (h)	t_{last} (h)
Controls										
1	9.3	6.8	2.9	0.5	11.2	6.3	5.2	1.6	0.5	23.6
2	6.1	5.1	2.9	1.0	8.1	10.8	7.4	1.7	3.0	30.8
3	3.1	2.9	1.4	1.0	11.0	6.1	4.1	1.9	1.4	11.0
4	6.0	0.8	0.5	1.5	5.0	6.0	2.2	0.5	1.0	23.1
5	10.1	8.6	3.6	1.0	30.4	11.2	5.0	1.0	1.5	30.4
6	5.1	6.5	2.3	0.8	11.0	6.8	7.6	4.5	4.5	11.0
Mean	6.6	5.1	2.3	1.0		7.9	5.2	1.9	2.0	
± SD	± 2.6	± 2.9	± 1.1	± 0.3		± 2.4	± 2.1	± 1.4	± 1.5	
Patients										
1	18.3	7.5	3.2	2.0	24.0	5.2	7.1	4.3	1.0	23.6
2	2.9	4.4	3.0	0.5	10.9	2.8	3.8	3.3	0.5	8.0
3	1.1	2.1	0.8	3.1	8.0	2.2	3.6	1.3	1.0	10.9
4	10.1	5.9	1.6	0.6	10.8	11.4	17.3	4.0	2.1	31.6
5	13.2	4.2	1.4	3.0	11.4	9.0	4.6	2.5	0.8	23.6
6	12.7	3.7	1.5	1.0	30.0	10.5	7.7	3.6	0.5	23.6
Mean	9.7	4.6	1.9	1.7		6.8	7.4	3.2	1.0	
± SD	± 6.6	± 1.9	± 1.0	± 1.2		± 4.0	± 5.2	± 1.1	± 0.6	

Abbreviations: $t_{1/2}$ = elimination half-life; C_{max} = peak plasma drug concentration; t_{max} = time to C_{max}.

in the two groups. The relationship between plasma nisoldipine and increases in heart rate was very similar in both groups. No differences were observed between the concentration-effect data after single-dose and short term nisoldipine.

Plasma concentrations of PTH and noradrenaline are given in table IV. Intact PTH levels were 5-fold higher in renal patients than in healthy control subjects. Plasma levels 1 hour after oral nisoldipine were not different from basal levels before drug dosing. No differences were observed between single-dose and short term nisoldipine. Basal plasma levels of noradrenaline did not differ in renal patients and healthy controls. In renal patients, however, the increase in plasma noradrenaline was greater than in the control group.

As shown in table V, headache was common on the first day of nisoldipine intake at home, but disappeared on continued treatment. In one of the control subjects pedal oedema developed during the study week.

Discussion

In the present study the pharmacokinetics of nisoldipine and effects on blood pressure, heart rate and plasma concentrations of intact parathyroid hormone and plasma noradrenaline are investigated. Single-dose data are compared with data obtained after multiple-dose administration.

Little nisoldipine is excreted unchanged in urine, and therefore it was anticipated that the plasma clearance of the drug would not be substantially influenced by renal impairment. Although it has been reported that the metabolism of nimodipine (Kirch et al. 1984) and nicardipine (Lee et al. 1986) was impaired in renal patients, it was shown that plasma clearance of the dihydropyridine calcium channel blockers nifedipine (Bogaert et al. 1984; Kleinbloesem et al. 1985), nitrendipine (Aronoff & Sloan 1985) and nisoldipine (Boelaert et al. 1988) was unaffected. In the present study the mean oral clearance showed no difference in patients and

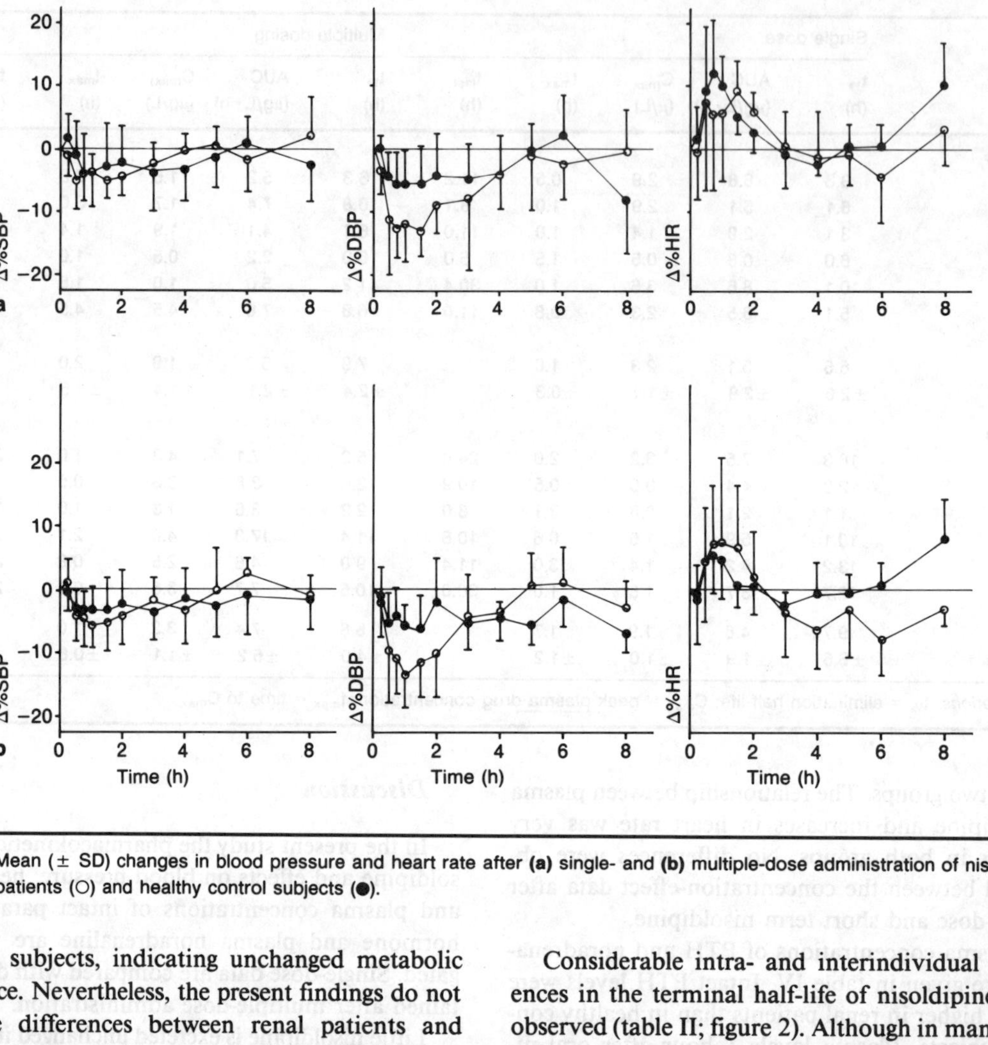

Fig. 3. Mean (± SD) changes in blood pressure and heart rate after **(a)** single- and **(b)** multiple-dose administration of nisoldipine to renal patients (○) and healthy control subjects (●).

control subjects, indicating unchanged metabolic clearance. Nevertheless, the present findings do not exclude differences between renal patients and healthy subjects, because of the limited study population and the considerable interindividual variability observed.

Volume of distribution of nifedipine was found to be increased in renal patients, and this was attributed to a decreased plasma protein binding of the drug. As a result, $t_{1/2}$ was increased in the patient group (Kleinbloesem et al. 1985). Plasma protein binding of nisoldipine, which has been reported to be 99.7% in healthy subjects (Ahr et al. 1987), seems to be similar in patients with renal disease (Boelaert et al. 1988).

Considerable intra- and interindividual differences in the terminal half-life of nisoldipine were observed (table II; figure 2). Although in many subjects concentrations could be measured up to at least 24 hours after dosing, in some cases this appeared to be impossible. This is caused by inability to measure the very low plasma concentrations of nisoldipine, and hence 'pre-terminal' half-lives are reported. In figure 2b the curves of the renal patient and the control subjects are identical, but due to inability to measure plasma nisoldipine beyond 11 hours in the control subject, the calculated $t_{1/2}$ was much shorter than in the renal patient. However, since no relationship was found between the calculated $t_{1/2}$ and the time when the last plasma concentration (see table II) could be measured, it was judged to be correct to give the mean half-lives in table II. The remaining AUC calculated from the data points from 11 hours onwards contributed to only a small extent (5 to 10%) to the total AUC, and therefore all data points (instead of points up to a certain cut-off time) were used in the calculations of the AUC in table II.

The haemodynamic effect profile of nisoldipine in patients and in healthy control subjects was

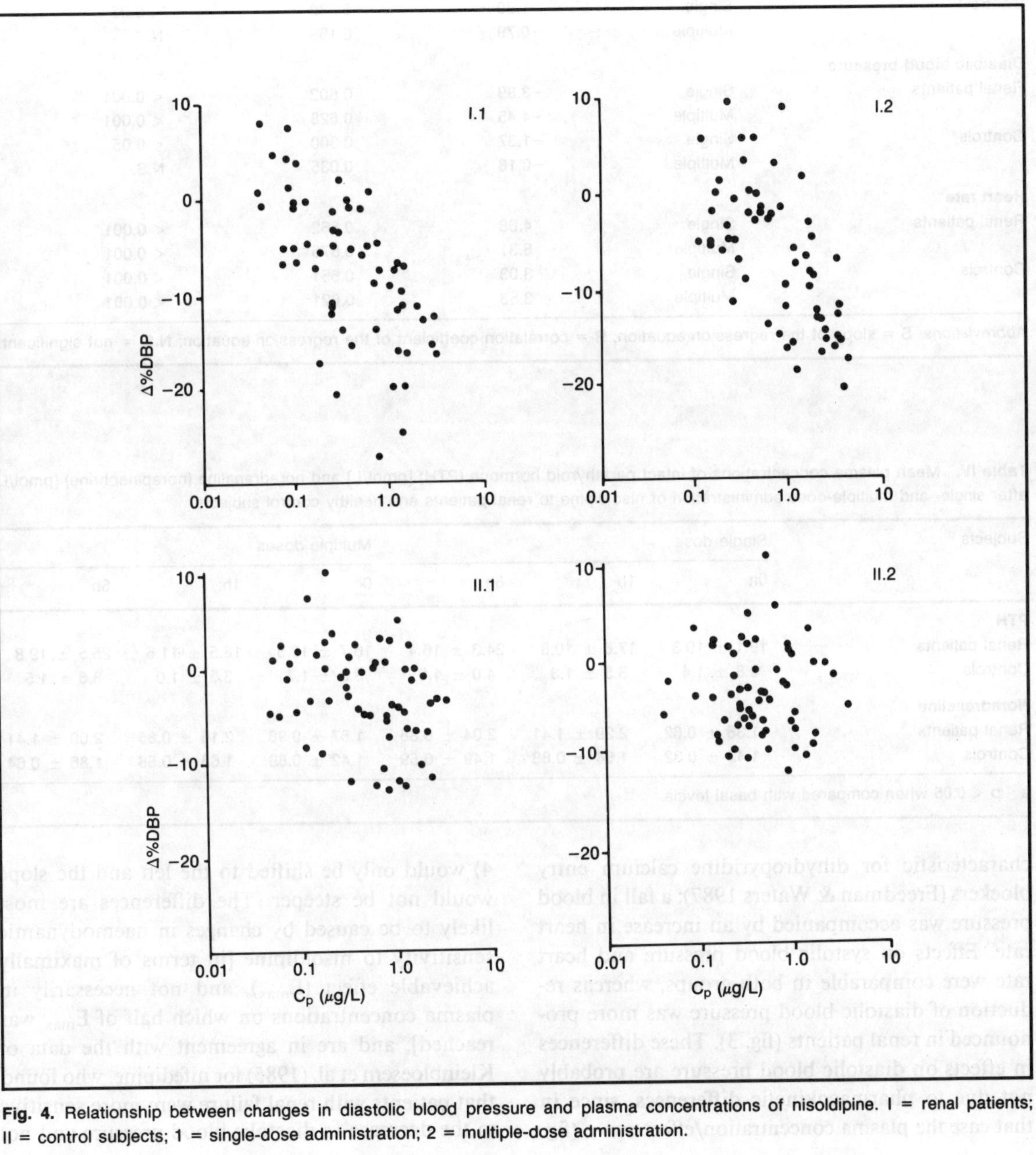

Fig. 4. Relationship between changes in diastolic blood pressure and plasma concentrations of nisoldipine. I = renal patients; II = control subjects; 1 = single-dose administration; 2 = multiple-dose administration.

Table III. Relationship between log plasma concentrations of nisoldipine and effects on blood pressure and heart rate in patients with renal failure and healthy control subjects

Subjects	Dose	S	R	p value
Systolic blood pressure				
Renal patients	Single	−1.30	0.417	< 0.01
	Multiple	−1.97	0.448	< 0.001
Controls	Single	−1.20	0.282	< 0.05
	Multiple	−0.79	0.159	N.S.
Diastolic blood pressure				
Renal patients	Single	−3.89	0.602	< 0.001
	Multiple	−4.45	0.628	< 0.001
Controls	Single	−1.37	0.300	< 0.05
	Multiple	−0.18	0.035	N.S.
Heart rate				
Renal patients	Single	4.66	0.662	< 0.001
	Multiple	5.31	0.575	< 0.001
Controls	Single	3.03	0.551	< 0.001
	Multiple	3.58	0.621	< 0.001

Abbreviations: S = slope of the regression equation; R = correlation coefficient of the regression equation; N.S. = not significant.

Table IV. Mean plasma concentrations of intact parathyroid hormone (PTH) [pmol/L] and noradrenaline (norepinephrine) [pmol/L] after single- and multiple-dose administration of nisoldipine to renal patients and healthy control subjects

Subjects	Single dose			Multiple doses		
	0h	1h	6h	0h	1h	6h
PTH						
Renal patients	19.1 ± 10.3	17.6 ± 10.8	24.3 ± 16.4	16.7 ± 10.5	16.5 ± 11.6	25.5 ± 19.8
Controls	3.8 ± 1.4	3.5 ± 1.3	4.0 ± 1.9	3.5 ± 1.7	3.5 ± 1.0	3.6 ± 1.5
Noradrenaline						
Renal patients	1.38 ± 0.62	2.29 ± 1.41	2.04 ± 0.88	1.57 ± 0.98	2.16 ± 0.85[a]	2.09 ± 1.41
Controls	1.42 ± 0.32	1.64 ± 0.68	1.49 ± 0.59	1.42 ± 0.69	1.63 ± 0.56	1.86 ± 0.64

a $p < 0.05$ when compared with basal levels.

characteristic for dihydropyridine calcium entry blockers (Freedman & Waters 1987): a fall in blood pressure was accompanied by an increase in heart rate. Effects on systolic blood pressure and heart rate were comparable in both groups, whereas reduction of diastolic blood pressure was more pronounced in renal patients (fig. 3). These differences in effects on diastolic blood pressure are probably not due to pharmacokinetic differences, since in that case the plasma concentration/effect curve (fig. 4) would only be shifted to the left and the slope would not be steeper. The differences are most likely to be caused by changes in haemodynamic sensitivity to nisoldipine [in terms of maximally achievable effect (E_{max}), and not necessarily in plasma concentrations on which half of E_{max} was reached], and are in agreement with the data of Kleinbloesem et al. (1985) for nifedipine, who found that patients with renal failure were more sensitive to the decrease in diastolic blood pressure and not to effects on systolic blood pressure and heart rate.

Basal plasma concentrations of PTH were much higher in renal patients than in controls. This finding is in agreement with the fact that renal disease is often accompanied by secondary hyperparathyroidism (Lindall et al. 1983; Nieuwenhuijzen Kruseman et al. 1987). In a previous study we found that basal levels of PTH in hypertensive patients were significantly increased after 4 weeks of oral treatment with nisoldipine (unpublished observations). In the present study, however, PTH levels were not influenced by nisoldipine. Further studies should elucidate whether nisoldipine influences plasma PTH, a hormone which not only influences bone metabolism (Habener et al. 1984), but also has hypotensive properties (Pang et al. 1980).

Since the increase in heart rate after administration of dihydropyridine calcium entry blockers is baroreflex mediated (Kunze et al. 1986; Stern et al. 1986), we measured plasma noradrenaline to correlate differences in reflex tachycardia with increases in plasma noradrenaline. Basal levels of noradrenaline were comparable in renal patients and control subjects, but in the healthy control subjects plasma noradrenaline increased only marginally after oral nisoldipine, whereas renal patients showed a significant increase. In these patients the stronger vasodilatation resulted in either stronger baroreflex activation or decreased peripheral noradrenaline metabolism (Chang et al. 1986), but this did not result in more reflex tachycardia. Clearly, haemodynamic sensitivity for reflex tachycardia is different in renal patients. For nifedipine it was also found that a greater decrease in diastolic blood pressure was accompanied by a greater increase in plasma noradrenaline, while reflex tachycardia was not altered (Kleinbloesem et al. 1985).

Remarkably, the occurrence of headache was limited to the first day of nisoldipine treatment, and this finding may explain the apparent discrepancy between the high incidence of adverse effects in single-dose studies with dihydropyridine calcium entry blockers and the more favourable adverse effect profile on continued administration (Ebner & Donath 1980).

Table V. Frequency of side effects (n = 6 for each group)

Effect	Renal patients		Controls	
	single dose	short term	single dose	short term
Headache	3		2	
Diuresis			2	2
Pedal oedema				1
Flushing	2	2	1	1

Therapeutic Implications

Since dihydropyridine calcium entry blockers are promising agents in the treatment of hypertension in patients with renal dysfunction, the pharmacokinetics and haemodynamic effects of nisoldipine were investigated in renal patients.

From the results obtained in this small study population it is concluded that nisoldipine is an effective, well-tolerated antihypertensive drug in patients with renal dysfunction. The pharmacokinetics of nisoldipine, after both single and multiple dosing, show no difference in renal patients compared with healthy subjects. Thus, the dosage regimen of nisoldipine does not need to be adjusted in renal patients.

Acknowledgements

The authors wish to thank Mrs J.W. Guyt-Scholten for analytical assistance, G.J. Blauw, M.D., for cooperation during the study, M. Frölich, M.D., for measurement of plasma parathyroid hormone, and Mr E. Kriek for measurement of plasma noradrenaline.

References

Ahr G, Wingender W, Kuhlmann J. Pharmacokinetics of nisoldipine. In Hugenholtz & Meyer (Eds) Nisoldipine 1987, pp. 59-66, Springer-Verlag, Berlin, Heidelberg, 1987

Aronoff GR, Sloan RS. Nitrendipine kinetics in normal and impaired renal function. Clinical Pharmacology and Therapeutics 38: 212-218, 1985

Bennet WN, Singer I, Golper TA, Feig T, Coggins CJ. Guidelines for drug therapy in renal failure. Annals of Internal Medicine 86: 754-783, 1977

Boelaert J, Valcke Y, Dammekens H, de Vriese G, Ahr G, et al.

Pharmacokinetics of nisoldipine in renal dysfunction. European Journal of Clinical Pharmacology 34: 207-209, 1988
Bogaert MG, Rosseel MT, Joos R, Boelaert J. Plasma concentrations of nifedipine in patients with renal failure. Arzneimittel-Forschung 34: 307-308, 1984
Chang PC, van der Krogt JA, Vermeij P, van Brummelen P. Norepinephrine removal and release in the forearm of healthy subjects. Hypertension 8: 801-809, 1986
Cockcroft DW, Gault MH. Prediction of creatinine clearance from serum creatinine. Nephron 16: 31-41, 1976
Danhof M, Hisaoka M, Levy G. Kinetics of drug action in disease states, II: effect of experimental renal dysfunction on phenobarbital concentrations in rats at onset of loss of righting reflex. Journal of Pharmacology and Experimental Therapeutics 230: 627-631, 1984
Deeg P, Weiss KH, Schmitz H. Nisoldipin in der Therapie der essentiellen Hypertonie. Deutsche Medizinische Wochenschrift 112: 429-433, 1987
Dettli L. Drug dosage in renal disease. Clinical Pharmacokinetics 1: 126-134, 1976
Dundee JW, Richards RK. Effect of azotemia upon the action of intravenous barbiturate anesthesia. Anesthesiology 15: 333-346, 1954
Ebner F, Donath M. Mode of action and efficacy of nifedipine. In Puech & Krebs (Eds) 4th International Adalat Symposium, pp. 25-34, Excerpta Medica, Amsterdam, 1980
Eliahou HE, Cohen D, Ben-David A, Herzog D, Serban I, et al. Nisoldipine delays progression of chronic renal failure in man irrespective of change in blood pressure. In Hugenholtz & Meyer (Eds) Nisoldipine 1987, pp. 151-158, Springer-Verlag, Berlin, Heidelberg, 1987
Freedman DD, Waters DD. 'Second generation' dihydropyridine calcium antagonists: greater vascular selectivity and some unique applications. Drugs 34: 578-598, 1987
Galeazzi RL, Gugger M, Weidmann P. Beta blockade with pindolol: differential cardiac and renal effects despite similar plasma kinetics in normal and uremic man. Kidney International 15: 661-668, 1979
Gibson TP. Influence of renal disease on pharmacokinetics. In Evans et al. (Eds) Applied Pharmacokinetics, principles of therapeutic drug monitoring, pp. 32-56, Applied Therapeutics Inc., San Francisco, 1980
Habener JF, Rosenblatt M, Potts JT. Parathyroid hormone: biochemical aspects of biosynthesis, secretion, action, and metabolism. Physiological Reviews 64: 985-1053, 1984
Keller F, Maiga M, Neumayer H-H, Lode H, Distler A. Pharmacokinetic effects of altered plasma protein binding of drugs in renal disease. European Journal of Drug Metabolism and Pharmacokinetics 9: 275-282, 1984
Kirch W, Rämsch KD, Dührsen U, Ohnhaus EE. Clinical pharmacokinetics of nimodipine in normal and impaired renal function. International Journal of Clinical and Pharmacological Research 4: 381-384, 1984
Kleinbloesem CH, van Brummelen P, van Harten J, Danhof M, Breimer DD. Nifedipine: influence of renal function on pharmacokinetic/pharmacodynamic relationship. Clinical Pharmacology and Therapeutics 37: 563-574, 1985
Kunze DL, Andresen MC, Torres LA. Do calcium antagonists act directly on calcium channels to alter baroreceptor function? Journal of Pharmacology and Experimental Therapeutics 239: 303-310, 1986
Lam J, Chaitman BR, Crean P, Blum R, Waters DD. A dose-ranging, placebo-controlled, double-blind trial of nisoldipine in effort angina: duration and extent of antianginal effects. Journal of the American College of Cardiology 6: 447-452, 1985
Lee SM, Williams R, Warnock D, Emmett M, Wolbach RA. The effects of nicardipine in hypertensive subjects with impaired renal function. British Journal of Clinical Pharmacology 22: 297S-306S, 1986
Lindall AW, Ells J, Elting J, Roos B. Estimation of biologically active intact parathyroid hormone in normal and hyperparathyroid sera by sequential *N*-terminal immunoextraction and mid-region radioimmunoassay. Journal of Clinical Endocrinology and Metabolism 57: 1007-1014, 1983
Lopez LM, Rubin MR, Holland JP, Mehta JL. Improvement in exercise performance with nisoldipine, a new second generation calcium blocker, in stable angina pectoris. American Heart Journal 110: 991-996, 1985
Müller FO, Hundt HKL, Luus HG, Joubert AL, Groenewoud G, et al. Estimation of the bioavailability of nisoldipine in man. Nisoldipine Workshop, Luxembourg, October 16-18 (Abstract), 1986
Neureth I, Szelezhi T. Enhanced drug metabolism and renal dysfunction. British Journal of Clinical Pharmacology 11: 92-93, 1981
Nieuwenhuijzen Kruseman AC, Frölich M, Walma ST, Valentijn RM. Diagnostic value of intact parathyroid hormone measurement. Netherlands Journal of Medicine 31: 10-15, 1987
Pang PKT, Tenner TE, Yee JA, Yang M, Janssen HF. Hypotensive action of parathyroid hormone preparations in rats and dogs. Proceedings of the National Academy of Science of the United States of America 77: 675-678, 1980
Peuler JD, Johnson GA. Simultaneous single isotope radioenzymatic assay of plasma norepinephrine, epinephrine and dopamine. Life Science 21: 625-636, 1977
Reidenberg MM. The biotransformation of drugs in renal failure. American Journal of Medicine 62: 482-485, 1977
Rosendorff C, Goodman C. Double-blind double-dummy crossover study of the efficacy and safety of nisoldipine (Bay k 5552) versus nifedipine. Current Therapeutic Research 37: 912-920, 1985
Scherling D, Ahr G, Karl W. Biotransformation of nisoldipine in man. In Hugenholtz & Meyer (Eds) Nisoldipine 1987, pp. 85-88, Springer-Verlag, Berlin, Heidelberg, 1987
Stern HC, Matthews JH, Belz GG. Intrinsic and reflex actions of verapamil and nifedipine: assessment in normal subjects by noninvasive techniques and autonomic blockade. European Journal of Clinical Pharmacology 29: 541-547, 1986
van Harten J, Lodewijks MThM, Guyt-Scholten JW, van Brummelen P, Breimer DD. Gas chromatographic determination of nisoldipine and one of its metabolites in plasma. Journal of Chromatography 423: 327-333, 1987
van Harten J, van Brummelen P, Lodewijks MThM, Danhof M, Breimer DD. Pharmacokinetics and hemodynamic effects of nisoldipine and its interaction with cimetidine. Clinical Pharmacology and Therapeutics 43: 332-341, 1988a
van Harten J, van Brummelen P, Zeegers RRECM, Danhof M, Breimer DD. The influence of infusion rate on the pharmacokinetics and haemodynamic effects of nisoldipine in man. British Journal of Clinical Pharmacology 25: 709-717, 1988b

Authors' address: *J. van Harten*, Center for Bio-Pharmaceutical Sciences, Division of Pharmacology, P.O. Box 9503, 2300 RA Leiden (The Netherlands).

Clinical Pharmacokinetics 16: 65-73 (1989)
0312-5963/89/0002-0065/$04.50/0

Protein Binding Drug Displacement Interactions
Fact or Fiction?

Janis J. MacKichan
College of Pharmacy, Ohio State University, Columbus, Ohio, USA

A drug displacement interaction is loosely defined as the reduction in extent of plasma protein binding of one drug caused by the presence of another drug. These interactions may be caused by competition between the drugs involved for a common binding site (competitive inhibition) or by the ability of the displacer to alter tertiary conformation of the binding protein (non-competitive inhibition). Regardless of the mechanism, the end result is an increased unbound fraction of the displaced drug.

In most early reports of adverse drug interactions that were known to involve binding displacement, observed toxicities were concluded to be a direct result of the displacement. More recently, the role of binding displacement as a cause of clinically important drug interactions has been questioned (D'Arcy & McElnay 1982; McElnay & D'Arcy 1983; Sellers 1979; Shand et al. 1975). With our present understanding of the influence of plasma protein binding on the distribution and elimination of drugs (Gillette 1973; MacKichan 1984; Shand et al. 1975; Yacobi et al. 1975), we now recognise that the adverse consequences of many interactions that were originally attributed to displacement were in fact caused by the effect of the displacers on the elimination of the displaced drugs.

Protein binding displacement interactions are 'clinically important' if they require a temporary or sustained reduction in the daily dose of the displaced drug. This will occur if the displacement results in a temporary or sustained increase in the unbound drug concentration in plasma. The goals of this article are to describe the theoretical effects of displacement on unbound concentrations of drug in plasma, and to review examples of drug displacement interactions for which the mechanisms are known. It is concluded that although drug displacement is common and sometimes predictable, it alone is rarely responsible for observations of adverse drug interactions.

1. *Drug Displacement*

The following general requirements must be satisfied for displacement of drug from plasma protein:

1. The displaced drug must be highly bound, so that a given decrease in its bound fraction will result in a large percentage increase in its unbound fraction.
2. The displacer and the displaced drug must share a common binding site (if competitive) or a common protein (if non-competitive).
3. For true competition to occur, the binding sites must be limited in number; hence, the molar concentration of the displacer must approach the concentration of protein binding sites.
4. The free concentration of the displacer must be higher than that of the displaced drug and/or the binding site affinity for the displacer must be higher than that for the displaced drug.

Because of these requirements, *in vitro* studies designed to examine the possibility of *in vivo* displacement must use physiological protein concentrations and drug concentrations that are seen following therapeutic doses. The use of unusually low protein concentrations or supra-therapeutic concentrations of displacer may produce displacement *in vitro* but not *in vivo*.

Additional consideration must be given to drugs that bind to more than one protein in plasma. Significant displacement of drug from one of the binding proteins may not result in a demonstrable increase in the unbound fraction in plasma, which contains all binding proteins. This is evident with drugs that are displaced from high affinity, low capacity proteins like α_1-acid glycoprotein, but not from high capacity, low affinity proteins such as albumin. Bupivacaine caused a 109% increase in the unbound fraction of mepivacaine in a solution of α_1-acid glycoprotein but only a 9% increase in the unbound fraction of mepivacaine in plasma containing the same α_1-acid glycoprotein concentration (Hartrick et al. 1984). Similarly, we have reported significant displacement by disopyramide of lignocaine (lidocaine) and propranolol from α_1-acid glycoprotein, but minimal displacement in human plasma (MacKichan 1984). This occurs because the high capacity albumin 'buffers' any change in unbound fraction caused by displacement of a relatively small amount of drug from the low capacity α_1-acid glycoprotein. Hence, increases in unbound fractions in plasma due to displacement from α_1-acid glycoprotein will be much more evident for drugs that are predominantly bound to this protein, such as disopyramide, than for drugs that are bound more to albumin, such as carbamazepine (Lima et al. 1981; MacKichan & Zola 1984). For the same reason, displacement interactions that are insignificant in healthy subjects may be pronounced in the plasma of patients with both hypoalbuminaemia and disease-induced elevations in α_1-acid glycoprotein concentrations, such as patients with cancer.

2. *Displacement of Drugs that are Restrictively Cleared*

2.1 Pharmacokinetic Consequences

Theoretical expectations for the displacement of restrictively cleared drugs in plasma have been extensively reviewed (Aarons & Rowland 1981; MacKichan 1984; McQueen & Wardell 1971; Rowland & Matin 1973). The intrinsic elimination processes responsible for the removal of these drugs are very weak, such that only drug which is unbound in plasma can be cleared. An increase in the unbound fraction in plasma will therefore increase body clearance, and reduce the total concentration of drug in plasma. As long as the intrinsic clearance of drug is not altered, i.e. by inhibition of enzyme or tubular secretion carrier activity, the unbound concentration of drug in plasma will be unaltered. Viewing this in another way, the unbound concentration does not change because the total concentration is lower and because the unbound fraction is higher.

An increase in the unbound concentration of drug in plasma will occur immediately after introduction of the displacing drug, but will gradually return to its predisplacement steady-state value after redistribution occurs. The significance of this transient rise in unbound concentration will depend on many factors, including the rate of displacer input and the pharmacokinetic characteristics of the displaced drug. Rapid intravenous infusion of the displacing drug will result in a higher peak unbound concentration of displaced drug than will slow input of the displacer (i.e. by slow intravenous infusion or oral administration) [Oie & Levy 1979]. The peak unbound concentration will be highest for displaced drugs with relatively small volumes of distribution (< 0.25 L/kg), and will remain high for longer periods for drugs with long elimination half-lives (Koch-Weser & Sellers 1976). It should also be noted that displacement will have no effect on the elimination half-life of displaced drugs with moderate to large volumes of distribution (> 0.4 L/kg), but will shorten the half-life of drugs with small volumes of distribution. This will result in greater fluctuation in unbound concentration of the displaced drug during a steady-state dosing interval.

All of the above predictions assume that the displacing drug does not affect the intrinsic activities of hepatic or renal elimination processes (intrinsic clearance). If the displacer also decreases the intrinsic clearance of the displaced drug, higher un-

Table I. Pure displacement interactions: restrictively cleared drugs

Displaced drug	Displacer	Effects on displaced drug	Reference
Phenytoin	Salicylate	*In vivo* increase in fu at high aspirin doses. Decreases in C_{tot}, no change in C_{free}. Transient increases in C_{free} not studied. No phenytoin toxicity observed	Fraser et al. (1980); Leonard et al. (1981); Olanow et al. (1981); Paxton (1980)
	Tolbutamide	*In vivo* increase in fu, decrease in C_{tot}, transient but slight increase in C_{free}. No report of toxicity	Wesseling & Mols-Thurkow (1975)
Tolbutamide	Sulphadimethoxine	*In vitro* increase in fu; *in vivo* decrease in C_{tot}, decrease in $t_{1/2}$	Kristensen (1976)
		No change in hypoglycaemic response seen in tolbutamide-treated diabetics after sulphadimethoxine administration	Christensen (1963)
Warfarin	Trichloroacetic acid (metabolite of chloral hydrate and triclofos)	*In vivo* increase in fu, decrease in C_{tot}, decrease in $t_{1/2}$	Sellers & Koch-Weser (1970)
		Potentiation of warfarin response early during combination therapy	Sellers & Koch-Weser (1970); Sellers et al. (1972); Udall (1974)
		No change in response after 1 week of combination therapy	Griner et al. (1971); Udall (1974, 1975)
		Clinically important, transient increase in response does not occur in all patients	Sellers & Koch-Weser (1977)
	Diflunisal	*In vivo* increase in fu, decrease in C_{tot}, no change in C_{free}. No change in response observed; lack of transient effect attributed to slow input of displacer	Serlin et al. (1980)

Abbreviations: fu = unbound fraction in plasma; C_{tot} = total (bound + unbound) concentration in plasma; C_{free} = unbound concentration in plasma; $t_{1/2}$ = elimination half-life.

bound concentrations will be sustained for the duration of displacer therapy. Total concentrations of the displaced drug can be higher, lower, or unchanged, depending on the relative magnitude of changes in the unbound fraction and intrinsic clearance.

No untoward effects will therefore be seen for most drug interactions that involve only displacement, since drug response and toxicity are usually closely related to the unbound concentration of a drug in plasma. Hence, no change in daily dose will be required. For those few drugs with small volumes of distribution and narrow therapeutic indices, exaggerated response or toxicity may occur transiently after initiation of displacer therapy, and a temporary reduction of the daily dose may be required. Once re-equilibration occurs, the use of a shorter dosing interval may be desirable to offset greater fluctuations in unbound concentrations during the interval.

2.2 Examples from the Literature

Examples of drug interactions that involve displacement of restrictively cleared drugs are presented in tables I and II. Only those interactions for which the mechanism(s) of interaction is clearly documented are reported.

Drug interactions involving only displacement in plasma are summarised in table I. None of the interactions results in a sustained increase in response or toxicity, and only one (trichloroacetic acid-warfarin interaction) results in a significant transient exaggeration of response. This is not surprising in light of warfarin's very small volume of distribution (0.1 L/kg), long elimination half-life,

Table II. Interactions involving displacement and decreased free drug clearance: restrictively cleared drugs

Displaced drug	Displacer	Effects on displaced drug	Reference
Carbamazepine	Valproate	*In vivo* increase in fu, increase in C_{free}, no change in C_{tot}, increase in $t_{½}$. Carbamazepine side effects reported to be more severe when valproate given concurrently	MacPhee et al. (1988)
		Carbamazepine total concentrations are increased, unchanged, or decreased during concurrent valproate administration to patients	Baciewicz (1986)
Ceftriaxone	Probenecid	*In vivo* increase in fu, decrease in C_{tot}. Increase in C_{free} due to decreased renal clearance of free drug. Of little clinical importance due to wide therapeutic index and unlikelihood of combination	Stoeckel et al. (1988)
Diazepam	Valproate	*In vivo* increase in fu, decrease in C_{tot}, increase in C_{free}. No report of side effects to single diazepam dose in presence of valproate	Dhillon & Richens (1982)
Ketoprofen	Probenecid	*In vivo* increase in fu, increase in C_{tot}. Increase in C_{free} caused by decreased conjugative metabolism and decreased renal clearance of free drug. No report of toxicity	Upton et al. (1982)
Methotrexate	Salicylate	*In vivo* increase in fu, increase in C_{tot}, increase in C_{free}	Liegler et al. (1969)
		Case reports and clinical observations of methotrexate toxicity when aspirin taken concurrently	Evans & Christensen (1985)
	Probenecid	*In vitro* increase in fu at high probenecid concentrations	Paxton (1984)
		Increase in C_{tot}, increase in $t_{½}$	Bourke et al. (1975)
		Reports of methotrexate toxicity with this combination	Kates et al. (1976)
	Sulphafurazole (sulfisoxazole)	*In vivo* increase in fu, increase in C_{tot}, increase in C_{free}	Liegler et al. (1969)
		No reports of clinical toxicity	
Phenytoin	Phenylbutazone	*In vivo* increase in fu. Initial decrease in C_{tot}, followed by increase above original values. Increase in C_{free} after 1 week of phenylbutazone. Phenytoin toxicity necessitated discontinuation of phenylbutazone in 1 of 13 patients	Neuvonen et al. (1979)

and narrow therapeutic index. Exaggeration of warfarin response occurs not only in situations where chloral hydrate or triclofos is initiated in a patient who is already stabilised on warfarin; lower warfarin doses may also be required for the first few days after initiation of that drug in a patient who is already taking chloral hydrate (Boston Collaborative Drug Surveillance Program 1982; Udall 1974). This 'initial effect' is consistent with expectations: the volume of distribution of unbound warfarin is smaller in the chloral hydrate/triclofos-treated patient, and will result in higher peak un-

Table II. Contd

Displaced drug	Displacer	Effects on displaced drug	Reference
Phenytoin	Valproate	*In vivo* increase in fu, decrease in C_{tot}. Increases in C_{free}, with some reports of phenytoin toxicity	Bruni et al. (1980); Perucca et al. (1980); Rodin et al. (1981)
		No change in C_{free} with no evidence of phenytoin toxicity	Mattson et al. (1978); Tsanaclis et al. (1984)
		Phenytoin fu and C_{free} vary as a function of valproate concentration during a valproate dosing interval; administration of smaller valproate doses at more frequent intervals recommended to avoid wide fluctuations in C_{free}	Knott et al. (1982)
Tolbutamide	Sulphaphenazole	*In vitro* increase in fu, increase in C_{tot}, and increase in $t_{½}$. Decrease in blood sugars seen after few days of sulphaphenazole treatment; return to baseline after discontinuation. Serious hypoglycaemic reactions have been reported	Christensen et al. (1963)
Valproate	Salicylate	Large *in vivo* increase in fu, decrease in C_{tot}, increase in C_{free}, and increase in $t_{½}$. No untoward effects noted after 1 day of concurrent aspirin	Orr et al. (1982)
		Inhibition of valproate metabolism confirmed in a separate study	Abbott et al. (1986)
Warfarin	Phenylbutazone	*In vivo* increase in fu	Sellers (1984)
		Stereoselective metabolic inhibition of more potent S(−) isomer	Lewis et al. (1974); O'Reilly et al. (1980)
		Many reports of serious haemorrhagic complications	Sellers (1984)

Abbreviations: fu = unbound fraction in plasma; C_{tot} = total (bound + unbound) concentration in plasma; C_{free} = unbound concentration in plasma; $t_{½}$ = elimination half-life.

bound concentrations of warfarin following the initial doses. Interestingly, no transient hypoprothrombinaemic response was detected when diflunisal was initiated in warfarin-treated subjects (Serlin 1980). This was attributed by the authors to slow accumulation of the displacing drug. Although transient increases in unbound phenytoin concentrations were observed when tolbutamide was co-administered, the increases were not of sufficient magnitude to result in toxicities (Wesseling & Mols-Thurkow 1975). This is also to be expected, since phenytoin has a moderately large volume of distribution.

Two well-known displacement interactions were not included in table I because of their unusual natures. The hypoprothrombinaemia seen when clofibrate is administered to warfarin-treated patients is not explained by displacement, but rather by an effect of clofibrate on the pharmacodynamics of warfarin (Bjornsson et al. 1977, 1979). The increased unbound fractions in plasma reported for many drugs following administration of heparin are now believed to be *in vitro* artefacts (Brown et al. 1981; Chou & Levy 1981; Giacomini et al. 1980a,b; Lohman et al. 1985). Heparin administration probably does not increase plasma free fatty acid concentrations to a degree sufficient to cause *in vivo* displacement.

As stated previously, sustained increases in unbound drug concentrations of restrictively cleared drugs are expected only if the displacing drug also inhibits either the metabolism or the renal tubular secretion of the displaced drug. Such interactions are more likely to lead to side effects and toxicities, as summarised in table II. Adverse effects were documented for 7 of the 12 reported drug interactions, with the warfarin-phenylbutazone interaction being especially serious in nature. The lack of reported side effects with the other interactions may be explained by (1) the wide therapeutic index for the affected drug (ceftriaxone-probenecid; ketoprofen-probenecid), (2) insufficient duration of combined therapy (valproate-aspirin), or (3) a study that is designed to examine pharmacokinetic rather than clinical consequences (diazepam-valproate). The lack of reported side effects for the methotrexate (amethopterim)-sulphafurazole (sulfisoxazole) combination remains an enigma; perhaps this combination is not commonly used.

The list of protein binding displacement interactions that also involve altered elimination of free drug (table II) is noticeably longer than the list of pure displacement interactions (table I). This is probably because most pure displacement interactions do not result in toxicities and therefore go undetected and unstudied. In contrast, drug interactions that result in sustained increases in unbound concentrations are more likely to be studied because of side effects and toxicities that are noted in the clinical setting.

3. Displacement of Drugs that are Non-Restrictively Cleared

3.1 Pharmacokinetic Consequences

Theoretical expectations for the displacement of non-restrictively cleared drugs have also been reviewed (MacKichan 1984). Drugs which are non-restrictively cleared are so avidly extracted by the liver or kidney that binding to plasma proteins does not limit their removal. Thus, body clearance is unaffected by alterations in plasma protein binding (Kornhauser et al. 1978). Because the total concentration of displaced drug in plasma is unaffected by displacement, an increase in unbound fraction will result in an immediate and sustained increase in the unbound concentration. This will be of clinical significance for drugs with narrow therapeutic indices. The half-life will be minimally prolonged for drugs with a small volume of distribution, and greatly prolonged for drugs with a large volume of distribution. Thus, although the average unbound concentration during a period of dosing will be higher, there will be less fluctuation.

3.2 Examples from the Literature

There are no clear examples of displacement interactions that involve non-restrictively cleared drugs (MacKichan 1984; Shand et al. 1975). There are several possible reasons for this. First, many of the drugs that are known to be non-restrictively cleared by the liver are weakly basic compounds that bind to both α_1-acid glycoprotein and albumin in plasma. As stated in section 1, and as confirmed by Svensson et al. (1986), significant displacement of these α_1-acid glycoprotein-binding drugs in plasma is rare. Secondly, many of the drugs that are cleared by non-restrictive mechanisms have wide therapeutic indices, or unclear relationships between concentration and response. For example, the penicillins are non-restrictively cleared by renal tubular secretion and are known to be displaced by other drugs. However, little effort has been dedicated to characterising the pharmacokinetic consequences of these displacement interactions because they cause no adverse effects. Finally, drugs that are highly extracted and non-restrictively cleared by the liver exhibit considerable interpatient variability in first-pass elimination after oral administration. The resulting interpatient variability in total drug concentration and response at a given dose rate will make any displacement difficult to detect (Shand et al. 1975).

The 2 examples of non-restrictive drug displacement described below demonstrate that the pharmacokinetic and clinical consequences of such interactions are consistent with theoretical expectations. Kunin (1966) reported *in vivo* displacement of several penicillins by concurrent administration of aspirin or sulpha drugs. The unbound fractions of the penicillins increased by as much as 88%, with no change in total penicillin concentration but an increase in the free concentration. Although these displacement interactions are of no clinical concern, due to the wide therapeutic ranges of the displaced drugs, such interactions could be important for other drugs.

The adverse effects caused by the acetazolamide-aspirin drug combination may also be explained by displacement of a non-restrictively cleared drug. Using the approach proposed by Gillette (1973) and the data of Sweeney et al. (1986), acetazolamide is determined to be non-restrictively cleared by renal tubular secretion. When aspirin is administered, the unbound fraction of acetazolamide increases by 170%, while free concentrations increase by approximately 100% (Sweeney et al. 1986). The magnitude of this increase in unbound concentration is consistent with expectations for a drug that is cleared by both filtration (a restrictive process) and secretion (non-restrictive). Although Sweeney et al. suggest that this interaction is caused by salicylate inhibition of both protein binding and renal tubular secretion of acetazolamide, their explanation ignores the non-restrictive nature of acetazolamide.

4. Conclusions

There is no question that pure protein binding displacement interactions occur. Of the interactions that have been fully characterised, however, most are clinically unimportant. For restrictively cleared drugs, transient increases in response will be of potential importance only for those drugs, such as warfarin, having a particular set of pharmacokinetic characteristics and a narrow therapeutic index. The clinical importance of by far the majority of drug interactions involving restrictively cleared drugs is caused by the displacer's effect on metabolism or renal tubular secretion. Although there are few documented examples of non-restrictive drug displacement, the potential significance of such interactions cannot be disregarded.

Finally, displacement interactions are always 'clinically significant' if plasma concentrations of the displaced drug are used as a guide to dosage adjustment. All drug displacement interactions will result in total drug concentrations of displaced drug that do not reflect the same level of response as that before addition of the displacer. Recognition of displacement is therefore necessary to avoid adverse reactions that can occur as a result of improper dosage adjustments.

References

Aarons LJ, Rowland M. Kinetics of drug displacement interactions. Journal of Pharmacokinetics and Biopharmaceutics 9: 181-190, 1981

Abbott FS, Kassam J, Orr JM, Farrell K. The effect of aspirin on valproic acid metabolism. Clinical Pharmacology and Therapeutics 40: 94-100, 1986

Baciewicz AM. Carbamazepine drug interactions. Therapeutic Drug Monitoring 8: 305-317, 1986

Bjornsson TD, Meffin PJ, Blaschke TF. Interaction of clofibrate with warfarin. I. Effect of clofibrate on the disposition of the optical enantiomorphs of warfarin. Journal of Pharmacokinetics and Biopharmaceutics 5: 495-505, 1977

Bjornsson TD, Meffin PJ, Swezey S, Blaschke TF. Clofibrate displaces warfarin from plasma proteins in man: an example of a pure displacement interaction. Journal of Pharmacology and Experimental Therapeutics 210: 316-321, 1979

Boston Collaborative Drug Surveillance Program. Interaction between chloral hydrate and warfarin. New England Journal of Medicine 286: 53-55, 1982

Bourke RS, Cheda G, Bremer A, Watanabe O, Tower DB. Inhibition of renal tubular transport of methotrexate by probenecid. Cancer Research 35: 110-116, 1975

Brown JE, Kitchell BB, Bjornsson TD, Shand DG. The artifactual nature of heparin-induced drug protein binding alterations. Clinical Pharmacology and Therapeutics 30: 636-643, 1981

Bruni J, Gallo JM, Lee CS, Perchalski RJ, Wilder BJ. Interactions of valproic acid with phenytoin. Neurology 30: 1233-1236, 1980

Chou RC, Levy G. Effect of heparin or salicylate infusion on serum protein binding and on concentrations of phenytoin in serum, brain and cerebrospinal fluid of rats. Journal of Pharmacology and Experimental Therapeutics 219: 42-48, 1981

Christensen LK, Hansen JM, Kristensen M. Sulphaphenazole-induced hypoglycaemic attacks in tolbutamide-treated diabetics. Lancet 2: 1298-1301, 1963

D'Arcy PF, McElnay JC. Drug interactions involving the displacement of drugs from plasma protein and tissue binding sites. Pharmacology and Therapeutics 17: 211-220, 1982

Dhillon S, Richens A. Valproic acid and diazepam interaction *in vivo*. British Journal of Clinical Pharmacology 13: 553-560, 1982

Evans WE, Christensen ML. Drug interactions with methotrexate. Journal of Rheumatology 12 (Suppl. 12): 15-20, 1985

Fraser DG, Ludden TM, Evens RP, Sutherland EW. Displacement of phenytoin from plasma binding sites by salicylate. Clinical Pharmacology and Therapeutics 27: 165-169, 1980

Giacomini KM, Giacomini JC, Blaschke TF. Absence of effect

of heparin on the binding of prazosin and phenytoin to plasma proteins. Biochemical Pharmacology 29: 3337-3340, 1980a

Giacomini KM, Swezey SE, Giacomini JC, Blaschke TF. Administration of heparin causes *in vitro* release of non-esterified fatty acids in human plasma. Life Sciences 27: 771-780, 1980b

Gillette JR. Overview of drug-protein binding. Annals of the New York Academy of Sciences 226: 6-17, 1973

Griner PF, Raisz LG, Rickles FR, Wiesner PJ, Odoroff CL. Chloral hydrate and warfarin interaction: clinical significance? Annals of Internal Medicine 74: 540-543, 1971

Hartrick CT, Dirkes WE, Coyle DE, Raj PR, Denson DD. Influence of bupivacaine on mepivacaine protein binding. Clinical Pharmacology and Therapeutics 36: 546-550, 1984

Kates RE, Tozer TN, Sorby DL. Increased methotrexate toxicity due to concurrent probenecid administration. Biochemical Pharmacology 25: 1485-1488, 1976

Knott C, Hamshaw-Thomas A, Reynolds F. Phenytoin-valproate interaction: importance of saliva monitoring in epilepsy. British Medical Journal 284: 13-16, 1982

Koch-Weser J, Seller EM. Binding of drugs to serum albumin (Part II). New England Journal of Medicine 294: 526-531, 1976

Kornhauser DM, Wood AJJ, Vestal RE, Wilkinson GR, Branch RA, et al. Biological determinants of propranolol disposition in man. Clinical Pharmacology and Therapeutics 23: 165-174, 1978

Kristensen MB. Drug interactions and clinical pharmacokinetics. Clinical Pharmacokinetics 1: 351-372, 1976

Kunin CM. Clinical pharmacology of the new penicillins. II. Effect of drugs which interfere with binding to serum proteins. Clinical Pharmacology and Therapeutics 7: 180-188, 1966

Leonard RF, Knott PJ, Rankin GD, Robinson DS, Melnick DE. Phenytoin-salicylate interaction. Clinical Pharmacology and Therapeutics 29: 56-60, 1981

Lewis RJ, Trager WF, Chan KK, Breckenridge A, Orme M, et al. Warfarin: stereochemical aspects of its metabolism and the interactions with phenylbutazone. Journal of Clinical Investigation 53: 1607-1617, 1974

Liegler DG, Henderson ES, Hahn MA, Oliverio VT. The effect of organic acids on renal clearance of methotrexate in man. Clinical Pharmacology and Therapeutics 10: 849-857, 1969

Lima JJ, Boudoulas H, Blanford MF. Concentration dependence of disopyramide binding to serum protein and its influence on kinetics and dynamics. Journal of Pharmacology and Experimental Therapeutics 219: 741-747, 1981

Lohman JJM, Hooymans PM, Koten MLP, Verhey MTJM, Merkus FWHM. Effect of heparin on digitoxin protein binding. Clinical Pharmacology and Therapeutics 37: 55-60, 1985

MacKichan JJ. Pharmacokinetic consequences of drug displacement from blood and tissue proteins. Clinical Pharmacokinetics 9 (Suppl. 1): 32-41, 1984

MacKichan JJ, Zola EM. Determinants of carbamazepine and carbamazepine 10,11-epoxide binding to serum protein, albumin and alpha-1-acid glycoprotein. British Journal of Clinical Pharmacology 18: 487-493, 1984

MacPhee GJA, Mitchell JR, Wiseman L, McLellan AR, Park BK, et al. Effect of sodium valproate on carbamazepine disposition and psychomotor profile in man. British Journal of Clinical Pharmacology 25: 59-66, 1988

Mattson RH, Cramer JA, Williamson PD, Novelly RA. Valproic acid in epilepsy: clinical and pharmacological effects. Annals of Neurology 3: 20-25, 1978

McElnay JC, D'Arcy PF. Protein binding displacement interactions and their clinical importance. Drugs 25: 495-513, 1983

McQueen EG, Wardell WM. Drug displacement from protein binding isolation of a redistributional drug interaction *in vivo*. British Journal of Pharmacology 43: 312-324, 1971

Neuvonen PJ, Lehtovaara R, Bardy A, Elomaa E. Antipyretic analgesics in patients on antiepileptic drug therapy. European Journal of Clinical Pharmacology 15: 263-268, 1979

Oie S, Levy G. Effect of sulfisoxazole on pharmacokinetics of free and plasma protein-bound bilirubin in experimental unconjugated hyperbilirubinemia. Journal of Pharmaceutical Sciences 68: 6-9, 1979

Olanow CW, Finn AL, Prussak C. The effects of salicylate on the pharmacokinetics of phenytoin. Neurology 31: 341-342, 1981

O'Reilly RA, Trager WF, Motley CH. Stereoselective interaction of phenylbutazone with ($^{12}C/^{13}C$)warfarin pseudoracemates in man. Journal of Clinical Investigation 65: 746-753, 1980

Orr JM, Abbott FS, Farrell K, Ferguson S, Sheppard I, et al. Interaction between valproic acid and aspirin in epileptic children: serum protein binding and metabolic effects. Clinical Pharmacology and Therapeutics 31: 642-649, 1982

Paxton JW. Effects of aspirin on salivary and serum phenytoin kinetics in healthy subjects. Clinical Pharmacology and Therapeutics 27: 170-178, 1980

Paxton JW. Interaction of probenecid with the protein binding of methotrexate. Pharmacology 28: 86-89, 1984

Perucca E, Hebdige S, Frigo GM, Gatti G, Lecchini S, et al. Interaction between phenytoin and valproic acid: plasma protein binding and metabolic effects. Clinical Pharmacology and Therapeutics 28: 779-789, 1980

Rodin EA, DeSousa G, Haidukewych D, Lodhi R, Berchou RC. Dissociation between free and bound phenytoin levels in presence of valproate sodium. Archives of Neurology 38: 240-242, 1981

Rowland M, Matin SB. Kinetics of drug-drug interactions. Journal of Pharmacokinetics and Biopharmaceutics 1: 553-567, 1973

Sellers EM. Plasma protein displacement interactions are rarely of clinical significance. Pharmacology 18: 225-227, 1979

Sellers EM. Drug displacement interactions: a case study of the phenylbutazone-warfarin interaction. In Reidenberg (Ed.) Drug protein binding, pp. 257-273, Praeger Publishers, New York, 1984

Sellers EM, Koch-Weser J. Potentiation of warfarin-induced hypoprothrombinemia by chloral hydrate. New England Journal of Medicine 283: 827-831, 1970

Sellers EM, Koch-Weser J. Kinetics and clinical importance of displacement of warfarin from albumin by acidic drugs. Annals of the New York Academy of Sciences 179: 213-224, 1977

Sellers EM, Lang M, Koch-Weser J, Colman RW. Enhancement of warfarin-induced hypoprothrombinemia by triclofos. Clinical Pharmacology and Therapeutics 13: 911-915, 1972

Serlin MJ, Mossman S, Sibeon RG, Tempero KF, Breckenridge AM. Interaction between diflunisal and warfarin. Clinical Pharmacology and Therapeutics 28: 493-498, 1980

Shand DG, Mitchell JR, Oates JA. Pharmacokinetic drug interactions. In Gillette et al. (Eds) Handbook of experimental pharmacology: concepts in biochemical pharmacology, Vol. 28/3, pp. 272-314, Springer-Verlag, New York, 1975

Stoeckel K, Trueb V, Buback UC, McNamara PJ. Effect of probenecid on the elimination and protein binding of ceftriaxone. European Journal of Clinical Pharmacology 34: 151-156, 1988

Svensson CK, Woodruff MN, Lalka D. Influence of protein binding and use of unbound (free) drug concentrations. In Evans et al. (Eds) Applied pharmacokinetics, 2nd ed., pp. 187-219, Applied Therapeutics Inc., Spokane, WA, 1986

Sweeney KR, Chapron DJ, Brandt L, Gomolin IH, Feig PU, et al. Toxic interaction between acetazolamide and salicylate: case reports and a pharmacokinetic explanation. Clinical Pharmacology and Therapeutics 40: 518-524, 1986

Tsanaclis LM, Allen J, Perucca E, Routledge PA, Richens A. Effect of valproate on free plasma phenytoin concentrations. British Journal of Clinical Pharmacology 18: 17-20, 1984

Udall JA. Warfarin-chloral hydrate interaction. Pharmacological activity and clinical significance. Annals of Internal Medicine 81: 341-344, 1974

Udall JA. Clinical implications of warfarin interactions with five sedatives. American Journal of Cardiology 35: 67-71, 1975

Upton RA, Williams RL, Buskin JN, Jones RM. Effects of probenecid on ketoprofen kinetics. Clinical Pharmacology and Therapeutics 31: 705-712, 1982
Wesseling H, Mols-Thurkow I. Interaction of diphenylhydantoin (DPH) and tolbutamide in man. European Journal of Clinical Pharmacology 8: 75-78, 1975
Yacobi A, Udall JA, Levy G. Serum protein binding as a determinant of warfarin body clearance and anticoagulant effect. Clinical Pharmacology and Therapeutics 19: 552-558, 1975

Author's address: Dr *Janis J. MacKichan,* The Ohio State University, College of Pharmacy, 217 Parks Hall, 500 West 12th Avenue, Columbus, OH 43210 (USA).

Clinical Pharmacokinetics 16: 74-85 (1989)
0312-5963/89/0002-0074/$06.00/0

Clinical Pharmacokinetics of Clofazimine
A Review

Mack R. Holdiness

Lakeside Hospital, Metairie (New Orleans), Louisiana, USA

Contents

Summary 74
1. Analytical Methods 75
2. Fundamental Pharmacokinetic Properties 76
   2.1 Absorption 76
   2.2 Distribution 77
   2.3 Metabolism 77
   2.4 Excretion 79
3. Pharmacokinetics in Various Pathophysiological States 80
   3.1 Pregnancy 80
4. Implications of the Pharmacokinetic Properties for Therapeutic Use 81
   4.1 Dose and Therapeutic Range 81
   4.2 Side Effects 82
   4.3 Biochemical and Haematological Side Effects 82
5. Pharmacokinetic Drug Interactions 82
   5.1 Dapsone 82
   5.2 Oestrogen 83
   5.3 Rifampicin 83
   5.4 Vitamin A 83
6. Conclusions 83

Summary

Clofazimine is useful in the treatment of Hansen's disease (leprosy) and some dermatological disorders, and is currently being used in drug regimens for patients with human immunodeficiency viral infections who are also infected with Mycobacterium avium *complex.*

After an oral dose, absorption is variable, but when given in an oil-wax suspension is approximately 70%. Administration with food appears to increase the peak plasma drug concentration and reduce the time to peak level. Data on the volume of distribution and percentage or type of protein binding are not available; however, the drug undergoes extensive tissue distribution. Clofazimine does not cross the blood-brain barrier, but does cross the placenta, and is found in human breast milk.

To date 3 urinary metabolites have been identified in man, but their biological activity is unknown. A substantial portion of the unchanged drug is excreted in faeces. The elimination half-life is variable, with values as long as 70 days being quoted in the literature.

Frequently reported side effects of clofazimine are hyperpigmentation of the skin and conjunctiva, and abdominal pain. These resolve upon cessation of therapy. Biochemical and haematological adverse effects have been reported, but are generally not clinically relevant. Pharmacokinetic drug interactions of potential clinical significance have been observed with dapsone, oestrogen, rifampicin and vitamin A.

Clofazimine [3-(p-chloroanilino)-10-(p-chlorophenyl)-2, 10-dihydro-2-isopropyliminophenazine] is an antimycobacterial agent which has been in use since 1962 for the treatment of *Mycobacterium leprae* (Browne & Hogerzeil 1962). Due to the development of primary resistance to monotherapy with dapsone (World Health Organization 1977; Zuidema et al. 1986), it is now recommended that combination drug therapy be used for all cases of Hansen's disease (leprosy) [World Health Organization 1982]. Clofazimine is also recommended in the treatment of *Mycobacterium avium* complex which is increasingly observed in individuals with human immunodeficiency virus (HIV) infections (Centers for Disease Control 1986; Woods & Washington 1987; Young 1988). Clofazimine is useful in a number of dermatological disorders such as pyoderma gangrenosum (Holdiness 1985a; Rosmusen 1983), lupus erythematosus (Mackey 1976), prurigo nodularis (Belaube et al. 1983) and pustular psoriasis (Chuaprapcislis & Piamphongsant 1978). However, its efficacy in the treatment of *Mycobacterium ulcerans* is questionable (deBergeyck et al. 1980; Revill et al. 1973). The mechanism of action of clofazimine in each of the above disorders has not yet been fully elucidated.

Based upon estimates by Sansirricq (1983), approximately 10 to 12 million individuals in the world are infected with the *Mycobacterium leprae* organism. Asia has highest incidence (62% of the total number of cases), followed by Africa (34%), South America (3%), with the rest of the world accounting for about 1%. Thus, about 1 billion people live in areas where the prevalence of Hansen's disease is approximately one per thousand of the population (Noorden 1985).

By March 1988 a total of 55,315 adults with HIV infections had been reported in the United States alone (Centers for Disease Control 1988). *Mycobacterium avium* complex, a frequent pathogen in these patients, has been observed to occur in up to 40% of those individuals autopsied at the National Institutes of Health (Masur et al. 1987). Thus, the potential number of patients who can benefit from clofazimine treatment is quite large.

Primary drugs available for treatment of Hansen's disease include dapsone, rifampicin, clofazimine and a combination of ethionamide/prothionamide. Secondary drugs consist of thioacetazone (amithiozone), thiambutosine, long acting sulphonamides such as sulphamethoxypridazine and certain aminoglycosides, especially streptomycin and kanamycin (Jacobson 1985). Most of these agents are also suitable for use against *Mycobacterium tuberculosis*.

This article deals with the clinical pharmacokinetics, therapeutic use, drug interactions and side effects of clofazimine. In addition, a review of the analytical techniques used to measure the drug in biological tissues is also presented.

1. Analytical Methods

Table I contains a list of analytical methods and their limits of detection. Early non-chromatographic procedures used spectrophotometric determination for clofazimine, at its wavelength of maximum absorption (530nm) [Barry et al. 1960]. Production of a fluorescent derivative by reduction with titanous chloride has also been performed (Dill et al. 1970).

Chromatographic procedures have also been used to analyse clofazimine. Lanyi and Dubois (1982) developed a thin layer chromatographic technique with densitometric detection. Using high performance liquid chromatography (HPLC), with ultraviolet detection, Gidoh and Tsutsumi (1981) separated clofazimine from dapsone, and rifampicin on a reversed phase column. However, the procedure involves a complicated extraction scheme, with the switching of 2 different mobile phases in order to allow complete resolution of clo-

Table I. Analytical techniques and detection limits for clofazimine

Method	Limit of detection (μg/L)	Medium	Reference
Spectrophotometric	100	Serum	Barry et al. (1960)
Spectrophotometric	100 mg/kg	Tissue	Mansfield (1974)
Fluorometric	100	Serum	Dill et al. (1970)
HPLC (UV detection)	10	Serum	Gidoh et al. (1981)
HPLC (UV detection)	10	Plasma	Peters et al. (1982)
TLC	5	Plasma	Lanyi & Dubois (1982)

Abbreviations: HPLC = high performance liquid chromatography; TLC = thin layer chromatography; UV = ultraviolet.

fazimine from related components. The latter assay was applied to animal models only. The HPLC method reported by Peters et al. (1982) involved separation of the drug into an organic solvent prior to chromatography. Mass spectrometry was used to confirm the specific separation of clofazimine from simultaneously administered antibiotics such as dapsone, rifampicin and ethionamide. Unfortunately, the disadvantage of all these chromatographic methods is that suitable internal standard(s) are not currently available.

2. *Fundamental Pharmacokinetic Properties*

2.1 Absorption

Studies on the human pharmacokinetics of clofazimine are limited. Plasma concentration data from a few reported studies are presented in table II. Absorption varies considerably from patient to patient. When the drug is administered as coarse crystals in a capsule only about 20% is absorbed, whereas, if it is taken orally, as a microcrystalline suspension in an oil-wax base, an absorption rate of 70% can be achieved (Yawalkar & Vischer 1979).

Schaad-Lanyi et al. (1987) studied the pharmacokinetics of single oral doses of clofazimine for 1 to 264 hours after administration. Following a 200mg tablet (after a breakfast of fats and proteins) the peak plasma drug concentation (C_{max}) was 0.41 mg/L, with a time to C_{max} (t_{max}) of 8 hours (fig. 1). In another experiment in the same study, the drug was administered to 3 volunteers either with or without food for a comparison of bioavailability. Mean area under the concentration/time curve (AUC) and C_{max} with food were 62 and 30% higher, respectively. The median t_{max} was 8 hours with food and 12 hours without food. This suggests the bioavailability of clofazimine is increased when concomitantly administered with food (fig. 2). Following the administration of clofazimine 50mg daily, steady-state plasma concentrations were not achieved by the 8th day (Schaad-Lanyi et al. 1987). This finding is consistent with the long elimination half-life estimated from a number of single-dose studies (see section 2.4). No data exist on steady-state concentrations. It is estimated to take approximately 70 days to achieve steady-state but this is purely an estimate. Data on loading dose are not available, nor as yet are established data on plasma concentration and therapeutic effect.

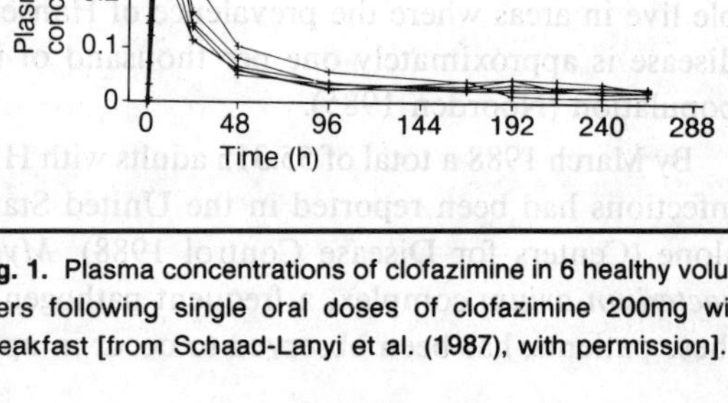

Fig. 1. Plasma concentrations of clofazimine in 6 healthy volunteers following single oral doses of clofazimine 200mg with breakfast [from Schaad-Lanyi et al. (1987), with permission].

There is currently no information on the pharmacokinetics of clofazimine following intravenous administration. In addition, it is not known how the absorption pharmacokinetics are altered in patients following administration of antacids or surgical procedures.

2.2 Distribution

There are no data available concerning volume of distribution or percentage or type of protein binding of clofazimine. Table III contains data of concentrations found in specific organs and tissues (the drug had been previously administered in a range of 200 to 300 mg/day for all studies, for undetermined variable lengths of time). Clofazimine does not appear to cross the intact blood-brain barrier (Desikan & Balakrishnan 1976; Mansfield 1974). Clofazimine crystals have been found in mesenteric lymph nodes of 1 patient 4 years after discontinuation of treatment (Jopling 1976). Cutaneous pigmentation usually disappears within 6 to 12 months as clofazimine leaches from the skin. Clofazimine is highly lipophilic and distributed principally to fatty tissue, and also taken up by macrophages throughout the body.

2.3 Metabolism

Limited information is available concerning the metabolism of clofazimine. Feng et al. (1981, 1982) used mass spectrometry to identify 3 urinary metabolites in humans: 3-(p-hydroxyanilino)-10-(p-chlorophenyl)-2,10-dihydro-2-isopropyliminophenazine (metabolite I), and two conjugated compounds, 3-(β-D-glucopyransiduronic acid)-10-(p-chlorophenyl)-2,10-dihydro-2-isopropyliminophenazine) [metabolite II] and 3-(p-chloroanilino)-10-(p-chlorophenyl)-4,10-dihydro-4-(β-D-glucopyranosiduronic acid)-2-isopropyliminophenazine (metabolite III) [fig. 3]. Metabolite I is believed to be formed by a hydrolytic dehalogenation reaction, metabolite II by hydrolytic deamination followed

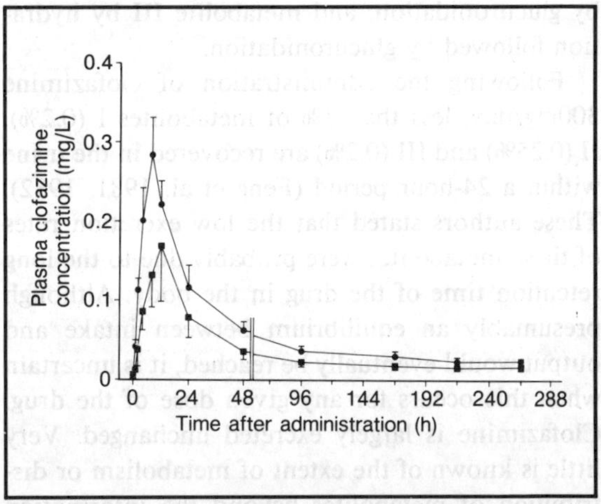

Fig. 2. Mean plasma concentrations of clofazimine after a single 200mg dose in healthy volunteers. ■ = fasted volunteers (n = 3); ● = 10 minutes after breakfast (n = 3) [from Schaad-Lanyi et al. (1987), with permission].

Table II. Fundamental pharmacokinetic properties of clofazimine: absorption and plasma concentration data

Dosage (mg)	No. of patients	Duration of treatment[a]	C_{max} (mg/L)	t_{max} (h)	Reference
100 × 3/week	17	4 years	0.50	1-6	Banerjee et al. (1974)
100 daily	17	4 years	0.70	1-6	
300 daily	17	4 years	1.00	1-6	
400 daily	17	4 years	1.40	1-6	
300 daily	5	197 days	1.30	NS	Levy (1974)
200 × 1 dose on empty stomach	3	Single dose on day 1	0.22	12	Schaad-Lanyi et al. (1987)
200 × 1 dose with breakfast	6	Single dose on day 1	0.41	8	

a Duration of treatment before measurement of plasma concentration.

Abbreviations: C_{max} = peak plasma concentration; t_{max} = time to C_{max}; NS = not stated.

by glucuronidation, and metabolite III by hydration followed by glucuronidation.

Following the administration of clofazimine 300mg/day, less than 1% of metabolites I (0.2%), II (0.25%) and III (0.2%) are recovered in the urine within a 24-hour period (Feng et al. 1981, 1982). These authors stated that the low excretion rates of these metabolites were probably due to the long retention time of the drug in the body. Although presumably an equilibrium between intake and output would eventually be reached, it is uncertain when this occurs for any given dose of the drug. Clofazimine is largely excreted unchanged. Very little is known of the extent of metabolism or distribution of metabolites beyond the information published by Feng et al. (1981, 1982). These authors did not investigate further, nor have any data been published since. No data exist on the pharmacological activity of metabolites, or whether they are found in faeces or bile.

Feng et al. (1981, 1982) have apparently demonstrated that metabolite III has been produced in the laboratory from metabolism by liver enzymes (not a model). However, it appears that they were unable to demonstrate the same hepatic conversion of clofazimine to metabolites I and II, although it is difficult to ascertain how rigorously they pursued this experiment. Therefore, they suggest the possibility exists that metabolites I and II may have been produced by degradation by bacteria in the intestine, before absorption and urinary excretion.

Table III. Fundamental pharmacokinetic properties of clofazimine (range 200 to 300 mg/day): tissue distribution

Organ	No. of patients	C_T (mg/g)	Reference
Liver	4	0.18-3.2	Desikan & Balakrishnan (1976); Mansfield (1974)
Spleen	3ᵃ	0.6-1.0	Desikan & Balakrishnan (1976); Mansfield (1974)
Small bowel	1	2.1	Desikan & Balakrishnan (1976)
Lung	4	0.17-1.4	Desikan & Balakrishnan (1976); Mansfield (1974)
Kidney	4	0.04-1.4	Desikan & Balakrishnan (1976); Mansfield (1974)
Omentum	1	0.35	Desikan & Balakrishnan (1976)
Mesenteric lymph nodes	3	1.0-3.30	Desikan & Balakrishnan (1976); Mansfield (1974)
Subcutaneous fat	4	2.1-5.3	Mansfield (1974)
Brain	4	Not detected	Desikan & Balakrishnan (1976); Mansfield (1974)
Adrenal glands	1	2.0	Mansfield (1974)
Gall bladder	2	2.0-3.6	Mansfield (1974)
Heart	3	0.3-1.5	Mansfield (1974)
Peripheral nerves	1	1.7	Mansfield (1974)
Pancreas	2	0.8	Mansfield (1974)
Eye (anterior chamber)	1	1.1	Mansfield (1974)
Skin (non-ichthyotic)	56	0.007-3.6	Mansfield (1974); Bharadwaj (1982)
Skin (ichthyotic)	53	0.014-0.070	Bharadwaj (1982)
Placenta; breast milk	15	Not detected	Farb et al. (1982); Holdiness (1988d)

Abbreviation: C_T = drug concentration in tissue.

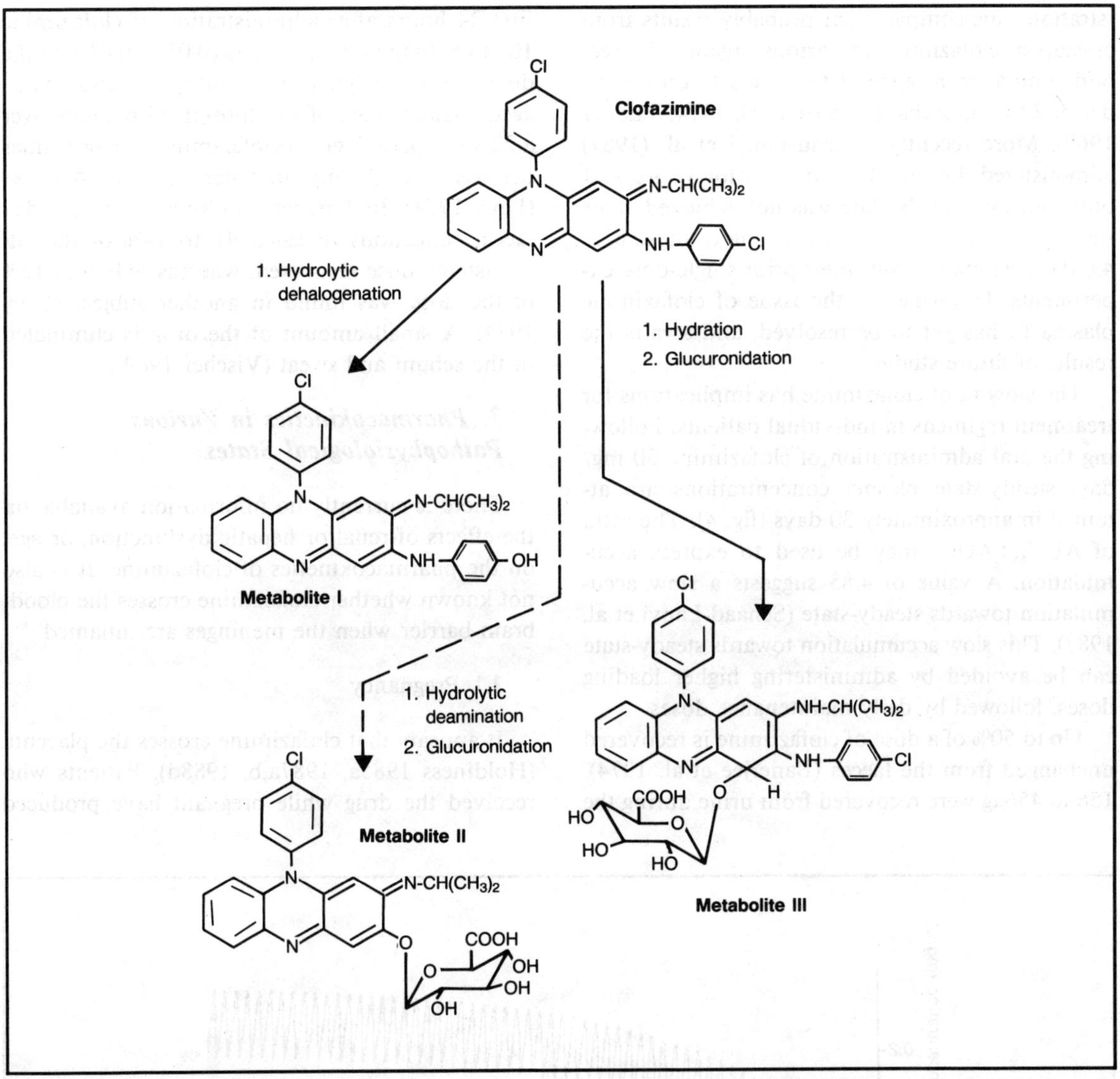

Fig. 3. Metabolic pathways of clofazimine in humans [from Feng et al. (1981, 1982), with permission].

2.4 Excretion

The elimination half-life ($t_{1/2}$) of clofazimine is a complex issue as yet unresolved. Clofazimine tends to remain for a long time in human tissues (fatty tissues, skin, lymph nodes, macrophages, intestines, adrenal glands and spleen), and is eliminated slowly. An earlier report indicates plasma $t_{1/2}$ to be approximately 70 days (Levy 1974). However, this figure must be considered with caution since it was only a rough estimate, based upon urinary excretion data. In experimental models, the drug appears to occupy 2 compartments, pharmacodynamically. One compartment is evident with relatively low-dose short term administration and has a plasma $t_{1/2}$ of approximately 1 week (Hastings et al. 1976; Levy 1974). A second compartment is evident with long term, high-dose administration; this compartment probably results from crystals of clofazimine in various organs. The second compartment appears to have a $t_{1/2}$ on the order of 2 to 3 months (Banerjee et al. 1974; Vischer 1969). More recently, Schaad-Lanyi et al. (1987) administered clofazimine 50 mg/day for 8 days, and observed that steady-state was not achieved. This finding was consistent with the long $t_{1/2}$ of 10.6 ± 4.0 days estimated from their prior single-dose experiments. Nevertheless, the issue of clofazimine plasma $t_{1/2}$ has yet to be resolved, and awaits the results of future studies.

The slow $t_{1/2}$ of clofazimine has implications for treatment regimens in individual patients. Following the oral administration of clofazimine 50 mg/day, steady-state plasma concentrations are attained in approximately 30 days (fig. 4). The ratio of $AUC_{SS}:AUC_1$ may be used to express accumulation. A value of 4.85 suggests a slow accumulation towards steady-state (Schaad-Lanyi et al. 1987). This slow accumulation towards steady-state can be avoided by administering higher loading doses, followed by daily maintenance doses.

Up to 50% of a dose of clofazimine is recovered unchanged from the faeces (Banerjee et al. 1974). 156 to 456μg were recovered from urine during the first 24 hours after administration of clofazimine 100 to 600mg in 2 volunteers (0.03 to 0.41% of the dose, respectively). Daily urinary excretion averaged 132μg (0.08% of the dose) in 17 patients over a 23-week period, given clofazimine 100mg 3 times per week to 1200mg once per week for 4 weeks (Levy 1974). In 1 patient multiple (n = 3) 3 day faecal collections revealed 41 to 74% of the administered dose recovered, whereas only 9 to 12% of the dose was found in another subject (Levy 1974). A small amount of the drug is eliminated in the sebum and sweat (Vischer 1969).

3. Pharmacokinetics in Various Pathophysiological States

There is currently no information available on the effects of renal or hepatic dysfunction, or age, on the pharmacokinetics of clofazimine. It is also not known whether clofazimine crosses the blood-brain barrier when the meninges are inflamed.

3.1 Pregnancy

It appears that clofazimine crosses the placenta (Holdiness 1985a, 1987a,b, 1988d). Patients who received the drug while pregnant have produced

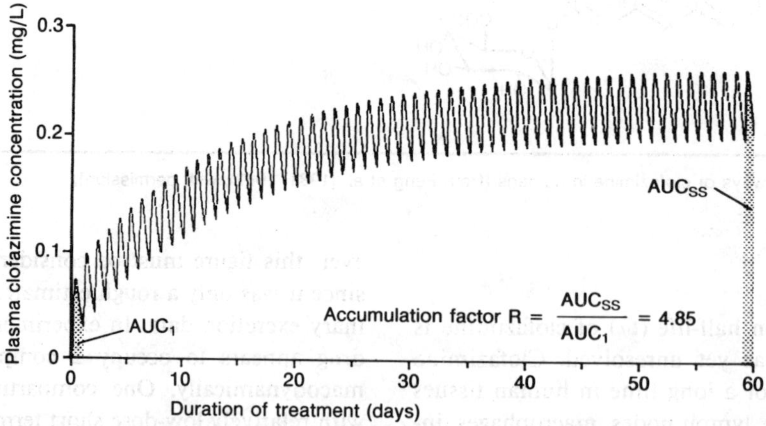

Fig. 4. Predicted clofazimine plasma concentration following single daily oral doses of 50mg [from Schaad-Lanyi et al. (1987), with permission].

offspring with a somewhat darker skin colour than could be accounted for by ethnic background (Farb et al. 1981; Holdiness 1988d; Karat 1975). In addition, mothers who did not breast-feed the neonates observed gradual fading of pigmentation over a 1-year period. In contrast, patients who received clofazimine after childbirth, and breast-fed their children, noted that the infants developed a ruddy colour to the skin (Browne & Hogerzeil 1962). The colour again faded following discontinuation of breast-feeding.

4. Implications of the Pharmacokinetic Properties for Therapeutic Use

4.1 Dose and Therapeutic Range

The World Health Organization (1982) has published guidelines for treatment of Hansen's disease. Dosage recommendations, for the most part, are not related to serum/plasma concentrations or pharmacokinetic data. Paucibacillary patients would be treated with dapsone 100mg daily, unsupervised, plus rifampicin 600mg once monthly, supervised, for 6 months; at that point all therapy would be discontinued. Multibacillary patients would be given dapsone 100mg and clofazimine 50mg daily, unsupervised, with rifampicin 600mg and clofazimine 300mg given once monthly under supervision. It is recommended that treatment be continued for at least 2 years, and preferably until the bacterial index becomes negative. The multibacillary regimen might also be supplemented by the addition of a supervised dose of ethionamide/prothionamide 500mg once monthly, but the efficacy of this has yet to be established. Patients refusing to take the clofazimine (because of its adverse cutaneous reaction) are recommended to replace it with ethionamide/prothionamide 250 to 375mg (Jacobson 1985; World Health Organization 1982).

Clofazimine has also been recommended for the treatment of HIV patients with disseminated *Mycobacterium avium* complex (Armstrong et al. 1985; Centers for Disease Control 1986; Greene et al. 1982; Hawkins et al. 1986; Holdiness 1984b; Horsburgh et al. 1984; Woods & Washington 1987; Yajko et al. 1987; Young 1988). Again, dosage was based upon empirical characteristics and clinical response. Greene et al. (1982) noted that the minimum inhibitory concentration of these isolates in 4 patients was 2.0 to 5.0 mg/L. Hawkins et al. (1986) observed 62 isolates from this type of patient to be 100% susceptible to a drug concentration of 1 mg/L. However, the potential benefit from use of this agent is still controversial. Some patients with disseminated *Mycobacterium avium* complex have responded poorly to treatment with clofazimine, despite a good *in vitro* response. Yajko et al. (1987) demonstrated with killing curve experiments that the concentration of clofazimine needed to kill 2 log units of *Mycobacterium avium* was at least 32 times greater than the concentrations needed to inhibit growth. Little or no killing occurred at concentrations achievable in plasma. Masur et al. (1987) reported results of the combined effects of clofazimine and ansamycin therapy on *Mycobacterium avium.* 13 individuals were given clofazimine 100mg daily with either 150 or 300mg of ansamycin each day. Combination therapy with these drugs, with or without other antimycobacterial agents such as amikacin, isoniazid, *para*-aminosalicylic acid, ethionamide, streptomycin, ethambutol, kanamycin, rifampicin, cycloserine and pyrazinamide, was not very effective in eradicating infection. In the study of Masur et al. (1987), bacteraemia persisted for a median of 92 days in all 13 patients. Only 2 of 13 patients ultimately demonstrated 2 or more consecutive negative blood cultures. The conversion to culture negativity correlated with clinical improvement (decreased fever, weight gain) in only 1 patient. Since clofazimine appears to require several weeks to months to saturate tissues, it may fail to reach inhibitory plasma concentrations during the initial months of therapy.

Recently, Young (1988) has identified a combination of clofazimine (50 to 100 mg/day) and amikacin (7.5 mg/kg intramuscularly or intravenously every 12 hours) to be an effective regimen when used concomitantly with conventional doses of ethambutol (15 to 25 mg/kg/day) and rifampicin (600 mg/day). Unfortunately, well-controlled study data are lacking in the literature at present. It is hoped that future studies will better define the role of clofazimine in combination chemotherapy as effective treatment for disseminated *Mycobacterium avium* complex in HIV patients.

4.2 Side Effects

The most frequently reported side effects of clofazimine therapy are red-brown hyperpigmentation of the skin and conjunctiva, and abdominal pain (Granstein & Sober 1981; Hastings et al. 1976; Jopling 1976; Moore 1983; Negrel et al. 1984; Venencie et al. 1986; Yawalkar & Vischer 1979). Skin and conjunctival pigmentation occurred in 64.6% and 49.2%, respectively, of 57 patients taking up to 700 mg/week (Moore 1983). Cutaneous pigmentation normally fades within 6 to 12 months, although a few examples have been reported to have lasted for as long as 5 years. Discoloration of sweat, hair, sputum, urine and faeces has also been observed (Yawalkar & Vischer 1979). Generalised xeroderma (30%), ichthyosis, pruritis, phototoxicity, acneiform eruptions, exfoliative dermatitis and nonspecific rashes have been reported (Pavithran 1985; Yawalkar & Vischer 1979). Negrel et al. (1984) monitored 57 patients treated with standard doses of the drug (100 to 300 mg/day) for 3 to 26 months. Apart from brown-red subepithelial pigmentation in the cornea, no other untoward effects on the eye were recorded. Interestingly, clofazimine crystals were found in the tears of 82% of the patients.

Gastrointestinal side effects (nausea, diarrhoea, anorexia, constipation and weight loss) have also been noted (Hastings et al. 1976; Moore 1983). The fact that this drug accumulates partly in a crystalline form has given rise to a number of cases of gastrointestinal and other complications. This has been reviewed extensively elsewhere (Jopling 1976). The true answer may never be known, but nonspecific granulomas have been noted in foreign body giant cell formation which may lead to extreme congestion of the mucosa and possibly produce these symptoms.

Giddiness and transient haematuria associated with a decrease in creatinine clearance have been noted (Working Party on B663, 1968). Clofazimine also displays anti-inflammatory effects which are clinically valuable in controlling erythema nodosum leprosum reactions occurring in the multibacillary forms of Hansen's disease (Browne et al. 1981; Yawalkar & Vischer 1979), and in patients with reactions in the borderline to tuberculoid forms of disease (Pfaltzgraff 1972).

4.3 Biochemical and Haematological Side Effects

Hastings et al. (1976) studied 51 patients receiving long term clofazimine therapy (50 to 300 mg/day for at least 24 months continuously) who had undergone systematic clinical laboratory testing for possible signs of toxicity. In approximately 220 patient-years of observations, no statistically significant abnormalities were noted in: aspartate aminotransferase (AST); thymol turbidity; serum globulins; uric acid; alkaline phosphatase; white blood cell count or differential count; haemoglobin; haematocrit; blood urea nitrogen; serum creatinine, cholesterol, albumin, potassium or calcium; stool for occult blood; routine urinalysis or reticulocyte count. Statistically significant changes towards abnormality were found in fasting blood sugar and total serum bilirubin. These changes were small in magnitude, and were not associated with related clinical signs or symptoms and did not appear to be of major clinical significance.

5. Pharmacokinetic Drug Interactions

Only a few pharmacokinetic drug interactions involving clofazimine have been observed to date. However, as the drug continues to be used in combination therapy for HIV patients, clinically relevant interactions may well be reported in the future.

5.1 Dapsone

The majority of studies suggest that clofazimine does not influence dapsone excretion (Venkatesan et al. 1980, 1986; Zuidema et al. 1986). However,

Grabosz and Wheate (1975) observed an increase in the urinary excretion of dapsone in 8 of 17 patients studied.

5.2 Oestrogen

Duncan and Oakey (1983) reported that clofazimine 300mg daily diminished oestrogen excretion in a pregnant patient concomitantly receiving dapsone and prednisolone. Furthermore, according to the same authors, in 3 other pregnant women receiving clofazimine (300 mg/week), assays indicated that 85% (5 of 6 assay values) of oestrogen levels were subnormal relative to the lower limit of excretion previously reported for healthy European women at the same gestational stage.

5.3 Rifampicin

The effect of clofazimine 300 mg/day and dapsone 50 to 100 mg/day on the pharmacokinetics of dapsone and rifampicin 600 mg/day in multibacillary and paucibacillary individuals has recently been reported by Mehta et al. (1986). No statistically significant differences were noted in the following pharmacokinetic parameters of rifampicin: Ke, Ka, AUC, Vd, t_{max}, metabolic clearance rate, plasma $t_{1/2}$, C_{max} and AUC/$t_{1/2}$, suggesting that the type of Hansen's disease had no effect upon the pharmacokinetic parameters of rifampicin. However, absorption of rifampicin was less in patients with Hansen's disease than in healthy human volunteers (Acocella 1978; Holdiness 1984a; Kenny & Strates 1981). Whether this difference was due to decreased absorption in the gastrointestinal tract in patients with Hansen's disease or to lower levels of plasma proteins is difficult to say, due to the paucity of data.

Clofazimine reduced rifampicin absorption significantly, resulting in delayed time to reach peak serum concentrations (3.84 ± 0.12 *vs* 2.95 ± 0.16h) and increased $t_{1/2}$ (4.23 ± 0.25 *vs* 3.8 ± 0.36h). However, no significant changes were seen in AUC or C_{max}. Further studies are needed to determine the interval required between administration of clofazimine and rifampicin to obviate interference with the absorption of the latter.

5.4 Vitamin A

Ichthyosis eventually developed in 53 patients with lepromatous Hansen's disease receiving clofazimine therapy over varying periods (Bharadwaj et al. 1982). Six individuals with ichthyosis who were not taking clofazimine were included for comparison. Clofazimine concentrations and vitamin A levels were estimated in ichthyotic and non-ichthyotic areas of the skin of these patients. Clofazimine concentrations in the skin increased with duration of treatment (at least up to 24 months) in both types of skin, with an average of 26.6 ± 8.1 μg/g wet tissue non-ichthyotic compared with 70.9 ± 25.9 μg/g wet tissue in healthy subjects. The levels of vitamin A, on the other hand, showed a decrease of 0.969 mg/100g wet tissue vitamin A (non-ichthyotic skin) *versus* 0.348 ± 0.05 mg/100g wet tissue (ichthyotic skin) at 24 months. Plasma levels of vitamin A also decreased with increased duration of treatment with clofazimine. The ichthyotic skin of patients who did not receive clofazimine therapy contained higher levels of vitamin A than those on clofazimine therapy. This experiment suggests that a decreased level of vitamin A occurs in the skin of Hansen's disease patients, and that this deficiency appears to be aggravated by clofazimine treatment.

Further studies are necessary to explain this inverse relationship between clofazimine and vitamin A in the skin.

6. Conclusions

Clofazimine has proved to be an invaluable agent in the treatment of Hansen's disease. Its spectrum of use has also included various dermatological disorders, and recently combination chemotherapy for *Mycobacterium avium* complex infections in HIV patients. Limited information is currently available concerning its metabolism and certain aspects of its pharmacokinetic nature in man. However, it is to be hoped that, as further studies are performed, the pharmacokinetics of clofazimine will be fully elucidated.

References

Acocella G. Clinical pharmacokinetics of rifampicin. Clinical Pharmacokinetics 3: 108-127, 1978

Armstrong D, Gold JWM, Dryjanski J, Whimbey E, Polsky B, et al. Treatment of infections in patients with the acquired immunodeficiency syndrome. Annals of Internal Medicine 103: 738-743, 1985

Baciewicz AM, Self TM. Rifampicin drug interactions. Southern Medical Journal 78: 714-718, 1985

Baciewicz AM, Self TM, Bekemeyer WB. Update on rifampicin drug interactions. Archives of Internal Medicine 147: 565-568, 1987

Bajaj AK, Gupta SC, Sinha SN, Govil DC, Gaur UC. Renal functional status in lepromatous leprosy. International Journal of Leprosy 49: 37-41, 1981

Banerjee DK, Ellard GA, Gammon PT, Waters MFR. Some observations on the pharmacology of clofazimine (B663). American Journal of Tropical Medicine and Hygiene 23: 1110-1119, 1974

Barry VC, Buggle K, Byrne J, Conalty ML, Winder F. Absorption, distribution and retention of amino-compounds in the experimental animal. Irish Journal of Medical Science 416: 345-352, 1960

Belaube P, Devaux J, Pizzi M, Boutboul R, Privat Y. Small bowel deposition of crystals associated with the use of clofazimine in the treatment of prurigo nodularis. International Journal of Leprosy 51: 328-330, 1983

Bharadwaj VP, Sritharan V, Venkatesan K, Girdhar A, Ramu G. Vitamin A levels of ichthyotic and non-ichthyotic skin and plasma of leprosy patients with and without clofazimine therapy. Indian Journal of Medical Research 75: 773-777, 1982

Browne SG, Harman DJ, Waudby A, McDougall AC. Clofazimine the treatment of lepromatous leprosy in the United Kingdom: a 12 year review of 31 cases, 1966-1978. International Journal of Leprosy 49: 167-176, 1981

Browne SG, Hogerzeil LM. B663 in the treatment of leprosy: preliminary report of a pilot trial. Leprosy Review 33: 6-16, 1962

Centers for Disease Control. Diagnosis and management of mycobacterial infection and disease in persons with human T-lymphotrophic virus type III/lymphadenopathy associated virus infection. Morbidity Mortality Weekly 35: 448-452, 1986

Centers for Disease Control. AIDS and HIV among health care workers. Morbidity Mortality Weekly 37: 229-234, 1988

Chuaprapcislis T, Piamphongsant T. Treatment of pustular psoriasis with clofazimine. British Journal of Dermatology 99: 303-305, 1978

deBergeyck E, Janssens PG, de Muynck A. Radiological abnormalities of the ileum associated with the use of clofazimine in the treatment of skin ulceration due to *Mycobacterium ulcerans*. Leprosy Review 51: 221-228, 1980

Desikan KV, Balakrishnan S. Tissue levels of clofazimine in a case of leprosy. Leprosy Reviews 47: 107-113, 1976

Dill WA, Chricot L, Glazkio AJ. A new analytical procedure for B663 (clofazimine). International Journal of Leprosy 38: 355-356, 1970

Duncan ME, Oakey RE. Reduced estrogen excretion due to clofazimine. International Journal of Leprosy 51: 112-113, 1983

Farb H, West DP, Pedvis-Leftick A. Clofazimine in pregnancy complicated by leprosy. Obstetrics and Gynecology 59: 122-123, 1982

Feng PCC, Fenselau CC, Jacobson RR. Metabolism of clofazimine in leprosy patients. Drug Metabolism and Disposition 9: 521-524, 1981

Feng PCC, Fenselau CC, Jacobson RR. A new urinary metabolite of clofazimine in leprosy patients. Drug Metabolism and Disposition 10: 286-288, 1982

Fenselau CC, Pallante S, Parikh I. Solid phase synthesis of drug glucuronides by immobilized glucuronosyltransferase. Journal of Medicinal Chemistry 19: 679-683, 1976

Grabosz JAJ, Wheate HW. Effect of clofazimine on the urinary excretion of dapsone. International Journal of Leprosy 43: 61-62, 1975

Granstein RD, Sober AJ. Drug and heavy metal-induced hyperpigmentation. Journal of the American Academy of Dermatology 5: 1-18, 1981

Greene JB, Sidhu GS, Lewin S, Levine JF, Masur H, et al. *Mycobacterium avium-intracellulare*: a cause of disseminated life threatening infection in homosexuals and drug abusers. Annals of Internal Medicine 97: 539-546, 1982

Gidoh M, Tsutsumi S. Determination of 3 main antileprosy drugs and their metabolites in serum by HPLC. Journal of Chromatography – Biomedical Applications 223: 379-392, 1981

Hastings RC, Jacobson RR, Trautman JR. Long term clinical toxicity studies with clofazimine in leprosy. International Journal of Leprosy 44: 287-293, 1976

Hawkins CC, Gold JWM, Whimbey E, Kiehn TE, Brannon P, et al. *Mycobacterium avium* complex infection in patients with the acquired immunodeficiency syndrome. Annals of Internal Medicine 105: 184-188, 1986

Holdiness MR. Clinical pharmacokinetics of the antituberculosis drugs: a review. Clinical Pharmacokinetics 9: 511-544, 1984a

Holdiness MR. *Mycobacterium avium-intracellulare* infection. Southern Medical Journal 77: 1614, 1984b

Holdiness MR. Adverse cutaneous reactions to antituberculosis drugs: a review. International Journal of Dermatology 24: 280-285, 1985a

Holdiness MR. Cerebrospinal fluid pharmacokinetics of the antituberculosis drugs. Clinical Pharmacokinetics 10: 532-534, 1985b

Holdiness MR. Rifampicin adverse cutaneous reactions. International Journal of Dermatology 25: 72-73, 1986a

Holdiness MR. Contact dermatitis to ethambutol. Contact Dermatitis 15: 96-97, 1986b

Holdiness MR. Contact dermatitis to the antituberculosis drugs: a review. Contact Dermatitis 15: 282-288, 1986c

Holdiness MR. Neurological manifestations and toxicities of the antituberculosis drugs: a review. Medical Toxicology 2: 33-51, 1987a

Holdiness MR. Teratology of the antituberculosis drugs: a review. Early Human Development 15: 61-74, 1987b

Holdiness MR. Transplacental pharmacokinetics of the antituberculosis drugs. Clinical Pharmacokinetics 13: 125-129, 1987c

Holdiness MR. A review of iatrogenic nutritional deficiencies induced by antituberculosis drugs. Nutrition Research 7: 891-900, 1987d

Holdiness MR. Rifampicin drug interactions. Archives of Internal Medicine 147: 1856, 1987e

Holdiness MR. Blood dyscrasias induced by the antituberculosis drugs: a review. Tubercle 68: 301-309, 1987f

Holdiness MR. Ethionamide. In Dollery C. (Ed.) Therapeutic drugs: a clinical pharmacopoeia, Churchill Livingstone, Edinburgh, 1988a

Holdiness MR. Prothionamide. In Dollery C. (Ed.) Therapeutic drugs: a clinical pharmacopoeia, Churchill Livingstone, Edinburgh, 1988b

Holdiness MR. Thiacetazone. In Dollery C. (Ed.) Therapeutic drugs: a clinical pharmacopoeia, Churchill Livingstone, Edinburgh, 1988c

Holdiness MR. Clofazimine in pregnancy. Early Human Development 16: in press, 1988d

Horsburgh CR, Mason UG, Farhi DC, Iseman MD. Disseminated infection with *Mycobacterium avium-intracellulare.* Medicine 64: 36-48, 1984
Jacobson RR. Treatment. In Hastings (Ed.) Leprosy, pp. 193-222, Churchill Livingstone, Edinburgh, 1985
Jopling WH. Complications of treatment of clofazimine. Leprosy Review 47: 1-3, 1976
Karat ABA. Long term follow up of clofazimine in the management of reactive phases of leprosy. Leprosy Review 46s: 105-109, 1975
Kenny MT, Strates B. Metabolism and pharmacokinetics of the antibiotic rifampicin. Drug Metabolism Review 12: 159-218, 1981
Lanyi Z, Dubois JP. Determination of clofazimine in human plasma by TLC. Journal of Chromatography – Biomedical Applications 232: 219-223, 1982
Levy L. Pharmacologic studies of clofazimine. American Journal of Tropical Medicine and Hygiene 23: 1097-1109, 1974
Mackey JP. Clofazimine in dermatology. International Journal of Dermatology 15: 140-141, 1976
Mansfield RE. Tissue concentrations of clofazimine in man. American Journal of Tropical Medicine and Hygiene 23: 1116-1119, 1974
Masur H, Tuazon C, Gill V, Grimes G, Baird B, et al. Effect of combined clofazimine and ansamycin therapy on *Mycobacterium avium-Mycobacterium intracellulare* bacteremia in patients with AIDS. Journal of Infectious Diseases 155: 127-129, 1987
Mehta J, Gandhi IS, Sane SB, Wamburkar MN. Effects of clofazimine and dapsone of rifampicin pharmacokinetics in multibacillary leprosy cases. Leprosy Review 57s: 67-76, 1986
Moore VJ. A review of side effects experienced by patients taking clofazimine. Leprosy Review 54: 327-335, 1983
Negrel AD, Chovet M, Baquillon G, Lagadec R. Clofazimine and the eye: preliminary communication. Leprosy Review 55: 349-352, 1984
Noorden SK. The epidemiology of leprosy. In Hastings R. (Ed.) Leprosy, pp. 15-30, Churchill Livingstone, Edinburgh, 1985
Parikh I, MacGlashan DW, Fenselau CC. Immobilized glucuronsyltransferase for the synthesis of conjugates. Journal of Medicinal Chemistry 19: 296-299, 1976
Pavithran K. Exfoliative dermatitis after clofazimine. International Journal of Leprosy 53: 645-646, 1985
Peters JH, Hamme KJ, Gordon GR. Determination of clofazimine in plasma by HPLC. Journal of Chromatography – Biomedical Applications 229: 503-508, 1982
Pfaltzgraff RE. The control of neuritis in leprosy with clofazimine. International Journal of Leprosy 40: 392-398, 1972
Revill WDL, Morrow RH, Pike MC, Ateng J. A controlled trial of the treatment of *Mycobacterium ulcerans* infection with clofazimine. Lancet 2: 873-877, 1973
Rosmusen I. Pyoderma gangrenosum treatment with clofazimine. Clinical evaluation of 7 cases. Acta Dermato-Venereologica 63: 552-553, 1983
Sansarricq H. Leprosy in the world today. Leprosy Review 54s: 7-16, 1983
Schaad-Lanyi Z, Dieterle W, Dubois JP, Theobald W, Vischer W. Pharmacokinetics of clofazimine in healthy human volunteers. International Journal of Leprosy 55: 9-15, 1987
Venencie PY, Cortez A, Orieux G, Jost JL, Chomette G, et al. Clofazimine enteropathy. Journal of the American Academy of Dermatology 15: 290-291, 1986
Venkatesan K, Bharadwaj VP, Ramu G, Desikan KV. Study on drug interactions. Leprosy in India 52: 229-236, 1980
Venkatesan K, Mathur A, Girdhan BK, Bharadwaj VP. The effect of clofazimine on the pharmacokinetics of rifampicin and dapsone in leprosy. Journal of Antimicrobial Chemotherapy 18: 715-718, 1986
Vischer WA. The experimental properties of G30,320 (B633). Leprosy Review 40: 107-111, 1969
Wallace JM, Hannah JB. *Mycobacterium avium* complex infection in patients with the acquired immunodeficiency syndrome. Chest 93: 926-932, 1988
Woods GL, Washington JA. Mycobacteria other than *Mycobacterium tuberculosis:* review of the microbiological and clinical aspects. Review of Infectious Diseases 9: 275-294, 1987
Working Party on B663: Symposium on B663 (Lamprene, Geigy) in the treatment of leprosy and leprosy reactions. International Journal of Leprosy 36: 560-561, 1968
World Health Organization. Expert committee on leprosy 1977 fifth report. World Health Organization Technical Report Series Number 607, 1977
World Health Organization. Chemotherapy of leprosy for control programs. Report of a WHO study group. World Health Organization Technical Series Number 675, 1982
Yajko DM, Nassos PS, Hadley WK. Therapeutic implications of inhibition versus killing of *Mycobacterium avium* complex by antimicrobial agents. Antimicrobial Agents and Chemotherapy 31: 117-120, 1987
Yawalkar SJ, Vischer W. Lamprene (clofazimine) in leprosy. Leprosy Reviews 50: 135-144, 1979
Young LS. *Mycobacterium avium* complex infection. Journal of Infectious Diseases 157: 863-867, 1988
Zuidema J, Hilbers-Modderman ESM, Merkus FWHM. Clinical pharmacokinetics of dapsone. Clinical Pharmacokinetics 11: 299-315, 1986

Author's address: Dr *Mack R. Holdiness*, Lakeside Hospital, Suite 207 – Medical Office Building, 4720 I-10 Service Road, Metairie, LA 70001 (USA).

Clinical Pharmacokinetics 16: 86-99 (1989)
0312-5963/89/0002-0086/$07.00/0

Clinical Pharmacokinetics and Therapeutic Use of Hydralazine in Congestive Heart Failure

John P. Mulrow and *Michael H. Crawford*

Department of Medicine, Division of Cardiology, University of Texas Health Science Center, San Antonio, Texas, USA

Contents

Summary ... 86
1. Pharmacological Effects ... 87
2. Pharmacokinetics ... 88
 2.1 Methods of Measurement of Hydralazine ... 88
 2.2 Absorption, Metabolism and Clearance ... 88
 2.3 Congestive Heart Failure ... 89
3. Clinical Efficacy ... 90
 3.1 Short Term Use: Haemodynamics ... 90
 3.2 Regional Blood Flow and Metabolic Effects ... 91
 3.3 Coronary Flow and Positive Inotropic Effect ... 93
 3.4 Prediction of Clinical Response ... 93
 3.5 Long Term Use of Hydralazine ... 94
4. Adverse Effects ... 95
5. Conclusions ... 95
6. Recommendations ... 97

Summary

Hydralazine (1-hydrazinophthalazine) has been used extensively in the treatment of hypertension and congestive heart failure and produces arteriolar vasodilation, in part mediated by prostaglandins. Its associated reflex baroreceptor-mediated responses of tachycardia and increased ejection velocity are attenuated in congestive heart failure. A direct inotropic effect has been attributed to the drug. Pharmacokinetic data indicate hydralazine is absorbed well from the gastrointestinal tract, and has an extensive and complex metabolism depending on acetylator status: slow acetylators undergo primary oxidative metabolism, while rapid acetylators are acetylated. Half-lives, clearances and bioavailability of the drug are not significantly altered in congestive heart failure compared with hypertensive patients. A wide range of dosages in heart failure has been noted (150 to 3000 mg/24h), and may relate to a saturation of the first-pass effect. Hydralazine improves haemodynamics in the short term in patients with increased peripheral vascular resistance, and has variable effects on pulmonary capillary wedge and left ventricular filling pressures. Prediction of the short term clinical response is difficult and appears to be independent of pharmacokinetics. A meta analysis did not demonstrate long term efficacy of hydralazine alone in heart failure, but combination therapy with nitrates has been shown to improve survival and exercise performance in patients with mild to moderate heart failure. Side effects are common and are dependent on dose, duration and acetylator status.

Chronic congestive heart failure is a very common and disabling clinical syndrome (Franciosa 1986). Vasodilators have been shown to relieve symptoms and improve functional status, and thus are accepted as important in the treatment of congestive heart failure (Abrams 1985; Braunwald & Colucci 1984; Chatterjee et al. 1980; Cohn 1986; Franciosa 1985; Levine 1985; Lipkin & Poole-Wilson 1985; Mason et al. 1980; Massie 1986; Packer 1983; Stanaszek et al. 1983; Sutton 1986). Recently, improved survival in patients with mild to moderate congestive heart failure treated with the combination of nitrates and hydralazine (Cohn et al. 1986) and in patients with severe congestive heart failure treated with enalapril (Consensus Trial Study Group 1987) has been reported. Hydralazine (1-hydrazinophthalazine) is an arteriolar dilator which has been used in the treatment of hypertension for about 30 years and more recently in the treatment of congestive heart failure. The use of hydralazine in congestive heart failure, its pharmacokinetics in both healthy individuals and those with heart failure, and its pharmacodynamics in both acute and chronic congestive failure are the subject of this review.

1. Pharmacological Effects

The major pharmacological action of hydralazine is in decreasing peripheral vascular resistance by relaxing arteriolar smooth muscle (Khayyal et al. 1981; Stunkaid et al. 1954). The cellular mechanism of this process is unknown, but may involve chelation of trace metals (Koch-Weser 1976) or activation of guanosine 3′5′ monophosphate (Anderson 1973).

More recent studies have implicated vasodilator prostaglandins as mediators of the hypotensive effect of hydralazine. The drug has been shown to increase production of the vasodilating substances prostacyclin and prostaglandin E_2 in both rabbit aorta strips (Greenwald et al. 1980) and smooth muscle cultures (Dyer et al. 1981; Morisaki et al. 1983). It can also diminish vasoconstriction via decreased synthesis of thromboxane A_2 *in vitro* or in hypertensive rabbits (Greenwald et al. 1980). Animal studies have indicated that the cyclo-oxygenase inhibitor indomethacin reverses or abolishes the hypotensive effect of hydralazine (Haeusler & Gerald 1979; Maekawa et al. 1984; Spokas & Wang 1980).

Clinical studies in healthy subjects have indicated that indomethacin decreases, but does not totally abolish, the intravenous hypotensive effect of hydralazine (Cinquegrani & Liang 1986). β-Adrenergic vasodilation (Maekawa et al. 1984) or a non-prostaglandin endothelial relaxing factor (Spokas et al. 1983) have also been postulated as being involved in the vasodilation caused by hydralazine. Peripheral vasodilation is not uniform, with greater dilation being produced in the coronary, cerebral, splanchnic and renal beds than in skin or muscle; non-vascular smooth muscle is not affected. The effect of hydralazine is also more marked on postcapillary capacitance than on precapillary resistance vessels. Blood flow is increased in the preferentially affected sites unless marked hypotension occurs (Packer 1983).

The effect of hydralazine on peripheral vascular resistance is to lower arterial blood pressure, which activates baroreceptor-mediated cardiovascular reflexes and increases adrenergic nervous activity. As a result, heart rate, left ventricular ejection velocity, stroke volume and cardiac output increase (Koch-Weser 1976). It is also likely that hydralazine has a direct positive inotropic effect on the myocardium (Gerschwin & Smith 1967; Khatri et al. 1977), which may involve increased calcium flow secondary to activation of β-adrenoceptors and a resultant increase in cyclic adenosine monophosphate (cAMP) [Azuma et al. 1987].

Hydralazine can cause sodium and water retention in hypertensive patients (Koch-Weser 1976) and increase peripheral plasma renin activity (Yeda et al. 1968, 1970). However, the latter does not appear to occur in congestive heart failure patients treated with hydralazine on a short term basis (Evans & White 1964; Yeda et al. 1970). The effects of long term treatment are less well known.

2. Pharmacokinetics

Despite the common clinical use of hydralazine, understanding of its metabolism and pharmacokinetics has been hampered by the lack of a specific assay and the complex metabolic pathways of the drug. As emphasised by Ludden et al. (1982), the instability of hydralazine, particularly in plasma samples, is also a major problem yet to be overcome. Since that review little additional research into the pharmacokinetics of hydralazine has been published and only the major properties of the drug are discussed here.

2.1 Methods of Measurement of Hydralazine

The first assay for plasma hydralazine was introduced in 1961 (Schulert 1961), but it and subsequent assays (Jack et al. 1975; Reidenberg et al. 1973; Schneck et al. 1978; Zacest & Koch-Weser 1972) were nonspecific and non-selective. Interference by acid-labile metabolites resulted in an 'apparent' hydralazine concentration which overestimated the true plasma level. Subsequently, more specific assays utilising gas chromatography and high pressure liquid chromatography have been developed (Ludden et al. 1979, 1980; Reece et al. 1980). A whole blood hydralazine assay has also been described using derivatisation with *p*-anisaldehyde (Ludden et al. 1983a). This method avoids the need for separation of plasma from the cellular components, and may reduce the risk of further metabolism of hydralazine.

2.2 Absorption, Metabolism and Clearance

Hydralazine shares with other drugs such as procainamide, isoniazid and some sulphonamides, the involvement of the genetically determined *N*-acetyltransferase enzyme in the liver, which is important in metabolising the parent compound (Melander et al. 1977). This has important implications for the pharmacokinetic profile of the drug.

2.2.1 Oral Administration

Carbon-14 labelling studies have shown that oral hydralazine is effectively absorbed from the gastrointestinal tract (Koch-Weser 1976). Less than 10% is recovered in the faeces, and 65 to 90% is excreted in the urine. Little of the parent drug is present in the urine, showing that it undergoes extensive metabolism.

The bioavailability of hydralazine is affected by concomitant food administration (Melander et al. 1977), which increases absorption 2- to 3-fold, although there are differences between standard and sustained release preparations in this regard (Shepherd et al. 1988). Bioavailability is also influenced by acetylator status (Ludden et al. 1982; Reece et al. 1980; Shepherd et al. 1980; Talseth 1976, 1977; Timbrell et al. 1981). Bioavailability is lower in the fast acetylator group than in the slow acetylator group.

The metabolism of hydralazine is complex, involving acetylation, aromatic, aliphatic and alicyclic oxidation, and loss of the hydrazino group (fig. 1). Two major pathways are available, depending on the acetylator status.

Slow acetylators metabolise less of the drug by the acetylation pathway and more by the oxidation pathways (Streeter & Timbrell 1983), with phthalazin-1-one as the major oxidation metabolite. A larger fraction of hydralazine escapes first-pass metabolism and reaches the systemic circulation in the slow acetylators. Hydralazine is then metabolised in the plasma with pyruvic acid to form hydralazine pyruvic acid hydrazone (HPAH).

Methyltriazolophthalazine and 3-hydroxymethyltriazolophthalazine are the major acetylated metabolites associated with the fast acetylator phenotype. This dichotomy in oral metabolism is important because the slow acetylator phenotype is a predisposing factor in the development of the major adverse effect of hydralazine, a lupus erythematosus-like syndrome. The syndrome is observed almost exclusively with the slow acetylator phenotype (Perry et al. 1970; Reece et al. 1980; Weinstein 1980).

2.2.2 Intravenous Administration

Significant differences occur when hydralazine is administered intravenously rather than orally. In bypassing first-transit metabolism in the liver, hydralazine reacts primarily with pyruvic acid in

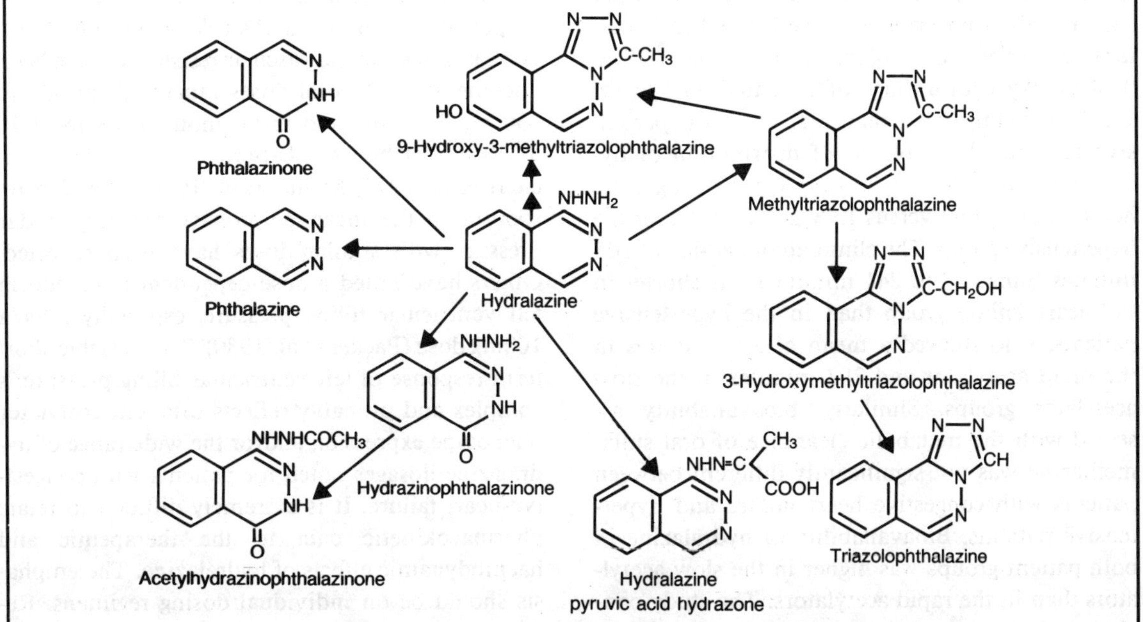

Fig. 1. Metabolic pathways for hydralazine.

plasma to form HPAH. Extrahepatic clearance occurs in plasma *in vitro*: some 55% of the clearance in rapid acetylators and 70% in slow acetylators appears to be extrahepatic. The rate at which this clearance occurs is independent of acetylator phenotype. An additional important difference is the demonstrated lack of significant dose dependency of systemic clearance over a range of intravenous doses (Ludden et al. 1983). Dose dependency does occur after oral administration and is likely to occur either at the level of the gastrointestinal mucosa or during first-pass metabolism in the liver. This implies that the acetylation process may be saturable during oral administration (Shepherd et al. 1984). Reece et al. (1980) found no correlation between the time course of hydralazine plasma concentration and its prolonged antihypertensive effect after intravenous dosing. While half-lives varied slightly between slow and fast acetylators, the hypotensive effect in both groups continues for several hours after dosing. Potential mechanisms postulated include persistence of an active metabolite with a prolonged half-life, prolonged binding, or the presence of an active metabolite which is bound to a deep compartment.

2.3 Congestive Heart Failure

The oral and intravenous pharmacokinetics previously discussed pertain to healthy volunteers and hypertensive patients with preserved left ventricular function. Based on the wide range of hydralazine dosages (150 to 3000 mg/day) used in early studies of heart failure, Crawford et al. (1985) investigated the determinants of systemic availability of oral hydralazine in severe congestive heart failure despite digoxin and more than 200 mg/day of frusemide (furosemide). A 75mg oral dose of hydralazine was used initially, but titrated up to 1000mg to achieve maximal haemodynamic improvement. The overall pharmacokinetics of hydralazine in congestive heart failure did not differ significantly from prior work performed in hypertensive patients. Mean blood clearance was 1.77 ± 0.48 L/h/kg with a range of 1.06 to 2.43 L/h/kg, which is slightly lower than that seen in hypertensive patients. The volume of distribution of hydralazine was 1.34 ± 0.79 L/kg for the congestive heart failure group versus 1.98 ± 0.22 L/kg for the hypertensive group. The elimination half-life at 105 minutes (range 57 to 241 minutes) was shorter in the heart failure group than in the hypertensive patients, who showed a mean of 200 minutes in the rapid acetylator and 297 minutes in the slow acetylator groups. Similarly, bioavailability assessed with the metabolic clearance of oral sulfamethazine was not significantly different between patients with congestive heart failure and hypertensive patients. Bioavailability of hydralazine in both patient groups was higher in the slow acetylators than in the rapid acetylators. The study concluded that congestive heart failure had only a modest effect on hydralazine concentrations after a single small oral dose. However, a saturation of the first-pass effect or of systemic clearance was suggested by a disproportionate rise in dose-normalised area under the curve from the first to the final doses of oral hydralazine (table I). Crawford et al. (1985) therefore emphasised the need for individual dose titration from 75 to 1000mg to achieve maximal haemodynamic benefits.

3. *Clinical Efficacy*

3.1 Short Term Use: Haemodynamics

Significant improvement in haemodynamic indices with the short term administration of oral (Chatterjee et al. 1976; Franciosa et al. 1977; Genks & Redwood 1980; Goldberg et al. 1983; Hindman et al. 1980; Mehta et al. 1978) and intravenous (Greenberg et al. 1978; Wilson et al. 1983b) hydralazine have been reported in patients with severe congestive heart failure refractory to treatment with diuretics, digitalis and nitrates (Chatterjee et al. 1976; Crawford et al. 1985; Franciosa et al. 1977; Genks & Redwood 1980; Goldbert et al. 1983; Hindman et al.1980; Mehta et al. 1978) [table II]. In the resting supine position, increases in cardiac output, stroke volume and stroke work index, with decreases in systemic vascular resistance, have been documented with oral doses ranging from 300 to 450 mg/24 hours and intravenous doses from 10 to 40 mg/24 hours (Chatterjee et al. 1976; Franciosa et al. 1977; Mehta et al. 1978). Variable responses in the mean pulmonary capillary wedge pressure with similar doses have been reported. Others have noted a dose-dependent reduction in left ventricular filling pressure, especially after a 100mg dose (Packer et al. 1980). The variable short term response of left ventricular filling pressure is complex and probably reflects different acetylator phenotype expression and/or the wide range of hydralazine dosages noted for patients with congestive heart failure. It is extremely difficult to relate pharmacokinetic data to the therapeutic and haemodynamic effects of hydralazine. The emphasis should be on individual dosing regimens. Reduction in the degree of mitral regurgitation and decreases in sympathetic tone may also account for this variation in response.

Similar significant and sustained haemodynamic improvement has been reported with exercise following the short term administration of hydralazine. Two studies (Genks & Redwood 1980; Hindman et al. 1980) reported administration of hydralazine 50 to 100mg orally to patients with severe congestive heart failure maintained on conventional therapy and investigation of the haemodynamic response at rest and during upright bicycle exercise. Both studies confirmed the previously reported effects of hydralazine on resting haemodynamics: increased cardiac output, decreased arterial venous oxygen difference, increased stroke volume, and a decrease in systemic vascular resistance. Again, a variable response to left ventricular filling pressure was found. With exercise, hydralazine increased cardiac output and stroke volume, and decreased the arterial venous oxygen difference and systemic vascular resistance compared with the drug's effect on resting haemodynamics. Both studies found a decrease in left ventricular filling pressures and mean pulmonary

Table I. Pharmacokinetics of hydralazine in patients with congestive heart failure (from Crawford et al. 1985 with permission)

Subject No.	CL_{smz} (ml/min)	CL_{hyd} (ml/min/kg)	Vd_{ss} (L/kg)	$t_{½}$ (min)	F (%)	Dose-normalised AUC (min/L × 10^3)		ICG clearance (ml/min)	
						initial	final	initial	final
1	239	37.9	2.060	158	2.4	5.1	10.2	632	667
2	54	25.6	0.656	102	12.2	47.4	303.0	403	471
3	224	26.1	0.912	135	8.2	27.9	115.0	322	255
4	22	21.6	0.797	102	28.7	139.0	443.0	276	532
5	106	40.5	2.470	89	19.8	30.8	200.0	182	260
6	10	36.5	0.766	57	42.9			1166	
7	116	37.9	2.030	112	13.4	31.6	370.0	100	100
8	110	17.7	0.442	94	9.2	39.7	100.0	283	366
9	220	26.4	0.904	109	6.6	18.8	31.6	720	1281
10	42	25.1	2.380	241	21.0	141.0	652.0	228	198
Mean	114.3	29.5	1.340	105[a]	16.4	53.5	247.2	305	459
±SD	±86.4	±8.0	±0.791		±12.1	±50.5	±213.4	±233	±356

a Harmonic mean.
Abbreviations: CL_{smz} = apparent metabolic clearance; CL_{hyd} = clearance of hydralazine; VD_{ss} = apparent volume of distribution at steady-state; $t_{½}$ = half-life; F = bioavailability; AUC = area under the concentration/time curve; ICG = indocyanine green.

artery pressures with exercise compared to the resting state. Overall, these studies demonstrated improved cardiac performance with hydralazine during upright exercise.

Radionuclide angiography was also used to study ejection fraction and filling volumes during rest and exercise by Hindman et al. (1980). No significant improvement in either ejection fraction or left ventricular diastolic volume was noted during exercise. Rubin et al. (1979) studied the haemodynamic responses at rest and during supine bicycle exercise after administration of hydralazine 50 to 100mg every 6 hours. Hydralazine significantly increased cardiac output and stroke volume while decreasing the arterial venous oxygen difference, mean arterial pressure, and systemic vascular resistance. During exercise, the increased stroke volume was maintained and further increases in cardiac output and decreases in arterial venous oxygen difference were observed. Thus hydralazine has demonstrated haemodynamic benefits in patients both at rest and during exercise in the short term doses tested.

3.2 Regional Blood Flow and Metabolic Effects

The resting supine regional haemodynamics of hydralazine were examined by Magorien et al. (1981) using doses of 75 and 100mg in patients with severe congestive heart failure despite diuretics, digitalis and nitrates. Upper extremity blood flow, hepatic plasma flow and renal plasma flow were determined using venous occlusive plethysmography, indocyanine green clearance and aminohippurate clearance, respectively. The increased cardiac output and decreased systemic vascular resistance associated with hydralazine dosing was associated with increased limb flow, unchanged hepatic flow and resistance, and increased renal blood flow with decreased resistance. Selective regional haemodynamic effects occur and may be influenced by coadministered drugs such as antiprostaglandin agents, or high-dose dopamine infusions.

Wilson et al. (1983a) investigated the effect of hydralazine on skeletal muscle oxygen delivery during upright bicycle exercise in patients with severe congestive heart failure. The total intravenous

Table II. Pharmacodynamics of hydralazine (from Crawford et al. 1985, with permission)

Subject No.	Treatment	D_{max} (mg tid)	HR (bpm)	SBP (mm Hg)	PAWP (mm Hg)	CO (L/min)	AoP (mm Hg)	RAP (mm Hg)	SVR (dyne · sec/cm^5)	Weight (kg)
1	Control	0	70	140	16	4.28	103	5	1832	63.8
	Hydralazine	75	65	162	11	4.36	101	2	1798	61.2
2	Control	0	108	170	47	3.14	137	8	3286	80.8
	Hydralazine	1000	88	120	29	5.01	93	7	1381	68.8
3	Control	0	104	120	34	7.20	75	21	600	126.6
	Hydralazine	225	96	136	18	9.90	104	6	792	105.2
4	Control	0	106	108	35	3.47	81	13	1579	75.4
	Hydralazine	1000	103	108	32	6.14	85	15	912	64.7
5	Control	0	88	126	45	4.38	95	35	1096	116.0
	Hydralazine	550	94	124	42	5.07	88	29	931	110.3
6	Control	0	92	100	28	2.11	85	14	2692	79.2
	Hydralazine	1000	96	98	24	4.63	73	12	1054	72.6
7	Control	0	83	148	27	4.27	107	17	1686	85.3
	Hydralazine	400	100	130	17	5.59	97	10	1245	80.2
8	Control	0	114	120	22	4.73	93	12	1370	98.2
	Hydralazine	100	110	110	13	6.74	82	6	902	94.3
9	Control	0	72	124	17	2.73	88	4	2476	56.5
	Hydralazine	100	72	114	15	3.15	81	10	1803	54.9
Control										
Mean		0	93	128	30	4.03	96	12	1846	86.9
±SD			±16	±21	±11	±1.50	±18	±10	±839	±23.0
Hydralazine										
Mean		494	92	122	22[a]	5.60[a]	89	10[b]	1202[b]	79.1[c]
±SD		±409	±15	±19	±10	±1.90	±10	±9	±385	±19.8

a $p < 0.005$.
b $p < 0.05$.
c $p < 0.01$ compared with control value.
Abbreviations: D_{max} = Hydralazine dose at maximum haemodynamic effects; HR = heart rate; SBP = systolic blood pressure; PAWP = pulmonary artery wedge pressure; CO = cardiac output; AoP = mean aortic pressure; RAP = mean right atrial pressure; SVR = systemic vascular resistance; tid = 3 times daily.

hydralazine dose averaged 32 ± 14mg, with a range of 15 to 60mg administered to achieve an increase in cardiac output of 30% or until systolic blood pressure was less than 100mm Hg. Measurements of cardiac output by the thermal dilution principle with sampling of the venous effluent for lactate and oxygen extraction were made in addition to central monitoring. In agreement with other studies these investigators demonstrated exercise-induced increases in cardiac output, decreases in systemic vascular resistance, and unchanged maximal oxygen uptake. Increased leg blood flow with exercise was found, but the proportion of cardiac output delivered to the leg was unchanged. The increased leg flow was not associated with either an increase in oxygen extraction or a decrease in peak femoral venous lactate concentration. These data suggest an anatomical shunting of increased limb blood flow rather than increased delivery to working skeletal muscle. Rubin et al. (1980) likewise found improved central haemodynamics with hydralazine 300 mg/day during supine exercise, without alterations in peak lactate production or rate of lactate disappearance. While the design was less rigid than that of Wilson et al. (1983a), it was speculated that maldistribution of increased cardiac output to non-working skeletal muscle or abnormal distribution within tissues was responsible for the poor metabolic response to exercise with hydralazine.

3.3 Coronary Flow and Positive Inotropic Effect

Investigations of short term hydralazine use have also evaluated coronary flow dynamics and the positive inotropic effect of hydralazine. Magorien et al. (1982) investigated the short term effects of oral hydralazine administered in a 1 mg/kg dose on coronary blood flow and myocardial energetics in patients with severe congestive heart failure. Central and coronary sinus haemodynamics and metabolic measurements were made before and after oral hydralazine. With modest decreases in mean arterial pressure, pulmonary capillary wedge pressure and systemic vascular resistance, there was an associated increase in cardiac index and left ventricular stroke work index. Coronary blood flow increased with decreases in coronary vascular resistance. Despite increases in myocardial oxygen consumption, the arterial-coronary sinus oxygen difference and myocardial oxygen extraction ratio decreased. These results suggest that hydralazine has a beneficial effect on the coronary circulation and improves the myocardial oxygen supply : demand ratio.

Since animal models (Gerschwin & Smith 1967; Khatri et al. 1977) have suggested a positive inotropic effect of hydralazine, Leier et al. (1980) investigated haemodynamic and echocardiographic parameters of left ventricular performance in patients with severe congestive heart failure before and after oral dosing with hydralazine 75 or 100mg. Hydralazine significantly shortened the pre-ejection period and increased the mean rate of rise of isovolumic pressure without a positive chronotropic effect. Thus, the mechanism for the positive inotropic effect is uncertain but Khatri et al. (1977) and Brunner et al. (1967) suggested that hydralazine may directly or indirectly stimulate β-adrenergic receptors. Increased calcium flow has also been suggested (Azuma et al. 1987).

3.4 Prediction of Clinical Response

Despite the demonstrated short term benefits of hydralazine, not all patients improve with the drug (Packer et al. 1980) and the need to predict clinical response becomes important. In general, however, pharmacokinetic studies have failed to produce a reliable method of predicting the short term clinical effects of hydralazine. Goldberg et al. (1983) attempted to use radionuclide angiography in place of Swan-Ganz monitoring to assess the efficacy of hydralazine in patients with severe congestive heart failure. Rest and supine bicycle exercise were assessed with Swan-Ganz monitoring and radionuclide angiography at baseline and after administration of hydralazine 50 to 100mg every 6 hours. When responders were defined as those having $\geqslant$ 20% decrease in systemic vascular resistance, radionuclide angiography was unable to predict hydralazine response on the basis of control left ventricular ejection fraction at rest or the percentage increase in ejection fraction with hydralazine at rest. Similar proven beneficial haemodynamic effects were substantiated: increased cardiac index, stroke volume index, left ventricular stroke work index and decreased systemic vascular resistance. Left ventricular filling pressures were unchanged with hydralazine at rest and during exercise. An increase in ejection fraction both at rest and during exercise was found in Goldberg's study, in contrast to the findings of Hindman et al. (1980). The lack of correlation between haemodynamics and radionuclide angiography in predicting response to hydralazine was attributed to either the insensitivity of radionuclide left ventricular ejection fraction technique or changes in the amount of concomitant mitral regurgitation by hydralazine.

Packer et al. (1980) examined the effect of left ventricular chamber size in determining the response to short term hydralazine therapy in patients with severe congestive heart failure. Hydralazine dosing was titrated to maximal haemodynamic benefit. Effective single doses ranged from 75 to

1000mg, with one patient requiring 20mg intravenously to obtain haemodynamic improvement. The daily dosing likewise ranged from 150 to 3000mg with the same patient requiring 60mg intravenously. Left ventricular end-diastolic dimension (LVEDD) determined echocardiographically correlated significantly with percent change in stroke volume, left ventricular filling pressure and stroke work index. In patients with a ⩾ 60mm LVEDD the decrease in systemic vascular resistance was accompanied by greater improvement in cardiac output, stroke work and left ventricular filling pressure and a minimal decrease in arterial blood pressure without a reflex tachycardia. In contrast, patients who had an LVEDD of less than 60mm had a decrease in systemic vascular resistance associated with less improvement in cardiac output, and no change in left ventricular filling pressure. Blood pressure decreased substantially in these patients and was associated with reflex tachycardia.

Wilson et al. (1983b) investigated the short term intravenous effect of hydralazine on vascular responsiveness and left ventricular pump function in an attempt to identify physiological factors accounting for the variable circulatory responses to hydralazine. Administration of 20mg intravenously had variable effects on peripheral vascular resistance, with 60% of patients decreasing systemic vascular resistance by ⩾ 20%. The initial systemic vascular resistance showed a linear correlation with the observed change in this parameter. Left ventricular pump responses to both a 20mg intravenous dose and a titration method to achieve a ⩾ 20% decrease in systemic vascular resistance also varied greatly. Changes in stroke work index were directly related to indices of left ventricular preload, end-diastolic wall stress and pulmonary capillary wedge pressure, and inversely related to stroke work index. Patients with the most severe degree of left ventricular dysfunction appeared to respond best to intravenous hydralazine, but correlations between initial haemodynamic parameters and response to hydralazine were not predictive of an individual patient's response. The close correlation between left ventricular end-diastolic dimension and haemodynamic response found by Packer et al. (1980) may have been due to more marked vasodilation produced by hydralazine in their study compared with that of Wilson et al. (1983b).

3.5 Long Term Use of Hydralazine

The relative efficacy of the various vasodilators is not known. Improved survival has been reported with mild to moderate congestive heart failure treated with combined hydralazine and nitrates (Cohn et al. 1986). The reduction in mortality in this trial was found to be inversely related to ejection fraction and oxygen consumption and directly related to the radiographic cardiothoracic ratio and a history of antiarrhythmic drug usage. Subgroup analysis indicated a 95% confidence interval which excluded zero in patients with lower ejection fractions, young age, hypertensive history, and no alcohol abuse (Cohn et al. 1987). Other vasodilating agents have not been associated with improved survival, probably due largely to the small numbers of subjects in the trials (Furberg & Yusuf 1985).

The determination of the relative efficacy of hydralazine in the long term treatment of congestive heart failure can only be achieved through the use of the meta analysis technique, owing to the paucity of studies with hydralazine and the small number of patients studied. Mulrow et al. recently published a meta analysis of the relative efficacy of 6 different vasodilators used in congestive heart failure drug regimens. The analyses involved randomised placebo-controlled trials with clinical endpoints of mortality, functional status and exercise capacity, with treatment durations of ⩾ 4 weeks, conducted between 1965 and 1987. 28 trials were found, involving 1976 patients, all of whom were symptomatic despite digitalis and diuretic treatment.

Hydralazine monotherapy accounted for 3 randomised placebo-controlled trials (Conradson 1981; Franciosa et al. 1982; Magorien et al. 1984), with a total of 114 patients treated for 12 to 52 weeks on doses ranging from 200 to 300mg administered on a three to four times daily dosing regimen. The patients' mean age was 61 and they had primarily ischaemic heart failure of > 3 to > 12 months' duration. They were classified as class III-IV (New York Heart Association). Hydralazine was also part of the combination of nitrates plus hydralazine *versus* prazosin *versus* placebo in the randomised placebo-controlled Veterans' Administration (VHeFT) study in mild to moderate congestive heart failure (Cohn et al. 1986). In this trial 459 patients were randomised to hydralazine plus nitrates for 120 weeks of treatment, with nitrates 160 mg/day and hydralazine 300 mg/day in a 4 times daily dosing regimen. VHeFT's patient population was similar: they were middle aged (mean age 58) men (100%) who had mixed ischaemic and non-ischaemic congestive heart failure which would be classified as New York Heart Association I-III. Of the remaining 24 trials angiotensin-converting enzyme inhibitors (ACE) comprised 13, nitrates alone 3, and α-antagonists 8. The population characteristics were similar to those in the hydralazine studies.

Mortality analyses indicated ACE inhibitors were the only class of vasodilator agent associated with a statistically significant protective effect against mortality (odds ratio 0.51, 95% confidence limits 0.34 to 0.75) [fig. 2]. A non-statistical point estimate of 0.81 was found with the combination therapy of nitrates and hydralazine (odds ratio 0.81, 95% confidence limits 0.55 to 1.18). This was consistent with the VHeFT study which showed a borderline statistically significant protective effect of the combination. Hydralazine alone did not improve survival (odds ratio 0.94, 95% confidence limits 0.35 to 2.56). Functional status results indicated an overall improvement in all patients given vasodilators compared to placebo (odds ratio 4.76, 95% confidence limits 3.74 to 6.54) [fig. 3]. All individual vasodilators examined improved functional status, with the exception of hydralazine. The hydralazine and nitrate combination in the VHeFT could not be assessed in this regard since the trial did not assess functional status.

Meta analysis results for exercise improvement could not be assessed because common units of comparison were not available for all 25 studies with exercise data. Of the 25 studies, however, 18 reported similar improvements in both exercise duration and functional status. Of the 3 hydralazine studies, 2 reported concordant improvement in exercise duration and functional status.

4. Adverse Effects

Adverse reactions to hydralazine are common and may be more frequent than with other vasodilator agents (Packer 1983). During short term administration headache and flushing are common, but these generally disappear after 2 weeks. In the VHeFT trial (Cohn et al. 1986) nausea and vomiting were the primary adverse reactions, accounting for the large withdrawal rate observed in that 120-week trial. Exacerbation of ischaemic events (Packer et al. 1981) and the development of a systemic lupus erythematosus-like syndrome (Perry 1973) have also been primary concerns with hydralazine therapy. Again in the large VHeFT trial with relatively low-dose hydralazine combined with nitrates, the reported incidences of both reactions were negligible and not clinically relevant. Predisposing factors to the development of adverse reactions include dose, duration of therapy and the slow acetylator phenotype (Timbrell et al. 1980).

5. Conclusions

Hydralazine is an arteriolar vasodilator which has been used extensively in the treatment of severe congestive heart failure. It has complex pharmacokinetics with both oral and intravenous dosing, and has a tendency to require higher daily dosing regimens in the treatment of congestive heart failure than have been observed for the treatment of hypertension. In general, the short term trials discussed titrated dosage based on the haemodynamic response, while the long term trials used fixed dosing. Salutory short term haemodynamic effects of increased cardiac output and stroke volume with decreases in systemic vascular resistance have been demonstrated. Variable short term effects on left ventricular filling pressures have been noted even though hydralazine does not affect preload. While central haemodynamics improve rapidly following

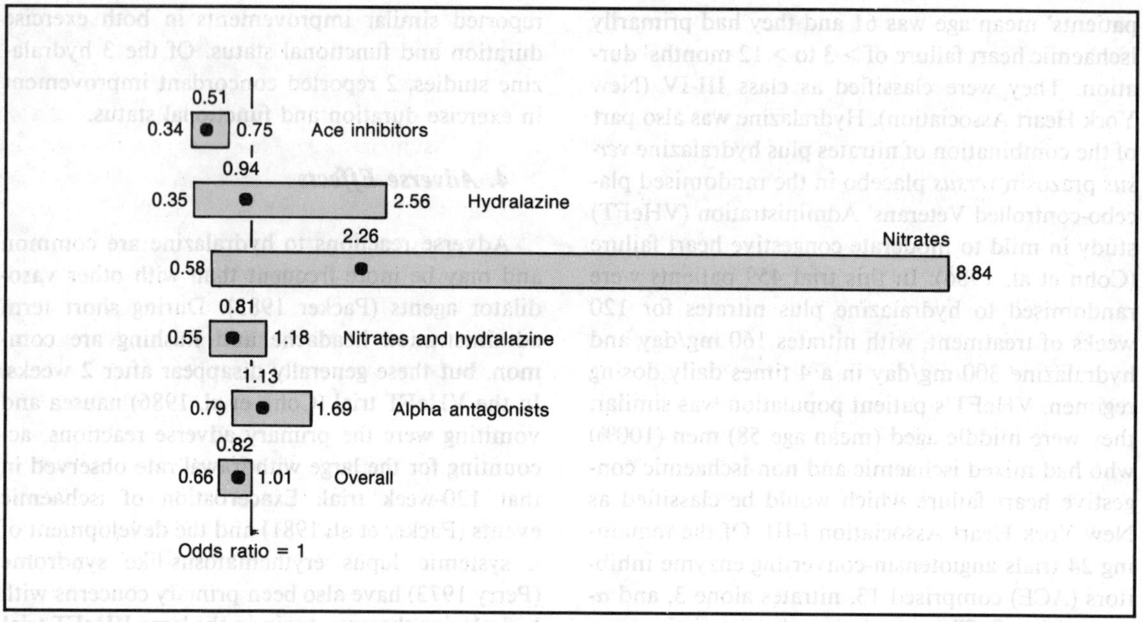

Fig. 2. Pooled mortality effect sizes of randomised trials of vasodilator agents. Agents whose 95% confidence limits cross the line representing an odds ratio of 1 are not statistically significant (i.e. $p > 0.05$). Confidence limits tending towards the right of the line reflect increased mortality, while those tending towards the left of the line reflect decreased mortality (from Mulrow et al. 1988, with permission).

single doses of hydralazine, both at rest and during exercise, regional variation in haemodynamics and metabolism is seen. At rest upper extremity and renal blood flows increase with no change in hepatic flow. Metabolic effects of hydralazine during upright or supine exercise do not appear to increase oxygen availability within working muscle, and anatomical shunting of increased limb flow probably occurs, rather than increased delivery to working muscle.

The haemodynamic improvement noted is not exhibited by all patients treated with short term administration of hydralazine. Attempts to predict individual responses to hydralazine using haemodynamics, radionuclide angiography or echocardiography have been undertaken with variable success, but suggest that hydralazine is most effective in patients with primary dilated cardiomyopathy. Long term clinical efficacy has been examined in a meta analysis investigating the relative efficacy of 5 different vasodilator agents with respect to clinical end-points of mortality, functional class improvement and exercise function. Hydralazine did not improve survival and was the only vasodilator agent examined which did not improve functional status. It is possible that the lack of beneficial effect seen in long term therapy was related to the low fixed doses used in these studies, since there is evidence indicating that higher doses are required in many patients.

Short term use of hydralazine does not appear to be limited by major side effects necessitating discontinuation. However, long term use is associated with a high rate of discontinuation. Headache and nausea are the most common side effects. The incidence of late toxicity to hydralazine resulting in a syndrome similar to systemic lupus erythematosus has been reported to be as high as 11%, but was neglible in the VHeFT trial, probably because of the low doses used.

Future work in the pharmacokinetics of hydralazine in the short term treatment of congestive heart failure is unlikely because of the proliferation of newer angiotensin-converting enzyme inhibitors under investigation, which may have fewer side effects, and the availability of inotropic agents such as dobutamine as well as inotropic/vasodilator agents such as amrinone or enoximone.

6. Recommendations

Our recommendations regarding hydralazine use in congestive heart failure are as follows. While hydralazine has demonstrated salutory short term effects haemodynamically when used as a sole agent, the existence of other agents with easier titratability, proven improvement in functional status, and increased survival, such as ACE inhibitors, argues against the first-line use of hydralazine. In a clinical situation in which ACE inhibitors are not recommended, such as worsening renal function, practitioners should institute treatment with a combination of hydralazine and nitrates.

Short term hydralazine doses should be started with 50 to 100mg orally every 8 hours and titrated to the haemodynamic response determined by Swan-Ganz monitoring. Doses up to 1000mg may be required to achieve an initial response in heart failure patients, but can usually be decreased later. While prediction of clinical response varies, patients with the severest haemodynamic compromise are likely to benefit most rapidly. The rare patient may require intravenous hydralazine in doses ranging from 20 to 60mg daily to obtain haemodynamic improvements.

Long term use of hydralazine in combination with nitrates should be dictated by the guidelines of the VHeFT study. The higher doses probably required in short term treatment will undoubtedly

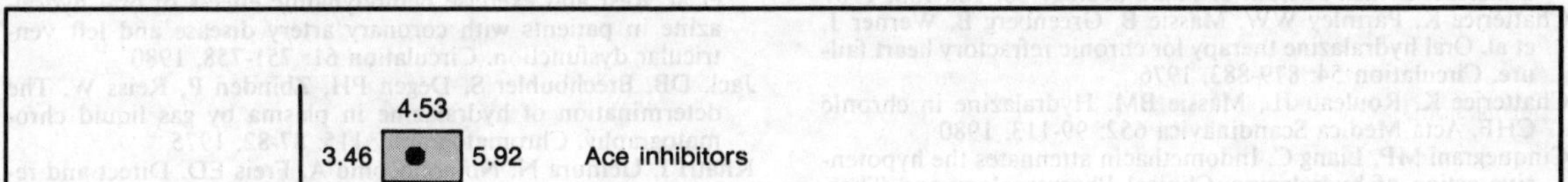

Fig. 3. Pooled functional status effect sizes of randomised trials of vasodilator agents. Estimates in dotted brackets are with non-homogeneous studies excluded. Agents whose 95% confidence limits cross the line representing an odds ratio of 1 are not statistically significant (i.e. > 0.05). Confidence limits tending towards the right of the line reflect improved functional status (from Mulrow et al. 1988, with permission).

be responsible for an unacceptable withdrawal rate should the doses be continued. The VHeFT oral dosage was 300mg daily. Despite this notably lower dose, a significant withdrawal rate was present in the trial. While survival improved with the combination, the effect on functional status is currently unknown.

References

Abrams J. Vasodilator therapy for chronic congestive heart failure. Journal of the American Medical Association 254: 3070-3074, 1985

Anderson R. Cyclic AMP as a mediator of the relaxing action of papaverine, nitroglycerin, diazoxide, and hydralazine in intestinal vascular smooth muscle. Acta Pharmacologica et Toxicologica 32: 321-336, 1973

Azuma J, Sawamura A, Harada H, Awata N, Kishimoto S, et al. Mechanism of direct cardiostimulating actions of hydralazine. European Journal of Pharmacology 135: 137-144, 1987

Braunwald E, Colucci WS. Vasodilation therapy of heart failure: has the promissory note been paid? New England Journal of Medicine 310: 459-461, 1984

Brunner H, Hedwall PR, Meier M. Influence of adrenergic beta receptor blockade in the acute cardiovascular effects of hydralazine. British Journal of Pharmacology 30: 123-133, 1967

Chatterjee K, Parmley WW, Massie B, Greenberg B, Werner J, et al. Oral hydralazine therapy for chronic refractory heart failure. Circulation 54: 879-883, 1976

Chatterjee K, Rouleau JL, Massie BM. Hydralazine in chronic CHF. Acta Medica Scandinavica 652: 99-113, 1980

Cinquegrani MP, Liang C. Indomethacin attenuates the hypotensive action of hydralazine. Clinical Pharmacology and Therapeutics 39: 564-570, 1986

Cohn JN, Archibald DG, Francis GS, Ziesche S, Franciosa JA, et al. Veterans' administration cooperative study on vasodilator therapy of heart failure: influence of pre-randomization variables on the reduction of mortality by treatment with hydralazine and isosorbide dinitrate. Circulation 75 (Suppl. IV): IV49-IV54, 1987

Cohn JN, Archibald DG, Ziesche S, et al. Effect of vasodilator therapy on mortality in chronic congestive heart failure. New England Journal of Medicine 314: 1547-1552, 1986

Cohn JN. Vasodilator therapy of dilated cardiomyopathy. Postgraduate Medical Journal 62: 599-600, 1986

Conradson TB. Hydralazine versus placebo in CHF – preliminary results from a multicenter long term study in Sweden. Acta Medica Scandinavica 652 (Suppl.): 177-180, 1981

Consensus Trial Study Group. Effects of enalapril on mortality in severe congestive heart failure: results of the Cooperative North Scandinavian Enalapril Survival Study. New England Journal of Medicine 316: 1429-1435, 1987

Crawford MH, Ludden TM, Kennedy GT. Determinants of systemic availability of oral hydralazine in heart failure. Clinical Pharmacology and Therapeutics 38: 538-543, 1985

Dyer RD, Huttner JJ, Tan SY, Mulrow PJ. Prostaglandin synthesis by vascular smooth muscle cells is stimulated by bradykinin, prazosin, and hydralazine. Progress in Lipid Research 20: 557-560, 1981

Evans DAP, White TA. Human acetylation polymorphism. Journal of Laboratory and Clinical Medicine 63: 394-403, 1964

Franciosa JA. Current indications for vasodilator therapy for left ventricular failure. Comprehensive Therapy 11: 39-46, 1985

Franciosa JA. Epidemiologic patterns, clinical evaluation, and long term prognosis in chronic congestive heart failure. American Journal of Medicine 80 (Suppl. 2B): 14-21, 1986

Franciosa JA, Pierpoint G, Cohn JN. Hemodynamic improvement after oral hydralazine in left ventricular failure. Annals of Internal Medicine 86: 388-393, 1977

Franciosa JA, Weber KT, Levine TB, et al. Hydralazine in the long term treatment of chronic heart failure: lack of difference from placebo. American Heart Journal 104: 587-594, 1982

Furberg CD, Yusuf S. Effect of vasodilators on survival in chronic congestive heart failure. American Journal of Cardiology 55: 1110-1113, 1985

Genks WR, Redwood DR. Haemodynamic effects of hydralazine at rest and during exercise in patients with chronic heart failure. British Heart Journal 44: 259-264, 1980

Gerschwin ME, Smith NT. Mode of action of hydralazine on guinea pig atria. Archives Internationales de Pharmacodynamie et de Therapie 170: 108-116, 1967

Goldberg MJ, Franklin BA, Rubenfire M, Kerin NZ, Willens HJ, et al. Hydralazine therapy in severe chronic heart failure: inability of radionuclide left ventricular ejection fraction measurement to predict the hemodynamics response. Journal of the American College of Cardiology 2: 887-893, 1983

Greenberg BH, Massie BM, Brundage BH, Botvinecik E, Parmley WW, et al. Beneficial effects of hydralazine in severe mitral regurgitation. Circulation 58: 273-279, 1978

Greenwald JE, Wong JL, Alexander M, Bianchine JR. *In vivo* inhibition of thromboxane biosynthesis by hydralazine. Advances in Prostaglandin and Thromboxane Research 6: 293-295, 1980

Haeusler G, Gerold M. Increased levels of prostaglandin-like material in the canine blood during arterial hypotension produced by hydralazine, dihydralazine and minoxidil. Naunyn-Schmiedebergs Archives of Pharmacology 310: 155-167, 1980

Hindman MC, Slosky DA, Peter RH, Newman GE, Jones RH, et al. Rest and exercise hemodynamic effects of oral hydralazine in patients with coronary artery disease and left ventricular dysfunction. Circulation 61: 751-758, 1980

Jack DB, Brechbuhler S, Degen PH, Zbinden P, Reiss W. The determination of hydralazine in plasma by gas liquid chromatography. Chromatography 115: 87-82, 1975

Khatri I, Uemura N, Notargiocomo A, Freis ED. Direct and reflex cardiostimulation effects of hydralazine. American Journal of Cardiology 40: 38-42, 1977

Khayyal M, Gross F, Kreye VA. Studies on the direct vasodilator effect of hydralazine in the isolated rabbit renal artery. Journal of Pharmacology and Experimental Therapeutics 216: 390-394, 1981

Koch-Weser J. Hydralazine. New England Journal of Medicine 295: 320-323, 1976

Leier C, Desch CE, Magorien RD, Triffon DW, Unverferth DV, et al. Positive inotropic effects of hydralazine in human subjects: comparison with prazosin in the setting of congestive heart failure. American Journal of Cardiology 46: 1039-1044, 1980

Levine TB. Role of vasodilators in the treatment of congestive heart failure. American Journal of Cardiology 55: 32A-35A, 1985

Lipkin DP, Poole-Wilson PA. Treatment of chronic heart failure: a review of recent drug trials. British Medical Journal 291: 993-996, 1985

Ludden TM, Goggin LK, McNay JL, Haegele, Shepherd AMM. High pressure liquid chromatographic assay for hydralazine in human plasma. Journal of Pharmaceutical Sciences 68: 423, 1979

Ludden TM, Ludden LK, McNay JL, Skrdlant HB, Swaggerty PJ, et al. Improved assays for hydralazine and hydralazine pyruvic acid hydrazone in human plasma. Analytica Chimica Acta 120: 297-304, 1980

Ludden TM, Ludden LK, Wade KE, Allerheiligen SRB. Determination of hydralazine in human whole blood. Journal of Pharmaceutical Sciences 72: 693-695, 1983

Ludden TM, McNay JL, Shepherd AMM, Lin MS. Clinical Pharmacokinetics of hydralazine. Clinical Pharmacokinetics 7: 185-205, 1982

Ludden TM, Shepherd AMM, McNay JL, Lin M-S. Effect of

intravenous dose on hydralazine kinetics after administration. Clinical Pharmacology and Therapeutics 34: 148-152, 1983b
Maekawa K, Liang C-S, Tsui A, Chen BT, Kawashima S. Vasodilative effect of hydralazine in awake dogs: the role of prostaglandins and the sympathetic nervous system. Circulation 70: 908-916, 1984
Magorien RD, Brown GP, Unverferth DV, Nelson S, Boudoulas H, et al. Effects of hydralazine on coronary blood flow and myocardial energetics in congestive heart failure. Circulation 65: 528-533, 1982
Magorien RD, Triffon DW, Desch CE, Bay WH, Unverferth DV, et al. Prazosin and hydralazine in congestive heart failure. Regional hemodynamic effects in relation to dose. Annals of Internal Medicine 95: 5-13, 1981
Magorien RD, Unverferth DW, Leier CV. Hydralazine therapy in chronic congestive heart failure. American Journal of Medicine 77: 267-274, 1984
Mason Dt, Awan NA, Hoye JA, et al. Treatment of acute and chronic congestive heart failure by vasodilator afterload reduction. Archives of International Medicine 140: 1577-1581, 1980
Massie B. Update, diagnosis and management of congestive heart failure. Geriatrics 41: 30-42, 1986
Mehta J, Pepine CJ, Conti CR. Haemodynamic effects of hydralazine and of hydralazine plus glyceryl trinitrate paste in heart failure. British Medical Journal 40: 845-850, 1978
Melander A, Danielson K, Hanson A, Rudell B, Schersten B, et al. Enhancement of hydralazine bioavailability by food. Clinical Pharmacology and Therapeutics 22: 104-107, 1977
Morisaki N, Lindsey JA, Milo Ge, Cornwell DG. Fatty acid metabolism and cell proliferation III: effect of prostaglandin biosynthesis either from exogenous fatty acid or endogenous fatty acid release with hydralazine. Lipids 18: 349-352, 1983
Mulrow CD, Mulrow JP, Linn WD, Aguilar C, Ramirez G. Relative efficacy of vasodilator therapy in chronic congestive heart failure: implications of randomized trials: relative efficacy of vasodilator therapy. Journal of the American Medical Association 259: 3422-3426, 1988
Packer M, Meller J, Medina N, Gorlin R, Herman MN. Importance of left ventricular chamber size in determining the response to hydralazine in severe chronic heart failure. New England Journal of Medicine 303: 250-255, 1980
Packer M, Miller J, Medina N, Yushak M, Garlin R. Provocation of myocardial ischaemia during creation of vasodilation therapy for chronic heart failure: clinical and hemodynamic evaluation of 52 consecutive patients with ischaemic cardiomyopathy. American Journal of Cardiology 48: 939-946, 1981
Packer M. Vasodilator and inotropic therapy for severe chronic congestive heart failure: passion and skepticism. Journal of the American College of Cardiology 2: 841-852, 1983
Perry HM. Late toxicity to hydralazine resembling systemic lupus erythematosus or rheumatoid arthritis. American Journal of Medicine 54: 58-72, 1973
Perry HM, Tan EM, Carmody S, Sakamoto A. Relationship of acetyltransferase activity to antinuclear antibodies and toxic symptoms in hypertensive patients treated with hydralazine. Journal of Laboratory and Clinical Medicine 76: 114-125, 1970
Reece PA, Cozamanis I, Zacest R. Kinetics of hydralazine and its main metabolites in slow and fast acetylators. Clinical Pharmacology and Therapeutics 28: 769-778, 1980
Reece PA, Cozamanis I, Zacest R. Selective high performance liquid chromatographic assay for hydralazine and its metabolites in plasma of man. Journal of Chromatography 181: 427, 1980
Reidenberg MM, Drayer D, De Marco AL, Bello CT. Hydralazine elimination in man. Clinical Pharmacology and Therapeutics 14: 970-977, 1973
Rubin SA, Chatterjee K, Parmley WW. Metabolic assessment of exercise in chronic heart failure treated with short term vasodilators. Circulation 61: 543-548, 1980
Rubin SA, Chatterjee K, Ports TA, Gilberg JH, Brundage BH, et al. Influence of short term oral hydralazine therapy on exercise hemodynamics in patients with severe chronic heart failure. American Journal of Cardiology 44: 1183-1189, 1979
Schenck DW, Sprouse JS, Miller K, Vary JE, Dewitt FD, et al. Plasma levels of free and acid labile hydralazine: effects of multiple dosing and procainamide. Clinical Pharmacology and Therapeutics 24: 714-719, 1978
Schulert AR. Physiologic disposition of hydralazine (1-hydrazinophthalazine) and a method for its determination in biological fluids. Archives Internationales de Pharmacodynamie et de Therapie 132: 1-15, 1961
Shepherd AMM, Irvine NA, Ludden TM, Lin M-S, McNay JL. Effect of oral dose size on hydralazine kinetics and vasodepressor response. Clinical Pharmacology and Therapeutics 36: 595-600, 1984
Shepherd AMM, Jackson SHD, Rogers D, Ludden TM, Woodworth J, et al. Effect of food on hydralazine levels in hypertension. Abstract PIIB-1. Clinical Pharmacology and Therapeutics 43: 147, 1988
Shepherd AM, Ludden TM, McNay JL, Lin M. Hydralazine kinetics after single and repeated oral doses. Clinical Pharmacology and Therapeutics 28: 804-811, 1980
Spokas EG, Folco G, Quilley J, Chander P, McGiff JC. Endothelial mechanism in the vascular action of hydralazine. Hypertension 5 (Suppl. 1): 107-111, 1983
Spokas EG, Wang H. Regional blood flow and cardiac responses to hydralazine. Journal of Pharmacology and Experimental Therapeutics 212: 294-303, 1980
Stanaszek WF, Kellerman D, Brogden RN, Romankiewicz JA. Prazosin update: a review of its pharmacological properties and therapeutic use in hypertension and congestive heart failure. Drugs 25: 339-384, 1983
Streeter AJ, Timbrell JA. Studies on the *in vivo* metabolism of hydralazine in the rat. Drug Metabolism and Disposition 11: 184-189, 1983
Stunkard A, Wertheimer L, Redisch W. Studies on hydralazine: evidence for a peripheral site of action. Journal of Clinical Investigation 33: 1047-1053, 1954
Sutton FJ. Vasodilator therapy. American Journal of Medicine 80 (Suppl. 2B): 54-58, 1986
Talseth T. Kinetics of hydralazine elimination. Clinical Pharmacology and Therapeutics 21: 715-720, 1977
Talseth T. Studies on hydralazine I serum concentrations of hydralazine in man after a single dose and at steady state. European Journal of Clinical Pharmacology 10: 183-187, 1976
Timbrell JA, Harland SJ, Facchini V. Effect of dose on acetylator phenotype distribution of hydralazine. Clinical Pharmacology and Therapeutics 29: 337-343, 1981
Timbrell JA, Harland SJ, Facchini V. Polymorphic acetylation of hydralazine. Clinical Pharmacology and Therapeutics 28: 350-355, 1980
Weinstein A. Drug induced systemic lupus erythematosus. Progress in Clinical Immunology 4: 1-21, 1980
Wilson JR, Martin JL, Ferraro N, Weber KT. Effect of hydralazine on perfusion and metabolism in the leg during upright bicycle exercise in patients with heart failure. Circulation 68: 425-432, 1983
Wilson JR, St John Sutton M, Schwartz JS, Ferraro N, Reichek N. Determinants of circulatory response to intravenous hydralazine in congestive heart failure. American Journal of Cardiology 52: 299-303, 1983b
Yeda H, Kaneko Y, Takeda T, et al. Observations on the mechanism of renin release by hydralazine in hypertensive patients. Circulation Research 27 (Suppl. 2): 201-206, 1970
Yeda H, Yagi S, Kaneko Y. Hydralazine and plasma renin activity. Archives of Internal Medicine 122: 387-391, 1968
Zacest R, Koch-Weser J. Relation of hydralazine plasma concentration to dosage and hypotensive action. Clinical Pharmacology and Therapeutics 13: 420-425, 1972

Authors' address: Dr *John P. Mulrow*, Department of Medicine, Division of Cardiology, University of Texas Health Science Center, 7703 Floyd Curl Drive, San Antonio, TX 78284 (USA).

Clinical Pharmacokinetics 16: 100-128 (1989)
0312-5963/89/0002-0100/$14.50/0

Pharmacokinetic-Pharmacodynamic Relationships of Oral Hypoglycaemic Agents

An Update

Piero Marchetti and *Renzo Navalesi*

Cattedra Malattie del Ricambio, Istituto di Clinica Medica II, Università di Pisa, Pisa, Italy

Contents

Summary ... 100
1. Treating Diabetes Mellitus ... 101
2. Sulphonylureas ... 102
2.1 Chemistry ... 102
2.2 Mechanisms of Action ... 102
2.3 Assay Methods ... 104
2.4 Pharmacokinetics ... 105
2.5 Drug Interactions ... 109
2.6 Clinical Use ... 110
2.7 Dose-Plasma Concentration-Therapeutic Effect Relationships ... 110
2.8 Dose-Plasma Concentration-Toxic Effect Relationships ... 112
3. Biguanides ... 113
3.1 Chemistry ... 113
3.2 Mechanisms of Action ... 114
3.3 Assay Methods ... 115
3.4 Pharmacokinetics ... 115
3.5 Drug Interactions ... 117
3.6 Clinical Use ... 117
3.7 Dose-Plasma Concentration-Therapeutic Effect Relationships ... 118
3.8 Dose-Plasma Concentration-Toxic Effect Relationships ... 118
4. Conclusions ... 120

Summary *Oral hypoglycaemic drugs, sulphonylureas and biguanides, occupy an important place in the treatment of Type II (non-insulin-dependent) diabetic patients who fail to respond satisfactorily to diet therapy and physical exercise. Although the precise mechanisms of action of these compounds are still poorly understood, there is sufficient agreement that sulphonylureas have both pancreatic and extrapancreatic effects, whereas biguanides have predominantly extrapancreatic actions. By using labelled compounds or measuring the circulating concentrations, the main pharmacokinetic properties of oral hypoglycaemic agents have been assessed and, in some cases, their pharmacokinetic-pharmacodynamic relationships have been evaluated. A correlation between diabetes control and plasma sulphonylurea or biguanide concentrations is generally lacking at the steady-state, with the possible exception of long-acting agents; after either oral or intravenous dosing, the reduction of plasma glucose is usually related to the increased circulating drug concentra-*

tions. The toxic effects of oral hypoglycaemic drugs are more frequent in the elderly and in the presence of conditions that may lead to drug accumulation or potentiation (increased dosage, use of long-acting compounds, hepatic and renal disease, interaction with other drugs); however, a relationship between toxic effects and drug plasma levels has been reported only for biguanides.

Two main classes of oral hypoglycaemic drugs are currently being used in the therapy of human diabetes mellitus (Foster 1983; Lebovitz & Feinglos 1983): the sulphonamide-derivative sulphonylureas and the guanidine-derivative biguanides (table I). Both sulphonylureas and biguanides, alone or in combination, can be usefully employed in properly selected patients with Type 2 (non-insulin-dependent) diabetes, when diet and physical exercise fail. Evidence has also been presented on the possible benefits of these drugs, in combination with insulin, in the management of Type 1 (insulin-dependent) diabetic patients (Goldman et al. 1984; Kabadi 1985). The mechanisms of action and the therapeutic and toxic effects of sulphonylureas and biguanides are discussed here in relation to their pharmacokinetic properties. Additional information is available in recently published reviews (Asmal & Marble 1984; Ferner & Chaplin 1987; Jackson & Bressler 1981; Lebovitz & Feinglos 1983; Melander 1987; Schafer 1983; Vigneri & Goldfine 1987). Newer hypoglycaemic agents which are at present under experimental and, in some cases, clinical investigation are not reviewed in this paper, and interested readers are referred to pertinent reports (Baron et al. 1987; Federlin et al. 1987; Kashiwagi et al. 1986).

1. Treating Diabetes Mellitus

Human diabetes mellitus is a heterogeneous disorder (Fajans et al. 1978). The most common types encountered clinically are Type 1 (insulin-dependent) diabetes mellitus (IDDM) and Type 2 (non-insulin-dependent) diabetes mellitus (NIDDM) (National Diabetes Data Group 1979). The former is mainly characterised by β-cell destruction, which leads to profound deficiency of insulin secretion (Cahill & McDevitt 1981); in NIDDM 2 major metabolic abnormalities contribute to the hyperglycaemic state: peripheral and hepatic insulin resistance (Rizza et al. 1981) and impaired insulin secretion (Savage et al. 1975).

The short term aim in treating diabetic patients is to control symptoms by restoring glycaemia to near normal levels. There is no doubt, however, that the most difficult goal is to prevent the long term micro- and macrovascular complications that affect both Type 1 and Type 2 diabetic patients. In this regard, effective treatment strategies must include control of blood pressure, regulation of plasma lipids, reduction of bodyweight, and modification of life-style (cigarette smoking, physical inactivity), together with the maintenance of blood glucose levels as near normal as possible, without major iatrogenic disturbances. Unfortunately, the levels of glucose intolerance which will increase the risk of development of micro- and macroangiopathy are not known. In Type 1 diabetic patients, data from prospective studies suggest that the progression of microangiopathic lesions can be delayed by maintaining fasting plasma glucose at or below a value of approximately 115 mg/dl and glycosylated haemoglobin (HbA_1) concentration not

Table I. Principal oral hypoglycaemic drugs

Sulphonylurea	Biguanide
Acetohexamide	Buformin
Chlorpropamide	Metformin
Glibenclamide (glyburide)	Phenformin
Gliclazide	
Glipizide	
Gliquidone	
Glisoxepide	
Tolazamide	
Tolbutamide	

higher than 9.0% (less than 15% greater than normal subjects) [Dahl-Jorgensen 1987]. It is not known whether the same figures are true for Type 2 diabetic patients.

It is noteworthy, however, that the risk of developing the specific microvascular lesions of diabetes does not appear to be great until the plasma glucose level 2 hours after oral glucose 75g is higher than 200 mg/dl (Jarrett & Keen 1976; National Diabetes Data Group 1979), a value that is approximately equivalent to the fasting plasma glucose level of 140 mg/dl (Pettit et al. 1980). Conversely, even minimal glucose intolerance (fasting plasma glucose ⩾ 110 to 120 mg/dl) is associated with accelerated macroangiopathy (Eschwege et al. 1980; Fuller et al. 1980). The risk of chronic diabetic macrovascular complications is absent until plasma glucose levels above 125 mg/dl are achieved 2 hours after an oral glucose 50g loading dose (Fuller et al. 1979).

In view of these findings, it is our opinion that diabetes control can be considered excellent if fasting and postprandial plasma glucose concentrations are below 115 mg/dl and 144 mg/dl, respectively. Diet therapy (Arky et al. 1982), weight reduction (Beck-Nielsen et al. 1979a) and physical exercise (Skyler 1984) can substantially reduce insulin resistance and improve insulin secretion in Type 2 diabetes. If good diabetes control is not achieved, or maintained, then an oral hypoglycaemic drug can be administered.

2. *Sulphonylureas*

2.1 Chemistry

During World War II, Janbon, a clinician from Montpelier, treating typhoid fever with a new sulphonamide derivative, glyprothiazole (2254 RP), noted that many patients developed hypoglycaemia (Janbon et al. 1942). The compound was extensively studied by Loubatieres (1957), and some derivatives were used in the treatment of diabetes mellitus in the mid-1950s. It was subsequently found that the elimination of an NH_2-moiety on the benzene ring and the opening of the heterocyclic nitrogen ring enhanced the therapeutic efficacy and reduced toxicity. The sulphonylurea drugs are derived from this latter molecule.

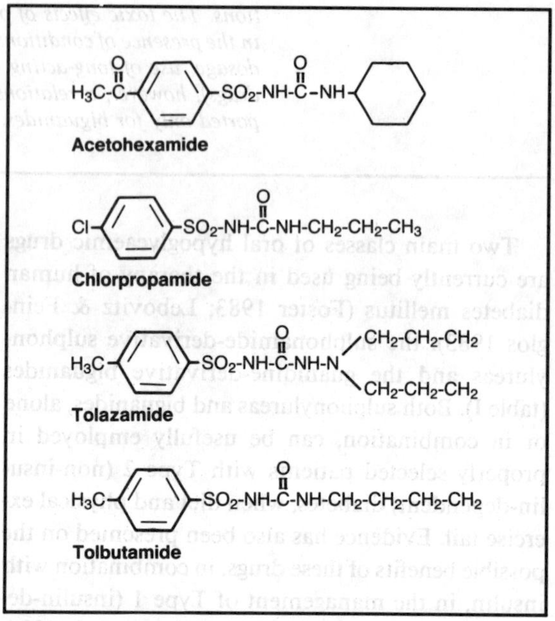

Fig. 1. Structural formulae of some first-generation sulphonylureas.

About 25 years after production of the original compounds [first-generation sulphonylureas (fig. 1)], the introduction of a cyclohesyl group instead of the aliphatic side-chain, and the addition of another ring structure linked to glycine in the other end of the molecule, led to the second-generation sulphonylureas (fig. 2). Compared with first-generation agents, the latter agents have similar mechanisms of action and much greater intrinsic activity.

2.2 Mechanisms of Action

Sulphonylurea agents improve glucose tolerance by increasing insulin secretion and enhancing insulin action. Thus, pancreatic and extrapancreatic mechanisms are involved in the hypoglycaemic effects of the drugs. However, despite much investigation, the exact site and mode of action of sulphonylureas remain unclear. In addition, although it is clear that these drugs show some similarities in their action, differences exist among first- and second-generation compounds (Melander 1987) and even among agents of the same generation (Groop et al. 1987). The already impressive amount of new information is being continually expanded and this section is merely an attempt to discuss some points of the issue.

2.2.1 Pancreatic Effects

The short term effect of sulphonylureas to stimulate insulin release from the pancreatic β-cells has been positively shown in hundreds of studies performed in healthy subjects, Type 2 diabetic patients, perfused animal pancreata and isolated islets of Langerhans (Cerasi et al. 1979; Goldfine et al. 1971; Grodsky et al. 1977; Hellman & Taljedal 1975; Hosker et al. 1985; Lebovitz 1987; Sussman et al. 1967). Glibenclamide and tolazamide also exert an inhibitory effect directly on glucagon-producing α-cells, this action not being due to a paracrine action of concomitant somatostatin release (Ostenson et al. 1986; Sako et al. 1986).

The action of the sulphonylureas on insulin secretion is more pronounced in the presence of glucose and is limited to the first phase of insulin release (Hellman & Taljedal 1975). In this regard, however, recent results obtained using the perfused rat pancreas indicate that tolbutamide and gliquidone, but not glibenclamide, stimulate both the first and second phase of insulin release in the absence of glucose (Santeusanio, personal communication). The cellular mechanisms of sulphonylurea-induced insulin secretion are still being actively investigated. Some studies support the hypothesis that the drugs exert their effect through an interaction with the β-cell membrane, without entering the cells (Gylfe et al. 1984; Kaubisch et al. 1982). The binding sites have high affinity and are multiple and saturable, and the rank order of potency of sulphonylurea-receptor interaction (evaluated for glibenclamide, glipizide and tolbutamide) reflects the biological activity of the drugs in either stimulating insulin secretion or inhibiting K^+ efflux from the cells (Gaines et al. 1988; Schmid-Antomerchi et al. 1957).

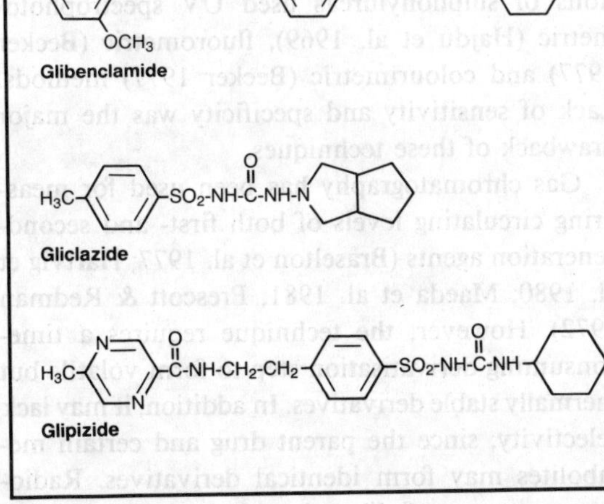

Fig. 2. Structural formulae of some second-generation sulphonylureas.

On the other hand, by using radiolabelled glibenclamide it has been demonstrated that approximately 80% of the radioactivity was localised in the cytoplasm of β-cells, associated with the insulin secretory granules (Carpentier et al. 1986).

In any case, it is believed that the interaction between sulphonylureas and the β-cell causes a sequence of events that includes a decrease in membrane potassium permeability, the depolarisation of membrane and the influx of calcium ions through voltage-dependent channels (Abrahamsson et al. 1985; Matthews & Shotton 1984). The increased cytosolic calcium level triggers the release of insulin from secretory granules; the effect is amplified by the increase of cyclic adenosine monophosphate (cAMP) due to the activation of adenylate cyclase (Sharpe 1979) and inhibition of 4′-5′ monophosphate diesterase (Goldfine et al. 1971). It is noteworthy that the non-sulphonylurea moieties of glibenclamide (Henquin et al. 1987) and gliquidone (Garrino et al. 1986), two second-generation sulphonylureas, have the same effects as the parent drugs on β-cells.

Despite maintenance of good metabolic control and improvement of glucose tolerance, both basal and glucose-induced plasma insulin levels have been found to be unchanged, or even decreased, during long term therapy with sulphonylureas. The phenomenon has been described with the use of most of the available sulphonylureas of both the first (Elkeles et al. 1982; Fineberg & Schneider 1980; Sheldon et al. 1966; Turtle 1970) and the second generation (Duckworth et al. 1972; Wajchenberg et al. 1980), with the possible exception of glipizide (Feinglos & Lebovitz 1980). Attention must be drawn to the fact that as plasma glucose levels fall during sulphonylurea therapy, peripheral insulin levels may return towards pretreatment values, thereby masking the improvement of β-cell function.

Interestingly, it has recently been observed that long term exposure of pancreatic β-cells to therapeutic concentrations of the sulphonylurea tolazamide induces a reversible state of refractoriness to acute intravenous stimulation from tolbutamine (Karam et al. 1986); this suggests that the insulinotropic effects of sulphonylureas might be more effective if these drugs are given either on an intermittent schedule or as 'pulse' therapy, using agents with short duration of action.

2.2.2 Extrapancreatic Effects

Successful treatment of Type 2 diabetes mellitus by sulphonylureas is associated with a decrease in basal hepatic glucose production and a return towards normal insulin suppression of hepatic glucose production (Amatruda et al. 1984; Kolterman et al. 1984). Sulphonylureas inhibit gluconeogenesis from lactate and pyruvate in experimental models, possibly by raising the intracellular content of fructose 2,6-bisphosphate (Cabello et al. 1987; Matsutani et al. 1984). Fructose 2,6-bisphosphate plays a key role in regulating the activity of enzymes of the glycolytic/gluconeogenic pathway (Hers & Hue 1983).

Another major extrapancreatic effect of sulphonylureas responsible for their hypoglycaemic action is the increase in insulin-mediated glucose uptake by peripheral tissues (Beck-Nielsen et al. 1979b; De Fronzo et al. 1983; Greenfield et al. 1982; Kolterman 1985; Lebovitz et al. 1977). Controversy exists about the mechanisms of the extrapancreatic effects of sulphonylureas at the cellular level. Despite many reports showing that sulphonylureas increase insulin binding to various cell types (Beck-Nielsen et al. 1979a,b; Feinglos & Lebovitz 1978; Hjollund et al. 1983; Joost et al. 1982; Prince & Olefsky 1980), most studies on insulin-sensitive cells indicate that the drugs do not have a direct effect on insulin receptors (Goldfine et al. 1984; Maloff & Lockwood 1981; Salhanick et al. 1983). Thus, it is currently believed that enhancement of insulin responsiveness occurs through post-binding mechanisms (Kolterman et al. 1984; Lockwood et al. 1983). In isolated human monocytes, the reduced intracellular degradation found in Type 2 diabetic patients (Trischitta et al. 1987) can be ameliorated by sulphonylurea treatment (Ciccarone et al. 1987). Recently, the improvement in peripheral glucose disposal has been ascribed to direct effects of sulphonylurea on glucose transport, in the absence of insulin (Rogers et al. 1987).

2.3 Assay Methods

To be able to accurately assess the relationships between the pharmacokinetic and pharmacodynamic properties of a drug, it is necessary to measure drug concentrations in plasma (and possibly other biological fluids) by sensitive, specific and precise analytical methods.

Early attempts to measure plasma concentrations of sulphonylureas used UV spectrophotometric (Hajdu et al. 1969), fluorometric (Becker 1977) and colourimetric (Becker 1977) methods. Lack of sensitivity and specificity was the major drawback of these techniques.

Gas chromatography has been used for measuring circulating levels of both first- and second-generation agents (Braselton et al. 1977; Hartvig et al. 1980; Maeda et al. 1981; Prescott & Redman 1972). However, the technique requires a time-consuming derivatisation step to form volatile but thermally stable derivatives. In addition, it may lack selectivity, since the parent drug and certain metabolites may form identical derivatives. Radioimmunoassays of glibenclamide (glyburide) [Glogner et al. 1973, 1977; Kawashima et al. 1979; Royer et al. 1976] and glipizide (Maggi et al. 1981) have been developed. These methods showed good sensitivity, but in some cases cross-reactivity between glibenclamide and its major metabolites was observed (Glogner et al. 1973, 1977; Royer et al. 1976). The cross-reaction among glipizide, glibenclamide and gliclazide (Maggi et al. 1981) should not create problems because the 3 sulphonylureas are not administered together. We are not aware of any commercially available kits for radioimmunoassay of sulphonylureas.

At present, it is our opinion that high performance liquid chromatographic (HPLC) methods represent the best choice for measuring sulphonylurea concentration in biological fluids because of their sensitivity, precision, specificity and ease of use (Charles & Ravenscroft 1984; Emilsson 1987; Emilsson et al. 1986; Keal et al. 1986; Kimura et al. 1980; Potter & Hulm 1983; Raghow & Mcyer 1981; Vihlein & Sistovaris 1982; Wahlin-Boll & Melander 1979).

In general, however, all the reported techniques suffer a common major drawback, i.e. they have been used almost exclusively to measure total (bound and unbound) drug concentration. In fact, as discussed below, sulphonylureas are largely bound to plasma proteins and only the free drug is pharmacologically active. As recently reviewed (Svensson et al. 1986), the most widely used methods to separate free and bound drug are equilibrium dialysis and ultrafiltration. For the sulphonylureas, the unbound drug has only occasionally been measured (Neuvonen et al. 1987). This fact must be carefully taken into account when evaluating the dose-plasma concentration-effect relationships. Of course, sensitivity problems become much more relevant when measuring the unbound fraction of sulphonylureas.

2.4 Pharmacokinetics

The available information on the pharmacokinetics of oral sulphonylureas (table II) has been obtained mainly in healthy subjects, during single-dose or short term administration, and the validity of extrapolation to diabetic patients is not clear. Many factors affecting absorption, distribution, excretion and metabolism of these agents require further investigation. Little is known on the effect of fibre administration (meals rich in fibre are advisable for diabetic patients) on absorption of sulphonylureas (Shima et al. 1983). In addition, absorption may be delayed in patients with diabetic autonomic neuropathy (Matikainen & Juntunen 1984). Sulphonylureas are largely employed in elderly patients, and age can profoundly modify the pharmacokinetics of a drug (Cohen 1986): much more information is needed in this regard. Renal and hepatic diseases can perturb the disposition of drugs (Gibson 1986). However, the second-generation agents have seldom been studied from this point of view. As recently discussed (Abernethy & Greenblatt 1986), drug disposition may be changed in obese individuals, and although oral hypoglycaemic drugs are often administered to overweight patients, data on this issue are lacking. Glucose itself may affect drug metabolism (Yau et al. 1987), as suggested in laboratory animals: the issue of whether this has a clinical relevance for the disposition of sulphonylureas given to patients with different degrees of hyperglycaemia might be an interesting field of research. Finally, genetic factors may play an important role in oral hypoglycaemic drug metabolism, as suggested for tolbutamide and phenformin (Oates et al. 1982; Scott & Poffenbarger 1979): the relevance of this issue for other agents requires investigation.

2.4.1 *Absorption*

Both first- and second-generation compounds are well absorbed after oral administration (Jackson & Bressler 1981; Shen & Bressler 1977). Time to peak plasma drug concentration varies among the different sulphonylureas, with the shortest values (2 to 3 hours) being observed for glipizide, gliquidone, glibenclamide and tolbutamide, and the longest (3 to 6 hours) for chlorpropamide and gliclazide (Ferner & Chaplin 1987; Holmes et al. 1984; Jackson & Bressler 1981; Melander 1987; Pearson 1985). Studying the absorption of glibenclamide from different sites of the gastrointestinal tract, it has been shown that the amount of drug absorbed

Table II. Pharmacokinetic properties of some sulphonylureas (adapted from Asmal & Marble 1984; Gerich 1985)

Drug	$t_{1/2}$ (h)	Vd (L/kg)	Protein binding	Duration of action (h)	Metabolism	Excretion	Daily dose range (mg)
Acetohexamide	0.8-2.4[a] 4-6[b]		Ionic	8-18	Hepatic	Renal	250-1500
Chlorpropamide	24-48	0.09-0.27	Ionic	24-72	Hepatic	Renal	100-500
Glibenclamide (glyburide)	1.4-3 10-16[c]	0.3	Non-ionic	16-24	Hepatic	Renal, biliary	2.5-20
Gliclazide	6-15	0.2	Non-ionic	24	Hepatic	Renal, biliary	40-320
Glipizide	1-7	0.16	Non-ionic	12-24	Hepatic	Renal	2.5-40
Tolazamide	4-7		Ionic	12-18	Hepatic	Renal	100-1000
Tolbutamide	3-28	0.1-0.15	Ionic	6-12	Hepatic	Renal	500-3000

a Parent drug.
b Active metabolite.
c Third phase.
Abbreviations: $t_{1/2}$ = elimination half-life; Vd = apparent volume of distribution.

was the same regardless of the site at which it was placed (i.e. stomach, duodenum and ascending colon). However, the rate of absorption from the colon was lower than from the other sites (Brockmeier et al. 1985).

Differences in absorption rate between tablets from different manufacturers have been described for tolbutamide (Olson et al. 1985; Rupp et al. 1975). Early glibenclamide tablets marketed in Europe also displayed incomplete absorption (Rupp et al. 1972); although it has been reported that recent formulations show 80 to 100% bioavailability (Pearson 1985), other authors demonstrated differences in the bioavailability of glibenclamide from 3 different tablet preparations (Chalk et al. 1986). These findings suggest that it might not be wise to assume the bioequivalence of different pharmaceutical preparations of the same agent. 'Fast' and 'slow' absorbers of gliclazide (peak plasma concentrations within 4 and 8 hours, respectively) [Campbell et al. 1980] and glibenclamide (peak plasma concentrations within 2 and 6 hours, respectively) [Ikegami et al. 1986] have been described. The delay in glibenclamide absorption was related to the presence of diabetic autonomic neuropathy.

Food delays the absorption of chlorpropamide (but not its bioavailability) and glipizide (Sartor et al. 1980c; Wahlin-Boll et al. 1980), but not of tolbutamide (Sartor et al. 1980c; Antal et al. 1982) and glibenclamide (Sartor et al. 1980a). It has, however, been reported that glibenclamide administration 2 hours after breakfast significantly delays the rate of drug absorption in Type 2 diabetic patients (Grill et al. 1986). Glucomannan, a dietary fibre, and activated charcoal delay the absorption of glibenclamide (Shima et al. 1983) and tolbutamide (Neuvonen et al. 1983), respectively. Age does not affect the rate of absorption of tolbutamide in healthy volunteers (Sartor et al. 1980c); on the other hand, gliclazide absorption decreases with age (Forette et al. 1982). The absorption of glipizide (Wahlin-Boll et al. 1980), but not of gliclazide (Kobayashi et al. 1981), is more variable in diabetic patients than in healthy subjects.

2.4.2 Protein Binding

Sulphonylureas are strongly bound to plasma proteins at concentrations within the normal therapeutic range. The high degree of binding may modify drug distribution and elimination, and displacement by other drugs with similar binding tendencies is also possible (see below). Albumin represents the class of protein to which sulphonylureas are bound to the greatest extent (Crooks &

Brown 1974; Judis 1972): acetohexamide also binds to fibrinogen (10%) and α-globulin IV-4 (7 to 16%). Chlorpropamide and tolbutamide bind to some extent to β-globulin III (13.5 and 15.8%, respectively) and α-globulin IV-4 (4 and 12.9%, respectively) [Judis 1972]. Among the various sulphonylureas, glibenclamide appears to be the most strongly bound, compared with tolbutamide, chlorpropamide and tolazamide (Crooks & Brown 1974). Scatchard analysis of the interaction between sulphonylureas and albumin suggests that glibenclamide binds with only 1 site, while tolbutamide, chlorpropamide and glipizide bind with 2 sites (Crooks & Brown 1974). Binding increases with rising drug concentration (Crooks & Brown 1974). In this regard, binding of glibenclamide is less sensitive to changes in concentration than tolazamide and chlorpropramide. The binding sites for first- and second-generation agents are different (Crooks & Brown 1975; Hsu et al. 1974). Interestingly, first-generation agents interact with proteins through ionic forces, whereas second-generation compounds bind to albumin by Van der Waals forces, as suggested by temperature dependence and pH independence of binding (Crooks & Brown 1974). This difference may be of relevance in that second-generation sulphonylureas might be more weakly displaced by drug anions such as phenylbutazone, warfarin and salicylate; however, the true clinical significance of this point is still to be assessed.

2.4.3 Metabolism and Excretion

Sulphonylureas are extensively metabolised in the liver, with the metabolites and the parent drug being eliminated mainly in the urine, but also in the faeces (table II). For this reason sulphonylureas are contraindicated in hepatic and renal disease. In particular, liver disease increases the frequency and severity of hypoglycaemic episodes (Seltzer 1979), due to the reduced metabolism of the drug and hypoalbuminaemia, which may lead to lower protein binding and higher plasma free drug concentrations. On the other hand, reduced renal function causes a prolongation of hypoglycaemic drug effect (Asplund et al. 1983; Berger 1971; Seltzer 1979).

Chlorpropamide is about 80% metabolised in the liver (Taylor 1972). The 3 main metabolites are *p*-chlorobenzene sulphonylurea, 2-hydroxychlorpropamide and 3-hydroxychlorpropamide: the derivatives partially possess hypoglycaemic activity and are eliminated in the urine. The elimination half-life of chlorpropamide is the longest (35 hours) among the sulphonylureas (Brotherton et al. 1969; Knaupf et al. 1959; Taylor 1972). Alkalinisation and acidification of the urine respectively increase and reduce urinary excretion of the drug (Neuvonen et al. 1987). Due to the long half-life, on continued dosing the drug will accumulate, reaching steady-state concentrations in about 5 to 7 half-lives, i.e. 7 to 10 days. Both glomerular and tubular diseases increase the half-life of chlorpropamide, with a more pronounced effect in cases of tubular damage (Petitpierre et al. 1972).

The first step in the hepatic metabolism of tolbutamide is hydroxylation by a microsomal oxidase system, followed by transformation to a carboxyl derivative by further oxidation in the cytosol (Purba et al. 1987; Scott & Poffenbarger 1979; Thomas & Ikeda 1966). Both hydroxy- and carboxy-tolbutamide are excreted in the urine (Thomas & Ikeda 1966). The metabolites have minimal hypoglycaemic effects (Feldman & Lebovitz 1969). In healthy volunteers, a wide variability of tolbutamide disappearance rates from plasma after intravenous injection has been reported (Scott & Poffenbarger 1979), suggesting that genetic factors may control the rate of tolbutamide metabolism. Smoking (Scott & Poffenbarger 1979) and age (Sartor et al. 1980c) do not affect the elimination rate of the drug. Elimination half-life of tolbutamide has been reported to be decreased (Ueda et al. 1963) or unchanged (Nelson 1964) in liver cirrhosis; however, the period of tolbutamide-induced hypoglycaemia is longer in cirrhotics (Ueda et al. 1963). Clearance of unbound tolbutamide was similar during and after the acute phase of viral hepatitis (Williams et al. 1977). Following intravenous injection of the drug, mean plasma half-life was found to be increased in patients with unconjugated hyperbilirubinaemia due either to Gilbert's syndrome or thalassaemia (Carulli et al. 1976). A significant positive correlation between tolbutamide half-life and either glomerular filtration or serum non-protein nitrogen was observed in patients with renal disease (Ueda et al. 1963). Asthma (Sonatiemi et al. 1971a) and respiratory failure (Sonatiemi et al. 1971b) reduce tolbutamide half-life.

Most of the activity of acetohexamide *in vivo* is due to its metabolite hydroxyhexamide, which is produced in the liver and cleared by the kidney (Galloway et al. 1967; Smith et al. 1965). The drug and its metabolites have a longer half-life in renal disease (Cohen et al. 1967).

Tolazamide is metabolised, most probably in the liver, to *p*-carboxytolazamide, 2-hydroxy-metabolites, *p*-toluensulphonamide and an unknown metabolite, with 7% of the parent drug excreted unchanged in the urine (Thomas et al. 1978). The metabolites may have some hypoglycaemic activity.

Glibenclamide is almost completely metabolised in the liver to 2 hydroxy-metabolites, *cis*-3-hydroxyglibenclamide and *trans*-4-hydroxyglibenclamide, and a third unidentified metabolite (Rupp et al. 1969). The different isomers of the hydroxyglibenclamide occur because of the different substitution position. The metabolites are relatively inactive, with the *trans*-4-hydroxyglibenclamide having about 15% of the hypoglycaemic activity of the parent drug when tested in rats (Balant et al. 1979), and are eliminated in the bile and urine (Rupp et al. 1969). A 2-compartment open model is generally sufficient to describe the time course behaviour of plasma glibenclamide after both intravenous and oral administration (Adams & Krueger 1979; Fuccella et al. 1973; Sartor et al. 1980b). However, following intravenous injection of radiolabelled glibenclamide, a third component to the elimination phase has been suggested (Rupp et al. 1969). In addition, a semilog plot with non-linear terminal phase definition has been provided (Balant et al. 1977). A more recent study (Pearson et al. 1986) indicates that both the third phase and the non-linear semilog plot are probably due to an insufficiently specific technique and incomplete analysis. Nevertheless, a third, slowly equilibrating 'deep' compartment may exist, which would be detectable only as the drug accumulates during long term administration giving rise to a measurable plasma concentration. Glibenclamide metabolites may accumulate in patients with renal failure (Balant et al. 1977) which might induce hypoglycaemia (Berger 1971). Glibenclamide half-life and clearance, however, do not correlate with creatinine clearance until the latter exceeds 5 ml/min/1.73m^2 (Pearson et al. 1986).

Hepatic metabolism accounts for transformation of glipizide to inactive 2-hydroxy-cyclohexyl derivatives and 2 unidentified metabolites (Fuccella et al. 1973; Schmidt et al. 1973). About 7% of the dose is excreted unchanged in the urine; the metabolites are also eliminated by the kidney (Fuccella et al. 1973; Schmidt et al. 1973). The terminal elimination half-life of glipizide is 1 to 4 hours after a single dose (Wahlin-Boll et al. 1982a) and increases to 2 to 5 hours after long term treatment (Wahlin-Boll 1986). Following intravenous administration, 2-compartment models fit the time course of plasma drug plus metabolite concentrations (Balant et al. 1978; Schmidt et al. 1973); more complicated models have been reported after oral dosing (Balant et al. 1978). No significant increase in glipizide half-life was found in 2 patients with renal impairment (Balant et al. 1973).

As recently reviewed (Holmes et al. 1984), gliclazide is metabolised in the liver to at least 8 metabolites, and less than 20% is excreted unchanged. The major metabolic pathways in humans involve oxidation with production of hydroxylated or *N*-oxygenated compounds and the corresponding alcohol and carboxylic acid. The most important gliclazide metabolite is an *N*-oxygenated derivative, which represents 1% of plasma drug-related compounds, has no hypoglycaemic action and possesses antiplatelet effect (Campbell et al. 1980). Studying the fate of ^{14}C-gliclazide in animals and humans, it has been reported that 60 to 70% of the drug dose is excreted in the urine, and the remainder in the faeces (Campbell et al. 1980; Miyazaki et al. 1983). There may be wide variation in the elimination half-life, which ranges from 6.1 to 14.3 hours in healthy volunteers; it is longer in males and in the elderly (Forette et al. 1982), and is increased in renal failure (Campbell et al. 1986). The existence of a 'gliclazide-degrading factor' in human serum has recently been suggested (Kobayashi et al. 1985).

The available information on gliquidone (Kaubish et al. 1979; Kopitar 1975; Kopitar & Koss 1975) can be summarised as follows. The drug is mainly deactivated in the liver by demethylation and parahydroxylation; the latter is pharmacologically active to some extent. Studies in experimental animals and in humans revealed a predominance of hepatic clearance, with renal excretion being only of secondary importance. A 2-compartment model with first-order absorption appeared to be appropriate for the mathematical description of the gliquidone plasma concentrations.

2.5 Drug Interactions

Numerous drugs have been reported to interact with sulphonylureas leading to either potentiation or attenuation of the latter's hypoglycaemic action, through pharmacokinetic and/or pharmacodynamic interactions. Potentiation of sulphonylurea action due to pharmacokinetic mechanisms may be achieved by displacement from plasma protein binding sites (phenylbutazone, antiepileptic drugs, salicylates, sulphonamides, clofibrate) [Berger 1971; Eckhardt et al. 1972; Ferrari et al. 1976; Field et al. 1967; Fernandez et al. 1985; MacKichan, this issue], inhibition of hepatic metabolism (sulphofenazone, pyrazolone derivatives, coumarin anticoagulants, propanolol, methyldopa, chloramphenicol, halofenate) [Berger 1971; Brunova et al. 1977; Gachalyi et al. 1980; Jain et al. 1975; Kristensen & Hansen 1972; Solomon & Schrogre 1967] or reduction of urinary excretion (probenecid, some sulphonamides, salicylates) [Christensen et al. 1963; Jumholtz et al. 1975]. Attenuation of sulphonylurea action has been observed during therapy with rifampicin and phenobarbitone, due to an increase in hepatic metabolism (Redman & Prescott 1973; Self & Morris 1980). Hepatic enzyme induction by these drugs is likely to minimise the possible potentiation of sulphonylurea effects which should theoretically exist, because of the displacement of the hypoglycaemic agents from the protein binding sites (see MacKichan, this issue). Hepatic enzyme induction of sulphonylurea metabolism is also caused by chronic alcoholism (Kater et al. 1969). Compounds which increase urine pH shorten chlorpropamide half-life, due to the positive correlation between chlorpropamide renal clearance and urine pH (Neuvonen & Karkkainen 1983).

Pharmacodynamic interactions have been claimed to explain the potentiation of sulphonylurea action by monoamine oxidase inhibitors (increased insulin secretion, decreased gluconeogenesis) [Conn 1965; Cooper & Ashcroft 1967], and short term ethanol administration (decreased gluconeogenesis) [Seltzer 1972]. Drugs which antagonise the action of oral hypoglycaemic agents through pharmacodynamic mechanisms include β-adrenergic blockers (regulation of substrate flow, interference with hormone secretion) [Hansten 1980; Verschoor et al. 1986], thiazide diuretics (decreased insulin release) [Conn 1965], glucocorticosteroids (Thorn 1966) and β-adrenoceptor agonists (increased gluconeogenesis and glycogenolysis) [Middleton & Finke 1968].

Some drugs have more complex interaction mechanisms. Besides the abovementioned action, for instance, salicylates increase glucose uptake by muscle (Randle & Smith 1958), inhibit gluconeogenesis (Woods et al. 1974), and increase insulin release (Giugliano et al. 1978). The potentiation of the action of chlorpropamide during sodium salicylate administration is achieved without any change in plasma sulphonylurea concentrations (Richardson et al. 1986). The combined interaction of displacement and metabolic inhibition has been claimed to explain the increased plasma concentration and potentiation of glipizide during indobufen administration (Elvander-Stahl et al. 1984). The calcium antagonist verapamil inhibits both glucose and sulphonylurea-stimulated insulin release *in vitro* (Devis et al. 1975); in many diabetic subjects, intravenous verapamil injection decreases insulin secretion following an oral dose of glibenclamide 5mg (De Marinis & Barbarino 1980). Concomitant oral dosing of verapamil and glibenclamide resulted in higher concentrations of the sulphonylurea, but not in a higher plasma insulin level, suggesting that verapamil may have an inhibitory effect on insulin release (Semple et al. 1986). Stockley et al. (1986) reported no effect by H_2-receptor antagonists on the disposition of tolbutamide in healthy subjects, while Cate et al. (1986) noted an increase. Thus, many agents through many mechanisms affect sulphonylurea action to different extents. It is noteworthy that the interaction is often bidirectional, so that particular caution is needed when prescribing any new medication in patients on sulphonylurea therapy as well as when starting treatment with oral hypoglycaemic agents in patients on therapy with other drugs.

2.6 Clinical Use

General considerations in the selection of patients who can be treated advantageously with hypoglycaemic agents are age at onset of diabetes (> 40 years), duration of diabetes (< 10 years), insulin dose (< 30 units/day) [Asmal & Marble 1984; Gunderson et al. 1975]. Additional criteria include obesity at time of presentation, absence of ketoacidosis, and fasting blood glucose levels < 200 mg/dl. It is possible that a more careful initial selection of patients to be treated with sulphonylureas might lower the high rates of primary failure of these drugs, which range from 5 to 36% (Bernhard 1965; Singer & Hurwitz 1967; Stowers & Bewsher 1962) and are similar with the use of both first- and second-generation agents. Sometimes patients unresponsive to first-generation sulphonylureas will respond to second-generation compounds (Beisswanger et al. 1987). Secondary failure may occur in approximately 5% of patients who initially have a response to sulphonylurea therapy (Krall 1985); in this regard, second-generation agents may offer some advantage over first-generation drugs (Lebovitz 1985).

2.7 Dose-Plasma Concentration-Therapeutic Effect Relationships

The relationship between sulphonylurea dose, plasma concentrations and therapeutic effects is not simple. Different conclusions may be drawn when considering the steady-state condition from those reached on consideration of the condition after dosing. Fasting plasma concentrations of sulphonylureas are generally very low, often below the detection limit, especially when agents with a short half-life are given, or during once-daily administration. Therefore, it is difficult to correlate fasting drug concentrations with drug dose and plasma glucose. Nevertheless, even when circulating sulphonylurea concentrations are undetectable, the hypoglycaemic effect is observed in comparison with placebo (Peterson et al. 1982). Melander et al. (1978) studied 37 diabetic patients on tolbutamide and 60 patients on chlorpropamide: fasting sulphonylurea concentrations ranged widely, from 0 to 370 μmol/L and from 0 to 882 μmol/L, respectively (fig. 3). No apparent correlation was found between the circulating drug and fasting blood glucose, nor between dosage (the variation of which was 4- to 6-fold) and serum drug concentrations. In a subgroup of 15 of 83 outpatients a relation was observed between predose serum chlorpropamide concentrations and fasting blood glucose (Bergman et al. 1980). Chlorpropamide dose was also correlated with serum drug concentrations. In 9 Type 2 diabetic patients, fasting chlorpropamide concentrations ranged from 90 to 466 μmol/L, and were inversely related to the blood glucose levels (Almer et al. 1982). Wahlin-Boll et al. (1982b) reported higher fasting chlorpropamide concentrations (but similar metabolic control) during a regimen consisting of chlorpropamide 431mg in comparison with 278mg given once daily.

Sartor et al. (1980a) studied 37 Type 2 diabetic patients treated with glibenclamide for at least 1 year; steady-state drug concentrations ranged from 0 to 1520 nmol/L (mean 478 nmol/L). No correlation was found between drug dose and serum levels, nor between drug concentrations and fasting blood glucose.

Fasting glipizide concentrations following a once-daily regimen or divided doses were found to range from 0 to 0.29 μmol/L and 0 to 0.56 μmol/L, respectively, in 9 diabetic patients (Almer et al. 1982); fasting plasma glucose was higher in patients with lower drug concentration. In a larger group

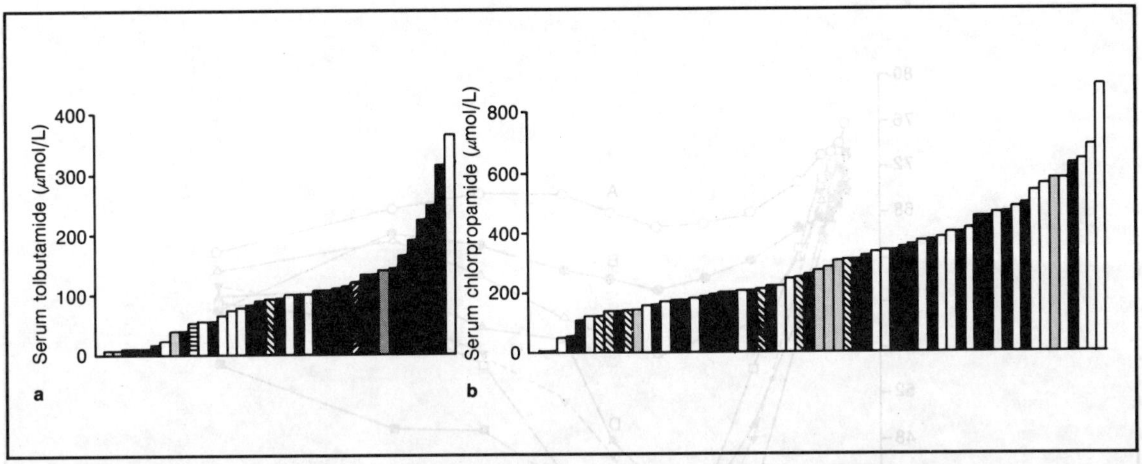

Fig. 3. Steady-state concentrations of (**a**) serum tolbutamide (▨ = 0.5g; ▤ = 0.75g; □ = 1.0g; ■ = 1.5g; ▧ = 2.0g; ▨ = 2.5g; ▩ = 3.0g; n = 37) and (**b**) serum chlorpropamide (▧ = 125mg; ■ = 250mg; □ = 375mg; ▩ = 500mg; n = 60) in patients with diabetes mellitus treated with daily doses of these drugs for at least a year. From Melander et al. (1978), with permission.

(n = 23) of diabetic patients, 2 crossover studies were performed to compare different schedules for glipizide treament (Wahlin-Boll et al. 1986). While demonstrating the therapeutic equivalence of glipizide given once or 3 times daily, the study also showed that at the steady-state, despite even double plasma drug concentrations, no difference in plasma glucose level could be found. Surprisingly, with administration of glipizide 25mg instead of 14.75mg in divided doses, despite higher fasting drug concentration at the high dose, impairment of metabolic control has been found (Wahlin-Boll et al. 1982b).

From these data one can reasonably conclude that, with the possible exception of chlorpropamide, which has a long half-life, fasting sulphonylurea concentrations do not generally correlate with dose and hypoglycaemic effects.

Conversely, after both oral and intravenous administration of sulphonylureas, a correlation can generally be found between dose, blood drug concentrations and effects. In the study by Sheldon et al. (1965), 55 diabetic patients treated with chlorpropamide, 40 with acetohexamide and 30 with tolbutamide were examined; patients were arbitrarily subdivided according to metabolic control (good, fair and poor). The serum concentrations of sulphonylureas 3 to 5 hours after the morning dose were correlated with drug dose and in good responders they were: tolbutamide 78 ± 18 ng/L; chlorpropamide 77 ± 38 ng/L; and acetohexamide 37 ± 12 ng/L. Many patients among fair and poor responders had drug concentrations within or above the therapeutic range. Age was not correlated with serum sulphonylurea concentrations.

After both oral and intravenous administration of glisoxepide, glibornuride and glibenclamide, a correlation between log dose and the fall in blood glucose levels was found in 5 healthy subjects (Haupt et al. 1972). In 12 healthy volunteers, following 3 different tablet preparations of glibenclamide, the decrease of plasma glucose paralleled the time course of plasma drug concentrations (Chalk et al. 1986). After intravenous tolbutamide (dose from 0.063g to 1.5g) a significant correlation between dose, serum tolbutamide, plasma insulin and fall in blood glucose was found in 4 healthy subjects (Ganda et al. 1975) [fig. 4]. However, when a single dose of tolbutamide 1g was given in 18 volunteers, the same correlations did not emerge, suggesting considerable biological variability of response in a given population sample.

In healthy subjects, following oral administration of gliclazide 80mg, a correlation was found

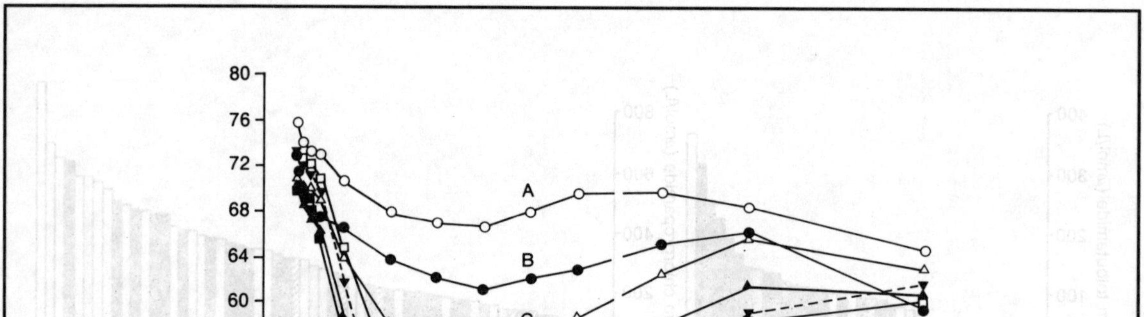

Fig. 4. Mean levels of blood glucose in 4 healthy subjects following different intravenous doses of tolbutamide [reproduced from Ganda et al. (1975), with permission].

between the fall in glucose levels and drug concentrations when the 0 to 4-hour period was considered (Campbell et al. 1980); the threshold sulphonylurea concentration to elicit the hypoglycaemic action appeared to be 0.25 g/L. Similar results were obtained in diabetic patients given gliclazide and oral glucose 50g, although the threshold concentration of gliclazide was found to be 1.5 g/L. Up to a dose of gliquidone 30mg, plasma drug concentrations rose proportionally with increasing doses, given intravenously; glucose levels decreased, as a consequence of the rise of insulin levels (Kaubisch et al. 1979). After oral dosing in Type 2 diabetic patients, the rise in plasma gliquidone was paralleled by a rise in plasma insulin and a decrease in blood glucose (Kaubisch et al. 1979).

In conclusion, the experimental design is the main determinant when searching for the relationships between sulphonylurea dose, plasma concentrations and action, the correlations usually being found when samples are drawn within a few hours after administration of the drug.

2.8 Dose-Plasma Concentration-Toxic Effect Relationships

Considering the large number of patients treated with sulphonylurea agents (1.8 million in the United States in 1980); the frequency of side effects and toxicity can be considered low. Allergic dermatitis and mild gastrointestinal disturbances occur in a percentage varying from 0.5 to 7.8% (Emanueli et al. 1972; Gunderson et al. 1975; O'Donovan 1959; Pannekock 1976), with a higher frequency for chlorpropamide. Chlorpropamide may also cause dilutional hyponatraemia (Weissman et al. 1971). These effects are usually dose-related and harmless, if the offending substance is discontinued or the dose reduced. Hypersensitivity reactions may occur during therapy with sulphonylureas (Clarke et al. 1974; Levitt 1987; Pannekock 1976): they include skin, blood, gastrointestinal and cardiovascular reactions, and their intensity is variable, with haematological dyscrasias being the most threatening. The relation between toxic effects and sulphonylurea dose and plasma concentrations has not been investigated.

Disulfiram-like reactions are an acute flushing of the skin surface and other vascular phenomena in patients using alcohol while on therapy with chlorpropamide. In a study by Groop et al. (1984), chlorpropamide concentrations were higher in patients with flushing (104 ± 4 μmol/L) than in patients without the reaction (79 ± 3 μmol/L).

The commonest adverse reaction due to sulphonylureas is hypoglycaemia. This can be considered a manifestation of relative or actual overdosage, as well as inadequate food intake. Severe hypoglycaemia occurs in approximately 1% of sulphonylurea-treated patients (Berger 1971), the mortality being about 11% for patients presenting in coma (Seltzer 1979). In a series of 57 cases of glibenclamide-associated hypoglycaemia, Asplund et al. (1983) reported 10 cases with fatal outcome. Chlorpropamide and glibenclamide account for the majority of cases, because of their long half-lives (Asplund et al. 1983; Seltzer 1979). Administration in the elderly, renal function impairment, liver disease or ingestion of other drugs known to potentiate the hypoglycaemic action of sulphonylureas represent well-assessed risk factors for sulphonylurea-induced hypoglycaemia. All these factors, as already discussed, modify the pharmacokinetic properties of the drugs, and this very probably causes inappropriate circulating sulphonylurea concentrations; nevertheless, the authors are not aware of any studies that evaluate plasma sulphonylurea levels during hypoglycaemic episodes in sulphonylurea-treated diabetic patients, so that this issue remains unsettled. Jordan et al. (1977) reported plasma drug concentrations in 2 cases of sulphonylurea-induced factitious hypoglycaemia: plasma chlorpropamide concentrations of 4 g/L and 2.4 g/L were found.

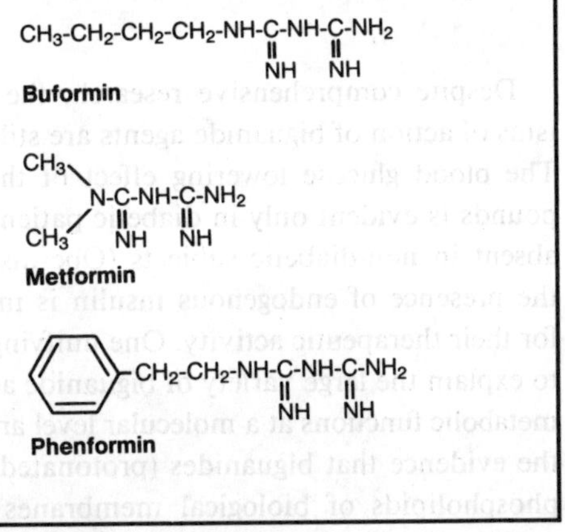

Fig. 5. Structural formulae of the biguanides.

3. Biguanides

3.1 Chemistry

Biguanide derivatives are constituted by 2 molecules of guanidine linked together with the elimination of an ammonia group, and a hydrocarbon side-chain of various types and lengths. There are more than 300 known biguanide derivatives (Beckmann 1977), but only 3 have clinical interest: phenethyl-biguanide (phenformin), dimethyl-biguanide (metformin) and butyl-biguanide (buformin) [fig. 5]. Biguanides are strong bases and at physiological pH values they exist in the form of positively charged protons. The apolar hydrocarbon side-chain allows these agents to bind to hydrophilic structures, such as the phospholipids of biological membranes.

3.2 Mechanisms of Action

Despite comprehensive research, the mechanisms of action of biguanide agents are still unclear. The blood glucose lowering effect of these compounds is evident only in diabetic patients, and is absent in non-diabetic subjects (Oberdisse 1977); the presence of endogenous insulin is mandatory for their therapeutic activity. One unifying concept to explain the large variety of biguanide actions on metabolic functions at a molecular level arises from the evidence that biguanides (protonated) bind to phospholipids of biological membranes (Schafer 1972); this causes a positive shift of membrane surface charges and a fluidity modification of membrane lipids. The consequence is a change in the biological membrane functions.

3.2.1 Pancreatic Effects

There is general agreement that biguanides do not stimulate insulin secretion (Hermann 1979; Schafer 1983); at high concentrations, they may even inhibit insulin release induced by glucose in isolated rat islets of Langerhans (Schatz et al. 1972b). Nevertheless, using the perfused pancreas of normal rats, a potentiating effect of metformin on insulin output in response to glucose and arginine has been observed (Bobbioni et al. 1979); in pigs, metformin enhances the arginine-induced insulin release (Kuhl et al. 1979). In preliminary experiments from this laboratory, insulin release from isolated pig islets in response to 4 g/L glucose is potentiated in the presence of metformin at therapeutic concentrations (Giannarelli et al. 1988). Early studies in man (Schatz et al. 1972a; Vermeulen & Rottius 1972) showed lower plasma glucose and normal (or even decreased) insulin levels after metformin treatment basally and during an oral glucose tolerance test in comparison to the pretreatment values. More recently, a lack of stimulation of insulin secretion by metformin has been claimed, using the measurement of plasma *C*-peptide levels (Prager & Schernthaner 1983).

3.2.2 Extrapancreatic Effects

As extensively discussed (Schafer 1972, 1976), binding of biguanides to biological membranes causes a change in the membrane potential with consequences for transport and other metabolic processes. This is the reason for the multifactorial mode of action of the biguanides, although it is not known to what extent the different single effects contribute to the overall antidiabetic activity. Possibly by inhibiting active cell processes (see below) biguanides reduce the intestinal absorption of sugar, calcium, vitamin B_{12} and folic acid (Caspary 1977; Czyzyk et al. 1986; Lorch 1971). These effects have been demonstrated mainly *in vitro* using isolated intestinal loops. In humans, high doses of phenformin reduce glucose absorption (Czyzyk et al. 1986); in other studies with humans, this effect was not demonstrated for buformin (Bratusch-Marrain et al. 1981).

Inhibition of gluconeogenesis from various precursors in the liver by biguanides has long been recognised (Cook et al. 1973; Dietze et al. 1978; Meyer et al. 1967; Searle & Fulli 1980); the degree of this effect varies with the experimental conditions, and appears to be significant only for phenformin, not for metformin (Kuhl et al. 1976) and buformin (Soling et al. 1967). In many *in vitro* experiments, however, phenformin concentrations needed to obtain reduction of gluconeogenesis were much higher than those usually found under therapeutic conditions. Carrying out direct measurements with catheterisation of the subhepatic vein, Tranquada et al. (1960) found no change in the output of sugar by the liver in diabetic patients treated with phenformin. More recently, using a double isotope technique, it has been demonstrated that metformin lowered the oral glucose tolerance curve in 10 Type 2 diabetic patients because of a fall in the basal glucose concentration (Jackson et al. 1987). As fasting plasma glucose levels are determined mainly by the rate of hepatic glucose production, and as insulin levels were unchanged by metformin therapy, the authors concluded that metformin induces an increase in hepatic insulin sensitivity, probably leading to inhibition of hepatic gluconeogenesis. The obvious conclusion from these studies is that the issue of whether biguanides inhibit hepatic gluconeogenesis under usual therapeutic schedules is still unsettled.

As far as the potentiation of peripheral glucose utilisation induced by biguanides is concerned (Butterfield & Whinchelow 1962; Hermann 1979; Nosadini et al. 1987), the effect of the drugs at the mitochondrial membrane may be inhibition of oxidative metabolism and an increase of anaerobic glycolysis (Butterfield & Whinchelow 1962; Hermann 1979; Schafer 1983). Thus, reduced gluconeogenesis and enhanced anaerobic glycolysis appear to be mediated by the same mechanism(s), and, again, the possible effect on anaerobic glycolysis is more marked with phenformin than with buformin and metformin.

Although studies at the cellular level indicate that biguanides potentiate insulin action, it is not known whether this effect occurs at the receptor or a post-receptor site. Binding to different cell types is increased by biguanides *in vitro*: erythrocytes (Holle et al. 1981), IM-9 lymphocytes (Purrello et al. 1982), human breast cells (Cohen et al. 1982), human fibroblasts (Goldfine et al. 1984), hepatocytes (Lord et al. 1983a) and isolated monocytes (Trischitta et al. 1983). However, when studying 10 obese Type 2 diabetic patients in a double-blind crossover study, Prager and Schernthaner (1983) did not find any effect of metformin on insulin receptor binding to mononuclear leucocytes, despite improved metabolic control. In another paper (Lord et al. 1983b) it was observed that after withdrawal of metformin, insulin binding to erythrocytes was still raised although metabolic control had returned to the pretreatment levels. These latter results suggest that the drug may have some effects at post-receptor sites of insulin action.

In human and rat adipose tissue *in vitro*, no metformin-induced changes in insulin binding were observed, although the drug stimulated glucose metabolism in the presence of insulin (Cigolini et al. 1984; Fantus & Brosseau 1986). In rat adipocytes (Jacobs et al. 1986) metformin potentiated the effect of insulin on glucose transport at a site beyond insulin receptor binding, without affecting receptor tyrosine kinase activity. In isolated human monocytes, metformin ameliorates the decreased insulin internalisation and degradation of Type 2 diabetic patients (Benzi et al. 1988). Therefore, it is our opinion that the potentiation of insulin action induced by biguanides involves mechanisms located at a post-receptor site.

Finally, metformin may have an insulin-like activity, as suggested by the increased glucose metabolism in rat adipocytes and IM-9 lymphocytes in the absence of insulin (Fantus & Brosseau 1986; Purrello et al. 1987).

3.3 Assay Methods

The development of methods for the measurement of biguanide concentrations in biological fluids has received little attention. This may be due, at least in part, to the high polarity of these drugs which makes their extraction from biological fluids and derivatisation difficult. Spectrophotometric methods (Garrett et al. 1972) suffer from their lack of specificity and low sensitivity; chromatographic-mass spectrometric methods for measuring the *S*-triazine derivative of phenformin and metformin have been developed (Bosisio et al. 1981; Sirtori et al. 1978) but the equipment required is not generally available in a routine analytical laboratory. Convenient quantitative determination by gas chromatography was achieved after derivatisation techniques, with and without pre-extraction of the biological material (Bailey et al. 1966; Brohon & Noel 1978; De Groot et al. 1980; Lennard et al. 1979; Matin et al. 1975). A sensitive radioimmunoassay has been developed to measure *p*-hydroxyphenformin and apparent phenformin in human plasma and urine (Alkalay et al. 1978). Again, however, HPLC probably represents the best solution of the problem due to its simplicity, rapidity, sensitivity and precision (Benzi et al. 1986; Charles et al. 1981; Hill & Chamberlain 1978; Keal & Somogyi 1986; Ross 1977).

3.4 Pharmacokinetics

Compared with sulphonylureas, little information is available on the pharmacokinetics of biguanides, and the lack of definitive data about factors affecting biguanide absorption, distribution, metabolism and elimination is evident. Some kinetic parameters of these drugs are summarised in table III.

3.4.1 Absorption

After oral administration, phenformin and buformin accumulate transiently in liver, kidney, pancreas and muscle, with 16% of the administered phenformin dose being found in the liver in rats (Beckmann 1971).

Metformin concentrates mainly in the walls of the oesophagus, stomach, duodenum and kidney (Beckmann 1971; Cohen & Costerousse 1961). After oral administration of metformin HCl 850mg in 4 volunteers 37.6 ± 10.6% of the dose was excreted after 48 hours (Sirtori et al. 1978). This result was not due to low bioavailability of the metformin tablets, as a value of 29.7 ± 10.3% was found when metformin HCl solution was given. In a more recent study (Pentikainen 1986), it has been confirmed that the bioavailability of metformin even from aqueous solution and rapidly dissolving tablets is relatively low (< 40%) and further deteriorates when metformin is given in sustained release form.

After a single oral dose in 4 healthy subjects and 12 Type 2 diabetic patients, peak plasma metformin concentrations were observed after 2 hours, with urinary and faecal recovery of unchanged drug of 30 to 50% (Tucker et al. 1981). The absolute oral bioavailability was 50 to 60% of the doses. Using ^{14}C-labelled metformin, Pentikainen et al. (1979) reported a similar bioavailability. In healthy subjects, it has been observed that with an increased dose (1.5 *versus* 0.5g), urinary recovery of metformin was lower (Tucker et al. 1981). After a short lag time the available oral dose is absorbed at an exponential rate over about 6 hours.

3.4.2 Protein Binding

Binding of phenformin to plasma proteins has been reported to range from not significant to 12 and 20% (Garrett et al. 1972; Shepherd & McDonald 1958). By using ^{14}C-phenformin and fresh human plasma, with biguanide concentration kept at about 130 μg/L, drug binding amounted to 18.7 ± 0.7%, as assessed by the equilibrium dialysis method (Alkalay et al. 1975). By the same method, the percentage of binding of ^{14}C-metformin to serum proteins (albumin concentrations ranging from 32 to 47 g/L) was found to be negligible (Sirtori et al. 1978). The lack of binding of metformin to plasma proteins has been confirmed (Tucker et al. 1981). These protein binding characteristics contribute to the short half-life of metformin and to the absent or very low interaction with other drugs at this level.

3.4.3 Metabolism and Excretion

The reported plasma half-lives for phenformin, buformin and metformin range from 7 to 15 hours, 1.5 to 3.8 hours, and 1.5 to 4.5 hours, respectively (Beckmann 1968; Hermann 1979; Schafer 1983). Phenformin is metabolised in the liver to its 4-hydroxy derivative (Alkalay et al. 1979; Beckmann 1968). Approximately 50% of the parent drug undergoes biotransformation (Alkalay et al. 1975;

Table III. Pharmacokinetic properties of biguanides (adapted from Hermann 1979; Schafer 1983)

Drug	$t_{1/2}$ (h)	Vd (L/kg)	Duration of action (h)	Excretion	Daily dose range (mg)
Buformin	2.6	3.1	6-10	Renal	50-300
Metformin	1-4.5	1	8-12	Renal	500-3000
Phenformin	5-15	5-10	8-14	Renal, biliary	12.5-100

Abbreviations: $t_{1/2}$ = elimination half-life; Vd = apparent volume of distribution.

Shah et al. 1980). A genetic polymorphism of phenformin hydroxylation has been described (Oates et al. 1982): in 195 individuals, variations in the urinary ratio of phenformin/4-hydroxyphenformin ranged from 1 to 184. As the metabolite is inactive, slow metabolisers are thought to be at higher risk of developing lactic acidosis because of the inhibition of mitochondrial respiration by the parent drug (Bosisio et al. 1981; Idle et al. 1981).

Buformin is metabolised in many laboratory animals to 4-hydroxybuformin, but this does not appear to be the case in humans (Beckmann & Schmidt-Bothelt 1971). The metabolite of buformin has no hypoglycaemic action.

With metformin, there is evidence that the drug is excreted unchanged in animal and human studies (Beckmann 1969; Sirtori et al. 1978); however, Tucker et al. (1981) could not account for 20% of the dose. The authors presumed that this represented drug which had been metabolised.

Biguanides are eliminated by the kidney, phenformin also being excreted in the bile (Alkalay et al. 1979; Mehnert 1969). When phenformin 50mg was administered orally to healthy subjects, approximately 54% of the administered drug was recovered in the urine (Beckmann 1966). The excretion of the drug and its phenolic metabolite in urine was reported to occur in a 2 : 1 ratio. In 2 volunteers, after an oral dose of phenformin 100mg, the amount of unchanged drug excreted in the urine was 29 and 41%, respectively, most of the elimination occurring within the first 24 hours after drug administration (Alkalay et al. 1975). During a 26-hour period, in 4 subjects with normal hydroxylation capacity and 3 subjects with reduced hydroxylation capacity, recovery of drug in urine (metabolised and unchanged) was 61 and 58%, respectively (Shah et al. 1980). After intravenous administration in healthy subjects, the renal clearance value of metformin has been reported to be higher than creatinine clearance (Sirtori et al. 1978; Pentikainen et al. 1979; Tucker et al. 1981), suggesting tubular secretion of this highly ionised drug as a major mechanism of urinary excretion. A correlation between metformin renal clearance and creatinine clearance has been clearly demonstrated (Sirtori et al. 1978; Tucker et al. 1981), explaining the increased risk of lactic acidosis by metformin in the presence of reduced renal function. The elimination pattern of metformin can be described by multiexponentials only, with a fraction of the drug appearing to be distributed into a 'deep compartment' with a slower elimination rate (Noel 1979; Tucker et al. 1981).

3.5 Drug Interactions

Although direct evidence is lacking, it is conceivable that the same drugs able to affect sulphonylurea action by pharmacodynamic mechanisms can also interact with biguanides. The low or absent protein binding and the lack of hepatic metabolism of buformin and metformin reduce the possibility of drug interactions through pharmacokinetic mechanisms. Alcohol, barbiturates, salicylate and phenothiazine derivatives may precipitate severe lactic acidosis by biguanides (Luft et al. 1978).

3.6 Clinical Use

There are three main conditions for the use of biguanides (Nattrass & Alberti 1978; Vigneri & Goldfine 1987): as primary drug (Clarke & Campbell 1977; UK Prospective Study 1983, 1985), in combination with sulphonylureas (Krall & Balodimos 1967) and after sulphonylurea failure (Clarke & Duncan 1965). Some authors have reported an improvement of metabolic control and a decrease of insulin requirement in Type 1 diabetic patients treated with insulin plus metformin (Gin et al. 1985; Pagano et al. 1983), but this issue is still uncertain. The overweight, insulin-resistant Type 2 diabetic patient is the ideal subject for treatment with biguanides (Nattrass & Alberti 1978; Vermeulen & Rottiers 1972). Lactic acidosis (see below) has been reported in patients taking biguanides (Luft et al. 1978); in most instances, such patients had a concomitant disease, i.e. uraemia, liver disease, alcoholism or cardiac respiratory insufficiency, or were taking drugs able to reduce the cellular redox potential (such as barbiturate, salicylate or phenothiazine derivatives): these conditions represent contraindications to biguanide therapy. Treatment with biguanides must be replaced by insulin therapy in cases of major surgery.

3.7 Dose-Plasma Concentration-Therapeutic Effect Relationships

Studying the pharmacokinetics of phenformin in 2 healthy volunteers, Alkalay et al. (1975) reported peak plasma drug values between 150 and 200 μg/L after oral phenformin 100mg. In 6 normal subjects given a sustained-release capsule of phenformin 50mg, the mean peak concentration occurred 3.5 hours after ingestion and was 0.19 ± 0.03 μmol/L (mean ± SEM); a significant correlation between plasma drug concentration and blood lactate, but not blood glucose or serum insulin, was found (Nattrass et al. 1980). In a group of 24 diabetic patients on combined phenformin and a sulphonylurea and with normal hepatic and renal function, Marchetti et al. (1987) found fasting biguanide concentrations ranging from 28 to 114 μg/L; plasma concentrations were not correlated with the dose of the drug or with its therapeutic effects and various clinical parameters.

Sirtori et al. (1978) studied a group of fasting patients treated with long term metformin for hyperlipidaemia or diabetes: the daily drug dose was 500mg in 6 patients, 1000mg in 4 patients, 1700mg in 13 patients and 2550mg in 12 patients. There was a correlation between doses administered and the steady-state plasma concentrations (which ranged from 60 to 2240 μg/L). In 13 Type 2 diabetic patients on medium metformin dose (1240 ± 560 mg/day) no correlation was found between drug dose, fasting plasma concentrations and hypoglycaemic effects (Marchetti et al. 1987). In this study, mean steady-state metformin values were 505 μg/L (range 236 to 718 μg/L).

In a study of 6 diabetic patients over a 14-hour period, significantly higher drug concentrations were found when metformin 850mg twice daily instead of 500mg twice daily was given (Marchetti et al. 1988b): peak concentration 1173 μg/L *versus* 809 ± 196 μg/L; averaged value: 825 ± 90 μg/L *versus* 605 ± 51 μg/L (fig. 6).

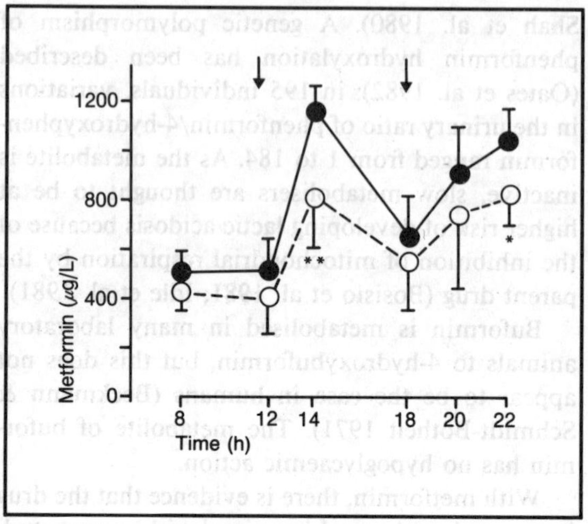

Fig. 6. Plasma concentrations of metformin in 6 Type 2 diabetic patients given metformin 500mg (○) and 850mg (●) twice daily. ↓ = Drug administration; * p = 0.05; ** p = 0.01.

As far as the action of biguanides on lipid metabolism is concerned, metformin has been demonstrated to have a lipid lowering effect in both non-diabetic and diabetic patients (Descovich et al. 1978; Sirtori et al. 1977). It has recently been found that plasma metformin concentrations are inversely correlated with circulating triglycerides and positively correlated with HDL_2-cholesterol in a group of Type 2 diabetic patients (Marchetti et al. 1988a).

Thus, the relationships between biguanide dose, fasting concentrations and hypoglycaemic effect are not evident, probably because of tissue accumulation, variable bioavailability and interindividual differences in the metabolism of these agents.

3.8 Dose-Plasma Concentration-Toxic Effect Relationships

The overall incidence of side effects due to biguanides ranges from 5 to 40% (Bergman et al. 1978; Schafer 1983). The drugs may cause gastrointestinal symptoms such as nausea, vomiting and diarrhoea, especially during the initial stage of treatment (Dandona et al. 1983); generally, the symptoms are transient. Gastrointestinal side effects are attributed to the high level of accumulation of biguanides in the intestinal mucosa cells.

Pruritus, urticaria and skin rashes occur rarely, and disappear after discontinuation or reduction of the drug dose. During long term therapy, malabsorption of vitamin B_{12} and folic acid has been described, and in elderly patients this may cause mild anaemia (Callaghan et al. 1980). Hyperlactic acidaemia generally (Nattrass et al. 1977; Waters et al. 1978), but not always (Fletcher et al. 1986; Gregorio et al. 1986), accompanies short or long term treatment with biguanides. Other metabolic abnormalities that may occur during biguanide therapy are an increase of blood alanine, pyruvate, total ketone bodies, lactate/pyruvate ratio and 3-hydroxybutyrate/acetoacetate ratio (Craug et al. 1960; Kattermann et al. 1968; Nattrass et al. 1976, 1977). Lactic acidosis is the most life-threatening adverse reaction of biguanides, with a mortality rate of approximately 40 to 50% (Luft et al. 1978; Misbin 1977). Inhibition of mitochondrial respiration (with increased lactate production by anaerobic glycolysis), and inhibition of glucose resynthesis from lactate, contribute to the development of this metabolic emergency.

Phenformin is associated with far more cases of lactic acidosis than metformin (Luft et al. 1978): the relative risk of the reaction was calculated to be 0.64 cases/1000 patients/year for phenformin and 0.05 cases for metformin. In a comparison of the risk of lactic acidosis caused by metformin with the risk of severe hypoglycaemia by chlorpropamide and other sulphonylureas, biguanides were calculated to be safer than the sulphonylurea agents (Campbell 1985). In almost all known cases of lactic acidosis, a pre-existing contraindication to the use of biguanide (see clinical use) was present, suggesting that correct use of these drugs may significantly lessen the risk of acidosis. Reviewing 330 cases of lactic acidosis in biguanide-treated patients, Luft et al. (1978) reported that the average daily doses of phenformin, buformin and metformin were 123 ± 4mg, 329 ± 30mg and 1595 ± 182mg, respectively. Abnormally elevated biguanide concentrations have been reported in a few cases of lactic acidosis. In 5 of 18 diabetic patients with lactic acidosis, plasma concentrations of phenformin were measured by a colorimetric method and were 50 ± 5 mg/L (approximately 10-fold higher than in patients treated with phenformin and without lactic acidosis) [Assan et al. 1974]. In 7 diabetic patients with lactic acidosis (Conlay et al. 1977), serum phenformin concentrations ranged from 20 to 625 μg/L; in 3 of these patients, serum drug concentrations were measured serially, and apparent half-lives of 5, 25 and 30 hours were found for corresponding serum creatinine concentrations of 17, 56 and 60 mg/L. In this report, phenformin dose is correlated to drug concentrations; the correlation between dosage, lactate and blood pH is not statistically significant. The dose of phenformin was also not correlated with blood lactate and pH in previous studies (Simpson et al. 1974). In patients with lactic acidosis during buformin therapy, circulating concentrations up to 55 mg/L have been reported (Berger et al. 1976; Deppermann et al. 1978; Verdonck et al. 1981); in a case of fatal lactic acidosis (Verdonck et al. 1981), postmortem concentrations were: in lung 2.8 ng/kg wet weight, in heart 3.0 ng/kg, in liver 5.2 ng/kg and in kidney 98 ng/kg. Studying 4 metformin-treated diabetic patients with lactic acidosis, Assan et al. (1977), using a colorimetric method, observed a guanidine substance in the plasma at concentrations of 45 to 110 mg/L. The doses of metformin in these patients (with known chronic renal failure) ranged from 1.6 to 2.4 g/day.

In an elderly patient with impaired renal function and lactic acidosis, plasma metformin was measured on admission and found to be 26.05 mg/L (Hermann et al. 1981). In conditions other than metabolic emergency, plasma phenformin concentrations have been reported to correlate with blood lactate in 24 Type 2 diabetic patients (Marchetti et al. 1987). Fasting plasma metformin did not correlate with lactate concentrations (Marchetti et al. 1987). However, studying 6 diabetic patients over a 14-hour period, we found a positive correlation between plasma metformin and blood lactate in 5 of 6 patients (Marchetti et al. 1988b): both parameters were evaluated at 12 time points, and at 2 different (1000 and 1700mg) daily metformin doses.

It can reasonably be concluded that the toxic effects of biguanide appear to be related to the circulating drug concentrations, so that all the factors able to increase plasma biguanide levels (large doses, renal impairment, liver and cardiovascular disease, age over 60 years, etc. (Luft et al. 1978), may increase the risk of lactic acidosis.

4. Conclusions

Taking into account the wide differences in pharmacokinetic properties of oral hypoglycaemic agents, it is possible to state the best schedule of treatment involves a single compound, so that Type 2 (non-insulin-dependent) diabetes mellitus can be successfully treated with any of the various sulphonylureas. Selected patients may benefit from administration of a biguanide (especially metformin), alone or in combination with a sulphonylurea.

The relationship between drug dose, plasma concentrations and effects on blood glucose is not obvious at steady-state, but becomes evident when evaluating the short term effect following oral or intravenous dosing. The toxicity of both sulphonylureas and biguanides is greatly dependent on the pharmacokinetics of the drugs: to minimise the risk of severe hypoglycaemia by sulphonylureas or lactic acidosis by biguanides, the use of short-acting agents is to be recommended, together with avoidance of administering highly potent compounds in the elderly. Obviously, all conditions that may lead to drug accumulation and/or potentiation (increased dosage, renal and hepatic disease, interaction with other drugs) must be carefully considered before initiating therapy with oral hypoglycaemic drugs. Evidence of a relationship between plasma drug concentrations and toxic effects has been reported for biguanides both during lactic acidosis and in conditions other than metabolic emergency. At present, it is not possible to define plasma ranges for sulphonylurea and biguanide concentrations beyond which either lack of therapeutic effect or toxic effects are to be expected.

Acknowledgement

The authors wish to express their thanks to Alberto di Carlo, M.D., for his assistance in the preparation of the manuscript.

References

Abernethy DR, Greenblatt DJ. Drug disposition in obese humans: an update. Clinical Pharmacokinetics 11: 199-213, 1986

Abrahamsson H, Berggren PO, Rorsmann P. Direct measurement of increased free cytoplasmic Ca^{2+} in mouse pancreatic β cells following stimulation by hypoglycaemic sulfonylureas. FEBS Letters 190: 21-24, 1985

Adams WJ, Krueger DS. Specific and sensitive high-performance liquid chromatographic determination of glyburide. Journal of Pharmaceutical Sciences 68: 1138-1140, 1979

Alkalay D, Khemani L, Bartlett MF. Radioimmunoassay determinations of p-hydroxyphenformin and of apparent phenformin in human plasma or serum. Analytical Letters B11: 741-751, 1978

Alkalay D, Khemani L, Wagner WE, Bartlett MF. Pharmacokinetics of phenformin in man. Journal of Clinical Pharmacology 15: 446-448, 1975

Alkalay D, Volk J, Roth W, Khemani L, Wagner WE, et al. Metabolism, plasma or serum levels, and elimination of phenformin in guinea-pigs, rats and dogs. Journal of Pharmaceutical Sciences 68: 160-165, 1979

Almer LO, Johansson E, Melander A, Wahlin-Boll E. Influence of sulfonylureas on the secretion, disposal and effect of insulin. European Journal of Clinical Pharmacology 22: 27-32, 1982

Amatruda JM, Salhanick AJ, Chang CL. Hepatic insulin resistance in non-insulin-dependent diabetes mellitus and the effects of a sulfonylurea in potentiating insulin action. Diabetes Care 7 (Suppl. 1): 47-53, 1984

Antal EJ, Gillespie WR, Phillips JP, Albert KS. The effect of food on the bioavailability and pharmacodynamics of tolbutamide in diabetic patients. European Journal of Clinical Pharmacology 22: 459-462, 1982

Arky R, Wylie-Rosett J, El-Beheri B. Examination of current dietary recommendations for individuals with diabetes mellitus. Diabetes Care 5: 59-63, 1982

Asmal AG, Marble A. Oral hypoglycaemic agents: an update. Drugs 28: 62-78, 1984

Asplund K, Wiholm BE, Lithner F. Glibenclamide-associated hypoglycaemia: a report on 57 cases. Diabetologia 24: 412-417, 1983

Assan R, Heuclin C, Ganeval G, Bismuth C, George J, et al. Metformin-induced lactic acidosis in the presence of acute renal failure. Diabetologia 13: 211-217, 1977

Assan R, Heuclin C, Girard JR, Le Maire F, Raymond A. Phenformin-induced lactic acidosis in diabetic patients. Diabetes 24: 791-800, 1974

Bailey RE, Under OM, Grettle DP. A method for determination of 3-phenethylbiguanide. Federation Proceedings 15: 557, 1966

Balant L, Fabre J, Loutan L, Samini H. Does 4-hydroxyglibenclamide show hypoglycaemic activity? Arzneimittel-Forschung 29: 162-163, 1979

Balant L, Fabre J, Zahnd GR. Comparison of the pharmacokinetics of glipizide and glibenclamide in man. European Journal of Clinical Pharmacology 8: 63-69, 1978

Balant L, Zahnd GR, Gorgia A, Schwarz R, Fabre J. Pharmacokinetics of glipizide in man: influence of renal insufficiency. Diabetologia 9 (Suppl.): 331-338, 1973

Balant L, Zahnd GR, Weber F, Fabre J. Behaviour of glibenclamide on repeated administration to diabetic patients. European Journal of Clinical Pharmacology 11: 19-25, 1977

Baron AD, Eckel RH, Schmeiser L, Kolterman OG. The effect of short-term α-glucosidase inhibition on carbohydrate and lipid metabolism in Type II (non-insulin dependent) diabetics. Metabolism Clinical and Experimental 36: 409-415, 1987

Becker R. Fluorimetrische Bestimmung von Glibornurid in Plasma und Serum mit 7-chlor-4-nitrobenzo-2-oxa-1,3-diazol. Arzneimittel-Forschung 27: 102-105, 1977

Beckmann R. Uber die Resorption und den biologischen Abbau von 1-(B-phenatyl)-biguanid (Phenformin). Diabetologia 3: 368-376, 1966

Beckmann R. The fate of biguanides in man. Annals of the New York Academy of Sciences 148: 820-832, 1968

Beckmann R. Resorption. Verteilung im Organismus und Ausscheidung von Metformin. Diabetologia 5: 318-324, 1969

Beckmann R. Biguanide. In Maske (Ed.) Handbuch der experimentellen Pharmakologie, Vol 24, pp. 43-592, Springer-Verlag, Berlin, Heidelberg, New York, 1971

Beckmann R. Pharmakologie und Wirkungmechanismus der Biguanide beim tier. In Oberdisse (Ed.) Handbuch der inneren Medizin. Bd 7/2 B, Diabetes Mellitus B, pp. 951-982, Springer-Verlag, Berlin, 1977

Beckmann R, Schmidt-Bothelt E. Evaluation of a sustained release form of the oral antidiabetic butylbiguanide (Silubin retard). European Journal of Clinical Pharmacology 3: 221-228, 1971

Beck-Nielsen H, Pedersen O, Lindskov HO. Normalization of the insulin sensitivity and the cellular insulin binding during treatment of obese diabetics for one year. Acta Endocrinologica 90: 103-112, 1979a

Beck-Nielsen H, Pedersen O, Lindskov HO. Increased insulin sensitivity and cellular insulin binding in obese diabetics following treatment with glibenclamide. Acta Endocrinologica 90: 451-462, 1979b

Beisswanger PJ, Dias N, Beckmann F. Evaluation of first-generation sulfonylureas and glipizide in non-insulin-dependent diabetes mellitus. American Journal of Medicine 83 (Suppl. 3A): 16-21, 1987

Benzi L, Marchetti P, Cecchetti P, Navalesi R. Determination of metformin and phenformin in human plasma and urine by reversed-phase high-performance liquid chromatography. Journal of Chromatography 375: 184-189, 1986

Benzi L, Trischitta V, Ciccarone AM, Cecchetti P, Brunetti A, et al. Metformin improves the reduced insulin-internalization and intracellular processing in obese diabetic patients but not in subjects with simple obesity. 24th EASD Meeting, Paris, 5-8 Sept, 1988

Berger W. 88 schwere Hypoglykamiezwischenfalle unter der Behandlung mit Sulfonylharnstoffer. Schweizerische Medizinische Wochenschrift 71: 1013-1022, 1971

Berger W, Mehnert-Aner S, Mully K, Heierli C, Ritz R. 10 Falle von Lactazidose under Biguanidtherapie (Buformin und Phenformin). Schweizerische Medizinische Wochenschrift 106: 1830-1834, 1976

Bergman U, Boman G, Wiholm BE. Epidemiology of adverse drug reactions to phenformin and metformin. British Medical Journal 2: 464-466, 1978

Bergman U, Christenson I, Jansson B, Wiholm BE, Ostnam J. Wide variation in serum chlorpropamide concentration in outpatients. European Journal of Clinical Pharmacology 18: 165-169, 1980

Bernhard H. Long-term observations on oral hypoglycaemic agents in diabetes. Diabetes 14: 50-70, 1965

Bobbioni E, Coscelli C, Zavaroni I, Alpi O. The effect of metformin on the insulin response *in vivo* and *in vitro* to arginine and glucose in the normal rat. Excerpta Medica 454: 353-358, 1979

Bosisio E, Kienle MG, Galli G, Ciconali M, Negri A, et al. Defective hydroxylation of phenformin as a determinant of drug toxicity. Diabetes 30: 644-649, 1981

Braselton WE, Brasome ED, Huff TA. Measurement of antidiabetic sulfonylureas in serum by gas-chromatography with electron-capture detection. Diabetes 226: 50-57, 1977

Bratusch-Marrain PR, Korn A, Waldhausl WK, Gasic S, Nowotny P. Effect of buformin on splanchnic carbohydrate and substrate metabolism in healthy man. Metabolism 30: 946-952, 1981

Brockmeier D, Grigoleit HG, Leonhardt H. Absorption of glibenclamide from different sites of the gastro-intestinal tract. European Journal of Clinical Pharmacology 29: 193-197, 1985

Brohon J, Noel M. Determination of metformin in plasma at therapeutic levels by gas-liquid-chromatography using a nitrogen detector. Journal of Chromatography 146: 148-151, 1978

Brotherton PM, Grievson P, McMartin C. A study of the metabolic fate of chlorpropramide in man. Clinical Pharmacology and Therapeutics 10: 505-514, 1969

Brunova E, Sldbochova Z, Platilova H, Paulik F, Grofneterova J, et al. Interaction of tolbutamide and chloramphenicol in diabetic patients. International Journal of Clinical Pharmacology and Biopharmacy 15: 7-12, 1977

Butterfield WJH, Whinchelow MJ. The hypoglycemic action of phenformin: effect of phenformin on glucose metabolism in peripheral tissue. Diabetes 18: 281-286, 1962

Cabello MA, Monge L, Ortega JL, Samper B, Feliu JE. Effect of glipizide on hepatic fructose-2,6-biphosphate concentration and glucose metabolism. Metabolism 36: 738-742, 1987

Cahill GF Jr, McDevitt HO. Insulin dependent diabetes mellitus: the initial lesions. New England Journal of Medicine 304: 1454-1465, 1981

Callaghan TS, Hadden DR, Tomkin GH. Megaloblastic anemia due to vitamin-B_{12} malabsorption associated with long-term metformin treatment. British Medical Journal 280: 1214-1215, 1980

Campbell DB, Adrianssen P, Hopkins YW, Gordon B, Williams JRB. Pharmacokinetics and metabolism of gliclazide: a review. In Keen et al. (Eds) Gliclazide and the treatment of diabetes. International Congress and Symposium Series No 20, pp. 71-82, Academic Press, Royal Society of Medicine, London, 1980

Campbell DB, Gordon BH, Ings RMJ, Beaufils M, Meynier A, et al. The effect of renal disease on the pharmacokinetics of gliclazide in diabetic patients. British Journal of Clinical Pharmacology 21: 572P, 1986

Campbell IW. Metformin and the sulfonylureas: comparative risks. Hormone and Metabolic Research 15 (Suppl.): 105-111, 1985

Carpentier JL, Sawano F, Ravazzola M, Malaisse WJ. Internalization of 3H-glibenclamide in pancreatic islet cells. Diabetologia 29: 259-261, 1986

Carulli N, Ponz de Leon M, Mauro E, Moneti F, Ferrari A. Alteration of drug metabolism in Gilbert's syndrome. Gut 17: 581-587, 1976

Caspary WF. Biguanides and intestinal absorptive function. Acta Hepato-Gastroenterologica 24: 473-480, 1977

Cate EW, Rogers JF, Powell JR. Inhibition of tolbutamide elimination by cimetidine but not ranitidine. Journal of Clinical Pharmacology 26: 372-377, 1986

Cerasi E, Efendic S, Thornqvist C, Luft R. Effect of two sulfonylureas on the dose kinetics of glucose-induced insulin release in normal and diabetic patients. Acta Endocrinologica 91: 282-293, 1979

Chalk JB, Patterson M, Smith MH, Eadie MJ. Correlations between *in vitro* dissolution, *in vivo* bioavailability and hypoglycaemic effect of oral glibenclamide. European Journal of Clinical Pharmacology 31: 177-182, 1986

Charles BG, Jacobsen NW, Ravenscroft PJ. Rapid liquid-chromatographic determination of metformin in plasma and urine. Clinical Chemistry 27: 434-436, 1981
Charles BG, Ravenscroft PJ. Measurement of gliclazide in plasma by radial compression reversed-phase liquid chromatography. Clinical Chemistry 30: 1789-1791, 1984
Christensen LK, Hansen JM, Kristensen M. Sulphaphenazole-induced hypoglycaemic attacks in tolbutamide-treated diabetics. Lancet 2: 1298-1300, 1963
Ciccarone AM, Benzi L, Cecchetti P, Trischitta V, Masoni A, et al. Effects of sulfonylureas on intracellular processing of insulin in monocytes from Type II (non-insulin-dependent) diabetic patients. Diabetologia 30: 507A, 1987
Cigolini M, Bosello O, Zancanaro C, Orlandi PG, Fezzi O, et al. Influence of metformin on metabolic effects of insulin in human adipose tissue *in vitro*. Diabetes & Metabolism 10: 311-315, 1984
Clarke BF, Campbell IW. Comparison of metformin and chlorpropamide in non-obese, maturity-onset diabetics uncontrolled by diet. British Medical Journal 2: 1576-1578, 1977
Clarke BF, Campbell IW, Ewing DJ, Beveridge GW, MacDonald MK. Generalized hypersensitivity reaction and visceral arteritis with fatal outcome during glibenclamide therapy. Diabetes 23: 739-742, 1974
Clarke BF, Duncan LJP. Combined metformin-chlorpropamide therapy in 108 diabetic sulphonylurea-failures. Lancet 1: 1248-1251, 1965
Cohen BD, Galloway JA, McMahon RE, Culp HW, Roost MA, et al. Carbohydrate metabolism in uremia: blood glucose response to sulfonylurea. American Journal of Medical Sciences 254: 608-618, 1967
Cohen D, Pezzino V, Vigneri R, Avola R, D'Agata R, et al. Phenformin increases insulin binding to human cultured breast cancer cells. Diabetes 29: 329-331, 1982
Cohen JL. Pharmacokinetic changes in aging. American Journal of Medicine 80 (Suppl. 5A): 31-38, 1986
Cohen Y, Costerousse O. Etude autoradiographique chez la souris d'un antidiabétique oral, le *NN*-dimethyl-biguanide marque en carbon 14. Thérapie 16: 109-120, 1961
Conlay LA, Karam JH, Matin SB, Loewenstein JE. Serum phenformin concentrations in patients with phenformin-associated lactic acidosis. Diabetes 26: 628-631, 1977
Conn J. Hypertension, the potassium ion and impaired carbohydrate tolerance. New England Journal of Medicine 273: 1135-1143, 1965
Cook DC, Blair JB, Landy HA. Mode of action of hypoglycemic agents. V. Studies with phenethylbiguanide in isolated perfused rat liver. Journal of Biological Chemistry 248: 5272-5277, 1973
Cooper AJ, Ashcroft G. Modification of insulin and sulfonylurea hypoglycaemia by monoamine-oxidase inhibitor drugs. Diabetes 16: 272-274, 1967
Craug JW, Miller M, Woodward H, Merk E. Influence of phenethylbiguanide on lactic, pyruvic and citric acids in diabetic patients. Diabetes 9: 186-193, 1960
Crooks MJ, Brown KF. The binding of sulfonylureas to serum albumin. Journal of Pharmacy and Pharmacology 26: 304-311, 1974
Crooks MJ, Brown KF. Interaction of glipizide with human serum albumin. Biochemical Pharmacology 24: 298-299, 1975
Czyzyk A, Tawak J, Sadowoki J, Possikowska I, Izczepanik Z. Effect of biguanides on intestinal absorption of glucose. Diabetes 17: 492-498, 1986
Dahl-Jorgensen K. Near-normoglycaemia and late diabetic complications: the Oslo Study. Acta Endocrinologica 115 (Suppl. 284): 1-38, 1987
Dandona P, Fonseca V, Mier A, Beckett AG. Diarrhea and metformin in a diabetic clinic. Diabetes Care 6: 472-474, 1983
De Fronzo RA, Ferrannini E, Koivisto V. New concepts in the pathogenesis and treatment of non-insulin dependent diabetes mellitus. American Journal of Medicine 74: 52-81, 1983
De Groot G, Maes RA, Songster B, van Heijst AN, Verdonck LF. Gas-chromatographic determination of buformin in body fluids and tissue using a nitrogen phosphorus detector: application to a postmortem case. Journal of Analytical Toxicology 4: 281-285, 1980
De Marinis L, Barbarino A. Calcium antagonists and hormone release. I. Effects of verapamil on insulin release in normal subjects and patients with islet cell tumour. Metabolism 29: 599-604, 1980
Depperman D, Heidland A, Ritz E, Hort W. Lactat-Azidose—eine mögliche Komplikation der Buformin-Therapie. Klinische Wochenschrift 56: 843-853, 1978
Descovich G, Montaguti V, Ceredi C, Cocuzza E, Sirtori CR. Long-term treatment with metformin in a large cohort of hyperlipidaemic patients. Artery 4: 348-359, 1978
Devis G, Somers G, Van Obberghen E, Malaisse WJ. Calcium antagonist and islet function, I: inhibition of insulin release by verapamil. Diabetes 24: 547-551, 1975
Dietze G, Wicklmayr M, Mehnert H, Czempiel H, Henftling HG. Effect of phenformin on hepatic balances of gluconeogenic substrates in man. Diabetologia 14: 243-248, 1978
Duckworth WC, Solomon SS, Kitabchi AE. Effect of chronic sulfonylurea therapy on plasma insulin and proinsulin levels. Journal of Clinical Endocrinology and Metabolism 35: 585-591, 1972
Eckhardt W, Rudolph R, Sauer H, Schubert WR, Underutsch D. Zur pharmakologischen Interferenz von Glibornurid mit Sulfaphenazol, Phenylbutazon, und Phenprocoumon beim Menschen. Arzneimittel-Forschung 22: 2212-2219, 1972
Elkeles RS, Heding LG, Paisey RB. The long-term effect of chlorpropamide on insulin, C-peptide and proinsulin secretion. Diabetes Care 5: 427-429, 1982
Elvander-Stahl E, Melander A, Wahlin-Boll E. Indobufen interacts with the sulfonylurea, glipizide, but not with the β-adrenergic receptor antagonists, propranolol and atenolol. British Journal of Clinical Pharmacology 18: 773-778, 1984
Emanueli A, Molari E, Pirola LC, Caputo G. Glipizide, a new sulfonylurea in the treatment of diabetes mellitus. Summary of clinical experience in 1064 cases. Arzneimittel-Forschung 22: 1881-1885, 1972
Emilsson H. High-performance liquid chromatographic determination of glipizide in human plasma and urine. Journal of Chromatography 421: 319-326, 1987
Emilsson H, Sjoberg S, Svedner M, Christenson I. High-performance liquid chromatographic determination of glibenclamide in human plasma and urine. Journal of Chromatography 383: 93-102, 1986
Eschwege E, Ducimetiere P, Papoz L, Claude JR, Richard JL. Blood glucose and coronary heart disease. Lancet 2: 472-473, 1980
Fajans SS, Cloutier MC, Crowther RL. Clinical and etiologic heterogeneity of idiopathic diabetes mellitus. Diabetes 27: 1112-1125, 1978
Fantus IG, Brosseau R. Mechanism of action of metformin: insulin receptor and postreceptor effects *in vitro* and *in vivo*. Journal of Clinical Endocrinology and Metabolism 63: 898-905, 1986
Federlin KF, Mehlburger L, Hillebrand I, Laube H. The effect of two new glucosidase inhibitors on blood glucose in healthy volunteers and in Type II diabetics. Acta Diabetologica Latina 24: 213-221, 1987
Feinglos MN, Lebovitz HE. Sulfonylureas increase the number of insulin receptors. Nature 276: 184-185, 1978
Feinglos MN, Lebovitz HE. Sulfonylurea treatment of insulin-dependent diabetes mellitus. Metabolism 29: 488-494, 1980
Feldman JM, Lebovitz HE. Biological activities of tolbutamide and its metabolites. Diabetes 18: 529-537, 1969

Fernandez MC, Erill S, Lucena MI, Pita E, Perez-Alferez O. Serum protein binding of tolbutamide in patients treated with antiepileptic drugs. Clinical Pharmacokinetics 10: 451-455, 1985
Ferner RE, Chaplin S. The relationship between the pharmacokinetic and pharmacodynamic efffects of oral hypoglycaemic drugs. Clinical Pharmacokinetics 12: 379-401, 1987
Ferrari C, Frezzati S, Testori GP, Bertazzoni A. Potentiation of hypoglycemic response to intravenous tolbutamide by clofibrate. New England Journal of Medicine 294: 1184, 1976
Field JB, Ohta M, Boyle C, Remer A. Potentiation of acetohexamide hypoglycemia by phenylbutazone. New England Journal of Medicine 277: 889-894, 1967
Fineberg SE, Schneider SH. Glipizide versus tolbutamide, an open trial: effects on insulin secretory patterns and glucose concentrations. Diabetologia 18: 49-54, 1980
Fletcher P, Hirji MR, Kuhn S, Alexander L, Muchlow JC. The effect of diabetes mellitus, exercise, and single doses of biguanides upon lactate metabolism in man. British Journal of Clinical Pharmacology 21: 691-699, 1986
Forette B, Rolland A, Hopkins Y, Gordon B, Campbell B. Gliclazide pharmacokinetics in the elderly. In Alberti et al. (Eds) 11th Congress of IDF, abstract p. 9. Excerpta Medica, Amsterdam, 1982
Foster DW. Diabetes mellitus. In Petersdorf et al. (Eds) Principles of internal medicine, pp. 661-679, McGraw Hill Inc., New York, 1983
Fuccella LM, Tamassia V, Valzelli G. Metabolism and kinetics of the hypoglycemic agent glipizide in man: comparison with glibenclamide. Journal of Clinical Pharmacology 13: 68-75, 1973
Fuller JH, McCartney P, Jarrett RJ, Keen H, Rose G, et al. Hyperglycemia and coronary heart disease: the Whitehall study. Journal of Chronic Disease 32: 721-728, 1979
Fuller JH, Shipley MJ, Rose G, Jarrett RJ, Keen H. Coronary heart disease risk and impaired glucose tolerance: the Whitehall study. Lancet 1: 1373-1376, 1980
Gachalyi B, Tornyossy M, Vas A, Kaldor A. Effect of alfamethyldopa on the half-lives of antitripsine, tolbutamide and D-glucaric acid excretion in man. International Journal of Clinical Pharmacology, Therapy and Toxicology 18: 133-135, 1980
Gaines KL, Hamilton S, Boyd III AE. Characterization of the sulphonylurea receptors on beta cell membranes. Journal of Biological Chemistry 263: 2589-2592, 1988
Galloway JA, McMahon RE, Culp HW, Marshall FJ, Young EC. Metabolism, blood levels and rate of excretion of acetohexamide in human subjects. Diabetes 16: 118-127, 1967
Ganda OP, Kahn CB, Soeldner JS, Gleason RE. Dynamics of tolbutamide, glucose and insulin interrelationships following varying doses of intravenous tolbutamide in normal subjects. Diabetes 24: 354-361, 1975
Garrett ER, Tsau J, Hinderling PH. Application of ion-pair methods to drug extraction from biological fluids II: quantitative determination of biguanides in biological fluids and comparison of protein binding estimates. Journal of Pharmaceutical Sciences 61: 1411-1418, 1972
Garrino MG, Meissner HP, Henquin JC. The non-sulfonylurea moiety of gliquidone mimics the effects of the parent molecule on pancreatic B-cells. European Journal of Pharmacology 124: 309-316, 1986
Gerich JE. Sulfonylureas in the treatment of diabetes mellitus, 1985. Mayo Clinic Proceedings 60: 439-443, 1985
Giannarelli R, Marchetti P, Zappella A, Masoni A, di Carlo A, et al. Metformin stimulates insulin release from porcine islets of Langerhans. 24th EASD Meeting, Paris, 5-8 Sept, 1988
Gibson TP. Renal disease and drug metabolism: an overview. American Journal of Kidney Disease 8: 7-17, 1986
Gin H, Messerchmitt C, Brottier E, Aubertin J. Metformin improved insulin resistance in Type I, insulin-dependent, diabetic patients. Metabolism 34: 923-925, 1985
Giugliano D, Torella R, Siniscalchi N, Improta L, D'Onofrio E. The effect of acetyl-salicylic acid on insulin response to glucose and arginine in normal man. Diabetologia 14: 359-362, 1978
Glogner P, Burmeister P, Heni N. Radioimmunologische Bestimmung von Glibenclamid in Serum. Klinische Wochenschrift 51: 352, 1973
Glogner P, Heni N, Nissen L. The radioimmunological determination of glibenclamide and its metabolites in serum. Arzneimittel-Forschung 27: 1703-1706, 1977
Goldfine ID, Iwamoto Y, Pezzino V, Trischitta V, Purrello F, et al. Effects of biguanides and sulfonylureas on insulin receptors in cultured cells. Diabetes Care 7 (Suppl. 1): 54-58, 1984
Goldfine ID, Periman R, Roth J. Inhibition of cyclic 3'5'-AMP phosphodiesterase in islet cells and other tissues by tolbutamide. Nature 234: 295-297, 1971
Goldman J, Tamayo RC, Whitehouse FW, Kahkonen DM. Effect of glyburide on metabolic control and insulin binding in insulin-dependent diabetes mellitus. Diabetes Care 7: 106-112, 1984
Greenfield M, Doberne L, Rosenthal M, Schutz B, Widstrom A, et al. Effect of sulfonylurea treatment on *in vivo* insulin secretion and action in patients with non-insulin dependent diabetes mellitus. Diabetes 31: 307-312, 1982
Gregorio F, Filipponi P, Angelici F, Carloni C, Cristallini S, et al. Effetti glico-metabolici di un trattamento con metformina a basse dosi. Recenti Progressi in Medicina 77: 549-553, 1986
Grill V, Efendic S, Regitz G. Potentiation by previous nutrients of glibenclamide-induced insulin release in man. An effect which is counteracted by meal-induced retardation of drug absorption. Scandinavian Journal of Clinical and Laboratory Investigation 46: 527-532, 1986
Grodsky GM, Epstein GH, Fanska R, Karam JH. Pancreatic action of the sulfonylureas. Federation Proceedings 36: 2714-2719, 1977
Groop L, Eriksson CJP, Wahlin-Boll E, Melander A. Chlorpropamide-alcohol flush: significance of body weight, sex and serum chlorpropamide level. European Journal of Clinical Pharmacology 26: 723-725, 1984
Groop L, Luzi L, Melander A, Groop PH, Ratheiser K, et al. Different effects of glyburide and glipizide on insulin secretion and hepatic glucose production in normal and NIDDM subjects. Diabetes 36: 1320-1328, 1987
Gunderson K, Molony BA, Crim JA, Hearron AE, Maile JP. Micronase (glyburide): a clinical overview. In Rifkin (Ed.) Micronase, pharmacology and clinical evaluation, pp. 254-264, Excerpta Medica, Amsterdam, 1975
Gylfe E, Hellman B, Sehlin J, Taljedal IB. Interaction of sulfonylureas with pancreatic β-cells. Experientia 40: 1126-1134, 1984
Hajdu P, Kohler KF, Schmidt FH, Spingler H. Physikalisch-chemische und analytische Untersuchungen an HB419. Arzneimittel-Forschung 19: 1381-1386, 1969
Hansten PD. Beta-blocking agents and antidiabetic drugs. Drug Intelligence and Clinical Pharmacy 14: 46-50, 1980
Hartvig P, Fagerlund C, Gyllenhall O. Electron-capture gas chromatography of plasma sulfonylureas after extractive methylation. Journal of Chromatography 181: 17-24, 1980
Haupt VE, Koberich W, Cordes V, Beyer J, Schoffling K. Untersuchungen, 2U dosis-wirkungs-Relationen werscheidener Sulfonylharnstoffderivate der alten und neuen Generation. Arzneimittel-Forschung 22: 2203-2208, 1972
Hellman B, Taljedal IB. Effects of sulfonylurea derivatives on pancreatic B-cells. In Hasselblatt and Bruchhausen (Eds) Handbook of Experimental Pharmacology, Vol. 32, Insulin, part 2, pp. 175-194, Springer-Verlag, Berlin, 1975
Henquin JC, Garrino MG, Henquin M. Stimulation of insulin release by benzoic acid derivatives related to the non-sulfonylurea moiety of glibenclamide: structural requirements and cellular mechanisms. European Journal of Pharmacology 141: 243-251, 1987

Hermann LS. Metformin: a review of its pharmacological properties and therapeutic use. Diabète et Métabolisme 5: 233-245, 1979

Hermann LS, Magnusson S, Moller B, Casey C, Tucker GT, et al. Lactic acidosis during metformin treatment in an elderly diabetic patient with impaired renal function. Acta Medica Scandinavica 209: 519-520, 1981

Hers HG, Hue L. Gluconeogenesis and related aspects of glycolysis. Annual Review of Biochemistry 52: 617-653, 1983

Hill HM, Chamberlain J. Determination of oral anti-diabetic agents in human body fluids using high-performance liquid chromatography. Journal of Chromatography 149: 349-358, 1978

Hjollund E, Richelsen B, Beck-Nielsen H, Pedersen O. The effect of glibenclamide on insulin receptors in normal man: comparative studies on insulin binding to monocytes and erythrocytes. Journal of Clinical and Endocrinological Investigation 57: 1257-1262, 1983

Holle A, Mangels W, Dreyer M, Kuhnau J, Rudiger HW. Biguanide treatment increases the number of insulin-receptor sites on human erythrocytes. New England Journal of Medicine 305: 563-566, 1981

Holmes B, Heel RC, Brogden RN, Speight TM, Avery GS. Gliclazide: a preliminary review of its pharmacodynamic properties and therapeutic efficacy in diabetes mellitus. Drugs 27: 301-327, 1984

Hosker JP, Burnett MA, Davies EG, Harris EA, Turner RC. Sulfonylurea therapy doubles β-cell response to glucose in Type 2 diabetic patients. Diabetologia 28: 809-814, 1985

Hsu PL, Ma JKH, Luzzi LA. Interaction of sulfonylureas with plasma proteins. Journal of Pharmaceutical Sciences 63: 570-573, 1974

Idle JR, Oates NS, Shah RR, Smith RL. Is there a genetic predisposition to phenformin-induced lactic acidosis? British Journal of Clinical Pharmacology 11: 418P-419P, 1981

Ikegami H, Shima K, Tanaka A, Tahara Y, Hirota M, et al. Interindividual variation in the absorption of glibenclamide in man. Acta Endocrinologica 111: 528-532, 1986

Jackson JE, Bressler R. Clinical pharmacology of sulfonylurea hypoglycaemic agents, part 1 and 2. Drugs 22: 211-245, 295-320, 1981

Jackson RA, Hawa MI, Jaspen JB, Sim BM, Di Silvio L, et al. Mechanism of metformin action in non-insulin-dependent diabetes mellitus. Diabetes 36: 632-640, 1987

Jacobs DB, Hayes GR, Truglia JA, Lockwood DM. Effects of metformin on insulin receptor tyrosine kinase activity in rat adipocytes. Diabetologia 29: 798-801, 1986

Jain AK, Ryan JR, McMahan FG. Potentiation of hypoglycaemic effect of sulfonylureas by halofenate. New England Journal of Medicine 293: 1283-1286, 1975

Janbon M, Chaptal J, Vedel A, Schaap J. Accidents hypoglycemiques graves par un sulfamidothiazol. Montpelier Medicine 21-22: 441-444, 1942

Jarrett RJ, Keen H. Hyperglycaemia and diabetes mellitus. Lancet 2: 1009-1012, 1976

Joost HG, Arend W, Holze SA. Effect of tolbutamide on insulin binding to isolated fat cells of the rat. Biochemical Pharmacology 31: 1227-1231, 1982

Jordan RM, Krammer H, Riddle MR. Sulfonylurea-induced factitious hypoglycaemia: a growing problem. Archives of Internal Medicine 137: 390-393, 1977

Judis J. Binding of sulfonylureas to serum proteins. Journal of Pharmaceutical Sciences 61: 89-93, 1972

Jumholtz B, Siershaek-Nielsen K, Skousted L, Kampmann J, Hansen J. Sulfamethizole-induced inhibition of diphenylhydantoin, tolbutamide, and warfarin metabolism. Clinical Pharmacology and Therapeutics 17: 731-734, 1975

Kabadi UM. Adjuvant therapy with tolazamide and insulin improves metabolic control in Type I diabetes mellitus. Diabetes Care 8: 440-446, 1985

Karam JH, Sanz N, Salamon E, Nolte M. Selective unresponsiveness of pancreatic β-cells to acute sulfonylurea stimulation during sulfonylurea therapy in NIDDM. Diabetes 35: 1314-1320, 1986

Kashiwagi A, Harano Y, Suzuki M, Kojima H, Harada M, et al. New α_2-adrenergic blocker (DG-5128) improves insulin secretion and *in vivo* glucose disposal in NIDDM patients. Diabetes 35: 1085-1089, 1986

Kater RMH, Tohon F, Iker FL. Increased rate of tolbutamide metabolism in alcoholic patients. Journal of the American Medical Association 207: 363-365, 1969

Kattermann R, Appels A, Muhich K, Proschek H, Soling HD, et al. Untersuchungen über die Wirkung von Diatt, Tolbutamid, und Buformin sowie deren Kombination auf Korpergewicht und verschiedene Stoffwechselgroben bei Diabetikern, II: Freie Fettsauren, Ketonkorper, Triglyceride und Cholesterin im Blut. Diabetologia 4: 221-228, 1968

Kaubisch N, Hammer R, Wollheim C, Renold AE, Offord RE. Specific receptors for sulfonylureas in brain and in a β-cell tumour of the rat. Biochemical Pharmacology 31: 1171-1174, 1982

Kaubisch N, Koss FW, Hammer R. The biochemistry of Glurenorm. In Piederse and Klarenbeck (Eds) New developments in the oral therapy of diabetes mellitus, pp. 37-50, Utrecht, 1979

Kawashima K, Kuzuja T, Matsuda A. Radioimmunoassay of glibenclamide. Diabetes 28: 221-226, 1979

Keal J, Somogyi A. Rapid and sensitive high-performance liquid chromatography assay for metformin in plasma and urine using ion-pair extraction techniques. Journal of Chromatography 378: 503-508, 1986

Keal J, Stockley C, Somogyi A. Simultaneous determination of tolbutamide and its hydroxy and carboxy metabolites in plasma and urine by high-performance liquid chromatography. Journal of Chromatography 378: 237-241, 1986

Kimura M, Kobayashi K, Hata M, Matsuaka A, Kitamura H, et al. Determination of gliclazide in human serum by high-performance liquid chromatography using an anion-exchange resin. Journal of Chromatography 183: 467-473, 1980

Knaupf RE, Fajans SS, Ramirez E, Conn JW. Metabolic studies of chlorpropamide in normal man and in diabetic subjects. Annals of the New York Academy of Sciences 74: 603-617, 1959

Kobayashi K, Hase A, Kimura M, Sakoguchi T, Shimosawa M, et al. Influence of blood proteins on biomedical analysis, VIII: attempts at purification of gliclazide-degrading factor in human serum. Life Sciences 37: 2015-2019, 1985

Kobayashi K, Kimura M, Sakoguchi T, Kitani Y, Mitsuo H, et al. Influence of blood proteins on biomedical analysis, III: pharmacokinetics and protein binding of gliclazide. Journal of Pharmacobio-Dynamics 4: 436-442, 1981

Kolterman OG. Longitudinal evaluation of the effects of sulfonylurea therapy in subjects with Type II diabetes mellitus. American Journal of Medicine 79 (Suppl. 3B): 23-33, 1985

Kolterman OG, Gray RS, Shapiro G, Scarlett JA, Griffin J, et al. The acute and chronic effects of sulfonylurea therapy in Type II diabetic subjects. Diabetes 33: 346-354, 1984

Kopitar Z. Human Pharmakokinetik und Metabolismus von ^{14}C-markiertem Gliquidone (AR-DF 26). Arzneimittel-Forschung 24: 1455-1460, 1975

Kopitar Z, Koss FW. Pharmacokinetic behaviour of ARDF 26, a new sulfonylurea. Proceedings of the International Conference on Glurenorm, 13-14 March, pp. 20-29, 1975

Krall LP. Oral hypoglycemic agents. In Marble et al. (Eds) Joslin's diabetes mellitus, pp. 412-452, Lea and Febiger, Philadelphia, 1985

Krall LP, Balodimos MC. Combined sulfonylurea-biguanide therapy of diabetes mellitus. In Butterfield and Westering (Eds)

Tolbutamide after 10 years, pp. 303-311, International Congress Series No. 149, Excerpta Medica, Amsterdam, 1967
Kristensen M, Hansen J. Potentiation of the tolbutamide effect by dicoumarol. Diabetes 16: 211-214, 1972
Kuhl C, Jensen SL, Nielsen OV, Pedersen J. The effect of dimethylbiguanide (DMB) on plasma insulin and glucagon concentrations. Diabetologia 12: 403, 1976
Kuhl C, Jensen SL, Nielsen OV, Pedersen J. The effect of metformin on the arginine induced insulin and glucagon release in pigs. Acta Pharmacologica et Toxicologica 44: 235-237, 1979
Lebovitz HE. Glipizide. A second-generation sulfonylurea hypoglycemic agent. Pharmacotherapy 5 (Suppl. 2): 63-77, 1985
Lebovitz HE. Oral hypoglycemic agents. In Alberti and Krall (Eds) The diabetes annual 3, pp. 72-93, Elsevier, Amsterdam, 1987
Lebovitz HE, Feinglos MN. The oral hypoglycemic agents. In Ellemberg and Rifkin (Eds) Diabetes mellitus, pp. 591-610, Medical Examination Publishing Co. Inc., New York, 1983
Lebovitz HE, Feinglos MN, Bucholtz HK, Lebovitz FL. Potentiation of insulin: a probable mechanism for the antidiabetic action for the sulfonylurea drugs. Journal of Clinical Endocrinology and Metabolism 45: 601-604, 1977
Lennard MS, Casey C, Tucker GT, Woods HF. Determination of metformin in biological samples. British Journal of Clinical Pharmacology 6: 183-185, 1979
Levitt LJ. Chlorpropamide-induced pure white cell aplasia. Blood 69: 394-400, 1987
Lockwood DH, Maloff BL, Nowak SM, McCaleb ML. Extrapancreatic effects of sulfonylureas. Potentiation of insulin action through post-binding mechanisms. American Journal of Medicine 74 (Suppl. 1A): 102-108, 1983
Lorch E. Inhibition of intestinal absorption and improvement of oral glucose tolerance by biguanides in the normal and in the streptozotocin-diabetic rat. Diabetologia 7: 195-203, 1971
Lord JM, Atkins TW, Bailey CJ. Effect of metformin on hepatocyte insulin receptor binding in normal, streptozotocin diabetic and genetically obese diabetic (ob/ob) mice. Diabetologia 25: 108-113, 1983a
Lord JM, White SD, Bailey CJ, Atkins TW, Fletcher RF, et al. Effect of metformin on insulin receptor binding and glycaemic control in type II diabetes. British Medical Journal 286: 830-831, 1983b
Loubatieres A. The hypoglycemic sulfonamides: history and development of the problem from 1942 to 1945. Annals of the New York Academy of Sciences 71: 4-11, 1957
Luft D, Schmulling RM, Eggstein M. Lactic acidosis in biguanide-treated diabetics: a review of 330 cases. Diabetologia 14: 75-87, 1978
MacKichan JJ. Protein binding drug displacement interactions: fact or fiction? Clinical Pharmacokinetics 16: 65-73, 1989
Maeda T, Yamaguchi T, Hasshimoto M. Gas chromatographic determination of hypoglycaemic agent gliclazide in plasma. Journal of Chromatography 223: 357-363, 1981
Maggi E, Pianezzola E, Valzelli G. Radioimmunoassay of glipizide in human plasma. European Journal of Clinical Pharmacology 21: 251-255, 1981
Maloff BL, Lockwood DH. Introductory effects of a sulfonylurea on insulin action in adipocytes: potentiation of insulin-stimulated hexose transport. Journal of Clinical Investigation 65: 85-90, 1981
Marchetti P, Benzi L, Cecchetti P, Giannarelli R, Ciociaro D, et al. Plasma biguanides levels are correlated with metabolic effects in diabetic patients. Clinical Pharmacology and Therapeutics 41: 450-454, 1987
Marchetti P, Benzi L, Cerri M, Cecchetti P, Giannarelli R, et al. Effects of plasma metformin concentrations on serum lipid levels in Type II diabetic patients. Acta Diabetologica Latina 25: 55-62, 1988a
Marchetti P, Benzi L, Gregorio F, Giannarelli R, Cecchetti P, et al. New findings on the metabolic effects of biguanides. Minerva Endocrinologica, in press, 1988b
Matikainen E, Juntunen J. Diabetic neuropathy: epidemiological, pathogenetic and clinical aspects with special emphasis on type 2 diabetes mellitus. Acta Endocrinologica 262 (Suppl.) 89-94, 1984
Matin SB, Karam JH, Forsham PH. Simple electron capture gas-chromatographic method for the determination of oral hypoglycemic biguanides in biological fluids. Analytical Chemistry 47: 545-548, 1975
Matsutani A, Kaku K, Kaneko T. Tolbutamide stimulated fructose-2,6-biphosphate formation in perfused rat liver. Diabetes 33: 495-498, 1984
Matthews EK, Shotton PA. The control of Rb85 efflux from rat isolated pancreatic islets by the sulfonylureas tolbutamide and glibenclamide. British Journal of Pharmacology 82: 689, 1984
Mehnert H. Pharmacokinetics of blood lowering biguanides. Acta Diabetologica Latina 1 (Suppl.): 137-142, 1969
Melander A. Clinical pharmacology of sulfonylureas. Metabolism 36 (Suppl. 1): 12-16, 1987
Melander A, Sartor G, Wahlin E, Schersten B, Bitzen PO. Serum tolbutamide and chlorpropamide concentrations in patients with diabetes mellitus. British Medical Journal 1: 142-144, 1978
Meyer F, Ipaktchi M, Clauser H. Specific inhibition of gluconeogenesis by biguanides. Nature 213: 203-204, 1967
Middleton E, Finke SR. Metabolic response to epinephrine in bronchial asthma. Journal of Allergy 42: 288-299, 1968
Misbin RI. Phenformin-associated lactic acidosis: pathogenesis and treatment. Annals of Internal Medicine 87: 591-595, 1977
Miyazaki H, Fujii T, Yoshida K, Arakawa S, Furukawa H, et al. Disposition and metabolism of ^{3}H gliclazide in rats. European Journal of Drug Metabolism and Pharmacokinetics 8: 117-131, 1983
National Diabetes Data Group. Classification and diagnosis of diabetes mellitus and other categories of glucose intolerance. Diabetes 28: 1039-1057, 1979
Nattrass M, Alberti KGMM. Biguanides. Diabetologia 14: 71-74, 1978
Nattrass M, Lloyd B, Todd PG. Metabolic effects of combined sulfonylurea and biguanide therapy. Diabetologia 12: 411, 1976
Nattrass M, Sizer K, Alberti KGMM. Correlation of plasma phenformin concentration with metabolic effects in normal subjects. Clinical Sciences 58: 153-155, 1980
Nattrass M, Todd PG, Hinks L, Lloyd B, Alberti KGMM. Comparative effects of phenformin, metformin and glibenclamide on metabolic rhythms in maturity-onset diabetics. Diabetologia 13: 145-152, 1977
Nelson E. Rate of metabolism of tolbutamide in test subjects with liver disease or with impaired renal function. American Journal of the Medical Sciences 248: 657-659, 1964
Neuvonen PJ, Kannisto H, Hirvisalo EL. Effect of activated charcoal on absorption of tolbutamide and valproate in man. European Journal of Clinical Pharmacology 24: 243-246, 1983
Neuvonen PJ, Karkkainen S. Effects of charcoal, sodium bicarbonate, and ammonium chloride on chlorpropamide kinetics. Clinical Pharmacology and Therapeutics 33: 386-393, 1983
Neuvonen PJ, Karkkainen S, Lehtovaara R. Pharmacokinetics of chlorpropamide in epileptic patients: effects of enzyme induction and urine pH on chlorpropamide elimination. European Journal of Clinical Pharmacology 32: 297-301, 1987
Noel M. Kinetic study of normal and sustained release dosage forms of metformin in normal subjects. Research and Clinical Forums 1: 35-50, 1979
Nosadini R, Avogaro A, Trevisan R. Effect of metformin on insulin-stimulated turnover and insulin binding to receptors in type II diabetes. Diabetes Care 10: 62-67, 1987
Oates NS, Shah RR, Idle JR, Smith RL. Genetic polymorphism of phenformin 4-hydroxylation. Clinical Pharmacology and Therapeutics 32: 81-89, 1982

Oberdisse K. Der Wirkungmechanismus der Biguanide auf Grund klinisch-experimenteller Untersuchungen und die klinische Anwendung der Biguanide. In Oberdisse (Ed.) Handbuch der inneren Medizin, Bd 712 B, Diabetes Mellitus, pp. 983-997, 999-1066, Springer-Verlag, Berlin, 1977

O'Donovan CJ. Analysis of long-term experience with tolbutamide (orinase) in the management of diabetes. Current Therapeutic Research 1: 69-75, 1959

Olson SC, Ayres JW, Antal EJ, Albert KS. Effect of food and tablet age on relative bioavailability and pharmacodynamics of two tolbutamide products. Journal of Pharmaceutical Sciences 74: 735-739, 1985

Ostenson CG, Nylen A, Grill V, Gutniak M, Efendic S. Sulfonylurea-induced inhibition of glucagon secretion from the perfused rat pancreas: evidence for a direct, non-paracrine effect. Diabetologia 29: 861-867, 1986

Pagano G, Tagliaferro V, Carta Q, Caselle MT, Fozzo C, et al. Metformin reduces insulin requirement in type 1 insulin-dependent diabetes. Diabetologia 24: 351-354, 1983

Pannekock JH. Insulin, glucagon and oral hypoglycemic drugs. In Dukas (Ed.) Meyler's side effects of drugs, Vol. 8, pp. 904-927, Excerpta Medica, Amsterdam, 1976

Pearson JC. Pharmacokinetics of glyburide. American Journal of Medicine 79 (Suppl. 3B): 67-71, 1985

Pearson JG, Antal EJ, Raehl GL, Gorsch HK, Craig WA, et al. Pharmacokinetic disposition of ^{14}C-glyburide in patients with varying renal function. Clinical Pharmacology and Therapeutics 39: 318-324, 1986

Pentikainen PJ. Bioavailability of metformin: comparison of solution, rapidly dissolving tablets, and three sustained release products. International Journal of Clinical Pharmacology, Therapy and Toxicology 24: 213-220, 1986

Pentikainen PJ, Neuvonen PJ, Penttila A. Pharmacokinetics of metformin after intravenous and oral administration to man. European Journal of Clinical Pharmacology 16: 195-202, 1979

Peterson CM, Sims RV, Jones RL, Rieders F. Bioavailability of glipizide and its effect on blood glucose and insulin levels in patients with non-insulin-dependent diabetes. Diabetes Care 5: 497-500, 1982

Petitpierre B, Perrin L, Reidhart M, Herrera A, Fabre J. Behaviour of chlorpropamide in renal insufficiency and under the effect of associated drug therapy. International Journal of Clinical Pharmacology 6: 120-124, 1972

Pettit DJ, Knowler WC, Lisse JR, Bennett PM. Development of retinopathy and proteinuria in relation to plasma glucose concentrations in Pima Indians. Lancet 2: 1050-1052, 1980

Potter H, Hulm M. Bestimmung von Glibenclamid mit hochleistungsflussigkeits-Chromatographie in Humanplasma. Journal of Chromatography 273: 217-222, 1983

Prager R, Schernthaner G. Insulin receptor binding to monocytes, insulin secretion, and glucose tolerance following metformin treatment. Diabetes 32: 1083-1086, 1983

Prescott LF, Redman DR. Gas-liquid chromatographic estimation of tolbutamide and chlorpropamide in plasma. Journal of Pharmacy and Pharmacology 24: 713-716, 1972

Prince MJ, Olefsky JM. Direct *in vitro* effect of a sulfonylurea to increase human fibroblast insulin receptors. Journal of Clinical Investigation 66: 608-611, 1980

Purba HS, Back DJ, Orme ML. Tolbutamide 4-hydroxylase activity of human liver microsomes: effect of inhibitors. British Journal of Clinical Pharmacology 24: 230-234, 1987

Purrello F, Gullo D, Brunetti A, Buscema M, Italia S, et al. Direct effects of biguanides on glucose utilization *in vitro*. Metabolism 36: 774-776, 1987

Purrello F, Trischitta V, Runello F, Vigneri R. Phenformin has opposite effects on insulin and growth-hormone binding to IM-9 lymphocytes. Metabolism 31: 1073-1076, 1982

Raghow G, Meyer MC. High-performance liquid chromatographic assay of tolbutamide and carboxytolbutamide in human plasma. Journal of Pharmaceutical Sciences 70: 1166-1167, 1981

Randle PJ, Smith GH. Regulation of glucose uptake by muscle, 1: the effect of insulin, anaerobiosis and cell poisons on the uptake of glucose and release of potassium by isolated rat diaphraghm. Biochemical Journal 70: 490-500, 1958

Redman DR, Prescott LF. Failure of induction of liver microsomal enzymes by tolbutamide in maturity-onset diabetes. Diabetes 22: 210-211, 1973

Richardson T, Foster J, Mawer GE. Enhancement by sodium salicylate of the blood glucose lowering effect of chlorpropamide – drug interaction or summation of similar effects? British Journal of Clinical Pharmacology 22: 43-48, 1986

Rizza RA, Mandarino LJ, Gerich JE. Mechanism and significance of insulin resistance in non-insulin-dependent diabetes mellitus. Diabetes 30: 990-995, 1981

Rogers BJ, Standaert ML, Pollet RJ. Direct effects of sulfonylurea agents on glucose transport in the BC 3H-1 myocyte. Diabetes 36: 1292-1296, 1987

Ross MJ. Determination of metformin in biological fluids by derivatization followed by high-performance liquid chromatography. Journal of Chromatography 133: 408-411, 1977

Royer ME, Ko H, Evans GS, Johnston KT. Radioimmunoassay for glyburide in human serum. Analytical Letters 9: 629-640, 1976

Rupp W, Christ O, Fulberth W. Untersuchungen zur Bioavailability von Glibenclamid. Arzneimittel-Forschung 22: 471-473, 1972

Rupp W, Christ O, Hepter W. Resorption, Ausscheidung und Metabolismus nach intravenoser und oraler Gabe von NB 419-14C an Menschen. Arzneimittel-Forschung 19: 1428-1434, 1969

Rupp W, Dibbern HW, Hajchu P, Ross G, Vander EE. Untersuchungen zur Bioaquivalenz von Tolbutamid. Deutsche Medizinische Wochenschrift 100: 690-695, 1975

Sako Y, Wasada T, Umeda F, Ibayashi H. Effect of glibenclamide on pancreatic hormone release from isolated perfused islets of normal and cysteamine-treated rats. Metabolism 35: 944-949, 1986

Salhanick AI, Konowitz P, Amatruda JM. Potentiation of insulin action by a sulfonylurea in primary culture of hepatocytes from normal and diabetic rats. Diabetes 32: 206-212, 1983

Sartor G, Melander A, Schersten B, Wahlin-Boll E. Serum glibenclamide in diabetic patients and influence of food on the kinetics and effects of glibenclamide. Diabetologia 18: 17-22, 1980a

Sartor G, Melander A, Schersten B, Wahlin-Boll E. Comparative single-dose kinetics and effects of four sulfonylureas in healthy volunteers. Acta Medica Scandinavica 208: 301-307, 1980b

Sartor G, Melander A, Schersten B, Wahlin-Boll E. Influence of food and age on the single-dose kinetics and effects of tolbutamide and chlorpropamide. European Journal of Clinical Pharmacology 17: 285-293, 1980c

Savage PJ, Dippe SE, Bennett PM, Gorden P, Roth J, et al. Hyperinsulinemia and hypoinsulinemia: insulin responses to oral carbohydrate over a wide spectrum of glucose tolerance. Diabetes 24: 362-368, 1975

Schafer G. Interaction of biguanides with mitochondrial and synthetic membranes. European Journal of Biochemistry 27: 364-375, 1972

Schafer G. Some new aspects on the interaction of hypoglycemia-producing biguanides with biological membranes. Biochemical Pharmacology 25: 2015-2024, 1976

Schafer G. Biguanides: a review of history, pharmacodynamics and therapy. Diabète et Métabolisme 9: 148-163, 1983

Schatz H, Doci S, Hofer R. The effect of dimethylbiguanide on glucose tolerance, serum insulin and growth hormone in obese patients. Diabetologia 8: 1-7, 1972a

Schatz H, Katsilambos N, Nierle C, Pfeiffer EE. The effect of biguanides on secretion and biosynthesis of insulin in isolated pancreatic islets of rats. Diabetologia 8: 402-407, 1972b

Schmid-Antomerchi H, De Weile J, Fosset M, Lezdunski M. The receptor for the antidiabetic sulphonylureas controls the activity of the ATP-modulated K^+ channel. Journal of Biological Chemistry 262: 15840-15844, 1987

Schmidt HAE, Schoog M, Schweer KM, Winkler E. Pharmacokinetics and pharmacodynamics as well as metabolism following orally and intravenously administered C14-glipizide, a new antidiabetic. Diabetologia 9 (Suppl.): 320-330, 1973

Scott J, Poffenbarger PL. Pharmacogenetics of tolbutamide metabolism in humans. Diabetes 28: 41-51, 1979

Searle GL, Fulli R. The mechanism of the acute hypoglycemic action of phenformin (DBI). Metabolism – Clinical and Experimental 29: 630-635, 1980

Self TH, Morris T. Interaction of rifampicin and chlorpropamide. Chest 77: 800-801, 1980

Seltzer HS. Drug induced hypoglycemia, a review based on 473 cases. Diabetes 21: 955-966, 1972

Seltzer HS. Severe drug-induced hypoglycemia: a review. Comprehensive Therapy 5: 21-29, 1979

Semple CG, Omile C, Buchanan KD, Beastall GH, Paterson KR. Effect of oral verapamil on glibenclamide stimulated insulin secretion. British Journal of Clinical Pharmacology 22: 187-190, 1986

Shah RR, Oates NS, Idle IR, Smith RL. Genetic impairment of phenformin metabolism. Lancet 1: 1147, 1980

Sharpe GWG. The adenylate cyclase-cyclic AMP system in islets of Langerhans and its role in the control of insulin release. Diabetologia 16: 287-296, 1979

Sheldon J, Anderson J, Stoner L. Serum concentration and urinary excretion of oral sulfonylurea compounds: relation to diabetic control. Diabetes 14: 362-367, 1965

Sheldon J, Taylor KW, Anderson J. The effects of the long-term acetohexamide treatment on pancreatic islet cell function in maturity-onset diabetes. Metabolism 15: 874-883, 1966

Shen SW, Bressler R. Clinical pharmacology of oral antidiabetic agents. First and second part. New England Journal of Medicine 296: 493-497, 787-793, 1977

Shepherd Jr HG, McDonald HJ. Binding affinity of purified plasma proteins for phenethylbiguanide, an oral hypoglycaemic compound. Clinical Chemistry 4: 496-498, 1958

Shima K, Tanaka A, Ikegami H, Tabata M, Sawazaki N, et al. Effect of dietary fiber, glucomannan, on absorption of sulfonylurea in man. Hormone and Metabolic Research 15: 1-3, 1983

Simpson IJ, Hanley JW, Sharpe DN. Lactic acidosis associated with phenformin therapy in diabetes mellitus. New Zealand Medical Journal 79: 645-648, 1974

Singer DL, Hurwitz D. Long-term experiences with sulfonylureas and placebo. New England Journal of Medicine 277: 450-456, 1967

Sirtori CR, Franceschini G, Galli-Kienle M, Cighetti G, Galli G. Disposition of metformin (N,N-dimethylbiguanide) in man. Clinical Pharmacology and Therapeutics 24: 683-693, 1978

Sirtori CR, Tremoli E, Sirtori M, Conti F, Paoletti R. Treatment of hypertriglyceridemia with metformin. Atherosclerosis 26: 583-592, 1977

Skyler JS. Non-insulin-dependent diabetes mellitus: a clinical strategy. Diabetes Care 7: 118-129, 1984

Smith DL, Vecchio TJ, Forist AA. Biological half-lives of the *p*-acetylbenzene-sulfonylureas U-18536 and acetohexamide and their metabolites. Metabolism 14: 229-240, 1965

Soling HD, Moshagen D, Skutella E, Kneer P, Creutzfeldt W. Die Wirkung von N19n-Butylbiguanide auf den Stoffwechsel der isolierten perfundierten Leber normaler und alloxandiabetischer Ketotischer Ratten. Diabetologia 3: 318-330, 1967

Solomon H, Schrogre J. Effect of phenyramidol and bishydroxycoumarol on the metabolism of tolbutamide in human subjects. Metabolism 116: 1029-1033, 1967

Sonatiemi E, Arvela P, Huhti E. Increased clearance of tolbutamide from the blood of asthmatic patients. Annals of Allergy 29: 139-141, 1971a

Sonatiemi E, Arvela P, Huhti E, Kovisto O. Half-life of tolbutamide in patients with chronic respiratory failure. European Journal of Clinical Pharmacology 4: 29-31, 1971b

Stockley C, Keal J, Rolan P, Bochner F, Somogyi A. Lack of inhibition of tolbutamide hydroxylation by cimetidine in man. European Journal of Clinical Pharmacology 31: 235-237, 1986

Stowers JM, Bewsher PD. The long-term use of sulfonylureas in diabetes mellitus. Lancet 1: 122-124, 1962

Sussman KE, Stjernholm M, Vaughan GD. Tolbutamide and its effect upon insulin secretion in the isolated perfused rat pancreas. In Butterfield and Westering (Eds) Tolbutamide after ten years, pp. 22-33 (International Congress Series No. 149). Excerpta Medica, Amsterdam, 1967

Svensson CK, Woodruff MN, Baxter JG, Laeka D. Free-drug concentration monitoring in clinical practice: rationale and current status. Clinical Pharmacokinetics 11: 450-469, 1986

Taylor JA. Pharmacokinetics and biotransformation of chlorpropamide in man. Clinical Pharmacology and Therapeutics 13: 710-718, 1972

Thomas RC, Duchamp DJ, Judy RW, Ikeda GJ. Metabolic fate of tolazamide in man and in the rat. Journal of Medicinal Chemistry 21: 725-732, 1978

Thomas RC, Ikeda GJ. The metabolic fate of tolbutamide in man and in the rat. Journal of Medicinal Chemistry 9: 507-510, 1966

Thorn G. Clinical considerations in the use of corticosteroids. New England Journal of Medicine 274: 775-781, 1966

Tranquada RE, Kleeman G, Brown J. Some effects of phenethylbiguanide on human hepatic metabolism as measured by hepatic vein catheterization. Diabetes 9: 207-214, 1960

Trischitta V, Benzi L, Brunetti A, Cecchetti P, Marchetti P, et al. Intracellular insulin processing is altered in monocytes from patients with Type II diabetes mellitus. Journal of Clinical Endocrinology and Metabolism 64: 914-920, 1987

Trischitta V, Gullo D, Pezzino V, Vigneri R. Metformin normalizes insulin binding to monocytes from obese non-diabetic subjects and obese type II diabetic patients. Journal of Clinical Endocrinology and Metabolism 57: 713-718, 1983

Tucker GT, Casey C, Phillips PJ, Connor H, Ward JD, et al. Metformin kinetics in healthy subjects and in patients with diabetes mellitus. British Journal of Clinical Pharmacology 12: 235-246, 1981

Turtle JR. Glucose and insulin secretory response patterns following diet and tolazamide therapy in diabetes. British Medical Journal 3: 606-610, 1970

Ueda H, Sakurai T, Ota M, Nakajima A, Kamiti K, et al. Disappearance rate of tolbutamide in normal subjects and in diabetes mellitus, liver cirrhosis, and renal disease. Diabetes 12: 414-419, 1963

Uihlein M, Sistovaris N. High-performance liquid column and thin-layer chromatographic determination of human serum glibenclamide at therapeutic levels. Journal of Chromatography 227: 93-101, 1982

UK Prospective Diabetes Study. II; Reduction in HbA1c with basal insulin supplement, sulfonylurea, or biguanide therapy in maturity-onset diabetes; a multicenter study. Diabetes 34: 793-798, 1985

UK Prospective Study of therapies of maturity-onset diabetes. I, Effect of diet, sulfonylurea, insulin or biguanide therapy on fasting plasma glucose and body weight over one year; multicenter study. Diabetologia 24: 404-411, 1983

Verdonck LF, Sangster B, van Heijst ANP, De Groot G, Maes RAA. Buformin concentrations in a case of fatal lactic acidosis. Diabetologia 20: 45-46, 1981

Vermeulen A, Rottiers R. Influence of dimethylbiguanide (metformin) on carbohydrate metabolism in obese, non-diabetic women. Diabetologia 8: 8-11, 1972

Verschoor L, Wolffenbuttel BHR, Weber RFA. β-blockade and carbohydrate metabolism: theoretical aspects and clinical implications. Journal of Cardiovascular Pharmacology 8 (Suppl. 11): 592-595, 1986

Vigneri R, Goldfine ID. Role of metformin in treatment of diabetes mellitus. Diabetes Care 10: 118-122, 1987

Wahlin-Boll E. Kinetics-effect relations of glipizide, Doctoral Thesis, University of Lund, Dalby, Sweden, 1986

Wahlin-Boll E, Almer LO, Melander A. Bioavailability, pharmacokinetics and effects of glipizide in Type 2 diabetics. Clinical Pharmacokinetics 7: 363-372, 1982a

Wahlin-Boll E, Groop L, Karhumaa S, Groop PH, Totterman KJ, et al. Therapeutic equivalence of once- and thrice-daily glipizide. European Journal of Clinical Pharmacology 31: 95-99, 1986

Wahlin-Boll E, Melander A. High-performance liquid chromatographic determination of glipizide and some other sulfonylurea drugs in serum. Journal of Chromatography 164: 541-546, 1979

Wahlin-Boll E, Melander A, Sartor G, Schersten B. Influence of food intake on the absorption and effect of glipizide in diabetics and in healthy subjects. European Journal of Clinical Pharmacology 18: 279-283, 1980

Wahlin-Boll E, Sartor G, Melander A, Schersten B. Impaired effect of sulfonylurea following increased dosage. European Journal of Clinical Pharmacology 22: 21-25, 1982b

Wajchenberg BL, Nery M, Leme CE, Silveira AA, Fioratti P, et al. Effect of prolonged gliclazide treatment on blood glucose and plasma insulin responses in obese patients with maturity-onset diabetes. Clinical Pharmacology and Therapeutics 27: 375-378, 1980

Waters AK, Morgan DB, Wales JK. Blood lactate and pyruvate levels in diabetic patients treated with biguanides with and without sulfonylureas. Diabetologia 11: 95-98, 1978

Weissman PN, Shenkman L, Gregerman RI. Chlorpropamide hyponatremia. Drug-induced inappropriate anti-diuretic hormone activity. New England Journal of Medicine 284: 65-71, 1971

Williams RL, Blaschke TF, Meflin PJ, Melmar KL, Rowland M. Influence of acute viral hepatitis on disposition and plasma binding of tolbutamide. Clinical Pharmacology and Therapeutics 21: 301-309, 1977

Woods HF, Stubbs WA, Johnson G, Alberti KGMM. Inhibition by salicylate of gluconeogenesis in the isolated and perfused rat liver. Clinical and Experimental Pharmacology and Physiology 1: 535-540, 1974

Yau LSK, Strother A, Buchboltz J, Abu-El-Haj S. Glucose effect on drug action, metabolism, and pharmacokinetic parameters in mice. Drug Nutrient Interactions 5: 9-20, 1987

Authors' address: Dr *Piero Marchetti*, Cattedra Malattie del Ricambio, Istituto di Clinica Medica II, via Roma 67, 56100 Pisa (Italy).

Leading Article

Clinical Pharmacokinetics 16: 129-133 (1989)
0312-5963/89/0003-0129/$02.50/0

Clinical Significance of Differences in Bioavailability of Medroxyprogesterone Acetate Preparations

A.D. Stockdale and *A.Y. Rostom*

Regional Centre for Radiotherapy and Oncology, St Luke's Hospital, Guildford, England

Synthetic progestational agents first became widely available in the early 1960s and were investigated for use in patients with hormone-responsive tumours, i.e. breast, kidney, uterine and prostate cancer. A range of different preparations was available, but their clinical use was limited by side effects including nausea and vomiting, masculinisation, Cushingoid effects and liver damage (Stoll 1967). An early study (Stoll 1967) of 6 orally active agents, including medroxyprogesterone acetate (MPA), concluded that all were active in breast cancer and that resistance to one agent did not necessarily imply resistance to others. However, response rates were disappointing, ranging from 16 to 22%, and over the ensuing years the use of medroxyprogesterone acetate was confined mainly to endometrial and kidney cancers.

1. High-Dose MPA in Carcinoma of the Breast

Interest in medroxyprogesterone acetate in carcinoma of the breast was rekindled by the work of Pannuti and colleagues, who investigated its maximum tolerated intramuscular dose, and reported greatly increased objective response rates of 44% with intramuscular doses of 1500mg daily for 30 days (Pannuti et al. 1978). Although the initial studies were troubled by a high incidence of sterile abscess formation at the injection site, investigators were impressed by a feeling of well being associated with increased appetite and weight gain due to the drug, which were thought to be of benefit to the patient. Prompt improvement of bone pain was also noted for many patients. These results implied a dose-response effect for medroxyprogesterone acetate, which became accepted on the basis of the historical results (Ganzina 1979). It might thus be assumed that differing bioavailability of medroxyprogesterone acetate preparations could be of significance. When radioimmunoassay (RIA) techniques became available to measure serum medroxyprogesterone acetate concentrations, attempts were made to rationalise dosage schedules and elucidate the pharmacokinetics of the drug.

2. Pharmacokinetics of Medroxyprogesterone Acetate

Following a single intramuscular injection, peak plasma concentrations of medroxyprogesterone acetate occur within several hours. However, due to the slow and prolonged absorption from the injection site, 'steady-state' concentrations are rapidly reached, as absorption is balanced by metabolism and excretion, with an apparent elimination half-life of approximately 5 to 6 weeks. This is in contrast to the same dose given by mouth, following which blood concentrations rise to a peak from 2 to 10 times higher before falling rapidly, with a half-life of 48 hours (Salimtschik et al. 1980). The pharmacology of prolonged administration is very different. Comparison of patients treated with equal daily doses of medroxyprogesterone acetate given by mouth or intramuscular injection for 30 days showed concentrations approximately 3 times higher following intramuscular therapy at the end of this period. Concentrations rose throughout the study when the intramuscular route was used, while steady-state was reached after approximately 10 days of oral therapy (Camaggi et al. 1983). It was predicted that steady-state would be reached after 6 to 8 months of continuous intramuscular therapy, and a schedule of daily intramuscular injections for 1 month to achieve a high blood concentration, followed by a once-weekly maintenance dose, was suggested (Tamassia et al. 1982). It was noted that there was a very wide variation in plasma concentrations between patients, particularly after oral administration, and it was thought that response might relate to the blood concentration achieved.

2.1 MPA Assays

The use of medroxyprogesterone acetate plasma concentrations became confused by the very wide range of values reported from different laboratories following effective treatment regimens. Some authors studying direct RIA techniques, prescribing 1500mg daily by mouth, reported blood concentrations of 1000 to 12,000 μg/L (Blossey et al. 1982), while others, prescribing an oral dose of 600mg daily, reported levels up to 1000-fold lower (Hedley et al. 1985). This effect can be explained by the specificity of the assay chosen and the inadvertent inclusion of metabolites. Antibodies to different portions of the medroxyprogesterone acetate molecule were raised in goats or rabbits. Those raised against C17 conjugates of the parent compound cross-reacted significantly less with metabolites of the A ring and C6 position than those raised against C11 conjugates, which estimated both medroxyprogesterone acetate and metabolites (Sturm & Schulz 1984). Ether extraction and enzymic hydrolysis techniques indicate that the majority of the drug *in vivo* is present as a glucuronide conjugate (Mathrubutham & Fotherby 1981). Recent and more specific chromatographic techniques which are able to distinguish the parent molecule from its metabolites showed concentrations 5 to 10 times lower than with RIA, confirming that a large proportion of the drug is present as metabolites (Mould et al. 1988). It is not known if these metabolites are biologically active.

2.2 Absorption and Metabolism

Scant pharmacological information exists relating to the absorption and metabolism of medroxyprogesterone acetate. As no intravenous single-dose studies are available, the best estimate of absorbed dose compares oral and intraperitoneal absorption in patients with ascites, assuming total absorption from the abdominal cavity and equivalent metabolism by the portal system. Such studies have implied an oral absorption of less than 10% of the dose administered (Camaggi et al. 1985). Absorption after oral administration is rapid, peak blood drug concentrations being achieved within several hours, but medroxyprogesterone acetate undergoes extensive first-pass hepatic metabolism. Adlercreutz et al. (1983) showed that 21% of a dose of medroxyprogesterone acetate was present as metabolite only 20 minutes after administration; after 1 hour the figure was 53%. Other authors have confirmed this very rapid metabolism (Gupta et al. 1979). Another group has also shown that medroxyprogesterone acetate is rapidly reduced by human faecal bacteria, and suggested that intestinal metabolism may be significant in man (Martin et al. 1980).

3. *Response to MPA Therapy in Breast Cancer*

The early dosage regimens requiring daily intramuscular injections were a daunting prospect and, not surprisingly, high-dose oral administration was investigated. As predicted from pharmacokinetic data, high blood concentrations can be achieved (Tamassia et al. 1982) and high response rates were reported. The question remained as to the optimum dosage and route of administration of medroxyprogesterone acetate to achieve maximum response.

3.1 Objective Response Criteria

Objective response criteria have been carefully defined by the International Union Against Cancer (UICC) [Hayward et al. 1977], but the pattern of metastatic disease most likely to respond to hormone manipulation is well recognised and response rates are greatly influenced by the choice of patient. Assessment of objective response in metastatic bone disease remains a very problematic area. Most recent papers require healing of lytic bone lesions confirmed on x-ray; thus, although many patients with bone disease benefit from undoubted reduction in pain whilst taking medroxyprogesterone acetate, the majority of these in practice can only be classed as stable disease. Criteria for response in some early papers were solely the lack of progression of bone disease over a 3-month period (Della Cuna et al. 1978; Pannuti et al. 1979). Thus, patient selection and interpretation of response can explain the improved percentages reported in series where the majority of patients have predominantly bone disease.

3.2 Correlation Between Blood Concentration and Response

There are conflicting reports in the literature on correlations between medroxyprogesterone acetate blood concentrations and response. Tamassia et al. (1982) predicted that blood concentrations should be between 100 and 200 μg/L, and others described appropriate thresholds of 100 μg/L and 150 μg/L (Johnson et al. 1984; Mahlke et al. 1985). However, objective responses and disease stasis have been shown with concentrations as low as 20 μg/L (Stockdale et al. 1987), while others have also found no correlation (Beex et al. 1987; Hedley et al. 1985). Thus, there is no consistent trend to suggest a threshold for effectiveness of medroxyprogesterone acetate therapy. Randomised studies comparing oral and intramuscular therapy have shown no advantage for the latter route, although doses by mouth needed to be approximately twice as large in the former to achieve equivalent blood concentrations (Beex et al. 1987; Paridaens et al. 1986).

Are then improved response rates with medroxyprogesterone acetate due to higher-dose therapy or patient selection and less rigorous response criteria?

3.3 Randomised Studies at High and Low Dose

Few randomised studies have been published comparing low- and high-dose treatment regimens. One study comparing intramuscular medroxyprogesterone acetate 1500mg daily for 30 days with 500mg twice weekly for 30 days in breast cancer patients showed equivalent objective response rates; a statistically significant difference in favour of the higher dose was noted only when disease stasis was included (Pannuti et al. 1979). A similar study found no difference between 500mg and 1000mg intramuscularly daily for 30 days, and discussed the advantages of low-dose therapy (Della Cuna et al 1978). Only Cavalli et al. (1984) have shown improved response rates associated with higher doses, but time to progression and survival were unaltered. Gallagher et al. (1987), comparing 1000mg with 300mg daily by mouth, showed equal response rates. Moreover, Goss et al. (1986), from the same institute, highlighted the toxicity of high-dose medroxyprogesterone acetate, particularly in patients with pulmonary disease. Responding patients who remain on high-dose therapy frequently develop Cushingoid side effects which may not be noted in non-responders who discontinue the drug (Stockdale & Rostom, unpublished data).

3.4 Choice of Preparation

Medroxyprogesterone acetate is poorly absorbed and rapidly metabolised when given orally, and it has been shown that significant differences occurred between peak and steady-state blood concentrations with 3 separate preparations (Stockdale et al. 1987). Other investigators have elegantly shown that both speed of dissolution and resultant particle size are important for optimum absorption (Johansson et al. 1986). A further group comparing intramuscular and oral preparations of medroxyprogesterone acetate have also shown significant differences (Miller et al. 1988).

Although it must surely be logical to choose the preparation which will maximise absorption of this expensive drug, the clinical significance of these observations is not clear. With so many potential variables the relevance, if any, of blood concentrations and thus of differences of bioavailability between preparations will only be established from properly conducted randomised studies.

References

Adlercreutz H, Eriksen PB, Christensen MS. Plasma concentration of megestrol acetate and medroxyprogesterone acetate after single oral administration to healthy subjects. Journal of Pharmacology and Bio-medical Analysis 1: 153-162, 1983

Beex L, Burghout SJ, Van Turnhout J, Breed W, Hillen H, et al. Oral *vs* IM administration of high dose medroxyprogesterone acetate in pre-treated patients with advanced breast cancer. Cancer Treatment Reports 71: 1151-1156, 1987

Blossey HC, Bartsch HH, Kanne D, Koebberling J, Nagel GA. The pharmacokinetics of high dose medroxyprogesterone acetate in the therapy of advanced breast cancer. Cancer Chemotherapy and Pharmacology 8: 77-81, 1982

Camaggi CM, Strocchi E, Constanti B, Beghelli P, Ferrari P, et al. Medroxyprogesterone acetate bioavailability after high dose intraperitoneal administration in advanced cancer. Cancer Chemotherapy and Pharmacology 14: 232-234, 1985

Camaggi CM, Strocchi E, Giovannini M, Angelelli B, Constanti B, et al. Medroxyprogesterone acetate (MPA) plasma levels after multiple high-dose administration in advanced cancer patients. Cancer Chemotherapy and Pharmacology 11; 19-22, 1983

Cavalli F, Goldhirsch A, Jungi F, Martz G, Mermillod B, et al. Randomised trial of low *versus* high dose medroxyprogesterone acetate in the induction treatment of post-menopausal patients with advanced breast cancer. Journal of Clinical Oncology 2: 414-419, 1984

De Lena M, Villa S, Di Fronzo G. Therapeutic activity of medroxyprogesterone acetate in metastatic breast cancer: a correlation between estrogen receptors and various dosages. Recent Results in Cancer Research 91: 243-247, 1984

Della Cuna GR, Calciati A, Strada MRB, Bumma C, Campio L. High dose medroxyprogesterone acetate (MPA) treatment in metastatic carcinoma of the breast: a dose response evaluation. Tumori 64: 143-149, 1978

Falkson G, Falkson HC. A phase II study of high dose medroxyprogesterone acetate in advanced breast cancer. Cancer Chemotherapy and Pharmacology 11: 16-18, 1983

Gallagher CJ, Cairnduff F, Smith IE. High dose *versus* low dose medroxyprogesterone acetate: a randomised trial in advanced breast cancer. European Journal of Cancer and Clinical Oncology 23: 1895-1900, 1987

Ganzina F. High dose medroxyprogesterone acetate (MPA) treatment in advanced breast cancer. A review. Tumori 65: 563-585, 1979

Goss PE, Ashley S, Powles TJ, Coombes RC. High dose medroxyprogesterone acetate in heavily pre-treated patients with metastatic breast cancer. Cancer Treatment Reports 70: 777-779, 1986

Gupta C, Osterman J, Santen R, Bardin CW. *In vitro* metabolism of progestins. V. The effect of protocol design on the estimated metabolic clearance rate and volume of distribution of medroxyprogesterone acetate in women. Journal of Clinical Endocrinology and Metabolism 48: 816-820, 1979

Hayward JL, Carbone PP, Heuson JC, Kumaoka S, Segaloff A, et al. Assessment of response to therapy in advanced breast cancer. A project of the Programme on Clinical Oncology of the International Union Against Cancer, Geneva, Switzerland. Cancer 39: 1289-1293, 1977

Hedley DW, Christie M, Weatherby RP, Caterson ID. Lack of correlations between plasma concentration of medroxyprogesterone acetate, hypothalamic-pituitary function and tumour response in patients with advanced breast cancer. Cancer Chemotherapy and Pharmacology 14: 112-115, 1985

Hortobagyi GN, Buzdar AU, Yap HY, Hug V, Pinnamaneni K, et al. Oral medroxyprogesterone acetate in the treatment of metastatic breast cancer. Breast Cancer Research and Treatment 5: 321-326, 1985

Johansson EDB, Johansen PB, Rasmussen SN. Medroxyprogesterone acetate pharmacokinetics following oral high dose administration in humans. A bioavailability evaluation of a new MPA tablet formulation. Acta Pharmacologica Toxicologica 58: 311-317, 1986

Johnson JR, Priestman TJ, Fotherby K, Kelly KA, Priestman SG. An evaluation of high-dose medroxyprogesterone acetate (MPA) therapy in women with advanced breast cancer. British Journal of Cancer 50: 363-366, 1984

Mahlke M, Grill HJ, Knapstein P, Wiegand U, Pollow K. Oral high-dose medroxyprogesterone acetate (MPA) treatment: control/MPA/ serum profiles in relation to breast cancer regression. Oncology 42: 144-149, 1985

Martin F, Jarvenpaa P, Kosunen K, Somers C, Lindstrom B, et al. Ring-A reduction of medroxyprogesterone acetate (17 alpha acetoxy-6-alpha methyl-4-pregnene-3,20-dione) (MPA) in biological systems. Journal of Steroid Biochemistry 12: 491-497, 1980

Mathrubutham M, Fotherby K. Medroxyprogesterone acetate in human serum. Journal of Steroid Biochemistry 14: 783-786, 1981

Miller AA, Becher R, Schmidt CG. Plasma concentrations of medroxyprogesterone acetate and megestrol acetate during long-term follow-up in patients treated for metastatic breast cancer. Journal of Cancer Research and Clinical Oncology 114: 186-190, 1988

Mould GP, Read J, Bye A. A comparison of the HPLC and RIA measurement of medroxyprogesterone acetate. Journal of Pharmaceutical and Biomedical Analysis, in press, 1988

Nemoto T, Patel J, Rosner D, Dao TL. Oral medroxyprogesterone acetate in the treatment of metastatic breast cancer. Journal of Surgical Oncology 32: 211-213, 1986

Pannuti F, Martoni A, Lenaz GR, Piana E, Nanni P. A possible new approach to the treatment of metastatic breast cancer: massive doses of medroxyprogesterone acetate. Cancer Treatment Reports 62: 499-504, 1978

Pannuti F, Martoni A, Dimarco AR, Piana E, Saccani F, et al. Prospective randomised clinical trial of two different high dosages of medroxyprogestrone acetate (MAP) in the treatment of metastatic breast cancer. European Journal of Cancer 15: 593-601, 1979

Paridaens R, Becquart D, Michel J, Vanderlinden B, Longueville J, et al. Oral *versus* intramuscular high-dose medroxyprogesterone acetate (HD-MPA) in advanced breast cancer. Anticancer Research 6: 1089-1094, 1986

Salimtschik M, Mouridsen HT, Loeber J, Johansson E. Comparative pharmacokinetics of medroxyprogesterone acetate ad-

ministered by oral and intramuscular routes. Cancer Chemotherapy and Pharmacology 4: 267-269, 1980
Stockdale AD, Chapman D, Mould GP, Rostom AY. Medroxyprogesterone acetate: variation in serum concentrations achieved with three commercially available preparations. Cancer Treatment Reports 71: 813-815, 1987
Stoll BA. Progestin therapy of breast cancer: comparison of agents. British Medical Journal 3: 338-341, 1967
Sturm G, Schulz KD. MPA assays: measurement of plasma MPA levels in high-dose MPA-treated patients. In Pellegrini et al. (Eds) Role of medroxyprogesterone in endocrine-related tumours, Vol. 3, pp. 23-42, Raven Press, New York, 1984
Tamassia V, Battaglia A, Ganzina F, Isetta AM, Sacchetti G, et al. Pharmacokinetic approach to the selection of dose schedules for medroxyprogesterone acetate in clinical oncology. Cancer Chemotherapy and Pharmacology 8: 151-156, 1982

Authors' address: Dr *A.D. Stockdale*, Regional Centre for Radiotherapy and Oncology, St Luke's Hospital, Warren Road, Guildford, Surrey GU1 3NT (England).

Clinical Pharmacokinetics 16: 134-161 (1989)
0312-5963/89/0003-0134/$14.00/0

Clinical Pharmacokinetics in Organ Transplant Patients

Raman Venkataramanan, Karen Habucky, Gilbert J. Burckart, and *Richard J. Ptachcinski*

School of Pharmacy, University of Pittsburgh, Pittsburgh, Pennsylvania, USA

Contents

Summary ... 134
1. Drug Absorption ... 135
2. Drug Distribution ... 135
3. Drug Elimination ... 136
4. Liver Transplant Patients ... 136
5. Renal Transplant Patients ... 140
6. Heart Transplant Patients ... 141
7. Bone Marrow Transplant Patients ... 142
8. Specific Drugs ... 143
9. Conclusions ... 155

Summary

Diseases of the liver, kidney and heart influence the pharmacokinetics of several drugs. Organ transplantation is an accepted therapeutic option for the treatment of several disease states associated with these organs. Recently, there has been an increase in both graft and patient survival after transplantation of the liver, heart, kidney and bone marrow. Such patients normally receive a wide range of drugs, and optimisation of drug therapy requires a thorough understanding of the pharmacokinetics and pharmacodynamics of these drugs in transplant patients. However, only limited studies have been carried out to characterise drug kinetics in these situations. Available information indicates that drug kinetics cannot be considered normal in transplant patients. Drug absorption generally appears to be similar to that in healthy subjects. The plasma protein binding of drugs that primarily bind to albumin increases after transplantation, but remains lower than that observed in healthy subjects. While the binding of certain basic drugs may increase after transplantation due to an increase in the concentration of α_1-acid glycoprotein, a lower albumin concentration may mask this effect. Oxidative and conjugative metabolism as measured by the kinetics of antipyrine (phenazone) and paracetamol (acetaminophen) is normal, while the metabolism of steroids may be impaired. Serum creatinine does not appear to be a good indicator of the functional status of the kidney in transplant patients. It is also important to realise that there will be time-dependent changes in several kinetic parameters of drugs due to improvement in the physiological function from that associated with the disease state to that of the normal state. Individualisation and close monitoring of drug therapy is necessary in transplant patients.

Organ transplantation is an accepted mode of therapy for diseases that result in chronic irreversible failure of kidney, liver and heart. In 1986, 185 transplant centres in the United States performed nearly 9000 kidney transplant operations. 90 centres transplanted 1427 hearts and 40 liver transplant centres carried out nearly 900 liver transplant operations. The number of heart-lung transplants performed is relatively small, and only a few multivisceral transplants have been performed so far. Significant improvements in experimental techniques and immunosuppressive therapy have also been reported in small bowel transplantation in animals. The current 1-year survival of transplant patients is remarkable when compared with the early days of transplantation: 95% for kidneys, 78% for hearts and 70% for livers. The longer patient and graft survival is attributed to the discovery of the immunosuppressive properties and the subsequent use of cyclosporin, use of low-dose combination therapy with cyclosporin, steroids and azathioprine, and the proper use of monoclonal antibodies against T-3 lymphocytes.

Optimisation of drug therapy is often very difficult in transplant patients. Patients must have long term maintenance on a variety of immunosuppressants, antihypertensives, antibiotics, antifungal agents, antiviral agents and other drugs. Immunosuppressive drug therapy consists of various combinations of cyclosporin, corticosteroids, azathioprine, antilymphocyte globulin (ALG) or monoclonal antibody (OKT3) therapy. In addition, a number of drugs such as thromboxane synthetase inhibitors, prostaglandin derivatives and platelet aggregating factor inhibitors are currently being tested in laboratory animals and humans to determine their effectiveness in preventing or minimising the nephrotoxic side effects of cyclosporin.

Following transplantation, patients undergo marked changes in the physiological functions associated with the transplanted organ. Each of the 3 major transplanted organs (heart, liver and kidney) is directly or indirectly involved in drug absorption and disposition. Drug absorption, distribution and elimination may undergo a time-dependent transition from that associated with organ failure to that of the normal state. While successful transplantation is expected to normalise drug kinetics, limited information is available on the pharmacokinetics or pharmacodynamics of drugs in transplant patients. The available information is primarily related to the kinetics of immunosuppressants such as cyclosporin, prednisolone, prednisone and azathioprine. A thorough understanding of the factors that may influence drug kinetics in transplant patients is essential for optimal drug therapy and for improving their long term survival. The objective of this review is to discuss various aspects of drug kinetics in transplant patients, and to identify areas for future studies.

1. *Drug Absorption*

Gastrointestinal motility, infections and diseases, altered splanchnic blood flow, changes in bile, acid or enzyme secretion, the presence of food and concomitant drug therapy can alter absorption of several drugs. A number of these factors play a role in the impaired absorption of drugs in patients with liver, renal or cardiac diseases. Following successful transplantation, drug absorption is expected to be similar to that observed in normal subjects. Because of postoperative ileus, intravenous drug therapy may be required during the immediate postoperative period. Once gastrointestinal function recovers, oral drug therapy can be instituted. Since transplant patients receive multiple drug therapy, drug interactions at the level of absorption may also be anticipated.

2. *Drug Distribution*

Organ blood flow, tissue partitioning and plasma protein binding influence the distribution of drugs. One or more of these factors may be altered in cardiac, hepatic and renal diseases. Decreased perfusion of certain tissues and impaired tissue uptake due to the disease state will result in a higher concentration of the drug in blood. Decreased plasma protein binding, on the other hand, will result in increased distribution of the drug outside the vascular system. While there is some information on the plasma protein binding of drugs in transplant patients, virtually nothing is known about the tissue binding of various drugs after transplantation.

It is known that the concentration of α_1-acid glycoprotein in plasma increases after surgery (Arunsen et al. 1972). In addition to surgery, the functional status of the transplanted organ and rejection or infection drug therapy (steroids, rifampicin) will also influence the concentration of several plasma proteins and, therefore, the plasma protein binding of drugs in transplant patients.

3. Drug Elimination

Liver, kidney and lung play an integral role in drug elimination; their contribution to the overall elimination depends on the specific drug. The intrinsic activity of the enzymes in the eliminating organ, the blood flow to the organ and the blood protein binding of the drugs are the major determinants of the drug elimination process in individual organs (Rowland et al. 1973). Disease states associated with these organs result in altered elimination of certain drugs, but in clinically stable transplant patients drug metabolism is expected to be similar to that observed in normal subjects. A complicating factor, however, is the ability of certain drugs used long term in transplant patients, such as cyclosporin (Augustine & Zemaitis 1986), steroids, rifampicin, erythromycin, phenytoin or phenobarbitone, to alter drug kinetics due to enzyme inhibition or induction.

4. Liver Transplant Patients

4.1 Absorption

The absorption of lipid and lipid-soluble compounds is impaired in patients with liver disease. This is related to the low concentration or lack of the bile salts that are necessary for solubilising lipid soluble materials prior to absorption (Hoffmann 1966). Plasma concentrations of fat soluble vitamins A and E are lower in patients with liver disease (0.46 ± 0.34 and 5.4 ± 4.2 mg/L, respectively) compared with normal subjects (0.72 ± 0.19 and 10.2 ± 2.9 mg/L, respectively). Following transplantation, the absorption of fat soluble compounds is considerably improved. In clinically stable (total serum bilirubin < 30 mg/L) liver transplant patients the plasma concentrations of vitamins A and E (1.39 ± 0.41 and 8.6 ± 1.5 mg/L, respectively) are similar to those observed in healthy subjects (Huang et al. 1986). Normalisation of these plasma vitamin concentrations indicates that the transplanted liver is able to produce sufficient quantities of bile salts for absorption of these vitamins. Vitamin E deficiency and the resulting neurological complications that are observed in children are also reversed after successful liver transplantation. Significant improvement in the absorption of the fat soluble immunosuppressant drug cyclosporin has also been documented in patients after liver transplantation (bioavailability = 28%) [Burckart et al. 1986a] when compared to patients with liver disease (bioavailability = 12%) [Venkataramanan et al. 1985a].

Following orthotopic liver transplantation, patients who had Laennec's cirrhosis or primary biliary cirrhosis have a bile duct to bile duct anastomosis, and a T-tube is inserted in the common bile duct to divert bile flow. The T-tubes may remain open for up to 2 months after transplantation, and drainage of bile away from the gut will result in poor absorption of lipid soluble compounds during this period. After clamping or removal of the T-tube, the absorption of lipid soluble compounds is expected to increase. A significant increase (276%) in the dose-normalised area under the plasma concentration-time curve (AUC) has been reported for cyclosporin after T-tube clamping in liver transplant patients (Mehta et al. 1988). The absolute bioavailability of cyclosporin in these patients increased from 10.6% to 28.1% after clamping (Tredger et al. 1988). Similarly, increased absorption of vitamins, such as A, D, E and K, and other drugs, such as tetracyclines and sulphadiazine, will be observed following T-tube clamping.

In paediatric liver transplant patients a loop of bowel is usually pulled up (Roux-en-Y) and the donor bile duct is anastomosed to the Roux-loop. This is either because of biliary atresia or because of the small size of the bile duct preventing duct to duct anastomosis. Roux-en-Y construction is also performed in adult patients who have had liver tumours or sclerosing cholangitis. Roux-en-Y construction results in shortening of the bowel and the bile mixes with the bowel content distally. These 2 factors will tend to decrease absorption of drugs which are primarily absorbed in the proximal intestine. The absorption of cyclosporin decreases in rats with a Roux-en-Y biliary enterostomy (Kehrer et al. 1988). While the effect of the T-tube on drug absorption is only temporary, the effect of Roux-en-Y is permanent.

Liver disease is also known to increase systemic bioavailability of drugs with intermediate or high extraction ratios. The systemic availability of orally administered drugs such as pethidine (meperidine) [Neal et al. 1979], propranolol (Wood et al. 1978), lignocaine (lidocaine) [Huet & Villeneuve 1983], chlormethiazole (Pentikainen et al. 1980), labetalol (Homeida et al. 1978), pentazocine (Neal et al. 1979) and salicylamide (Neal et al. 1979) is substantially increased in patients with liver disease. This is related to the decreased intrinsic clearance and the development of portosystemic vascular shunts. Systemic bioavailability of high extraction drugs has not been studied in liver transplant patients. In clinically stable liver transplant patients the bioavailability of high clearance drugs is expected to be similar to that observed in normal subjects. However, drug therapy in this patient population may alter the intrinsic clearance and, therefore, the bioavailability of certain high clearance drugs.

4.2 Distribution

The liver is the major organ for the synthesis of albumin, α_1-acid glycoprotein and other macromolecules involved in drug binding. In patients with hepatic dysfunction, the binding of a number of drugs such as salicylic acid, phenytoin, warfarin and diazepam is impaired (Blaschke 1977). This may be related to decreased concentrations of the drug binding proteins, accumulation of endogenous binding inhibitors and/or qualitative changes in the drug binding proteins. Earlier studies have documented the ability of the newly transplanted liver to synthesise various plasma proteins (Mueller & Lie 1973). Studies in dogs indicate that albumin synthesis is normal within 2 hours of graft revascularisation (De Riborolles et al. 1975). In a liver transplant patient the concentrations of ceruloplasmin, the copper binding protein, and α_1-acid glycoprotein are persistently elevated after surgery but return to normal by day 56. During a subsequent chronic rejection the acute phase proteins [proteins in plasma (such as α_1-acid glycoprotein) whose concentrations are elevated during inflammatory processes] are elevated, although no specific information on the time course is available (Murray-Lyon et al. 1971). In patients with Wilson's disease, the concentration of ceruloplasmin is very low, although it increases to normal values after transplantation (Groth et al. 1972). Recent studies in clinically stable liver transplant patients indicate the plasma concentration of albumin (34 ± 7 mg/L) to be lower than that seen in healthy subjects (43 ± 3 mg/L) [Huang et al. 1988]. Consequently, the binding of the marker drugs diazepam and salicylic acid, which bind primarily to albumin, is lower in transplant patients than in healthy subjects (table I). However, when compared to patients with chronic liver disease, the binding of diazepam and salicylic acid is significantly increased in stable liver transplant patients; this is presumably related to the removal of endogenous binding inhibitors or a change in the affinity of albumin for the drug (Huang 1987). Similar changes are also expected for other drugs such as warfarin, cephalosporins, phenytoin and frusemide (furosemide), which primarily bind to albumin.

The concentration of α_1-acid glycoprotein (420 ± 220 mg/L) is below or near normal in patients prior to transplantation, although immediately after the transplantation there is a significant increase in α_1-acid glycoprotein concentrations. Even as long as 21 to 146 days after surgery, α_1-acid glycoprotein concentrations (1210 ± 280 mg/L) are ele-

Table I. Plasma protein binding of drugs in transplant patients

Drug	% Unbound			Drug concentration	Reference
	healthy subjects	patients with liver/renal disease	transplant patients		
Liver transplant patients					
Diazepam	1.8 ± 0.3	4.8 ± 1.5	3.5 ± 1.5	208 μg/ml	Huang (1987)
Salicylic acid	15.6 ± 1.3	56.1 ± 13.7	35.2 ± 14.5	551 ng/ml	Huang (1987)
Lignocaine (lidocaine)	30-50		22-41	0.1-16 μg/ml	Huang (1987)
Propranolol	10.9 ± 1.2		10.8 ± 1.2	20 ng/ml	Huang (1987)
Renal transplant patients					
Diazepam	1.64	3.23	2.11	4 ng/ml	Grossman et al. (1982)
Frusemide (furosemide)	1.2 ± 0.2	5.64 ± 0.77	1.7 ± 0.3		Smith & Benet (1982)
Lignocaine	30.7	20.8	24.6	3 μg/ml	Grossman et al. (1982)
Morphine	64.9 ± 5.8	70.7 ± 14.5	65.9 ± 7.4		Olsen et al. (1975)
Phenytoin	11.9	17.4-25.4	15.0-18.2	4.4 μg/ml	Odar-Cederlof (1977)
Salicylic acid	24.2 ± 3.3	>30	About 20.0	300 μg/ml	Levy et al. (1976)
Sulphafurazole (sulfisoxazole)	8.3-11.3	>25	About 10.0	100 μg/ml	Levy et al. (1976)
Warfarin		1.3-1.99	0.89-1.1	9.2 μg/ml	Odar-Cederlof (1977)

vated. Elevated α_1-acid glycoprotein concentrations are seen in some liver transplant patients as much as 5 months after surgery. Correspondingly, the unbound fraction of lignocaine is 24% in plasma of stable liver transplant patients and 34% in that from healthy subjects (Huang 1987). While there is a small reduction in the α_1-acid glycoprotein-lignocaine affinity constant, the constant for the albumin-lignocaine interaction is not significantly different from that in healthy subjects. There is a significant correlation between the bound fraction of lignocaine and α_1-acid glycoprotein concentration (r = 0.94) in liver transplant patients.

In contrast to the results obtained from lignocaine binding studies, the unbound fraction of propranolol was not significantly different between healthy subjects (10.1 ± 1.1%) and stable liver transplant patients (10.9 ± 1.2%) [Huang 1987]. There was no significant difference in the affinity constant between α_1-acid glycoprotein and propranolol in healthy subjects (2.1×10^{-5} mol/L) and in liver transplant patients (2.5×10^{-5} mol/L). It appears that a simultaneous increase in α_1-acid glycoprotein concentration and a reduction in albumin contributes to the lack of difference in the binding of propranolol in these 2 groups. Thus, it may be concluded that the binding of basic drugs may or may not be altered in liver transplant patients, depending on the relative contribution of albumin to the overall binding of the drug.

The plasma concentration of transcortin, the

protein responsible for steroid binding, is normal in stable liver transplant patients (Huang 1987).

Since drug binding to plasma proteins influences the clearance of low clearance drugs, the clearance of total drug will be altered in transplant patients, but minimal or no change will be observed in the steady-state unbound concentration of such drugs. Consequently, the dosing regimen of such drugs need not be changed because of altered drug binding (Gibaldi & Perrier 1982). In the case of high clearance drugs, the clearance will be unaltered by changes in drug binding, but the steady-state unbound concentration and therefore the pharmacological response attributed to a given total concentration will be different in transplant patients from that in healthy subjects. The dosing regimen of these drugs will have to be changed in the presence of altered drug binding.

Drug binding to plasma proteins and tissue proteins also influences the volume of distribution (Vd) of drugs. Decreased plasma protein binding that is observed in patients with liver disease results in an increase in the steady-state volume of distribution of several drugs such as diazepam (Klotz et al. 1975) and lignocaine (Thompson et al. 1973). Circulatory alterations associated with the liver disease and the presence of ascites may also alter drug distribution. Subsequent to successful transplantation, drug distribution will be determined by the net effect of changes in plasma and tissue binding of the drugs. The Vd of drugs that primarily bind to albumin is expected to be increased in liver transplant patients compared with healthy subjects, since binding appears to be lower in these patients. The Vd of drugs that are primarily bound to α_1-acid glycoprotein may or may not be altered in transplant patients.

4.3 Metabolism

It is the liver that is primarily responsible for drug metabolism, and its metabolising capacity is compromised in patients with liver disease (Wilkinson 1986; Williams 1983). Alterations in drug elimination in patients with liver disease may be the result of a reduction in hepatic blood flow, extrahepatic or intrahepatic shunting of blood, hepatocyte dysfunction or changes in plasma protein binding of drugs. It is not completely known whether all these functions are normalised in stable liver transplant patients. Recent studies indicate that the oxidative drug metabolising capacity of the liver in clinically stable liver transplant patients, as determined by antipyrine clearance, is similar to that observed in healthy subjects (2.2 *versus* 2.27 L/h/kg) [Mehta et al. 1986]. The clearance of cyclosporin [high performance liquid chromatography (HPLC) assay of whole blood], which is primarily metabolised by hepatic *N*-demethylation and hydroxylation, is similar in stable liver and renal transplant patients (Ptachcinski et al. 1986a). However, clinically stable liver transplant patients have a reduced ability (69% lower) to metabolise prednisolone. The clearance of unbound prednisolone is 0.33 L/h/kg in liver transplant patients compared with 1.05 L/h/kg in healthy subjects (Huang 1987; Rose et al. 1981).

The conjugative metabolism of paracetamol (acetaminophen) in liver transplant patients resembles that observed in healthy subjects, indicated by similar half-lives (2.7 ± 0.9 hours *versus* 2.8 ± 0.8 hours). At therapeutic doses, long term combination therapy with cyclosporin and prednisolone does not appear to have any effect on conjugative drug metabolism in stable liver transplant patients (Venkataramanan et al. 1989). The effect of other immunosuppressants on drug metabolism is not completely characterised.

Hepatic blood flow, measured by indocyanine green clearance, significantly improves after liver transplantation (personal observation). In general, one would expect drug metabolism to be normal in clinically stable liver transplant patients. However, due to decreased plasma protein binding of acidic drugs and increased plasma protein binding of certain basic drugs, the total clearance of highly protein bound drugs is expected to differ between transplant patients and healthy subjects.

4.4 Urinary Excretion

Renal impairment is common in liver transplant patients, primarily due to drug-induced nephrotoxicity. Serum creatinine, which is a common clinical marker of renal function and used for drug dosing adjustments in renal failure, does not appear to be of any predictive value in liver transplant patients. The clearance of ceftizoxime and cefotaxime is lower in liver transplant patients compared with healthy subjects, and the impairment is not proportional to the change in serum creatinine concentrations (Burckart et al. 1987). Similarly, the half-lives of gentamicin and vancomycin are also elevated in liver transplant patients with near normal serum creatinine concentrations (Howrie, personal communication).

4.5 Biliary Excretion

The functional status of the biliary excretory pathways has not been studied in liver transplant patients. Initial observations indicate some impairment in biliary excretory function during the immediate postoperative period. In liver transplant patients, relatively large amounts of cyclosporin metabolites are present in the blood during the immediate postoperative period [measured by the difference in radioimmunoassay (RIA) and HPLC concentrations], indicating a deficiency in the biliary excretion pathway of these metabolites (Burckart et al. 1985). Biliary excretion of cyclosporin and its metabolites depends on the functional status of the liver (Burckart et al. 1986b). Patients with normal liver function excrete more parent drug and more metabolites than patients with poor liver function.

5. Renal Transplant Patients

5.1 Absorption

In patients with renal failure altered gastric pH, nausea, vomiting, diarrhoea, oedematous changes in the gastrointestinal tract, uraemic colitis, gastritis and pancreatitis may alter drug absorption. While altered concentrations of propranolol and digoxin are observed in patients with renal failure, the absolute bioavailability of propranolol (Wood et al. 1980) and digitoxin (Ohnhaus et al. 1979) is reported to be normal. Decreased bioavailability has been reported for frusemide (Tilstone & Fine 1978), pindolol (Chaun et al. 1977) and D-xylose (Craig et al. 1983) in this patient population. In contrast, the oral bioavailability of dextropropoxyphene (propoxyphene) is increased in patients with renal failure, presumably due to decreased presystemic metabolism (Gibson et al. 1980). In renal transplant patients, the absorption of frusemide (Smith et al. 1981) and prednisolone (Frey et al. 1981; Gambertoglio et al. 1980a,b) is similar to that observed in normal subjects, while cyclosporin absorption is similar to that observed in other patient populations such as liver, bone marrow and heart transplants (Ptachcinski et al. 1986a). The absolute bioavailability of high first-pass drugs such as dextropropoxyphene, which undergo extensive first-pass metabolism, has not been studied in renal transplant patients.

5.2 Distribution

Impaired drug binding to plasma proteins in patients with renal failure is well documented (Reidenberg 1976). After renal transplantation, the abolition of the uraemic state, the change from a restricted to a normal diet, the immunosuppressive therapy used and complications such as rejection episodes, may influence the concentrations of serum proteins and drug binding. Serum albumin concentrations tend to increase after transplantation but remain significantly lower than those observed in healthy volunteers. The mean half-life of albumin in 5 renal transplant patients was 14.3 hours compared to a range of 14 to 23 hours in normal subjects (Wells 1969). The fractional turnover rate of albumin is normal in these patients. During acute rejection of renal allografts, the concentration of albumin is decreased (Weeke et al. 1971a). Concentrations of transferrin are also low in renal transplant patients (Weeke et al. 1971b). Transcortin concentration appears to be normal in renal transplant patients (0.62 ± 0.23 μmol/L) compared with patients with autoimmune disease (0.65 ± 0.12 μmol/L) [Frey & Frey 1982]. α_1-Acid glycoprotein and retinol binding proteins, on the other hand, are elevated in stable renal transplant patients (Frey et al. 1977; Grossman et al. 1982; Weeke et al. 1971b). Based on this information, one would anticipate altered drug binding in renal transplant patients.

The plasma protein binding of sulphafurazole (sulfisoxazole), salicylic acid, frusemide, phenytoin, warfarin, diazepam and morphine increases after renal transplantation (table I). Increased drug binding is seen within a few days in some patients, while it may take several months in others. The initial increase in drug binding generally observed in renal transplant patients may be related to the removal of the endogenous drug binding inhibitors in the plasma. This phase is followed by a slow increase in the binding related to the synthesis of new plasma proteins. Despite significant increase in drug binding, the unbound fraction of many drugs that bind primarily to albumin is higher in renal transplant patients than in normal subjects. The binding capacity of methyl orange in the serum from uraemic patients and post-renal transplant patients is lower than in normal serum (Dromgoole 1972). On the other hand, the binding of lignocaine in renal transplant patients has been reported to be higher than that observed in normal subjects and is related to the higher concentration of the α_1-acid glycoprotein which is the major lignocaine binding plasma protein (Grossman et al. 1982).

Drug binding to plasma proteins improves after liver or renal transplantation. However, transplant patients cannot be considered normal with regard to drug binding. The effect of altered drug binding on the kinetics of drugs in renal transplant patients will be similar to that described for liver transplant patients (section 4.2).

5.3 Elimination

The effect of uraemia on drug metabolism has not been well studied. Drug metabolism is generally not impaired in renal disease, although some metabolic pathways can be altered. While the metabolism of antipyrine is increased, that of hydrocortisone is decreased in patients with renal failure (Gambertoglio 1984). In addition, active metabolites may accumulate in patients with end stage renal failure if their elimination is dependent on renal excretion (Szeto et al. 1976). If these metabolites are pharmacologically active or toxic, there will be an increase in the contribution of the metabolites to the observed pharmacological effect or the toxicity of the drug (Drayer 1977). Subsequent to successful renal transplantation the oxidative drug metabolising capacity of renal transplant patients as measured by antipyrine clearance is reported to be similar to that of normal subjects (Roberts et al. 1986). It is not known whether other metabolic pathways are normal in this patient group.

5.4 Urinary Excretion

Very little information is available on the kinetics of drugs that are primarily excreted via the renal route. Renal impairment is common in renal transplant patients due to either poor graft function or drug-induced nephrotoxicity. In stable renal transplant patients receiving cyclosporin, a serum creatinine concentration at or near the upper limit of the normal range may indicate marked renal impairment (Rose et al. 1987). Dosing regimens of drugs based on the serum creatinine will tend to overestimate the actual dose requirement in these patients. The dosing regimen of renally eliminated drugs such as aminoglycosides and cephalosporins must be closely evaluated in this patient group.

The renal clearance of frusemide in kidney transplant patients is lower than that in healthy subjects (Smith et al. 1981). The attenuated renal clearance indicates potential impairment in the secretory component of the organic acid transport system in renal transplant patients.

6. Heart Transplant Patients

6.1 Absorption

The effect of cardiac disease on drug absorption is not well characterised. Cardiac disease can alter drug absorption through delayed gastric emptying, decreased gastric motility, decreased splanchnic blood flow, changes in intraluminal pH of the gut, changes in gastric secretion, alterations in gastric or intestinal metabolism, changes in the gastric epithelial permeability due to mucosal oedema and decreased hepatic first-pass metabolism (Benowitz & Meister 1976). Earlier studies have documented malabsorption of neutral fat and fatty acids in patients with chronic congestive heart failure (Berkowitz et al. 1963). Decreased bioavailability of metolazone (Tilstone et al. 1974) and hydrochlorothiazide (Anderson et al. 1961), and delayed absorption of procainamide (Koch-Weser 1971) and quinidine (Crouthamul 1975), have been reported in patients with cardiac disease. During the immediate postoperative period (within 2 days after surgery) drugs are not well absorbed in transplant patients. However, absorption does not appear to be a problem in stable heart transplant patients. The absolute bioavailability of cyclosporin is similar in stable heart, liver and renal transplant patients (Venkataramanan et al. 1986). No studies have been conducted to specifically determine the absolute bioavailability of other drugs in heart transplant patients.

6.2 Distribution

In patients with myocardial infarction the concentration of α_1-acid glycoprotein is elevated, resulting in increased binding of basic drugs such as lignocaine (Routledge et al. 1980). Decreased Vd of several drugs, such as dihydroquinidine, disopyramide, lignocaine, procainamide, quinidine and theophylline, has been reported in patients with cardiac disease (Benowitz 1984). Increased Vd of water-soluble drugs such as amidopyrine (aminopyrine) in patients with cardiac disease has been attributed to fluid retention (Hepner et al. 1978). Although the concentration of α_1-acid glycoprotein has not been reported in cardiac transplant patients it is likely to be elevated, based on observations in other transplant patients, and consequently the Vd of basic drugs is expected to be decreased in this patient population. The overall effect of changes in drug binding on the kinetics of drugs will be similar to that discussed in section 4.2.

6.3 Metabolism and Elimination

Due to the limited size of the patient population, no studies have been carried out on the metabolism of drugs in heart transplant patients. The clearance of cyclosporin is lower in this group than in renal or liver transplant patients (Venkataramanan et al. 1986).

7. Bone Marrow Transplant Patients

7.1 Absorption

In bone marrow transplant patients who develop chemoirradiation-induced intestinal dysfunction or in the presence of acute graft-versus-host disease (GVHD) of the intestine, the absorption of cyclosporin is impaired (Atkinson et al. 1984). The extent of absorption of cyclosporin and other drugs in clinically stable bone marrow transplant patients is expected to be similar to that observed in renal, liver and cardiac transplant patients.

7.2 Distribution

There is no documentation available on plasma protein concentrations in bone marrow transplant patients. In general, these patients tend to have a lower plasma albumin concentration and therefore will have a decreased binding of some acidic drugs. The effect of altered drug binding on the kinetics of drugs used in this patient population will be similar to that described in section 4.2.

7.3 Metabolism and Elimination

Studies have not been carried out to characterise drug metabolism in bone marrow transplant patients. Clinically stable bone marrow transplant patients appear to clear cyclosporin similarly to other transplant patients.

8. Specific Drugs

8.1 Cyclosporin

Cyclosporin has significantly contributed to the improvement of patient and graft survival following transplantation of the liver, kidney and heart. A wide variability in the clinical response to a given dose of cyclosporin is seen in transplant patients. This may be a result of variability in the pharmacokinetic and pharmacodynamic factors. In order to achieve therapeutic concentrations of 700 to 1200 μg/L (based on whole blood RIA concentrations), doses ranging from 6 to 57 mg/kg/day are required in liver transplant patients (fig. 1). In renal transplant patients, doses ranging from 6 to 30 mg/kg are required to maintain the blood HPLC concentrations between 200 and 800 μg/L. Figure 2 illustrates interpatient variability in blood cyclosporin concentrations after oral administration. The presence of pharmacodynamic differences between patients may be related to differences in the sensitivity of lymphocytes to cyclosporin (Zeevi et al. 1988).

The pharmacokinetics of cyclosporin have been reviewed recently by several groups (Burckart et al. 1986c,d; Grevel 1986; Kahan 1985; Kahan et al. 1986a; Maurer 1985; Ptachcinski et al. 1986a,b; Venkataramanan et al. 1985b; Vine & Bowers 1987; Wood & Lemaire 1985; Yee & Kennedy 1986). Almost all the pharmacokinetic studies of cyclosporin have been carried out in patients pre- or post-transplantation.

Several methods (HPLC, RIA and fluorescence polarisation immunoassay) are available for estimation of cyclosporin in biological fluids (Hassan & Al-Yahya 1987; Shaw et al. 1987). The advantages and disadvantages of these methods have been

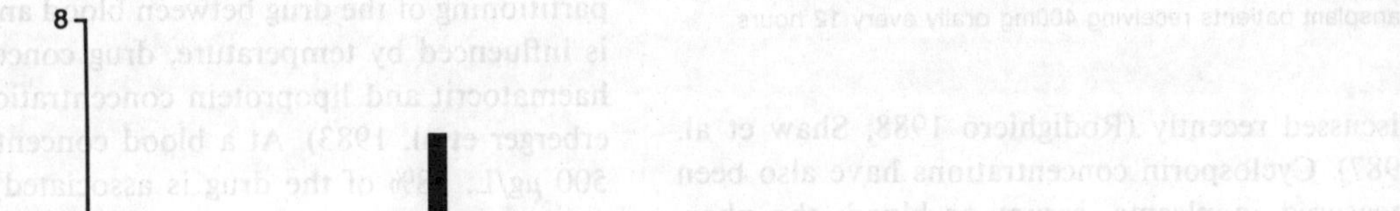

Fig. 1. Histogram of number of patients *vs* dose of cyclosporin required to maintain therapeutic whole blood RIA concentrations. ■ = stable liver transplant patients (700-1200 μg/L); ▨ = stable kidney transplant patients (200-800 μg/L).

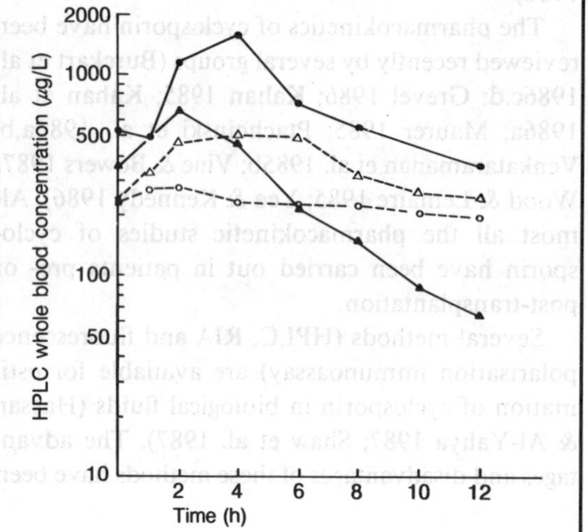

Fig. 2. HPLC blood cyclosporin concentration *vs* time in 4 liver transplant patients receiving 400mg orally every 12 hours.

discussed recently (Rodighiero 1988; Shaw et al. 1987). Cyclosporin concentrations have also been measured in plasma, serum or blood; the pharmacokinetic parameters estimated are dependent on the method and the biological medium used (Frey et al. 1988; Reynolds et al. 1988). Since the partitioning of cyclosporin between blood cells and plasma is temperature dependent (Wenk et al. 1983), physiologically meaningful kinetic parameters can be obtained only from blood samples or plasma separated at 37°C.

8.1.1 Absorption

The oral absorption of cyclosporin is slow, erratic and incomplete. Peak blood or plasma concentrations are normally reached in 2 to 6 hours after oral administration. Various factors have been shown to alter absorption of the drug (table II). The mean bioavailability of cyclosporin is about 30%. Immediately after liver transplantation the extent of absorption is frequently less than 5%. This improves with time after the transplant and reaches a mean value of approximately 30%. Improving liver function and increased bile flow may be responsible for the improvement in cyclosporin absorption. In renal transplant patients cyclosporin bioavailability increases 3- to 5-fold over a 3-month period (Kahan et al. 1983). The mean bioavailability of cyclosporin in bone marrow, renal and heart transplant patients is about 30% (Ptachcinski et al. 1986a).

Studies in animals indicate that lymphatics play a minimal role in cyclosporin absorption (Ueda et al. 1983), and that exogenous bile salts can improve it (Erickson et al. 1987). Cyclosporin does not undergo enterohepatic recirculation in humans (Venkataramanan et al. 1985c). In some patients the absorption of cyclosporin can be characterised by a zero-order process (Grevel et al. 1986).

8.1.2 Distribution

Cyclosporin is highly bound to erythrocytes and plasma proteins (Lemaire & Tillement 1982). The partitioning of the drug between blood and plasma is influenced by temperature, drug concentration, haematocrit and lipoprotein concentration (Niederberger et al. 1983). At a blood concentration of 500 µg/L, 58% of the drug is associated with the erythrocytes, 4% in the granulocytes, 5% in the lymphocytes and 32% in the plasma. In plasma, 57% of the drug is associated with low density lipoprotein, 25% with high density lipoprotein, 2% with very low density lipoprotein and about 10% with albumin (Lemaire & Tillement 1982).

The blood-to-plasma ratio is 2 in normal subjects. In renal and liver transplant patients the ratio is 1.36 and 1.32, respectively, and is due to the lower haematocrits in these patients (Rosano 1985). The blood-to-plasma ratio is also dependent on the drug concentration. While the plasma protein binding is independent of the concentration over the range of 20 to 3000 µg/L (Legg & Rowland 1987; Lemaire & Tillement 1982), the red blood cell uptake is saturable (Legg & Rowland 1988) and the binding capacity is variable between patients (Agarwal et al. 1985). The average maximum binding capacity in renal transplant patients is 2560 µg/L (2.1×10^{-6} mol/L) and the dissociation constant is reported to be 66.9 µg/L (5.6×10^{-8} mol/L). Using the charcoal adsorption technique, a binding

Table II. Factors affecting cyclosporin absorption

Factor	Observation	Comment	Reference
Chenodeoxycholic acid	Increases absorption		Personal observation
Cholestyramine	No change in absorption		Keogh et al. (1988)
Diabetes	Decreases peak plasma concentration	Presumably due to gastroparesis	Wadhwa et al. (1987a)
Diurnal variation	AUC is greater during resting cycle than active period		Canafax et al. (1988)
External biliary drainage (T-tube)	Decreases aborption	Loss of bile required in absorption	Mehta et al. (1988) Tredger et al. (1988)
Food	Increases absorption No change	Effect depends on the nature of the food and time of administration with respect to drug intake	Ptachcinski et al. (1985a) Keown et al. (1984)
Gastrointestinal dysfunction (diarrhoea)	Decreases absorption	Extent of impairment depends on volume of diarrhoea (liver and bone marrow transplant patients)	Atkinson et al. (1984) Burckart et al. (1985)
Liver disease	Poor bioavailability	Lack of bile and bile salts required for absorption	Venkataramanan et al. (1985b)
Time post transplant	Increased absorption with time	Improved bile flow to the gut Improved gastrointestinal function recovery from ileus	Burckart et al. (1985) Kahan et al. (1983)
Vehicle	No effect	Large variability obscures any potential vehicle effect	Johnston et al. (1986)

constant of 1.9×10^7 mol/L has been reported (Agarwal et al. 1987) for cyclosporin and the red blood cell binding protein. These observations indicate the possibility of non-linear cyclosporin kinetics in transplant patients due to saturable red blood cell uptake. A cyclosporin binding protein that is distinct from haemoglobin, carbonic anhydrase, calmodulin and cytochrome b_5 has been isolated from erythrocytes (Agarwal et al. 1986).

Temperature alters the binding of cyclosporin to plasma proteins and to erythrocyte proteins. The binding constant to erythrocytic protein increases with a decrease in the temperature, but the saturation capacity is independent of temperature (Agarwal et al. 1987). On the other hand, while 70% of cyclosporin is bound to plasma proteins at 4°C, 93% is bound at 24°C and 98% is bound at 37°C (Lemaire & Tillement 1982). The above 2 factors are responsible for the increase in the blood-to-plasma ratio with a decrease in temperature.

In transplant patients the unbound fraction of cyclosporin is highly variable (Legg & Rowland 1987; Zaghloul et al. 1987). The unbound fraction in plasma obtained from liver transplant patients is 0.08 ± 0.01 and in renal transplant patients is 0.09 ± 0.05, compared with 0.017 ± 0.03 in healthy subjects (Zaghloul et al. 1987). Lindholm et al. (1988) have reported the unbound fraction of cyclosporin in renal transplant patients to vary from 0.005 to 0.042 with a mean of 0.0137. The wide variation in the unbound fraction is thought to contribute to the variability in the kinetics of cyclosporin. Variations in the unbound fraction of cyclosporin may be the result of an altered lipoprotein profile secondary to the functional status of the transplanted organs. Increased blood protein binding due to increased haematocrit and lipopro-

Table III. Pharmacokinetic parameters [arithmetic mean (± SD) or harmonic mean (range)] for cyclosporin after intravenous administration

Reference	Patient population	No. of subjects	Dose (mg/kg)	Dosing interval (h)	K_e (h^{-1})	$t_{1/2}$ (h)	CL (ml/min/kg)	Vd_{ss} (L/kg)
HPLC of whole blood								
Ptachcinski et al. (1987a)	Healthy volunteers	5	2.2 (± 0.2)	48	0.112 (± 0.04)	6.2 (4.7-9.5)	3.9 (2.9-5.5)	1.3 (± 0.3)
Follath et al. (1983)	Renal failure	4	2.1-3.5	48	0.057 (± 0.04)	12.2 (6.4-26.9)	5.9 (4.5-6.4)	3.5 (± 2.7)
Venkataramanan	Liver failure	8[a]	2.0	48	0.034 (± 0.015)	20.4 (10.8-48)	2.8 (1.9-4.8)	3.9 (± 1.8)
Ptachcinski et al. (1985b)	Adult renal transplant	41	4.7	24	0.065 (± 0.04)	10.7 (4.3-53.4)	5.7 (0.6-23.9)	4.5 (± 3.6)
Ptachcinski et al. (1986c)	Paediatric renal transplant	7	4.5 (± 1.3)	12-24	0.095 (± 0.02)	7.3 (8.1-16.6)	11.8 (9.8-15.5)	4.7 (± 1.5)
Burckart et al. (1986)	Adult liver transplant	6	1.8 (± 0.5)	12			5.5 (4.9-7.6)	
Burckart et al. (1985)	Paediatric liver transplant	26	Variable	8			8.4 (1.9-13.9)	
Venkataramanan et al. (1986)	Heart transplant	4[e]	0.8 (± 0.4)	12	0.105 (± 0.029)	6.4 (5.2-9.3)	4.0 (2.1-5.3)	1.3 (± 0.2)
Frey et al. (1988)	Renal transplant	58	5.0	24		15.1 (± 4.7)	5.7 (± 1.8) (3.0-13)	3.6 (± 1.4) (1.8-10.4)
Reynolds et al. (1988)	Uraemic	30	3.0	Single dose		6.5 (± 1.7)	8.4 (4.3-17.9)	
Tredger et al. (1988)	Liver transplant	11	1.5-3.5	24			7.31 (pre-clamping) 5.47 (post-clamping)	
Lindberg et al. (1986)	Uraemic	21	5.0	Continuous infusion	26.9 (± 10.8)		4.9 (2.3-7.1)	11.1 (± 4.6)
Myre et al. (1988)	Heart transplant	15	2.4-3.7	Continuous infusion			5.13 (3.6-7.3)	
RIA of whole blood								
Ptachcinski et al. (1987a)	Healthy volunteers	5	2.2 (± 0.2)	48	0.089 (± 0.42)	7.8 (4.9-19.1)	2.8 (2.2-3.4)	1.5 (± 0.6)
Follath et al. (1983)	Renal failure	4	2.1-3.5	48	0.043 (± 0.01)	16.5 (± 3.1) 16.1 (14.1-20.9)	4.8 (± 1.3)	3.2 (± 1.3)
Venkataramanan[a]	Liver failure	8	2.0	48	0.029 (± 0.017)	23.9 (10.6-47.6)	1.2 (0.8-3.6)	2.9 (± 0.6)
Stewart et al. (1985)	Liver disease	9	5.0	20		8.7 (± 3.3)	30.4 (± 15.5)	13.8 (± 11.2)
Reynolds et al. (1988)	Uraemic	30	3.0	Single dose		7.4 (± 2.8)	5.8 (2.6-16.3)	
Tredger et al. (1988)	Liver transplant	11	1.5-3.5	24			3.25 (pre-clamping) 2.44 (post-clamping)	

Table III. Contd

Reference	Patient population	No. of subjects	Dose (mg/kg)	Dosing interval (h)	K_e (h)	$t_{1/2}$ (h)	CL (ml/min/kg)	Vd_{ss} (L/kg)
Frey et al. (1988)	Renal transplant	58	5.0	24		13.8 (± 4.5)	2.9 (± 1.0) (1.6-6.3)	1.8 (± 0.5) (0.9-3.7)
HPLC of serum								
Yee et al. (1984)	Bone marrow transplant	10[c]	1.4-2.5	12		6.7 (± 1.6)	12.8 (± 1.6)	4.3 (± 0.9)
Yee et al. (1984)	Bone marrow transplant	11[d]	1.4-2.5	12		12.7 (± 6.1)	9.8 (± 2.1)	3.5 (± 1.1)
Vernillet et al. (1988)	Nephrotic syndrome	8	4		0.056 (± 0.046)	18.2 (± 10.2)	6.65 (4.19-9.02)	3.0 (± 3.1)
Gupta et al. (1987)	Renal transplant	5	7	Continuous infusion			10.07 (± 2.5)	4.62 (± 2.29)
RIA of serum/plasma								
Yee et al. (1984)	Bone marrow transplant	10[c]	1.4-2.5	12		7.4 (± 2.0)	8.3 (± 0.9)	3.1 (± 0.8)
Yee et al. (1984)	Bone marrow transplant[d]	11[d]	1.4-2.5	12		10.3 (± 1.6)	4.8 (± 1.6)	3.1 (± 0.9)
Lockiec et al. (1983)	Bone marrow transplant	38[b]	4.0	12		6.8 (± 2.5)	5.2 (1.5-10)	
Newberger & Kahan (1983)	Renal transplant (pre-transplant)	3[b]	2.1	24	0.223	2.9 (2.6-5.0)		
Newberger & Kahan (1983)	Renal transplant (post-transplant)	2[b]	2.1	24	0.164	4.2		
Kahan et al. (1986b)	Renal transplant, 14 days after surgery	212				8.6 (± 4.6)	12.3 (± 8.2)	
Reynolds et al. (1988)	Uraemic	30	3.0	Single dose		6.4 (± 2.0)	13.0 (4.4-38.6)	
Kahan et al. (1986b)	Renal transplant	232	Variable	24		8.6 (± 4.6)	12.3 (± 8.2)	8.7 (± 6.2)
Kahan et al. (1986b)	Cardiac transplant	78	Variable	24		8.2 (± 4.9)	10.7 (± 16.4)	6.0 (± 6.7)
Lockiec et al. (1986)[e]	Paediatric transplant	71	4.0	12		10.1 (± 12.6)	31 (6-88)	21.2 (± 35.2)
Lockiec et al. (1986)[e]	Adult bone marrow	127	4.0	12		6.5 (± 5.4)	14.0 (2-79)	4.4 (± 4.2)
Bertault-Peres et al. (1985)	Adult bone marrow	15				16.8 (6-25)	10.44 (1.6-23.3)	

a Unpublished observation.
b Assuming 70kg bodyweight.
c Serum bilirubin < 12 mg/L.
d Serum bilirubin > 20 mg/L.
e Patients not receiving enzyme-inducing drugs.

Abbreviations: K_e = elimination rate constant; $t_{1/2}$ = elimination half-life; CL = clearance; Vd_{ss} = apparent volume of distribution at steady-state; HPLC = high performance liquid chromatography; RIA = radioimmunoassay.

teins has been suggested as a reason for the increase in blood drug concentrations with time post transplantation (Kasiske et al. 1988).

Due to its lipophilicity cyclosporin is extensively distributed in the body, and drug concentrations in fat, liver, pancreas, kidney, lungs, spleen and lymph nodes exceed the concentration in serum/plasma (Atkinson et al. 1983; Ried et al. 1983). Very low concentrations of cyclosporin are found in the brain and none is detectable in the CSF, indicating that the drug does not penetrate the blood-brain barrier. The cause of the cyclosporin-associated neurotoxicity that is reported in some patients is not clear at this time.

The binding of cyclosporin to blood proteins retards uptake by the kidney and the salivary glands but does not alter hepatic uptake of the drug in rats (Lemaire et al. 1988). This indicates that binding to red blood cells or plasma proteins may not limit the extraction of cyclosporin. The effect of various disease states on the plasma protein binding and the distribution of cyclosporin and its metabolites in various tissues requires further study.

During pregnancy, cyclosporin and its metabolites pass through the placenta and are found in the amniotic fluid and the cord blood (Fletchner et al. 1985; Venkataramanan et al. 1988). Although cyclosporin concentrations are low in breast milk, breast feeding is not recommended for infants of mothers receiving the drug.

8.1.3 Metabolism and Excretion

Cyclosporin undergoes extensive hepatic metabolism (Maurer et al. 1984). The primary metabolic pathways include hydroxylation at various amino acids and *N*-demethylation. More than 25 metabolites have been identified in human blood, bile and urine. In blood obtained from liver, kidney, heart and bone marrow transplant patients, metabolite 17 [numbering scheme as used by Maurer et al. (1984)] is in higher concentrations than the parent compound (Wang et al. 1988). Low concentrations of metabolites 1, 18 and 21 are present in the blood. In plasma from patients with end stage renal disease, cyclosporin is found in the highest concentration, while very little metabolite 17 and metabolite 1 is observed (Alexander et al. 1988). Cyclosporin metabolites are primarily excreted in the bile (Wood et al. 1983). A carboxy metabolite of cyclosporin has been identified and appears to be the primary metabolite in human and animal bile (Hartman et al. 1985; Lensmeyer et al. 1988). Large quantities of metabolites 8 and 17 are also excreted in the bile, but less than 1% of the dose administered is excreted unchanged by this route (Venkataramanan et al. 1985c). Urinary excretion accounts for less than 6% of the dose administered and less than 1% of the unchanged drug is excreted in the urine. Metabolites 17, 18, 8 and 26 and the carboxy metabolites are the primary metabolites in the urine (Lensmeyer et al. 1988).

Cyclosporin has a low to intermediate extraction ratio in humans (Ptachcinski et al. 1986a; Venkataramanan et al. 1985d). The pharmacokinetic parameters of cyclosporin are listed in table III. Various factors are known to alter the kinetics of the drug (table IV).

8.1.4 Drug Interactions

A number of drugs have been shown to interact with cyclosporin (table V), although some of these are based on only a few patient observations. Some of the drug interactions (erythromycin, ketoconazole and diltiazem) may be used to advantage, since a lowering of cyclosporin dose can be achieved in transplant patients; however, such combinations should be carefully monitored. While some of the drugs alter cyclosporin concentrations, cyclosporin also appears to alter the kinetics of several drugs. This information is of importance since transplant patients often receive multiple drug therapy. Concomitant drug therapy in transplant patients must be closely monitored.

8.2 Prednisone/Prednisolone

Low dose prednisone/prednisolone is used long term in transplant patients in combination with cyclosporin and azathioprine. Glucocorticoids vary in their potency and duration of action as a result of differences in steroid-receptor interactions,

Table IV. Factors affecting cyclosporin elimination

Factor	Observation	Comment	Reference
Age	Higher CL in paediatric liver transplant patients		Burckart et al. (1985)
	Higher CL in paediatric renal transplant patients		Ptachcinski et al. (1986c); Kahan et al. (1986)
	Inverse relationship between age *vs* CL and Vd		Yee et al. (1987)
Haemodialysis	Does not alter cyclosporin kinetics	High molecular weight; highly bound to plasma proteins	Venkataramanan et al. (1984)
Liver disease	Decreased elimination in patients with liver disease	Cyclosporin is eliminated by hepatic metabolism	Venkataramanan (1985e)
	Decreased elimination in renal transplant patients with liver dysfunction		Kahan et al. (1986a)
	Decreased elimination in bone marrow transplant patients with liver impairment		Yee et al. (1984)
Obesity	No significant difference in kinetics between obese and non-obese patients when normalised to ideal bodyweight or body surface area		Yee et al. (1988)
	Significant differences in kinetic parameters normalised to actual bodyweight		
Renal failure	No change in kinetics	Renal pathway is a minor component of cyclosporin elimination	Follath et al. (1983); Lindberg et al. (1986)
Time after transplantation	Decreased CL with time		Frey et al. (personal communication)

Abbreviations: CL = clearance; Vd = apparent volume of distribution.

binding to plasma proteins and metabolic clearance (Meikle & Tyler 1977).

The pharmacokinetics of prednisone and prednisolone have been reviewed in the literature (Frey 1987; Gambertoglio et al. 1980a; Jubiz & Meikle 1979; Jusko & Rose 1980; Pickup 1979). A summary of the pharmacokinetic parameters of prednisone and prednisolone in transplant patients is given in table VI.

8.2.1 Absorption

The absorption of prednisone appears to be normal in transplant patients. The time to peak prednisolone concentration and the peak prednisolone concentrations following oral administration of prednisone were comparable in renal transplant patients and healthy subjects (Gambertoglio et al. 1982; Uribe et al. 1978). In renal transplant patients, the fraction of prednisolone and prednisone absorbed is similar to that in healthy subjects (Gambertoglio et al. 1982). There is also no difference in the extent of absorption of prednisolone in Cushingoid and non-Cushingoid renal transplant patients (Frey et al. 1981). The fraction of prednisolone absorbed after oral administration of prednisone in stable liver transplant patients (68 ± 10%) is not significantly different compared with healthy subjects (Huang 1987). Prednisolone absorption has also been evaluated in orthotopic liver transplant patients by measurement of metabolites

Table V. Reported drug interactions with cyclosporin (based on 4 or more patient case reports except where otherwise indicated)

Drug	Proposed mechanism(s)	Reference
Drugs that decrease CsA concentration		
Carbamazepine	Induction of P450 enzymes	Lele et al. (1985)[a]
Isoniazid	Increased elimination of CsA	Langhoff & Madsen (1983)[a]
Nafcillin	Induction of CsA metabolism	Veremis et al. (1987)[a]
Phenobarbitone	Enhanced metabolism of CsA	Carstensen et al. (1986)[a]
Phenytoin	Accelerated metabolism of CsA	Keown et al. (1984)
	Reduced absorption	Freeman et al. (1984)[b]
		Rowland et al. (1987)[b]
Rifampicin	Increase rate of elimination	Cassidy et al. (1985)[a]
	Changes in bioavailability	
Somatostatin analogue	Alters intestinal absorption of CsA	Landgraf et al. (1987)[a]
Drugs that increase CsA concentration		
Danazol	Impairment of CsA metabolism	Ross et al. (1986)[a]; Koneru et al. (1988)
Diltiazem	Interference with CsA metabolism	Pochet & Pirson (1986)[a]; Henricsson & Lindholm (1988)[c]; Wagner et al. (1988)[b]
Erythromycin	Inhibition of hepatic elimination	Henricsson & Lindholm (1988)[c]
		Murray et al. (1987)
	Increased absorption of CsA	Wadhwa et al. (1987)[b]
		Gupta et al. (1988)[b]
Ketoconazole	Inhibition of hepatic metabolism of CsA	Ferguson et al. (1982)[a]
		Henricsson & Lindholm (1988)[c]
Methyltestosterone	Inhibition of metabolism of CsA	Moller & Ekelund (1985)[a]
Methylprednisolone	Inhibition of metabolism of CsA	Klintmalm et al. (1985); Henricsson & Lindholm (1988)[c]
Metoclopramide	Increased absorption of CsA	Wadhwa et al. (1987a)[b]
Nicardipine	Increased trough CsA levels	Bourbigot et al. (1986)[a]
Nifedipine	Decreased metabolism of CsA	Henricsson & Lindholm (1988)[c]
Oral contraceptive	Decreased metabolism of CsA	Deray et al. (1987)[a]
Verapamil	Inhibited metabolism of CsA	Lindholm & Henricsson (1987)
Drugs that do not affect CsA concentration		
Cimetidine	No *in vitro* inhibition	Henricsson & Lindholm (1988)[c]
	No *in vivo* effect	
Ranitidine	No change in CsA concentration	Zazgornik et al. (1985)[b]
Effect of CsA on other drugs		
Digoxin	Diminished renal clearance	Dorian et al. (1986)[a]
	Decreased Vd of digoxin	
Lovastatin	Increased toxicity of lovastatin due to decreased CL or decreased first-pass extraction	East et al. (1988); Norman et al. (1988)[a]
Drug interactions with increased toxicity		
Aminoglycosides	Increased nephrotoxicity	Kennedy et al. (1983)[a]
Amphotericin B	Increased nephrotoxicity	Hows et al. (1983)[a]
Cimetidine/ranitidine	Increased nephrotoxicity	Jarowenko et al. (1986)
Co-trimoxazole (trimethoprim + sulphamethoxazole)	Deteriorates renal function	Thompson et al. (1983)[a]
		Ringden et al. (1984)[a]
Trimethoprim	Deteriorates renal function	Thompson et al. (1983)

a Case report – single patients.
b Kinetic study.
c *In vitro* test.
Abbreviations: CsA = cyclosporin; Vd = apparent volume of distribution; CL = clearance.

and parent compound in the urine. It was concluded that the absorption was not influenced by a shortage of bile acids in the gastrointestinal tract, or by steatorrhoea (Koopman et al. 1986).

An important consideration in the use of prednisone is the variability in the systemic availability of prednisolone from prodrugs of prednisone such as prednisolone phosphate and prednisolone phthalate. In renal transplant patients nearly 50% of prednisolone phthalate is excreted or metabolised prior to its conversion to the biologically active prednisolone (Frey et al. 1985), while the phosphate ester has higher bioavailability. Therapeutic inequivalence is expected between these 2 products. Enteric-coated prednisolone tablets have been reported to exhibit erratic absorption in kidney transplant recipients (Henderson et al. 1979). The abovementioned factors must be kept in mind in the use of a proper dosage form of prednisone since malabsorption or incomplete bioavailability may precipitate rejection episodes.

8.2.2 Distribution

Prednisolone is primarily bound to transcortin and is also bound to albumin. Since the binding affinity to transcortin is high and the capacity is low, the glucocorticoids exhibit concentration-dependent binding (Rose et al. 1981). The plasma protein binding of prednisolone in liver transplant patients has been reported to be lower than in normal subjects (Townsend et al. 1983). Recent studies in stable liver transplant patients, however, indicate the binding affinity of prednisolone ($1.71 \pm 0.75 \times 10^{-7}$ mol/L) to transcortin to be comparable with that in normal subjects ($1.88 \pm 0.28 \times 10^{-7}$ mol/L) [Frey et al. 1981; Huang 1987]. The binding characteristics of prednisolone immediately following transplantation have not been evaluated. Since the liver contributes to the production of these proteins and they are often lower in concentrations immediately post transplant, the free fraction of prednisolone would be expected to be higher, possibly leading to a given dose of steroid producing variable effects when compared to stable patients. The binding capacity and the affinity of prednisolone to transcortin ($2.2 \pm 0.45 \times 10^{-7}$ mol/L) is not significantly different between renal transplant patients and normal subjects (Frey et al. 1981). The binding capacity for albumin and prednisolone does not differ significantly between patients with oral disease and renal transplant patients (Frey et al. 1981). However, renal transplant patients and patients with oral disease both have an albumin affinity constant that is approximately 10 to 40% lower than that of normal volunteers ($2.69 \pm 0.25 \times 10^{-3}$ mol/L). A recent study indicates a 3-fold increase in the affinity constant for prednisolone binding to transcortin (47.3 ± 14.7 *vs* 15.1 ± 10.1 μmol/L) post renal transplantation compared to pretransplant values. No changes in the transcortin or albumin concentration or albumin-prednisolone affinity constant were observed after transplantation (Rocci et al. 1988).

The volume of distribution at steady-state (Vd_{ss}) has also been reported in transplant patients. There appears to be no difference in the Vd_{ss} in non-Cushingoid renal transplant patients *versus* healthy subjects, although there does appear to be a significant difference between Cushingoid renal transplant patients and healthy subjects (Gambertoglio et al. 1980b). In a subsequent report no difference in the Vd_{ss} was reported between Cushingoid and non-Cushingoid patients (Benet et al. 1982). The Vd of prednisolone in liver transplant patients is significantly lower than in healthy subjects (Huang 1987). This lower Vd may be attributed to changes in tissue binding of prednisolone in these patients.

8.2.3 Metabolism

Prednisone is converted *in vivo* to the active moiety prednisolone by 11-β hydroxy dehydrogenase. This transformation is believed to be rapid due to the fact that equal doses of prednisone and prednisolone produced similar prednisolone concentration time profiles (Powell & Axelsen 1972). Prednisolone is extensively metabolised with greater than 90% of the radioactivity administered (^{14}C prednisolone) being recovered in the urine (Sandberg & Slaunwhite 1957). Approximately 7 to 15% of the orally administered dose is excreted unchanged in the urine (English et al. 1975). One study evaluated the amount of prednisolone excreted in

Table VI. Mean (± SD) pharmacokinetic parameters of prednisone and prednisolone in transplant patients

Reference	Patient population	No. of subjects	Dose (mg/kg)	Amount absorbed		$t_{1/2}$ (h)		Vd_{ss} (L/kg)		CL (ml/min/kg)	
				P	PN	total	unbound	total	unbound	total	unbound
Gambertoglio et al. (1982)	Stable kidney transplant	9	0.22 ± 0.07	86.1 ± 9.1		3.4 ± 0.3	2.7 ± 0.3				
		9	0.22 ± 0.07		93.6 ± 9.2	3.3 ± 0.5	2.6 ± 0.3				
Benet et al. (1982)	Non-Cushingoid kidney transplant	7	0.33 ± 0.07	80.0 ± 0.09				0.46 ± 0.07	1.30 ± 0.30	1.70 ± 0.29	7.5 ± 1.3
	Cushingoid kidney transplant	8	0.21 ± 0.08	86.0 ± 0.09				0.36 ± 0.06	1.21 ± 0.13	1.34 ± 0.36	6.3 ± 1.4
Gambertoglio et al. (1980b)	Non-Cushingoid kidney transplant	6	0.31 ± 0.062		82.2 ± 24.3	2.8 ± 0.6		0.52 ± 0.08		2.44 ± 0.46	
	Cushingoid kidney transplant	6	0.26 ± 0.061		58.7 ± 23.6	3.5 ± 0.5		2.77 ± 0.12		1.13 ± 0.41	
Huang (1987)	Stable liver transplant	10	0.31 ± 0.08	68.0 ± 10		3.5 ± 0.6	2.5 ± 0.6	0.48 ± 0.12	0.82 ± 0.2	1.43 ± 0.37	5.50 ± 2.33
Langhoff et al. (1985)	Kidney transplant	8[a]	0.16 ± 0.03			4.3 ± 0.6					
Langhoff et al. (1985)	Kidney transplant	8[b]	0.16 ± 0.02			2.9 ± 0.6					
Frey et al. (1987)	Renal transplant	25[a]	20[c] ± 7	82.3 ± 13.4				0.68 ± 0.08	1.48 ± 0.40	2.33 ± 0.46	8.20 ± 2.93
Frey et al. (1987)	Renal transplant	25[b]	25[c] ± 8	75.7 ± 24				0.61 ± 0.08	1.46 ± 0.37	2.20 ± 0.47	8.32 ± 2.05
Rocci et al. (1988)	Pre-renal transplant	6				4.0 ± 1.1	2.7 ± 0.4	0.78 ± 0.26	2.1 ± 1.2	2.67 ± 1.0	10.33 ± 5.5
	Post-renal transplant	6[a]				4.3 ± 1.7	2.4 ± 0.7	0.72 ± 0.1	1.6 ± 0.3	2.17 ± 0.67	8.5 ± 2.0

a Cyclosporin treated.
b Azathioprine treated.
c mg/day dosage.

Abbreviations: P = prednisone; PN = prednisolone; $t_{1/2}$ = elimination half-life; Vd_{ss} = apparent volume of distribution at steady-state; CL = clearance.

the urine of orthotopic liver transplant patients and reported the metabolic profile to be identical to that of healthy subjects (Koopman et al. 1986).

Since plasma protein binding of prednisolone is non-linear, the clearance does not increase in proportion to the dose (Legler et al. 1982). The pharmacokinetics of prednisolone prior to, 2 weeks to 1 month and 3 to 6 months after renal transplantation have been evaluated. The clearance and half-lives of total prednisolone were not significantly different in any of the trial periods (Ost et al. 1984). The clearance of unbound prednisolone in patients with oral disease was significantly higher than that in renal transplant patients. Reduced kidney function cannot account for the difference since less than 20% of the drug is excreted in the urine unchanged (Frey et al. 1981). Further studies are needed to investigate the mechanisms for decreased clearance of prednisolone in renal transplant patients. Similarly, the mean clearance of prednisolone in liver transplant patients is 63% lower than that of healthy subjects. The half-lives were also longer than normal values (4.9 ± 1.2 *versus* 3.2 ± 1.0 hours) [Huang 1987]. The decrease in intrinsic clearance may be a result of decreased enzymatic activity due to cyclosporin therapy. In all the studies the reported clearance values reflect only an apparent clearance estimate due to the interconversion of prednisone and prednisolone. Absolute clearance values can only be estimated after intravenous administration of prednisone and prednisolone to transplant patients. Diurnal variation in the clearance and bioavailability of prednisolone has also been reported (English et al. 1983). Therefore, the timing of any kinetic study must be carefully controlled.

8.2.4 Drug Interactions

Interactions that affect the pharmacokinetics or pharmacodynamics of prednisolone may adversely affect the status of the graft. Various drug interactions involving prednisone and prednisolone have been reported in transplant patients. In renal transplant patients, enzyme-inducing agents such as phenobarbitone, rifampicin and phenytoin have been reported to have deleterious effects on graft survival (Buffington et al. 1976; Wassner et al. 1976). Rifampicin has also been reported to reduce the bioavailability of prednisolone in healthy subjects (McAllister et al. 1983). Oral contraceptives decrease the clearance of prednisone (Boekenoogen et al. 1983; Kozower et al. 1974). Other drug interactions involving prednisolone that have been reported in healthy subjects are also expected to occur in transplant patients (Jubiz & Meikle 1979).

At present, prednisone is used primarily in combination with cyclosporin. A 25% reduction in the total body clearance of prednisolone and an increase in the half-life from 2.9 to 4.3 hours was observed in renal transplant patients receiving cyclosporin when compared with patients on azathioprine (Langhoff et al. 1985). A competitive inhibition of prednisolone metabolism has been suggested as the possible mechanism for such an observation. Another study, however, reported no difference in unbound prednisolone clearance and bioavailability between patients receiving prednisolone with cyclosporin and those receiving prednisolone with azathioprine early after transplantation (Frey et al. 1987).

The effect of steroids on the kinetics of other drugs used in transplant patients must also be recognised. Steroids are known to induce the metabolism of salicylic acid and increase the urinary excretion of metronidazole (Eradiri et al. 1988; Graham et al. 1977). The use of pancuronium with prednisone causes rapid termination of the muscular blockade (Laflin 1977). The effect of long term treatment with low-dose steroids on metabolism of other drugs is not known, but since transplant patients receive long term treatment, the potential for such interactions should be kept in mind.

8.3 Methylprednisolone

Methylprednisolone is administered in high doses to treat acute rejection episodes. This glucocorticosteroid appears to be primarily bound to albumin (Ebling et al. 1986). The kinetics of methylprednisolone have not been characterised in any transplant patients. The pharmacokinetics of methylprednisolone in renal, liver and cardiac transplant patients will be determined by the plasma protein binding and the intrinsic clearance in those patients. While the plasma protein binding will be influenced by the concentration of the binding proteins in the plasma, the intrinsic clearance may be influenced by other drugs used in transplant patients.

High-dose methylprednisolone treatment has been shown to increase serum cyclosporin concentrations as measured by a nonspecific RIA, due to inhibition of cyclosporin metabolism (Klintmalm et al. 1985). However, evaluation of this interaction using a specific HPLC method indicates a small increase in cyclosporin clearance (Ptachcinski et al. 1987b). This suggests a potential inhibition of the biliary excretion or further metabolism of cyclosporin metabolites by methylprednisolone. Further studies are needed to examine the metabolic profiles of cyclosporin during high-dose steroid treatment.

8.4 Azathioprine

Azathioprine has been extensively used for immunosuppression in autoimmune diseases and in organ transplant patients. The kinetics of azathioprine have been reviewed by Chan et al. (1987), Van Scoik (1985) and Benet et al. (1981). However, only limited information is available on the pharmacokinetics and pharmacodynamics of this drug in transplant patients. The dosage of azathioprine is determined empirically in transplant patients.

8.4.1 Absorption

Azathioprine is rapidly converted to 6-mercaptopurine after oral administration. The absorption of azathioprine is poor and variable. The bioavailability based on plasma drug concentration is 18% in uraemic patients (Odlind et al. 1986). This is the result of first-pass conversion to 6-mercaptopurine and other components. The reported bioavailability of 6-mercaptopurine after oral administration of azathioprine in kidney transplant patients is 60 ± 31% (Ding et al. 1980) and 41 ± 19% (Odlind et al. 1986).

8.4.2 Distribution

The distribution of azathioprine in humans has not been completely characterised. Based on animal studies it appears that while liver and intestine contain higher azathioprine concentrations, kidneys, lung, spleen and muscle contain concentrations similar to that in plasma (Elion & Hitchings 1975).

8.4.3 Metabolism and Excretion

Both azathioprine and 6-mercaptopurine are rapidly metabolised and exhibit large interindividual variation in their half-lives (table VII). Further metabolism results in 6-thioinosinic acid and 6-thioguanine nucleotides. There is high interpatient variability in the concentration of azathioprine metabolites in plasma while the intrapatient variability appears to be minimal (Lennard et al. 1984). Impaired renal function does not affect the pharmacokinetics of azathioprine or 6-mercaptopurine (Lin et al. 1980; Odlind 1986). Decreased hepatic biotransformation in the presence of hepatic dysfunction results in reduced rosette-inhibiting activity of the sera from patients (Bach & Dardenne 1972). This is due to the lack of formation of the active metabolites. The functional status of the liver in transplant patients will therefore influence the activity of azathioprine.

8.4.4 Drug Interactions

Allopurinol inhibits the first-pass metabolism of 6-mercaptopurine (Zimm et al. 1983). It also potentiates the pharmacological activity of orally administered azathioprine or 6-mercaptopurine (Elion et al. 1963). The increased dosing requirement of non-depolarising muscle relaxants such as pancuronium in surgical patients has been attributed to azathioprine.

Further studies of the kinetics and pharmacodynamics of azathioprine and 6-mercaptopurine and their metabolites in transplant patients are necessary for optimising azathioprine therapy in these patients.

Table VII. Pharmacokinetic parameters [arithmetic mean (± SD) or harmonic mean (range)] of azathioprine and 6-mercaptopurine in transplant patients

Reference	Patient population	No. of subjects	Dose[a] (mg)	Amount absorbed (%) AZA	Amount absorbed (%) MP	$t_{1/2}$ (min) AZA	$t_{1/2}$ (min) MP	Vd_{ss}[a] (L/kg)	CL[a] (ml/min/kg)
Ding et al. (1980)	Renal transplant	8	50-100		60 ± 31	9.7 ± 4.0	62.6 ± 24.4	0.81 ± 0.7	57.3 ± 31.0
Maddocks (1978)	Renal transplant	14	50			11-52			
		30	50				24-450		
Lin et al. (1980)	Renal transplant	14	100-150			12.5 ± 3.0			
		10	100-150				38.4 ± 16.7		
Odlind et al. (1986)	Uraemic	15	100	18 (1.8-72)	41 (19-67)	49.5 ± 31	73.6 ± 58.0		112 (68-240)

a Intravenous administration of azathioprine.
Abbreviations: AZA = azathioprine; MP = 6-mercaptopurine; $t_{1/2}$ = elimination half-life; Vd_{ss} = apparent volume of distribution at steady-state; CL = clearance.

8.5 OKT3

OKT3 is an IgG_{2A} murine monoclonal antibody that is effective in reversing the rejection of transplanted kidney, liver and heart. The therapeutic effect of this monoclonal antibody is related to its effect in blocking the killing of the allograft cells by cytotoxic T cells. *In vitro*, the effect of OKT3 is dependent on its concentration in the medium (Chang et al. 1981). In adult renal transplant patients, a daily dose of 5mg IV for 14 days provides a steady-state trough OKT3 concentration of 837 ± 160 μg/L in 3 days (Goldstein et al. 1986). This trough concentration is consistent with the *in vitro* inhibitory concentration of about 1000 μg/L and is maintained over the duration of the therapy. After cessation of therapy the plasma concentration declines to less than half its initial value, indicating a half-life of less than 24 hours. The primary mechanism of removal of OKT3 from the circulation is due to its binding to the T3 antigen of the circulating T cells and their removal by the reticuloendothelial system. Host antibodies to OKT3 that are developed during therapy are another mechanism of removal of circulating OKT3. Development of such antibodies can potentially limit repeated or prolonged use of the agent. It is essential to include immunological monitoring that consists of measurement of plasma OKT3 concentration, lymphocyte subpopulation and human antimurine antibodies.

9. Conclusions

It is clear that very few systematic studies have been carried out to characterise drug kinetics in transplant patients. It can generally be concluded that transplant patients are not normal with regard to drug kinetics. The kinetics of drugs in transplant patients will depend on the nature of the organ transplanted, time post transplantation, drug therapy, the inherent pharmacokinetics of the drug such as the extent of plasma protein binding, the intrinsic clearance of the drug and the elimination pathway (hepatic or renal), and the physicochemical properties of the drug such as lipid solubility.

It is important to realise that there will be time-dependent changes in the various biochemical markers such as serum creatinine, blood urea nitrogen, serum bilirubin and liver enzymes in transplant patients. This implies that during the immediate postoperative period these markers cannot be relied upon as a meaningful measure of the function of the various organs, and therefore cannot be used for adjusting the dosing regimens of drugs. Even in stable kidney and liver transplant patients, serum creatinine does not appear to be a good indicator of renal function. In addition, there will be time-dependent changes in the concentration of the plasma proteins and the activity of the drug-metabolising enzymes which will alter drug kinetics. Until a thorough understanding of drug kinetics in transplant patients is achieved, drug therapy should be closely monitored and individualised in transplant patients.

References

Agarwal RP, McPherson RA, Threatte GA. Assessment of cyclosporin A in whole blood and plasma in five patients with different hematocrits. Therapeutic Drug Monitoring 7: 61-65, 1985

Agarwal RP, McPherson RA, Threatte GA. Evidence of a cyclosporine binding protein in human erythrocytes. Transplantation 42: 627-632, 1986

Agarwal RP, Threatte GA, McPherson RA. Temperature dependent binding of cyclosporine to an erythrocyte protein. Clinical Chemistry 23: 481-485, 1987

Alexander DF, Horning L, Bowers LD. Cyclosporine metabolic disposition after oral administration in pretransplant end stage renal disease patients. Transplantation Proceedings 20: 499-508, 1988

Anderson KV, Brettell HR, Alkawa JK. C^{14}-labelled hydrochlorothiazide in human beings. Archives of Internal Medicine 107: 736-742, 1961

Arunsen KF, Ekelund G, Kindmark W, Laurell CB. Sequential changes of plasma proteins after surgical trauma. Scandinavian Journal of Clinical Laboratory Investigation 29 (Suppl. 124): 127-136, 1972

Atkinson K, Biggs JC, Britton E, Short R, Mrongovius R, et al. Oral administration of cyclosporine A for recipients of allogenic marrow transplants: implications of clinical gut dysfunction. British Journal of Haematology 56: 223-231, 1984

Atkinson K, Boland J, Britton K, Biggs J. Blood and tissue distribution of cyclosporine in humans and mice. Transplantation Proceedings 15: 2430-2449, 1983

Augustine JA, Zemaitis MA. The effect of cyclosporine A on hepatic microsomal drug metabolism in rat. Drug Metabolism and Disposition 14: 73-78, 1986

Bach JF, Dardenne M. Serum immunosuppressive activity of azathioprine in normal subjects and patients with liver disease. Proceedings of the Royal Society of Medicine 64: 260-263, 1972

Benet LZ, Frey BM, Frey FJ, Ding TL, Tsang S, et al. Immunopharmacokinetics. In Breimer & Speiser (Eds) Topics in pharmaceutical sciences, pp. 19-32, Elsevier, North Holland, 1981

Benet LZ, Frey FJ, Amend WJC, Lozada F, Frey BM. Endogenous and exogenous glucocorticoids in Cushingoid patients. Drug Intelligence and Clinical Pharmacy 16: 863-868, 1982

Benowitz NL. Effect of cardiac disease on pharmacokinetics. In Benet et al. (Eds) Pharmacokinetic basis for drug treatment, pp. 89-103, Raven Press, New York, 1984

Benowitz NL, Meister W. Pharmacokinetics in patients with cardiac failure. Clinical Pharmacokinetics 1: 389-405, 1976

Berkowitz ID, Croll MN, Likoff W. Malabsorption as a complication of congestive heart failure. American Journal of Cardiology 11: 43-47, 1963

Bertault-Peres P, Maraninchi D, Carcassunne Y, Cano JP, Barbet J. Clinical pharmacokinetics of ciclosporin A in bone marrow transplant patients. Cancer Chemotherapy and Pharmacology 15: 76-81, 1985

Blaschke TF. Protein binding and kinetics of drugs in liver disease. Clinical Pharmacokinetics 2: 32-44, 1977

Boekenoogen SJ, Szefler SJ, Jusko WJ. Prednisolone disposition and protein binding in oral contraceptive users. Journal of Clinical Endocrinology and Metabolism 56: 702-709, 1983

Bourbigot B, Guiserix J, Airiau J, Bressollette L, Morin JF, et al. Nicardipine increases cyclosporin blood levels. Lancet 1: 1447, 1986

Buffington GA, Dominguez JH, Piering WF, Hebert LA, Kauffman HM, et al. Interaction of rifampin and glucocorticoids – adverse effect on renal allograft function. Journal of the American Medical Association 236: 1958-1960, 1976

Burckart GJ, Ptachcinski RJ, Jones DH, Howrie DL, Venkataramanan R, et al. Impaired clearance of ceftizoxime and cefotaxime after orthotopic liver transplantation. Antimicrobial Agents and Chemotherapy 31: 323-324, 1987

Burckart GJ, Starzl TE, Venkataramanan R, Hashim H, Wong L, et al. Excretion of cyclosporine and its metabolites in human bile. Transplantation Proceedings 18: 46-49, 1986b

Burckart G, Starzl T, Williams L, Sanghvi A, Gartner C, et al. Cyclosporine monitoring and pharmacokinetics in pediatric liver transplant patients. Transplantation Proceedings 17: 1172-1175, 1985

Burckart GJ, Venkataramanan R, Ptachcinski RJ. Cyclosporine. In Taylor et al. (Eds) A textbook for the clinical application of therapeutic drug monitoring, pp. 339-352, Abbott Laboratories, Texas, 1986d

Burckart GJ, Venkataramanan R, Ptachcinski RJ, Starzl TE, Gartner CJ, et al. Cyclosporine absorption following orthotopic liver transplantation. Journal of Clinical Pharmacology 26: 647-651, 1986a

Burckart GJ, Venkataramanan R, Ptachcinski RJ, Starzl TE, Griffith BP, et al. Cyclosporine pharmacokinetic profiles in liver, heart and kidney transplant patients as determined by high performance liquid chromatography. Transplantation Proceedings 18: 129-136, 1986c

Canafax DM, Cipolle RJ, Hrushesky WJM, Rabatin JT, Graves NM, et al. The chronopharmacokinetics of cyclosporine and its metabolites in recipients of pancreas allografts. Transplantation Proceedings 20: 471-477, 1988

Carstensen H, Jacobsen N, Dreperink H. Interaction between cyclosporine A and phenobarbital. British Journal of Clinical Pharmacology 21: 550, 1986

Cassidy MJD, Van Zyl-Smit R, Pascoe MD, Swanepoel CR, Jacobson JE. Effect of rifampicin on cyclosporin A. Blood levels in a renal transplant recipient. Nephron 41: 207-208, 1985

Chan GLC, Canafax PM, Johnson CA. The therapeutic use of azathioprine in renal transplantation. Pharmacotherapy 7: 165-177, 1987

Chang TW, Kung PC, Gingran SP, Goldstein G. Does OKT3 monoclonal antibody react with an antigen recognition structure on human T cells. Proceedings of the National Academy of Sciences 78: 1805, 1981

Chaun P, Weiss YA, Safar ME, Lavene DE, Georges DR. Pindolol availability in hypertensive patients with normal and impaired renal function. Clinical Pharmacology and Therapeutics 22: 505-510, 1977

Craig RM, Murphy P, Gibson TP, Quintanilla A, Chao GC. Kinetic analysis of d-xylose absorption in normal subjects and in patients with chronic renal failure. Journal of Laboratory Clinical Medicine 101: 496-506, 1983

Crouthamul WG. The effect of congestive heart failure on quinidine pharmacokinetics. American Heart Journal 90: 335-339, 1975

Deray G, LeHoang P, Cacoub P, Assogba U, Grippon P, et al. Oral contraceptive interaction with cyclosporin. Lancet 1: 158-159, 1987

DeRiberolles C, Franco D, Lecompte Y, Blondeau B, Chauvaud S, et al. Early recovery of albumin synthesis after liver transplantation. European Surgical Research 7: 164-169, 1975

Ding TL, Gambertoglio JG, Amend WJC, Birnbaum J, Benet LZ. Azathioprine (AZA) bioavailability and pharmacokinetics in kidney transplant patients. Clinical Pharmacology and Therapeutics 27: 250, 1980

Dorian P, Strauss M, Ogilvie RI, David T, Cardella CJ. Cyclosporine induced digoxin toxicity – a new drug interaction. XI International Congress on Transplantation, Helsinki, pp. 32-45, 1986

Drayer DE. Active drug metabolites and renal failure. American Journal of Medicine 62: 486-489, 1977

Dromgoole SH. The effect of uremia and kidney transplantation on the binding capacity of albumin. Clinica Chimica Acta 52: 301-303, 1974

East C, Alivizatos PA, Grundy SM, Jones PH, Farmer JA. Rhabdomyolysis in patients receiving lovastatin after cardiac transplantation. New England Journal of Medicine 318: 47-48, 1988

Ebling WF, Milsap RL, Szefler SJ, Jusko WJ. 6α methylprednisolone and 6α methylprednisone plasma protein binding in humans and rabbits. Journal of Pharmaceutical Sciences 75: 760-763, 1986

Elion GB, Callahan S, Nathan H, Bieber S, Rundles BW, et al. Potentiation by inhibition of drug degradation: 6 substituted purines and xanthine oxidase. Biochemical Pharmacology 12: 85-93, 1963

Elion GB, Hitchings GH. Azathioprine. In Eichler et al. (Eds) Handbook of experimental pharmacology, Vol. 38, pp. 404-425, Springer-Verlag, New York, 1975

English J, Chakraborty J, Marks V, Trigger DJ, Thomson AG. Prednisolone levels in the plasma and urine. A study of two preparations in man. British Journal of Clinical Pharmacology 2: 327-332, 1975

English J, Dunne M, Marks V. Diurnal variation in prednisolone kinetics. Clinical Pharmacology and Therapeutics 33: 381-385, 1983

Eradiri O, Jamili F, Thomson A. Interaction of metronidazole with phenobarbital, cimetidine, prednisone and sulfasalazine in Crohn's disease. Biopharmaceutics and Drug Disposition 9: 219-227, 1988

Erickson BG, Todo S, Lynch S, Kam I, Ptachcinski RJ, et al. Role of bile and bile salts on cyclosporine absorption in dogs. Transplantation Proceedings 19: 1248-1249, 1987

Ferguson RM, Sutherland DER, Simmons RL, Najarian JS. Ketoconazole, cyclosporin metabolism and renal transplantation. Lancet 2: 882-883, 1982

Fletcher SM, Katz AR, Rogers AJ, Van Buren C, Kahan BD. The presence of cyclosporine in body tissues and fluids during pregnancy. American Journal of Kidney Diseases 1: 60-65, 1985

Follath F, Wenk M, Vozeh S, Thiel G, Brunner F, et al. Intravenous cyclosporine kinetics in renal failure. Clinical Pharmacology and Therapeutics 34: 638-643, 1983

Freeman DJ, Laupacis A, Keown PA, Stiller CR, Carruthers SG. Evaluation of cyclosporin-phenytoin interaction with observation on cyclosporin metabolites. British Journal of Clinical Pharmacology 18: 887, 1984

Frey BM, Frey FJ. Estimation of transcortin concentration by measurements of plasma protein binding of prednisolone and by electroimmunodiffusion. British Journal of Clinical Pharmacology 13: 245-248, 1982

Frey BM, Frey FJ, Wegmuller E, Holder J. Proteinurie nach Nierentransplantation. Schwiezerische Medizinische Wochenschrift 107: 1181-1190, 1977

Frey BM, Seeberger M, Frey FJ. Pharmacokinetics of 3 prednisolone prodrugs – evidence of therapeutic inequivalence in renal transplant patients with rejection. Transplantation 39: 270-274, 1985

Frey FJ. Kinetics and dynamics of prednisolone. Endocrine Reviews 8: 453-473, 1987

Frey FJ, Amend WJC, Lozada F, Frey BM, Holford NHG, et al. Pharmacokinetics of prednisolone and endogenous hydrocortisone levels in Cushingoid and non-Cushingoid patients. European Journal of Clinical Pharmacology 21: 235-242, 1981

Frey FJ, Horber FF, Frey BM. Trough levels and concentration time curve of cyclosporine in patients undergoing renal transplantation. Clinical Pharmacology and Therapeutics 43: 55-62, 1988

Frey FJ, Schnetzer A, Horber FF, Frey BM. Evidence that cyclosporine does not affect the metabolism of prednisolone after renal transplantation. Transplantation 43: 494-498, 1987

Gambertoglio JG. Effects of renal disease: altered pharmacokinetics. In Benet et al. (Eds) Pharmacokinetic basis for drug treatment, pp. 149-172, Raven Press, New York, 1984

Gambertoglio JG, Amend WJC, Benet LZ. Pharmacokinetics and bioavailability of prednisone and prednisolone in healthy volunteers and patients: a review. Journal of Pharmacokinetics and Bioipharmaceutics 8: 1-52, 1980a

Gambertoglio JG, Frey FJ, Holford NH, Birnbaum JL, Lizak PS, et al. Prednisone and prednisolone bioavailability in renal transplant patients. Kidney International 21: 621-626, 1982

Gambertoglio JG, Vincenti F, Feduska NJ, Birbaum J, Salvetierra O, et al. Prednisolone disposition in Cushingoid and non-Cushingoid kidney transplant patients. Journal of Clinical Endocrinology and Metabolism 51: 561-565, 1980b

Gibaldi M, Perrier D. Pharmacokinetics, 2nd ed., pp. 319-354, Marcel Dekker, Inc., New York, 1982

Gibson GG, Giacomini KM, Briggs WA, Whitman W, Levy G. Propoxyphene and norpropoxyphene plasma concentrations in the anephric patients. Clinical Pharmacology and Therapeutics 27: 665-670, 1980

Goldstein G, Fucello AJ, Norman DJ, Shield CF, Colvin RB, et al. OKT3 monoclonal antibody plasma levels during therapy and the subsequent development of host antibodies to OKT3. Transplantation 42: 507-511, 1986

Graham GG, Champion CD, Day RO, Paull PD. Patterns of plasma concentrations and urinary excretion of salicylate in rheumatoid arthritis. Clinical Pharmacology and Therapeutics 22: 410-420, 1977

Grevel J. Absorption of cyclosporine A after oral dosing. Transplantation Proceedings 18 (Suppl. 5): 9-15, 1986

Grevel J, Neusch E, Abische E, Kutz K. Pharmacokinetics of oral cyclosporin A (Sandimmune) in healthy subjects. European Journal of Clinical Pharmacology 31: 211-216, 1986

Grossman SH, Davis D, Kitchell BB, Shand DG, Routledge RA. Diazepam and lidocaine plasma protein binding in renal disease. Clinical Pharmacology and Therapeutics 31: 350-357, 1982

Groth CG, Kashiwagi W, Torisu M, Schroter G, Gustafsson A, et al. Protein metabolism in human liver transplant recipients. Erstes Internationales Bonner Leber Transplantations-Symposium, Bonn 23-25 June, 1972

Gupta SK, Bakran A, Johnson WG, Rowland M. Erythromycin enhances the absorption of cyclosporin. British Journal of Clinical Pharmacology 25: 401-402, 1988

Gupta SK, Legg B, Solomon LR, Johnsson RWG, Rowland M. Pharmacokinetics of cyclosporin: influence of rate of constant intravenous infusion in renal transplant patients. British Journal of Clinical Pharmacology 24: 519-526, 1987

Hartman NR, Trimble LA, Vederas JC, Jardine I. An acid metabolite of cyclosporine. Biochemical Biophysical Research Communication 133: 964-971, 1985

Hassan MMA, Al-Yahya MA. Cyclosporine. In Florey (Ed.) Analytical Profiles of Drug Substances, pp. 147-206, Academic Press, Inc., New York, 1987

Henderson RG, Wheatley T, English J, Chakraborty J, Marks V. Variation in plasma prednisolone concentrations in renal transplant recipients given enteric coated prednisolone. British Medical Journal 1: 1534-1536, 1979

Henricsson S, Lindholm A. Inhibition of cyclosporine metabolism by other drugs *in vitro*. Transplantation Proceedings 20: 569-571, 1988

Hepner GW, Veseue S, Tantum KR. Reduced drug elimination in congestive heart failure. Studies using aminopyrine and model drug. American Journal of Medicine 65: 271-276, 1978

Hoffman AF. A physicochemical approach to the intraluminal phase of fat absorption. Gastroenterology 50: 56-64, 1966

Homeida M, Jackson L, Roberts CJC. Decreased first pass metabolizing of labetalol in chronic liver disease. British Journal of Medicine 2: 1048-1050, 1978

Hows JM, Chipping PM, Fairhead S, Smith J, Baughan A, et al. Nephrotoxicity in bone marrow transplant recipients treated with cyclosporin A. British Journal of Haematology 54: 69-78, 1983

Huang ML. Drug disposition in liver transplant patients. A dissertation submitted to the University of Pittsburgh in partial fulfillment of the degree of Doctor of Philosophy, 1987

Huang ML, Burckart GJ, Venkataramanan R. Sensitive high performance liquid chromatographic analysis of vitamin E and vitamin A using ampherometric and ultraviolet detection. Journal of Chromatography 380: 321-338, 1986

Huang ML, Venkataramanan R, Burckart GJ, Ptachcinski RJ, Van Thiel DH, et al. Drug binding proteins in liver transplant patients. Journal of Clinical Pharmacology, in press, 1988

Huet PM, Villeneuve JP. Determinants of drug disposition in patients with cirrhosis. Hepatology 3: 913-918, 1983

Jarowenko MV, Van Buren CT, Kramer WG, Lorber MI, Flechner SM, et al. Ranitidine, cimetidine and the cyclosporine treated patient. Transplantation 42: 311, 1986

Johnston A, Marsden JT, Hla K, Henry JA, Holz DW. The effect of vehicle on the oral absorption of cyclosporine. British Journal of Clinical Pharmacology 21: 331-333, 1986

Jubiz W, Meikle AW. Alterations of glucocorticoid actions by other drugs and disease states. Drugs 12: 113-121, 1979

Jusko WJ, Rose JQ. Monitoring prednisone and prednisolone. Therapeutic Drug Monitoring 2: 169-176, 1980

Kahan BD. Individualization of cyclosporine therapy – using pharmacokinetic and pharmacodynamic parameters. Transplantation 5: 457-476, 1985

Kahan BD, Reid M, Newburger J. Pharmacokinetics of cyclosporine in human renal transplantation. Transplantation Proceedings 15: 446-453, 1983

Kahan B, Kramer WG, Wideman C, Flechner SM, Lorber MI, et al. Demographic factors affecting the pharmacokinetics of cyclosporine estimated by radioimmunoassay. Transplantation 41: 459-463, 1986a

Kahan B, Kramer WG, Wideman CA, Frazier OH, Lorber MI, et al. Analysis of pharmacokinetic profile in 232 renal and 87 cardiac allograft recipients treated with cyclosporine. Transplantation Proceedings 18: 115-119, 1986b

Kasiske BL, Awni WM, Duthoy-Heim KL, Rose M, Rao VK, et al. Alterations in cyclosporine pharmacokinetics after renal transplantation are linked to rapid increases in hematocrit, lipoproteins and serum protein. Transplantation Proceedings 20: 485-486, 1988

Kehrer BH, Whitington PF, Black AD. The effect of roux-en-y biliary enterostomy on the absorption of cyclosporine: relevance to poor drug bioavailability in children after orthotopic liver transplantation. Transplantation Proceedings 20: 523-528, 1988

Kennedy MS, Deeg HJ, Siegel M, Crowley JJ, Storb R, et al. Acute renal toxicity with combined use of amphotericin B and cyclosporine after marrow transplantation. Transplantation 35: 211-215, 1983

Keogh A, Day R, Critchley L, Duggin G, Baron D. The effect of food and cholestyramine on the absorption of cyclosporin in cardiac transplant recipients. Transplantation Proceedings 20: 27-30, 1988

Keown PA, Laupacis A, Carruthers G, Stawecki M, Koegler J. Interaction between phenytoin and cyclosporine following organ transplantation. Transplantation 38: 304-306, 1984

Klintmalm G, Sawe J, Ringden O. Cyclosporine plasma levels in renal transplant patients. Transplantation 39: 132-137, 1985

Klotz U, Avant GR, Hoyumpa A, et al. The effect of age and liver disease on the disposition and elimination of diazepam in adult man. Journal of Clinical Investigation 55: 347-359, 1975

Koch-Weser J. Pharmacokinetics of procainamide in man. Annals of the New York Academy of Science 179: 370-382, 1971

Koneru B, Hartner C, Iwatsuki S, Starzl TE. Effect of danazol on cyclosporine pharmacokinetics. Transplantation 45: 1001, 1988

Koopman BJ, van der Molen JC, Haagsma EB, Huizenga JR, Krom RAF, et al. Measurement of prednisolone and some of its metabolites in urine of patients after orthotopic liver transplantation as a means of monitoring prednisolone absorption. Journal of Clinical Chemistry and Clinical Biochemistry 28: 831-839, 1986

Kozower M, Veatch L, Kaplan MM. Decreased clearance of prednisolone, a factor in the development of corticosteroid side effects. Journal of Clinical Endocrinology and Metabolism 38: 407-412, 1974

Laflin MJ. Interaction of pancuronium and corticosteroids. Anesthesiology 47: 471-472, 1977

Landgraf R, Landgraf-Leurs MMC, Nusser J, Hillebrand G, Illner WD, et al. Effect of somatostatin analog (SM5201-995) on cyclosporine levels. Transplantation 44: 724-725, 1987

Langhoff E, Madsen S. Rapid metabolism of cyclosporin and prednisone in kidney transplant patient receiving tuberculostatic treatment. Lancet 2: 1031, 1983

Langhoff E, Madsen S, Flachs H, Olgaard K, Ladefoged J, et al. Inhibition of prednisolone metabolism by cyclosporine in kidney transplanted patients. Transplantation 39: 107-109, 1985

Legg B, Rowland M. Cyclosporin: measurement of fraction unbound in plasma. Journal of Pharmacy and Pharmacology 39: 599-603, 1987

Legg B Rowland M. Saturable binding of cyclosporine A to erythrocyte. Estimation of binding parameters in renal transplant patients and implications for bioavailability assessment. Pharmaceutical Research 5: 80-85, 1988

Legler UF, Frey FJ, Benet LZ. Prednisolone clearance at steady state in man. Journal of Clinical Endocrinology and Metabolism 55: 762-767, 1982

Lele P, Peterson P, Yang S, Jarrell B, Burke JF. Cyclosporine and tegretol – another drug interaction. Kidney International 27: 541, 1985

Lemaire M, Pardridge WM, Chaudhuri G. Influence of blood components on the tissue uptake indices of cyclosporine in rats. Journal of Pharmacology and Experimental Therapeutics 244: 740-744, 1988

Lemaire M, Tillement JP. Role of lipoproteins and erythrocytes in the *in vitro* binding and distribution of cyclosporine A in the blood. Journal of Pharmacy and Pharmacology 34: 715-718, 1982

Lennard L, Braun CB, Fox M, Maddocks JL. Azathioprine metabolism in kidney transplant recipients. British Journal of Clinical Pharmacology 18: 673-700, 1984

Lensmeyer GL, Wiebe DA, Carlson IH. Deposition of nine me-

tabolites of cyclosporine in human tissues, bile, urine and whole blood. Transplantation Proceedings 20: 614-622, 1988
Levy G, Baliah T, Procknal JA. Effect of renal transplantation on protein binding of drugs in serum of donor and recipient. Clinical Pharmacology and Therapeutics 20: 512-516, 1976
Lin SN, Jessup K, Floyd M, Wang TF, Van Buren CT, et al. Quantitation of plasma azathioprine and 6-mercaptopurine levels in renal transplant patients. Transplantation 29: 290-294, 1980
Lindberg A, Odlind B, Tufveson G, Lindstrum B, Gabrielsson J. The pharmacokinetics of cyclosporine A in uremic patients. Transplantation Proceedings 18: 146-152, 1986
Lindholm A, Henricsson S. Verapamil inhibits cyclosporin metabolism. Lancet 1: 1262-1263, 1987
Lindholm A, Henricsson S, Gang P. The free fraction of cyclosporine in plasma. Clinical findings with a new method. Transplantation Proceedings 20: 377-381, 1988
Lockiec F, Devergie A, Poirier O, Gluckman E. Pharmacologic monitoring and the clinical use of cyclosporine. Transplantation Proceedings 15: 2442-2445, 1983
Lockiec F, Fischer A, Gluckman E. A safer approach to the clinical use of cyclosporine. The predose calculation. Transplantation Proceedings 18: 194-199, 1986
Maddocks JL. Clinical pharmacological observations on azathioprine in kidney transplant patients. Clinical Science and Molecular Medicine 55: 20P, 1978
Maurer G. Metabolism of cyclosporine. Transplantation Proceedings 17 (Suppl.): 19-26, 1985
Maurer G, Loosli HR, Schreier E, Keller B. Disposition of cyclosporine in several animal species and man. Drug Metabolism and Disposition 12: 120-126, 1984
McAllister WAC, Thompson PJ, Al-Habet SM, Rogers HJ. Rifampin reduces effectiveness and bioavailability of prednisolone. British Medical Journal 286: 923-925, 1983
Mehta MU, Venkataramanan R, Burckart GJ, Ptachcinski RJ, Delamos B, et al. Effect of bile on cyclosporine absorption in transplant patients. British Journal of Clinical Pharmacology 25: 579-584, 1988
Mehta MU, Vankataramanan R, Burckart GJ, Ptachcinski RJ, Yang SL, et al. Antipyrine kinetics in liver disease and transplantation. Clinical Pharmacology and Therapeutics 39: 372-377, 1986
Meikle AW, Tyler FH. Potency and duration of action of glucocorticoids – effects of hydrocortisone, prednisone and dexamethasone on human pituitary-adrenal function. American Journal of Medicine 63: 200-207, 1977
Moller BB, Ekelund B. Toxicity of cyclosporine during treatment with androgens. New England Journal of Medicine 312: 1416, 1985
Mueller HE, Lie TS. The metabolism of 28 serum proteins in a human liver transplantation. Zeitschrift für Immunitätsforschung, Experimentelle und Klinische Immunologie 145: 250-274, 1973
Murray BM, Edwards L, Morse GD, Kohli PR, Venuto RC. Clinically important interaction of cyclosporine and erythromycin. Transplantation 43: 602-604, 1987
Murray-Lyon IM, Williams R, Freeman T, Clarke HGM. Serum proteins after a liver transplant. Nature 231: 45-46, 1971
Myre SA, Schroeder TJ, Melvin DB, Clardy CW, Pesce AJ, et al. Use of cyclosporine by constant rate infusion immediately after heart transplantation. Transplantation Proceedings 20: 316-322, 1988
Neal EA, Meffin PJ, Gregory PB, Blaschke TF. Enhanced bioavailability and decreased clearance of analgesics in patients with cirrhosis. Gastroenterology 77: 96-102, 1979
Newberger J, Kahan BD. Cyclosporine pharmacokinetics in man. Transplantation Proceedings 15: 2413-2415, 1983
Niederberger W, Lemaire M, Maurer G, Nussbaumer K, Wagner O. Distribution and binding of cyclosporine in blood and tissues. Transplantation Proceedings 15: 2419-2421, 1983
Norman DJ, Illingworth DR, Munson J, Hosenpud J. Myolysis and acute renal failure in a heart transplant recipient receiving lovastatin. New England Journal of Medicine 318: 46-47, 1988
Odar-Cederlof I. Plasma protein binding of phenytoin and warfarin in patients undergoing renal transplantation. Clinical Pharmacokinetics 2: 147-153, 1977
Odlind B, Hartvig P, Lindstrom B, Lonnerholm G, Tufveson G, et al. Serum azathioprine and 6-mercaptopurine levels and immunosuppressive activity after azathioprine in uremic patients. International Journal of Immunopharmacology 8: 1-11, 1986
Ohnhaus EE, Vozeh S, Neusch E. Absolute bioavailability of digoxin in chronic renal failure. Clinical Nephrology 11: 302-306, 1979
Olsen GD, Bennett WM, Porter GA. Morphine and phenytoin binding to plasma proteins in renal and hepatic failure. Clinical Pharmacology and Therapeutics 17: 677-684, 1975
Ost L, Bjorkhem I, van Bahr C. Clinical value of assessing prednisolone pharmacokinetics before and after renal transplantation. European Journal of Clinical Pharmacology 26: 363-369, 1984
Pentikainen PJ, Neuvonen PJ, Jostell KG. Pharmacokinetics of chlormethiazole in healthy volunteers and patients with cirrhosis of the liver. European Journal of Clinical Pharmacology 17: 225-284, 1980
Pickup ME. Clinical pharmacokinetics of prednisone and prednisolone. Clinical Pharmacokinetics 4: 111-128, 1979
Pochet JM, Pirson Y. Cyclosporin-diltiazem interaction. Lancet 2: 979, 1986
Powell LW, Axelsen E. Corticosteroids in liver disease: studies on the biological conversion of prednisone to prednisolone and plasma protein binding. Gut 13: 690-696, 1972
Ptachcinski RJ, Burckart GJ, Rosenthal JT, Venkataramanan R, Howrie D, et al. Cyclosporine pharmacokinetics in children following cadaveric renal transplantation. Transplantation Proceedings 18: 766-767, 1986c
Ptachcinski RJ, Burckart GJ, Venkataramanan R. Cyclosporine concentration determinations for monitoring and pharmacokinetic studies. Journal of Clinical Pharmacology 26: 358-366, 1986b
Ptachcinski RJ, Venkataramanan R, Burckart GJ. Clinical pharmacokinetics of cyclosporine. Clinical Pharmacokinetics 11: 107-132, 1986a
Ptachcinski RJ, Venkataramanan R, Burckart GJ, Gray JA, Van Thiel DH, et al. Cyclosporine kinetics in healthy volunteers. Journal of Clinical Pharmacology 27: 243-248, 1987a
Ptachcinski RJ, Venkataramanan R, Burckart GJ, Hakala TR, Rosenthal JT, et al. Cyclosporine-high dose steroid interaction in renal transplant recipients: assessment by HPLC. Transplantation Proceedings 19: 1728-1729, 1987b
Ptachcinski RJ, Venkataramanan R, Rosenthal JT, Burckart GJ, Taylor RJ. Cyclosporine kinetics in renal transplantation. Clinical Pharmacology and Therapeutics 38: 296-300, 1985b
Ptachcinski RJ, Venkataramanan R, Rosenthal JT, Burckart GJ, Taylor RJ, et al. The effect of food on cyclosporine absorption. Transplantation 40: 174-176, 1985a
Reidenberg MM. The binding of drugs to plasma proteins from patients with poor renal function. Clinical Pharmacokinetics 1: 121-125, 1976
Reynolds KL, Grevel J, Gibbons SY, Welsh MS, Rutzky LP, et al. Cyclosporine pharmacokinetics in uremic patients. Influence of different assay methods. Transplantation Proceedings 20: 462-465, 1988
Rodighiero V. Therapeutic drug monitoring of cyclosporin: practical applications and limitations. Clinical Pharmacokinetics 16: 27-37, 1989
Ried M, Gibbons S, Kwok D, Van Buren CT, Fletchner S, et al. Cyclosporine levels in human tissues of patients treated for

one week to one year. Transplantation Proceedings 15: 2434-2637, 1983
Ringden O, Myrenfors P, Klintmalm G, Tyden G, Ost L. Nephrotoxicity by co-trimoxazole and cyclosporin in transplanted patients. Lancet 1: 1016-1017, 1984
Roberts DE, Allen E, Routledge PA, Webb DB, Salaman JR. Are clearance pathways impaired in patients with cyclosporine nephrotoxicity. Transplantation Proceedings 18: 631-632, 1986
Rocci ML, Tietze KJ, Lee J, Harris H, Danzeisen J, et al. The effect of cyclosporine on the pharmacokinetics of prednisolone in renal transplant patients. Transplantation 45: 656-659, 1988
Rosano TG. Effect of hematocrit on cyclosporine (cyclosporin A) in whole blood and plasma of renal transplant patients. Clinical Chemistry 31: 410-412, 1985
Rose EA, Wilkinson A, Hawkins RA, Danovitch GM. The plasma creatinine concentration is not an accurate reflection of the glomerular filtration rate in stable renal transplant patients receiving cyclosporine. American Journal of Kidney Diseases 10: 113-117, 1987
Rose J, Yurchak A, Jusko W. Dose dependent pharmacokinetics of prednisone and prednisolone in man. Journal of Pharmacokinetics and Biopharmaceutics 9: 389-417, 1981
Ross WB, Roberts D, Griffin PJA, Salaman JR. Cyclosporin interaction with danazol and norethiderone. Lancet 2: 330, 1986
Routledge PA, Stargel WW, Wagner GS, Shand DG. Increased alpha 1 acid glycoprotein and lidocaine disposition in myocardial infarction. Annals of Internal Medicine 93: 701-704, 1980
Rowland M, Benet LZ, Graham GG. Clearance concepts in pharmacokinetics. Journal of Pharmacokinetics and Biopharmaceutics 1: 123-136, 1973
Rowland M, Gupta SK. Cyclosporin-phenytoin interaction: reevaluation using metabolite data. British Journal of Clinical Pharmacology 24: 329-334, 1987
Sandberg AA, Slaunwhite WR. Differences in metabolism of prednisolone C^{14} and Cortisol-C^{14}. Journal of Clinical Endocrinology 17: 1040-1050, 1957
Shaw LS, Bowers L, Demers L, Freeman D, Moyer T, et al. Critical issues in cyclosporine monitoring: report to the task force on cyclosporine monitoring. Clinical Chemistry 33: 1269-1288, 1987
Smith DE, Benet LZ. Plasma protein binding of furosemide in kidney transplant patients. Journal of Pharmacokinetics and Biopharmaceutics 10: 663-674, 1982
Smith DE, Gambertaglio JG, Vincenti F, Benet LZ. Furosemide kinetics and dynamics after kidney transplant. Clinical Pharmacology and Therapeutics 30: 105-113, 1981
Stewart LF, Cochran E, Williams SJ. Cyclosporine disposition in patients with liver disease. Drug Intelligence and Clinical Pharmacy 19: 451, 1985
Szeto H, Inturrisi C, Houde R, Saal S, Cheigh J. Accumulation of normeperidine (N) an active metabolite of meperidine (M) in patients with renal failure or cancer. Clinical Research 24: 258A, 1976
Thompson JF, Chalmers DH, Hunnisett AG, Wood RFM, Morris PJ. Nephrotoxicity of trimethoprim and cotrimoxazole in renal allograft recipients treated with cyclosporine. Transplantation 36: 204-206, 1983
Thompson PD, Melmon KL, Richardson JA, et al. Lidocaine pharmacokinetics in advanced heart failure, liver disease and renal failure in humans. Annals of Internal Medicine 78: 499-508, 1973
Tilstone WJ, Dargie H, Dargie EN, Morgan HG, Kennedy AC. Pharmacokinetics of metolazone in normal subjects and in patients with cardiac or renal failure. Clinical Pharmacology and Therapeutics 16: 322-329, 1974
Tilstone WJ, Fine A. Furosemide kinetics in renal failure. Clinical Pharmacology and Therapeutics 23: 644-650, 1978
Townsend RJ, Albert KS, Gibson FM, Sakman E, Wagner JG. Prednisone and prednisolone kinetics – observations after liver transplantation. Clinical Pharmacy 2: 103-104, 1983
Tredger JM, Naoumov NV, Steward CM, O'Grady JG, Grevel J, et al. Influence of biliary T-tube clamping on cyclosporine pharmacokinetics in liver transplant recipients. Transplantation Proceedings 20: 512-515, 1988
Ueda CT, Lemaire M, Gsell G, Nussbaumer K. Intestinal lymphatic absorption of cyclosporin A following oral administration in an olive oil solution in rats. Biopharmaceutics and Drug Disposition 4: 113-124, 1983
Uribe M, Schalm SW, Summerskill WHJ, Go VLW. Oral prednisone for chronic active liver disease: dose responses and bioavailability studies. Gut 19: 1131-1135, 1978
Van Scoik KG, Johnson CA, Porter WA. The pharmacology and metabolism of the thiopurine drugs 6-mercaptopurine and azathioprine. Drug Metabolism and Reviews 16: 157-174, 1985
Venkataramanan R, Burckart GJ, Ptachcinski RJ. Pharmacokinetics and monitoring of cyclosporine following orthotopic liver transplantation. Seminars in Liver Disease 5: 357-368, 1985b
Venkataramanan R, Burckart GJ, Ptachcinski RJ, Lee A, Hardesty RL, et al. Cyclosporine pharmacokinetics in heart transplant patients. Transplantation Proceedings 18: 768-770, 1986
Venkataramanan R, Kalp K, Rabinovitch M, Cuellar R, Ptachcinski RJ, et al. Conjugative drug metabolism in liver transplant patients. Transplantation Proceedings, in press, 1989
Venkataramanan R, Koneru B, Wang CP, Burckart GJ, Caritis SN, et al. Cyclosporine and its metabolites in mother and baby. Transplantation 46: 468-469, 1988
Venkataramanan R, Ptachcinski RJ, Burckart GJ, et al. Extraction ratio of cyclosporine in a liver transplant patient with organ rejection. Journal of Pharmaceutical Sciences 74: 901-902, 1985d
Venkataramanan R, Ptachcinski RJ, Burckart GJ, Gray J, Starzl TE. Cyclosporine bioavailability in liver disease. Drug Intelligence and Clinical Pharmacy 19 (Abstract): 451, 1985a
Venkataramanan R, Ptachcinski RJ, Burckart GJ, Yang SL, Starzl TE, et al. The clearance of cyclosporine by hemodialysis. Journal of Clinical Pharmacology 24: 528-531, 1984
Venkataramanan R, Ptachcinski RJ, Gray J, Burckart GJ, Van Thiel DH, et al. Cyclosporine kinetics in liver disease. Clinical Pharmacology and Therapeutics 37: 234, 1985e
Venkataramanan R, Starzl TE, Yang S, Burckart GJ, Ptachcinski RJ, et al. Biliary excretion of cyclosporine in liver transplant patients. Transplantation Proceedings 17: 286-289, 1985c
Veremis SA, Maddox MS, Pollak R, Mozes MF. Subtherapeutic cyclosporine concentrations during nafcillin therapy. Transplantation 43: 913-915, 1987
Vernillet L, Moulin B, Dadoun C, LeBigot JF, Fillastre JP. Pharmacokinetics of cyclosporine A in patients with nephrotic syndrome. Transplantation Proceedings 20: 529-535, 1988
Vine W, Bowers L. Cyclosporine: structure, pharmacokinetics, therapeutic drug monitoring. Critical Reviews in Clinical Laboratory Science 25: 275-311, 1987
Wadhwa NK, Schroeder TJ, O'Flaherty E, Pesce AJ, Myre SA, et al. The effect of oral metoclopramide on the absorption of cyclosporine. Transplantation 43: 211, 1987a
Wadhwa NK, Schroeder TJ, O'Flaherty E, Pesce AJ, Myre SA, et al. Interaction between erythromycin and cyclosporine in a kidney and pancreas allograft recipient. Therapeutic Drug Monitoring 9: 123-125, 1987b
Wagner K, Henkel M, Heinemeyer G, Neumayer HH. Interaction of calcium blockers and cyclosporine. Transplantation Proceedings 20(2): 561-568, 1988
Wang CP, Burckart GJ, Ptachcinski RJ, Venkataramanan R, Schwinghammer T, et al. Cyclosporine metabolite concentrations in blood of liver, heart, kidney and bone marrow transplant patients. Transplantation Proceedings 20: 571-596, 1988
Wassner SJ, Pennisi AJ, Malekz MH, Fine RN. The adverse ef-

fect of anticonvulsant therapy on renal allograft survival. Journal of Pediatrics 88: 134-137, 1976
Weeke B, Weeke E, Bendiner G. The variation in twenty one serum proteins before and after renal transplantation. Acta Medica Scandinavica 189: 113-118, 1971a
Weeke B, Weeke E, Bendiner G. The variation in twenty one serum proteins before and after renal transplantation. II. Changes during acute rejection. Acta Medica Scandinavica 189: 119-123, 1971b
Wells JV. Albumin metabolism in patients after renal transplantation. Clinical Science 37: 221-229, 1969
Wenk M, Follath F, Abisch E. Temperature dependency of apparent cyclosporin A concentrations in plasma. Clinical Chemistry 29: 1865, 1983
Wilkinson GR. Influence of hepatic disease on pharmacokinetics. In Evans et al. (Eds) Applied pharmacokinetics, pp. 116-138, Raven Press, New York, 1986
Williams RL. Drug administration in hepatic disease. New England Journal of Medicine 309: 1616-1622, 1983
Wood AJJ, Kornhauser DM, Wilkinson GR, Shand DG, Branch RA. The influence of cirrhosis on steady state blood concentrations of unbound propranolol after oral administration. Clinical Pharmacokinetics 3: 478-487, 1978
Wood AJJ, Vestal RE, Spannuth CL, Stone WJ, Wilkinson GR, et al. Propranolol disposition in renal failure. British Journal of Clinical Pharmacology 10: 561-566, 1980
Wood AJ, Lemaire M. Pharmacologic aspects of cyclosporine therapy: pharmacokinetics. Transplantation Proceedings 17 (Suppl.): 27-32, 1985
Wood AJ, Maurer G, Niederberger W, Beveridge T. Cyclosporine: pharmacokinetics, metabolism and drug interaction. Transplantation Proceedings 15: 2409-2412, 1983
Yee GC, Kennedy MS. Cyclosporine. In Evans et al. (Eds) Applied pharmacokinetics, 2nd edition, pp. 826-851, Applied Therapeutics, Inc., Spokane, Washington, 1986
Yee GC, Kennedy MS, Storr R, Thomas ED. Pharmacokinetics of intravenous cyclosporine in bone marrow transplant patients. Transplantation 38: 511-513, 1984
Yee GC, Lennon TP, Gmur DJ, Cheney CL, Oeser D. Effect of obesity on cyclosporine disposition. Transplantation 45: 649-651, 1988
Yee GC, Lennon TP, Gmar DJ, Kennedy MS, Deeg HJ. Effect of age on cyclosporine kinetics in marrow transplant recipients. Transplantation Proceedings 19: 1704-1705, 1987
Zaghloul I, Ptachcinski RJ, Burckart GJ, Van Thiel DH, Starzl TE, et al. Blood protein binding of cyclosporine in transplant patients. Journal of Clinical Pharmacology 27: 240-242, 1987
Zazgornik J, Schindler J, Gremmel F, Balcke P, Kopsa H, et al. Ranitidine does not influence the blood cyclosporin levels in renal transplant patients. Kidney International 27: 401, 1985
Zeevi A, Eiras G, Burckart G, Makowka L, Venkataramanan R, et al. Immunosuppressive effect of cyclosporine metabolites from human bile on alloreactive T cells. Transplantation Proceedings 20: 115-121, 1988
Zimm S, Collins JM, O'Neill D, Chabner BA, Poplock DG. Inhibition of first pass metabolism in cancer chemotherapy: interaction of 6-mercaptopurine and allopurinol. Clinical Pharmacology and Therapeutics 34: 810-816, 1983

Authors' address: Dr *R. Venkataramanan*, Clinical Pharmacokinetics Laboratory, Department of Pharmaceutical Sciences, University of Pittsburgh, 807 Salk Hall, Pittsburgh, PA 15261 (USA).

Clinical Pharmacokinetics 16: 162-179 (1989)
0312-5963/89/0003-0162/$09.00/0

Food Interactions with Sustained-Release Theophylline Preparations[1]

A Review

J.H.G. Jonkman

Pharma Bio-Research International B.V., Assen, and State University, Department of Analytical Chemistry & Toxicology, Groningen, The Netherlands

Contents

Summary 162
1. Twice-Daily Theophylline Preparations 165
   1.1 'Theo-Dur' 165
   1.2 'Theo-Dur Sprinkle' 166
   1.3 'Theolair SR' 167
   1.4 'Somophyllin CRT' 168
   1.5 'Sabidal' 168
   1.6 'Theograd' 168
   1.7 'Slo-Phyllin Gyrocaps' 169
   1.8 'Slo-Bid Gyrocaps' 169
   1.9 'Theobid Duracap' 170
   1.10 'Phyllocontin' 170
   1.11 'Euphyllin CR' 170
2. Once-Daily Theophylline Preparations 170
   2.1 'Theo-24' 170
   2.2 'Uniphyl' 172
   2.3 'Theo-Dur' 174
   2.4 'Dilatrane AP' 174
   2.5 'Euphylong' 175
   2.6 Riker Once-Daily Controlled-Release Theophylline 175
3. Discussion 175
4. Conclusion 176

Summary

Currently, theophylline is being used predominantly as sustained-release capsules or tablets. In the mid-seventies the first preparations for use with a dosage interval of 12 hours (twice-daily preparations) were introduced. Since 1983, theophylline preparations that can be given with an interval of 24 hours (once-daily preparations) have become available.

The release of theophylline from some of these products can be influenced (either increased or decreased) by concomitant intake of food. With some preparations the composition of the meal (especially the fat content) has an influence on the degree of effect.

1 All products in quotes (e.g. 'Theo-Dur') are registered trade marks of the manufacturers listed.

The consequence may be an effect on the rate of absorption or on the amount absorbed, or both simultaneously. This could result in an unexpected shift of the plasma theophylline concentration. Such a shift is therapeutically undesirable, because theophylline has a fairly narrow therapeutic range.

A review is given of those food interactions with the sustained-release theophylline preparations, both twice-daily and once-daily products, that are currently on the world market.

Special attention is paid to the specific (bio)pharmaceutical characteristics of the different products, and to the influence of the composition and timing of the meals. For each preparation the effect of food on the following pharmacokinetic parameters is discussed: area under the plasma concentration-time curve, peak plasma drug concentration and time to reach this peak. Where possible, the results for both adults and children are discussed. There are indications that children are more susceptible to food-effects than adults.

The regulatory aspects are mentioned briefly.

Clinically important effects of food have been observed with the following twice-daily products: 'Theo-Dur Sprinkle', 'Theolair SR' (= 'Nuelin SR') and 'Theograd'. Pronounced effects could have an even greater impact with once-daily preparations, as the total daily dose will be given at a single time. A particularly sudden release of a major part of the dose ('dose-dumping') may result in toxic plasma concentrations. Among these products, clinically important effects in children have been reported with 'Theo-24' and 'Uniphyl'.

The absorption of any drug after oral administration in a particular form can be considerably influenced by concomitant (or almost concomitant) intake of food or fluids (Melander 1978). There are several indications that concomitant food intake can have an effect on the rate and/or extent of absorption of theophylline, a bronchodilator.

Theophylline has a fairly narrow therapeutic range (Hendeles & Weinberger 1983; Hendeles et al. 1984). Thus, a decreased rate of release from a sustained-release theophylline product can easily result in possibly subtherapeutic plasma concentrations. Conversely, an increased rate of release, particularly when it occurs suddenly (e.g. due to a meal), can result in potentially toxic plasma concentrations. In order to keep the plasma theophylline concentration within the therapeutic range it is important to avoid unexpected situations, and therefore the clinician should be familiar with the effect of food on a particular brand of sustained-release theophylline.

Generally speaking, food can affect drug absorption and elimination in several ways; for example, by changing the gastric (and maybe intestinal) transit time, by changing the levels of pancreatic enzymes and bile, by stimulation of hepatic oxidative enzymes and by preferential binding of drugs to food (Boxenbaum 1982; Welling 1977). Furthermore, food intake can result in changes in splanchnic blood flow and changes in osmolality and influx of water into the gastrointestinal tract.

An important part of a food-drug interaction is the result of a *physiological* effect: filling of the stomach with food (plus a dose in some form) will result in a digestion period followed by gastric emptying after 2 to 3 hours. For drugs that are predominantly absorbed from the small intestine (e.g. theophylline), this means a delay of about 2 to 3 hours before absorption becomes effective (Jonkman et al. 1985; Welling et al. 1975) [fig. 1].

The composition of the diet also has an effect on the *pharmacokinetics* (disposition) of theophylline. Kappas and others (Anderson & Kappas 1984; Anderson et al. 1979; Kappas et al. 1976) found that theophylline was more rapidly eliminated during a high protein dietary period than with high carbohydrate or high fat diets. This suggests that theophylline is metabolised more rapidly with a high protein diet.

Similar effects were found by Feldman et al. (1980, 1982) in children. The effect is in the order

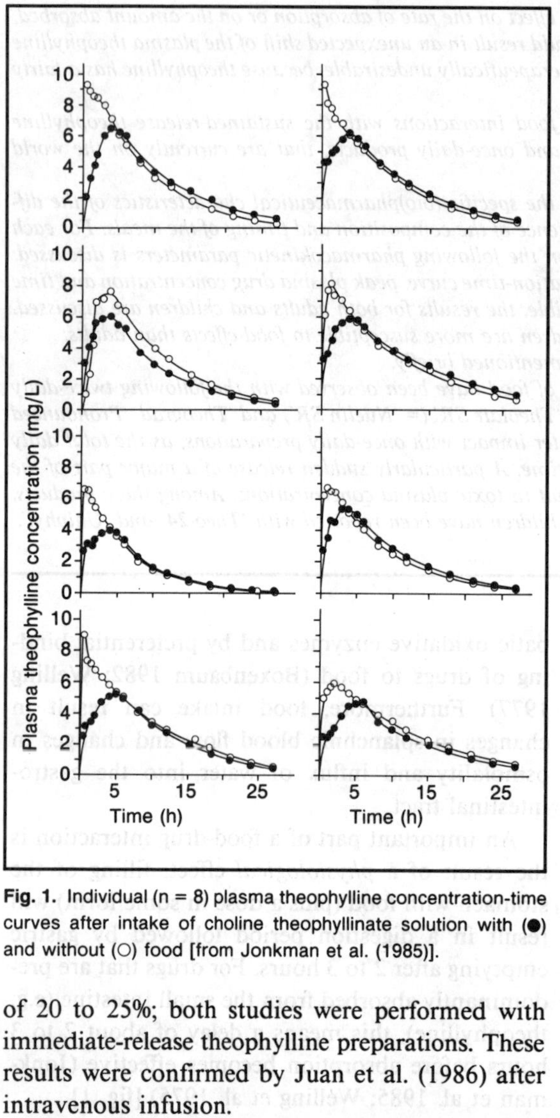

Fig. 1. Individual (n = 8) plasma theophylline concentration-time curves after intake of choline theophyllinate solution with (●) and without (○) food [from Jonkman et al. (1985)].

of 20 to 25%; both studies were performed with immediate-release theophylline preparations. These results were confirmed by Juan et al. (1986) after intravenous infusion.

Thompson et al. (1983) studied the effect of different diets on the disposition of a sustained-release theophylline preparation ('Theolair SR'). In contrast to the 2 previous studies, no significant effect on the elimination half-life was detected after changing from a high carbohydrate/low protein to a high protein/low carbohydrate diet. The authors suggested that the discrepancy may be caused by the difference in absorption site for theophylline after intake of an immediate-release formulation compared with a sustained-release one.

Another dietary cause of changes in drug elimination is that of charcoal broiling of meats. Kappas et al. (1978) found that a 5-day period of eating charcoal-broiled meat increased the elimination rate of theophylline by about 20%.

The physiological effects of concomitant food intake and the influence of diet on the pharmacokinetics of theophylline described above are important for optimal dosing of patients. These effects of diet on the metabolism of theophylline, although of importance with long term administration, will generally not result in sudden changes in plasma theophylline concentrations, and thus will probably not cause unexpected changes in effectiveness of the drug. However, the situation is different where it is the release of theophylline from a sustained-release preparation which is influenced (either increased or decreased); in this case the bioavailability is being changed, and the plasma concentration can alter quite suddenly. It is therefore important to realise that the possibility of a *biopharmaceutical* interaction exists. The degree of such an effect depends on the susceptibility of a particular preparation to such influences as pH, motility and solubility.

The absorption of a drug from a sustained-release product is intended to occur at a constant rate during the dosing interval. So, for twice-daily products this period of constant release and absorption would be 12 hours; for once-daily products it is 24 hours.

It is obvious that products with a 24-hour exposure to the gastrointestinal tract are more vulnerable than twice-daily preparations. Modern pharmaceutical technology provides many methods to prepare slow- or ultra-slow-release products, and with different methods of manufacture the rate of release can be programmed quite accurately. In practice, however, it appears that some slow-release products are sensitive to concomitant intake of food.

In this review we discuss food interactions with sustained-release theophylline products because such products are being used extensively, both as twice-daily and, more recently, as once-daily preparations (Hendeles & Weinberger 1985, 1986; Hendeles et al. 1985).

There is a substantial variation in gastrointestinal transit times, but the average is about 24 hours. It could be expected that there would be large variations in disposition of once-daily theophylline preparations; however, in practice it has been found that the absorption of such products is quite reliable.

1. Twice-Daily Theophylline Preparations

1.1 'Theo-Dur'

The manufacturer of 'Theo-Dur' is Key Pharmaceuticals Inc., US. This product is also sold by Pfizer Laboratories Division, US, under the name 'Sustaire' (100 and 300mg tablets only). In West Germany it is named 'Pulmo-Dur' and in The Netherlands 'Theolin Retard'.

'Theo-Dur' is a tablet that consists of 2 compartments: a matrix of compressed theophylline crystals, and coated theophylline granules which are embedded in this matrix. One-third of the dose is in the matrix, the remainder in the pellets (Golub et al. 1986).

In contact with fluid, the theophylline matrix disintegrates and dissolves. Next, theophylline diffuses slowly through the wall of the free granules. Finally, the granules dissolve completely. There are 3 dosage strengths, 100, 200 and 300mg, which do not necessarily have the same biopharmaceutical characteristics (Hendeles & Weinberger 1985).

In general, the release from 'Theo-Dur' (especially from the 200 and 300mg tablets) is relatively slow, slightly biphasic and almost independent of the pH of the medium. There is a slight intertablet variability in the *in vitro* release rate.

'Theo-Dur' has been on the market in the US since 1977 as a twice-daily preparation, where it is now the market leader with 60% of the sales of sustained-release theophylline products. It is also widely used in Europe. In 1984 it was approved by the FDA as a once-daily preparation for use in the same population of patients as the other 2 once-daily products, but the manufacturer still recommends that the product be administered twice a day for optimal therapy.

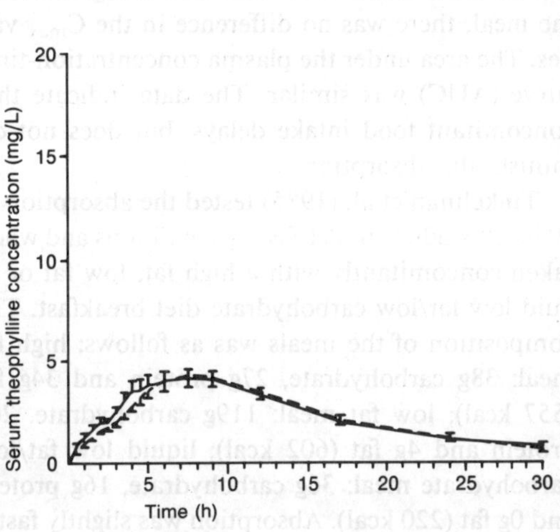

Fig. 2. Mean (± SEM) serum theophylline concentration-time curves in 10 subjects after a single dose of 'Theo-Dur' 300mg under fasting conditions (—) and after a standardised breakfast (---) [from Sips et al. (1984), with permission].

Most food interaction studies have been performed with the 300mg tablet. Sips et al. (1984) studied the absorption of theophylline after intake of a 'Theo-Dur' tablet, with or without breakfast, in 10 subjects. The breakfast consisted of 58g carbohydrate, 17g protein and 17g fat: 1910 kJ (= 455 kcal). An intravenous infusion of aminophylline was given as a reference.

When taken with breakfast, time to peak concentration (t_{max}) was decreased by about 0.5 hour. However, the total profile of the serum theophylline *versus* time curves indicated slightly slower absorption in the presence of food. The peak plasma concentration (C_{max}) was almost unchanged, as was the bioavailability. The absence of statistically significant differences in these parameters indicates that food has no effect on the absorption of 'Theo-Dur' (fig. 2). Leeds et al. (1982) also found a decrease in the rate of absorption in the presence of food. The meal consisted of 2 poached eggs, toast, margarine and 4oz skimmed milk (440 kcal). Although the t_{max} occurred at 6 hours under fasting conditions and at 8 hours after intake together with the meal, there was no difference in the C_{max} values. The area under the plasma concentration-time curve (AUC) was similar. The data indicate that concomitant food intake delays, but does not diminish, the absorption.

Tinkelman et al. (1985) tested the absorption in 10 healthy adults under fasting conditions and when taken concomitantly with a high fat, low fat or liquid low fat/low carbohydrate diet breakfast. The composition of the meals was as follows: high fat meal: 38g carbohydrate, 27g protein and 34g fat (557 kcal); low fat meal: 119g carbohydrate, 20g protein and 4g fat (602 kcal); liquid low fat/low carbohydrate meal: 36g carbohydrate, 16g protein and 0g fat (220 kcal). Absorption was slightly faster with preprandial administration; C_{max} seems to occur slightly later with the high fat meal, but no statistically significant difference was found when C_{max} and t_{max} values were compared by analysis of variance (at a level of $p = 0.05$).

Spector and colleagues (Spector 1985, 1986; Spector et al. 1985) found retarded absorption of theophylline when 'Theo-Dur' was taken once a day by asthmatics together with a high fat breakfast (t_{max} shifted from 6 to 8h).

Osman et al. (1983), using the 200mg tablet, also observed slightly slower absorption of theophylline from 'Theo-Dur' when taken with breakfast. The breakfast consisted of 1 cup of cornflakes with milk, 2 poached eggs with 2 slices of buttered toast and 1 cup of caffeine-free coffee. Nine healthy adults participated in the study. With preprandial administration t_{max} occurred at about 7 hours; postprandial it was 2 hours later. The values for C_{max} and AUC were not significantly different. When 'Theo-Dur' 200mg tablets were taken in the fasted state with only 25ml of water instead of 250ml, hardly any effect was found.

It can be concluded that concomitant food intake does cause a slightly slower absorption of theophylline when taken as a 'Theo-Dur' tablet. As this delay was similar to that observed after administration by solution, it is probably of a physiological nature and not related to the biopharmaceutical characteristics of the formulation.

1.2 'Theo-Dur Sprinkle' (Key Pharmaceuticals Inc., US)

This form is made by the same manufacturer as 'Theo-Dur' but there is no similarity in (bio)pharmaceutical properties. The product is primarily intended for paediatric use.

'Theo-Dur Sprinkle' is a hard gelatin capsule, filled with coated beads, and is available at strengths of 50, 75, 125 and 200mg. The *in vitro* dissolution rate is slightly faster than that of 'Theo-Dur' tablets. The release is almost independent of the pH of the medium.

Pedersen and Møller-Petersen (1984) found that this sustained-release product was well absorbed by 12 asthmatic children under fasting conditions. However, the rate and extent of absorption were severely affected by concomitant intake of a substantial, but rather dry, breakfast. The slower absorption resulted in a reduction of the bioavailability from 91.2 ± 9.2% to 44.1 ± 3.7% (mean ± SEM) [fig. 3]. Considerable differences were found under varying food conditions. Pronounced effects were particularly found with 'dry meals' (cornflakes, rye bread, butter, salami and 180ml of low fat milk; 70% carbohydrate, 10% protein and 20% fat; approximately 12 kcal/kg). On the other hand, a 'wet meal' (300g of apple sauce and milk) had

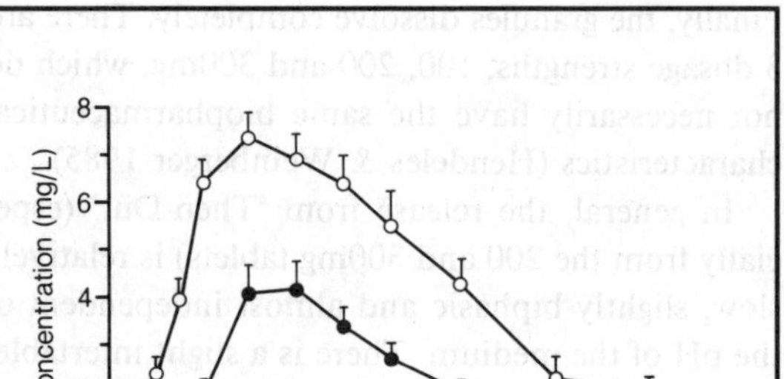

Fig. 3. Mean (± SEM) serum theophylline concentration-time curves in 12 asthmatic children after a single dose of 'Theo-Dur Sprinkle' under fasting conditions (○) and after breakfast (●) [from Pedersen & Møller-Petersen (1984), with permission].

less effect. Karim et al. (1985b) observed a similar phenomenon in adults. Food (a high fat breakfast comprising 58g carbohydrate, 33g protein and 58 to 75g fat; 870 to 1020 kcal) reduced the bioavailability to 53 ± 9% (mean ± SD) of that in the fasting state.

Leeder et al. (1986) evaluated steady-state (> 72h) serum theophylline concentrations following administration of 'Theo-Dur Sprinkle' in apple sauce to 12 asthmatic pre-school children aged 1 to 6 years. The daily dose was 23.4 ± 2.0 mg/kg (mean ± SD). Therapeutic concentrations were achieved with C_{max} of 15.1 ± 4.1 mg/L after 5.5 ± 1.5 hours. Peak-trough fluctuations were less than 100%. They were calculated according to the formula:

$$\% \text{ Fluctuation} = \frac{C_{max} - C_{min}}{C_{min}} \times 100$$

The authors concluded that the 'sprinkle technique' on apple sauce is a simple and effective method, but no comparison with the fasted state was made. It also should be realised that a small amount of apple sauce cannot be considered as a meal, and the volume of fluid might be too small to dissolve the poorly water-soluble theophylline effectively.

It can be concluded from these studies that care should be taken when giving this drug product together with food, particularly if the liquid content is low.

1.3. 'Theolair SR' (outside the US also called: 'Theolair Retard', 'Nuelin Retard', 'Nuelin SR'; Riker Laboratories Inc., USA)

This product is a tablet consisting of a matrix of cellulose acetate phthalate. In contact with the gastrointestinal medium a gel-like barrier is created, which slowly erodes under the influence of motility. It is available as tablets of 175 (not in US), 200 (US only), 250, 300 (US only), 350 (not in US) and 500mg.

The *in vitro* release of theophylline from 'Theolair SR' has been found to be pH-dependent (Jonkman et al. 1981): at pH 1.2 the dissolution rate is low, but at higher pH values (e.g. 6.8) the release rate is much faster.

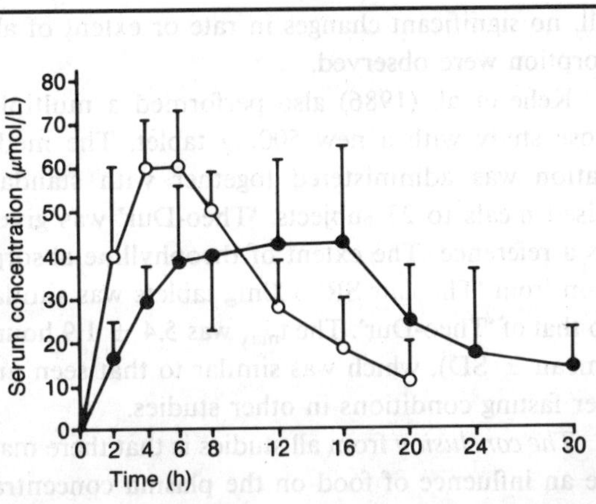

Fig. 4 Mean (± SD) serum theophylline concentration-time curves in 6 adults after a single dose of 'Theolair SR', under fasting conditions (○) and after breakfast (●) [from Pedersen & Møller-Petersen (1982), with permission].

Under fasting conditions absorption is usually complete (Jonkman et al. 1981). However, Pedersen and colleagues (Pedersen 1981; Pedersen & Møller-Petersen 1982) reported a significantly reduced absorption rate when 'Theolair SR' was given with breakfast to children or adults. The t_{max} was 16 hours longer in children and 10 hours longer in adults when the dosage form was taken with breakfast. The extent of absorption of theophylline was unaffected (fig. 4). Thompson et al. (1983), on the other hand, found that t_{max} was not influenced by food but the AUC was about 10% lower when the dose was taken with food.

Coulthard et al. (1983) found that absorption from 'Theolair SR' was much delayed in children at night, and bioavailability was significantly reduced. The cause is probably a combination of a food interaction and diurnal variation in absorption, which is probably caused by reduced gastrointestinal tract mobility at night.

Shenfield et al. (1984) reported that food appeared to delay the peak plasma concentration in 4 subjects; in another 4 C_{max} occurred earlier, and no change was observed in the remaining 4. Overall, no significant changes in rate or extent of absorption were observed.

Kehe et al. (1986) also performed a multiple-dose study with a new 500mg tablet. The medication was administered together with standardised meals to 23 subjects. 'Theo-Dur' was given as a reference. The extent of theophylline absorption from 'Theolair SR' 500mg tablets was similar to that of 'Theo-Dur'. The t_{max} was 5.4 ± 1.9 hours (mean ± SD), which was similar to that seen under fasting conditions in other studies.

The conclusion from all studies is that there may be an influence of food on the plasma concentration profile after intake of 'Theolair SR'. This preparation therefore should preferably be taken at the same time in relation to food intake every day in order to obtain optimal therapy.

1.4 'Somophyllin CRT' (Fisons plc, UK; Fisons Corporation, US)

'Somophyllin CRT' is a hard gelatine capsule filled with coated granules. It is available in strengths of 50 (not in US), 100, 200, 250, 300 and 350mg (not in US). The *in vitro* release of theophylline is fairly fast, but pH-independent and with very low intercapsule variability.

Under fasting conditions the bioavailability is usually about 100% (Pedersen & Møller-Petersen 1985). Food (breakfast) did reduce the rate of absorption in adults but only during the first 2 hours after drug intake, probably to delayed gastric emtying (Pedersen & Møller-Petersen 1985). After that time food had no effect upon the absorption characteristics of the preparation, and bioavailability was complete (fig. 5).

In other studies in children (Birkett et al. 1984; Pedersen & Steffensen 1986) similar results were found.

It can be concluded that the absorption of theophylline from 'Somophyllin CRT' is not influenced by concomitant intake of food, apart from a slight delay probably due to physiological reasons (delayed gastric emptying).

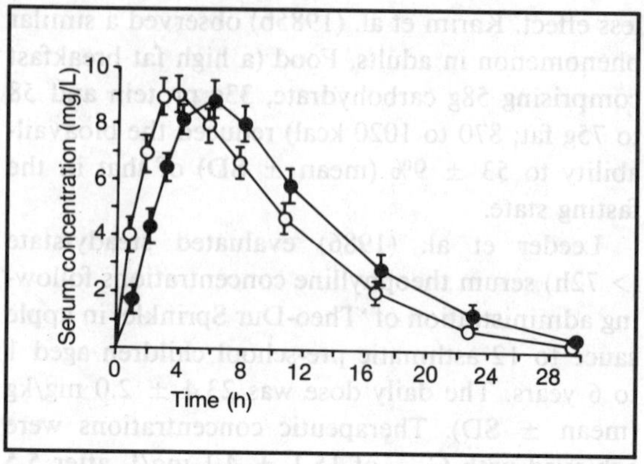

Fig. 5. Mean (± SEM) serum theophylline concentration-time curves in 10 asthmatic children after a single dose of 'Somophyllin CRT' under fasting conditions (○) and after breakfast (●) [from Pedersen & Steffensen (1986), with permission].

1.5 'Sabidal' (Zyma SA, Switzerland, 'Teovent' Ferrosan, Sweden)

This sustained-release theophylline product consists of a polymer shell filled with a salt of theophylline (theophylline cholinate) which readily dissolves and diffuses through the microporous membrane of the shell. The latter appears undissolved in the stool. It is available in three strengths: 90, 180 and 270mg. The *in vitro* release is fairly fast, pH-independent and with very small intertablet variability. The absolute bioavailability is 102 ± 10% (Jonkman et al. 1984).

Concomitant intake of an evening meal did not influence the rate or the extent of absorption (Jonkman et al. 1985). The bioavailability after intake with supper was 90.0 ± 13.8% compared with intake under fasting conditions (fig. 6).

The conclusion is that 'Sabidal' can be taken at any time in relation to food intake.

1.6 'Theograd' (Abbott Laboratories, UK)

'Theograd', the first sustained-release theophylline product to be developed, was introduced in the United Kingdom in 1974. The tablet consists of a matrix of a methylacrylate/methylmethacrylate copolymer. The granulated polymer is mixed with theophylline and compressed into 250 and 350mg tablets.

The release of theophylline *in vitro* is fairly fast; it is pH-independent (Crombeen & De Blaey 1983; Lagas & Jonkman 1986) but there is some dependence on the rotation speed.

When the 250mg tablets were taken together with breakfast, the rate of absorption decreased (t_{max} was 6.9 ± 1.0h *vs* 4.0 ± 1.7h in fasting conditions) but the amount absorbed increased from 64 ± 22% to 90 ± 13% [with an aminophylline solution as standard (Lagas & Jonkman 1983)]. A similar phenomenon was found with the 350mg tablet (Lagas & Jonkman 1985) [fig. 7]. With food, C_{max} occurred at 7.4 ± 1.4 hours (fasting: 3.4 ± 1.2h), and the postprandial bioavailability was 87 ± 14% compared with 65 ± 8% preprandial.

Therefore, it is recommended that 'Theograd' sustained-release tablets be taken after a meal.

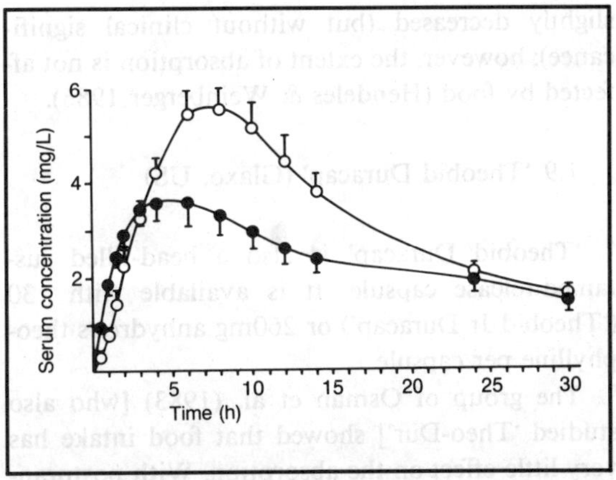

Fig. 7. Mean (± SD) serum theophylline concentration-time curves in 7 adults after ingestion of a 'Theograd' 350mg tablet under fasting conditions (●) and after breakfast (○) [from Lagas & Jonkman (1985), with permission].

1.7 'Slo-Phyllin Gyrocaps' (Rorer Pharmaceuticals, US)

This is a hard gelatine capsule filled with coated granules, available in strengths of 60, 125 and 250mg. It is one of the fastest-releasing twice-a-day theophylline products (Hendeles & Weinberger 1985). The relatively rapid absorption results in complete bioavailability.

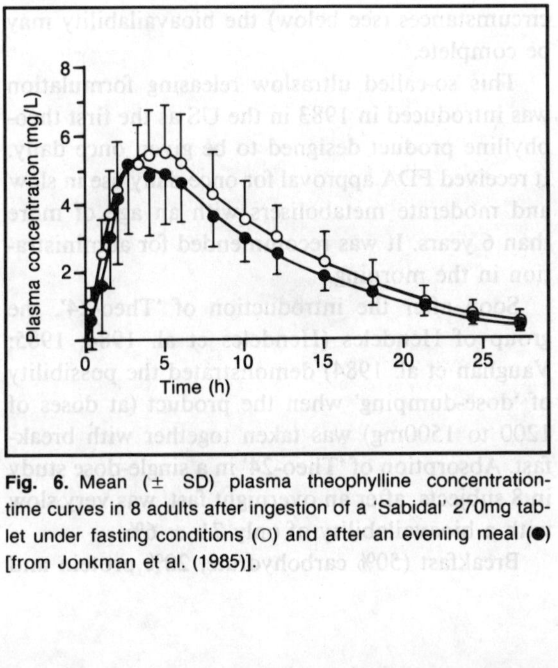

Fig. 6. Mean (± SD) plasma theophylline concentration-time curves in 8 adults after ingestion of a 'Sabidal' 270mg tablet under fasting conditions (○) and after an evening meal (●) [from Jonkman et al. (1985)].

Green et al. (1981) studied the absorption characteristics of 'Slo-Phyllin Gyrocaps' 250mg when the capsule was swallowed whole with 240ml of water and also in a crossover design when taken with water but with the capsule contents emptied and mixed with two teaspoonfuls of apple sauce. An oral solution was used as reference and 12 non-smoking adults aged 20 to 31 years participated in the study. The calculated total fraction absorbed (mean ± SEM) of the intact capsule and capsule contents in apple sauce compared with the liquid reference was 1.01 ± 0.02 and 0.86 ± 0.04, respectively. It was concluded that the 'sprinkle technique' could be used for this preparation, but as two teaspoonfuls cannot be considered as a meal, this study gives no information on the effect of food on the absorption.

1.8 'Slo-Bid Gyrocaps' (Rorer Pharmaceuticals, US)

'Slo-Bid' is also a hard gelatine capsule filled with coated granules with 50, 100, 200 and 300mg capsules available. It is an effective slow-releasing preparation. The rate of release is independent of the pH of the medium. The rate of absorption is slightly decreased (but without clinical significance); however, the extent of absorption is not affected by food (Hendeles & Weinberger 1986).

1.9 'Theobid Duracap' (Glaxo, US)

'Theobid Duracap' is also a bead-filled sustained-release capsule. It is available with 130 ('Theobid Jr Duracap') or 260mg anhydrous theophylline per capsule.

The group of Osman et al. (1983) [who also studied 'Theo-Dur'] showed that food intake has very little effect on the absorption. With postprandial administration the peak occurred slightly later (about 1.5h) and the AUC was slightly higher, but the differences were not significant (fig. 8). Similarly, there was no significant difference when the drug was taken in the fasted state with only 20ml of water instead of 250ml.

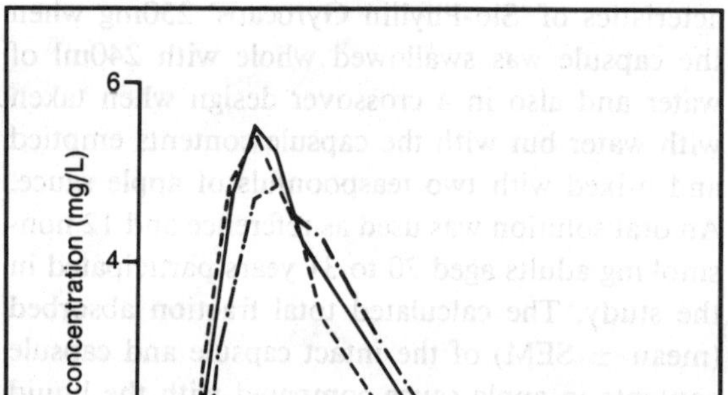

Fig. 8. Mean plasma theophylline concentration-time curves in 9 adults after ingestion of 1 'Theobid' capsule. — = with 20ml of water following overnight fast; --- = with 250ml of water following overnight fast; — · — = with 250ml of water immediately after a standard breakfast [from Osman et al. (1983), with permission].

1.10 'Phyllocontin' (Napp Laboratories, UK)

Although 'Phyllocontin' is widely used, especially in the United Kingdom, no specific data on the influence of food on the absorption of theophylline from this product are available.

1.11 'Euphyllin CR' (Byk Gulden Pharmaceuticals, Federal Republic of Germany)

'Euphyllin CR' was one of the first sustained-release preparations (a bead-filled capsule) to be launched in Europe, and is now widely used in Germany and Austria. However, no information is available on the effect of food on the absorption of theophylline from this product.

2. *Once-Daily Theophylline Preparations*

2.1 'Theo-24' (outside the US also called: 'Pulmo' Timelets; G.D. Searle & Co, US)

'Theo-24' is a hard gelatine capsule filled with coated beads available in strengths of 100, 200 and 300mg. The formulation is pH-dependent: theophylline is released more rapidly at basic pH than at acid pH, and much more rapidly at pH 7.4 than at pH 6.8 (personal observation). Under certain circumstances (see below) the bioavailability may be complete.

This so-called ultraslow releasing formulation was introduced in 1983 in the US as the first theophylline product designed to be given once daily. It received FDA approval for once-daily use in slow and moderate metabolisers with an age of more than 6 years. It was recommended for administration in the morning.

Soon after the introduction of 'Theo-24', the group of Hendeles (Hendeles et al. 1984, 1985; Vaughan et al. 1984) demonstrated the possibility of 'dose-dumping' when the product (at doses of 1200 to 1500mg) was taken together with breakfast. Absorption of 'Theo-24' in a single-dose study in 8 subjects, after an overnight fast, was very slow with a bioavailability of only 71 ± 6%.

Breakfast (50% carbohydrate, 20% protein and

30% fat; approximately 900 kcal) caused 'dose-dumping', resulting in peak concentrations that were, on average, 2.3 times higher than after a fasting dose. When taken with breakfast about half of the dose was absorbed in a 4-hour period, generally beginning 6 to 8 hours after intake. Complete absorption occurred within 24 hours. It was hypothesised that increased dissolution of the formulation might occur from exposure to the alkaline bile salts or pancreatic enzymes (or both) that are secreted following postprandial gastric emptying.

Karim and colleagues (1985a) studied the importance of meal composition and dosing time relative to meal intake when administering 'Theo-24'. They found that the serum concentration *versus* time curves were almost identical (12 subjects; 900mg) when the drug was taken under fasting conditions or immediately after a low fat breakfast (51g carbohydrate, 12g protein, 1g fat: 253 kcal) or after a medium fat breakfast (103g carbohydrate, 17g protein and 8g fat; 583 kcal), although it is questionable if a breakfast with only 8g of fat can be considered as a medium fat meal (fig. 9a).

When the drug was taken with a high fat breakfast (58g carbohydrate, 33g protein and 58 to 75g fat; 870 to 1020 kcal), C_{max} was significantly increased (mean: 13.0 mg/L, compared with 8.1 mg/L under fasting conditions). The AUC was also increased from 233 to 272 mg/L • h (fig. 9b).

In a separate study these investigators studied the importance of dosing time relative to meal intake. A dose of 'Theo-24' 900mg was given 0.5, 1.0 and 1.5 hours before and immediately after the high fat breakfast as described above. Taking the drug after the meal resulted in peak serum theophylline concentrations that were significantly higher than those achieved with the other treatments. The same observation applies to the AUC, although t_{max} was similar under all conditions. The authors conclude that if a high fat breakfast (> 55g fat) is taken, 'Theo-24' should be administered at least 1 hour before the meal.

Saccar et al. (1986) also found that the mean absorption time was significantly increased when 'Theo-24' was taken with a high fat meal.

From the studies discussed above, it can be concluded that both the rate and extent of absorption of 'Theo-24' can be significantly increased by concomitant intake of a fat breakfast. This difference might be explained by the fact that *in vitro* dissolution is dependent on the pH value (slow at low pH; fast at higher pH) and that the rate of release is correlated with the speed of rotation (which theoretically correlates with gastrointestinal motility). Although it might be preferable – based on chronopharmacological data – to administer a once-daily theophylline preparation in the evening, there

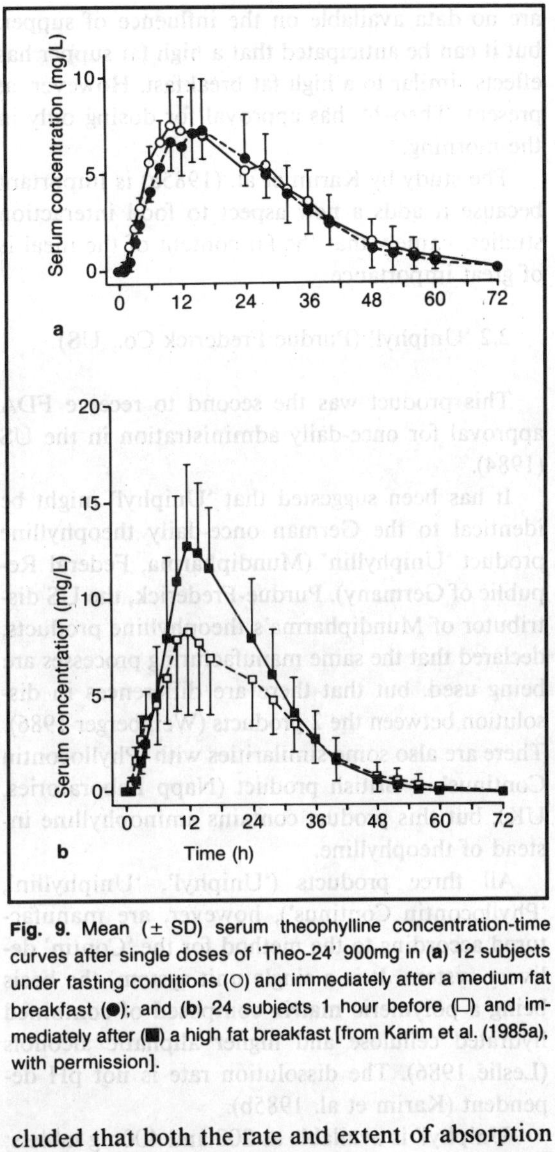

Fig. 9. Mean (± SD) serum theophylline concentration-time curves after single doses of 'Theo-24' 900mg in **(a)** 12 subjects under fasting conditions (○) and immediately after a medium fat breakfast (●); and **(b)** 24 subjects 1 hour before (□) and immediately after (■) a high fat breakfast [from Karim et al. (1985a), with permission].

are no data available on the influence of supper; but it can be anticipated that a high fat supper has effects similar to a high fat breakfast. However, at present 'Theo-24' has approval for dosing only in the morning.

The study by Karim et al. (1985a) is important because it adds a new aspect to food interaction studies, namely that the fat content of the meal is of great importance.

2.2 'Uniphyl' (Purdue Frederick Co., US)

This product was the second to receive FDA approval for once-daily administration in the US (1984).

It has been suggested that 'Uniphyl' might be identical to the German once-daily theophylline product 'Uniphyllin' (Mundipharma, Federal Republic of Germany). Purdue-Frederick, the US distributor of Mundipharma's theophylline products, declared that the same manufacturing processes are being used, but that there are differences in dissolution between the 2 products (Weinberger 1986). There are also some similarities with 'Phyllocontin Continus', a British product (Napp Laboratories, UK), but this product contains aminophylline instead of theophylline.

All three products ('Uniphyl', 'Uniphyllin', 'Phyllocontin Continus'), however, are manufactured according to the method for the 'Contin' delivery system. It is a single unit system, the basis being a polymeric matrix composed of combined hydrated cellulose and higher aliphatic alcohols (Leslie 1986). The dissolution rate is not pH dependent (Karim et al. 1985b).

'Uniphyl' is available as 200 and 400mg tablets; 'Uniphyllin' tablets contain 200 or 400 of anhydrous theophylline; and 'Phyllocontin Continus' tablets contain 100, 225 or 350mg of aminophylline. The manufacturers advise administration in the morning.

Karim et al. (1985b) studied the effect of food (breakfast) on the absorption of the US version of this product ('Uniphyl'). The composition of the breakfast was identical to the one described as 'high fat' in the section on 'Theo-24'. In 12 healthy adults

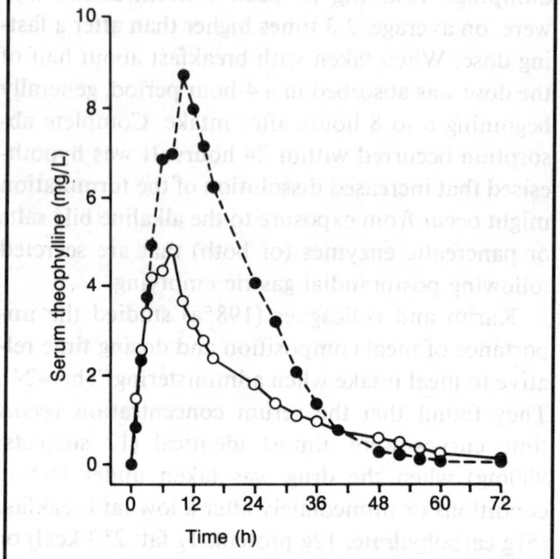

Fig. 10. Mean serum theophylline concentration-time curves in 12 subjects after a dose of 'Uniphyl' 800mg under fasting conditions (○) and immediately after a high fat breakfast (●) [from Karim et al. (1985b), with permission].

the bioavailability, relative to an immediate-release aminophylline product, increased from 53 ± 23% (mean ± SD) to 96 ± 46% when two 400mg 'Uniphyl' tablets were taken concomitantly with the high fat breakfast. The peak serum theophylline concentration increased by almost 100% (preprandial: 4.50 ± 0.92 mg/L; postprandial: 8.62 ± 2.73 mg/L). Time to peak was also almost doubled (fig. 10).

Milavetz et al. (1986) studied the bioavailability of 'Uniphyl' under fasting and non-fasting conditions in 8 adults. The extent of absorption was 68 ± 7% (mean ± SEM) following single doses and 61 ± 4% during multiple doses when taken in the fasting state. When the drug was taken immediately after a large breakfast the values were 83 ± 4% and 86 ± 4%, respectively, confirming the findings of Karim et al. (1985b).

Steffensen and Pedersen (1986) studied the European version of the drug. 'Uniphyllin' was given to 8 adults and 8 children under fasting conditions in the morning, and after a standardised breakfast (68% carbohydrate, 12% protein and 20% fat). The preparation was also administered to the adults under fasting conditions in the evening. Intravenous theophylline was used as the reference. In adults, the rate and extent of absorption were similar after all treatments. The mean C_{max} was slightly but significantly higher after administration with food (preprandial: 12.6 mg/L and postprandial: 14.4 mg/L). The bioavailability was 103 and 100%, respectively. The values for t_{max} were also comparable under both conditions (fig. 11). Thus, the findings are different from the observations of Karim et al. (1985b) and Milavetz et al. (1986) with the US version of the drug. At night, both rate and extent of absorption were found to be similar to those observed in the morning under fasting conditions. This observation is identical to the findings of Rivington et al. (1985).

The results from the adult studies were quite different from those in children at the same dose per kilogram of bodyweight. In children, food delayed the absorption of theophylline when taken as 'Uniphyllin'. The fraction absorbed at the time of each measurement was significantly lower during the first 4 hours after administration, when the drug was taken with food. The value of C_{max} was found to be about 50% higher after ingestion with food (11.1 mg/L *vs* 16.2 mg/L). The mean bioavailability was 114% in the fed state and 101% in the fasted state. In some children a high value (> 100%) was found, probably due to non-linear kinetics. Time to peak was fairly similar, except in one child (fig. 12a).

In 3 of 8 children a 'dose-dumping' phenomenon was observed (defined as more than 50% of the total dose absorbed in less than 2 hours), re-

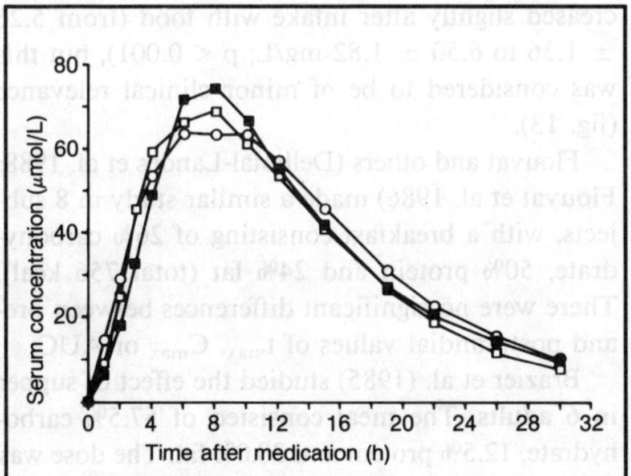

Fig. 11. Mean serum theophylline concentration-time curves after a single dose of 'Uniphyllin' under fasting conditions in the morning (○), after a standardised breakfast (■) and under fasting conditions in the evening (□) [from Steffensen & Pedersen (1986), with permission].

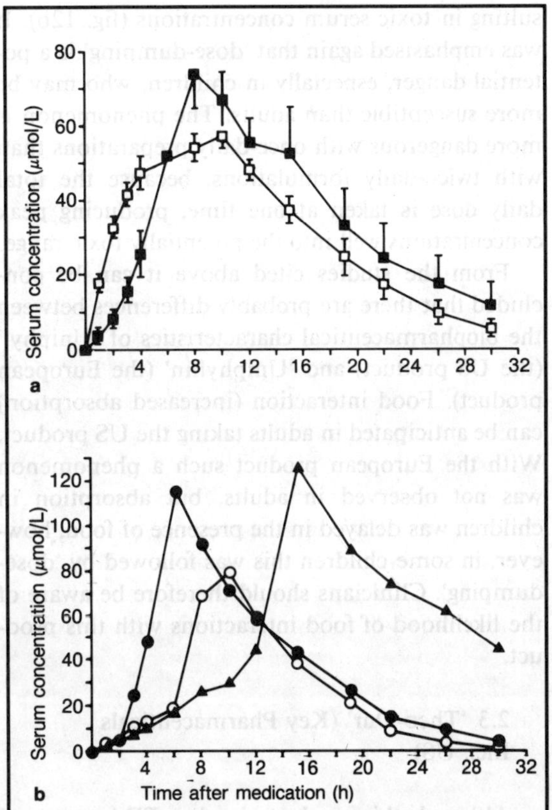

Fig. 12. Serum theophylline concentration-time curves after single doses of 'Uniphyllin' (a) in 8 children under fasting conditions (□) [mean ± SD] and after a standard breakfast (■); and (b) in 3 children in whom 'dose-dumping' was observed when the dose was ingested with a standard breakfast. (Note the different scales on the y axis) [from Steffensen & Pedersen (1985), with permission].

sulting in toxic serum concentrations (fig. 12b). It was emphasised again that 'dose-dumping' is a potential danger, especially in children, who may be more susceptible than adults. The phenomenon is more dangerous with once-daily preparations than with twice-daily formulations, because the total daily dose is taken at one time, producing peak concentrations well into the potentially toxic range.

From the studies cited above it can be concluded that there are probably differences between the biopharmaceutical characteristics of 'Uniphyl' (the US product) and 'Uniphyllin' (the European product). Food interaction (increased absorption) can be anticipated in adults taking the US product. With the European product such a phenomenon was not observed in adults, but absorption in children was delayed in the presence of food; however, in some children this was followed by 'dose-dumping'. Clinicians should therefore be aware of the likelihood of food interactions with this product.

2.3 'Theo-Dur' (Key Pharmaceuticals Inc., US)

Although this product also has FDA approval for once-daily use in the same population of patients as the other 2 products, the manufacturer still recommends the product be taken twice a day for optimal therapy. The studies dealing with the effects of food in theophylline absorption after intake of 'Theo-Dur' have been discussed in the section on twice-daily preparations.

2.4 'Dilatrane AP' (Fisons plc, UK)

'Dilatrane AP' is a hard gelatine capsule, filled with coated beads. It was introduced by the French subsidiary of Fisons plc, UK, and as yet is on the market only in France. It is available in strengths of 200, 350 and 400mg.

The *in vitro* release is quite rapid when compared with 'Theo-24', but is almost pH independent (personal observation).

In a single-dose crossover experiment the influence of breakfast on the bioavailability was studied in 12 healthy adults (Jonkman et al. 1986). The breakfast consisted of 47% carbohydrate, 16% protein and 37% fat (total 2000 kJ = 476 kcal). When taken with the breakfast, the mean values of t_{max} increased slightly (not significantly). A similar result was found for the AUC. The mean C_{max} increased slightly after intake with food (from 5.26 ± 1.36 to 6.50 ± 1.82 mg/L; $p < 0.001$), but this was considered to be of minor clinical relevance (fig. 13).

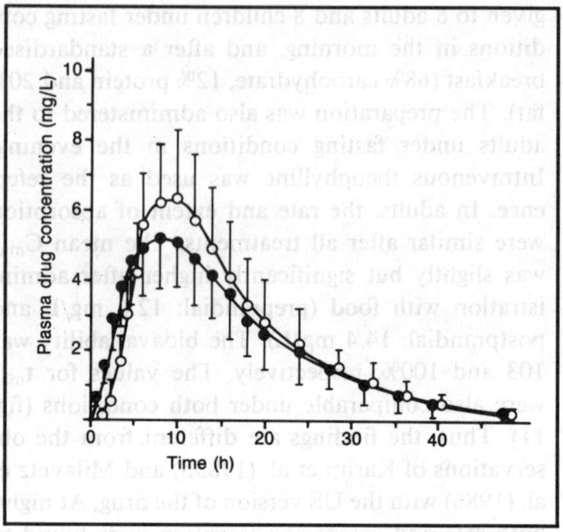

Fig. 13. Mean (± SD) plasma theophylline concentration-time curves in 12 subjects after a dose of 'Dilatrane AP' 400mg under fasting conditions (●) and after a standardised breakfast (○) [from Jonkman et al. (1987)].

Flouvat and others (Delhotal-Landes et al. 1988; Flouvat et al. 1986) made a similar study in 8 subjects, with a breakfast consisting of 26% carbohydrate, 50% protein and 24% fat (total 756 kcal). There were no significant differences between pre- and postprandial values of t_{max}, C_{max} or AUC.

Brazier et al. (1985) studied the effect of supper in 6 adults. The meal consisted of 57.5% carbohydrate, 12.5% protein and 30.0% fat. The dose was taken at 8 p.m. and the meal was taken at 6 p.m., 8 p.m. and midnight on 3 separate occasions. In comparison with the fasted state (meal 4h after drug intake) both t_{max} and C_{max} increased when the drug was taken 2 hours after or concomitant with the meal. The peak was delayed about 2.5 to 3.0 hours by food and C_{max} was increased by 8 to 10%. The AUC was identical during all 3 treatments.

It can be concluded that concomitant intake of 'Dilatrane AP' and food (breakfast or supper) caused only a slight delay of the absorption, probably due to physiological reasons. No indications of 'dose-dumping' were found with this once-daily theophylline preparation.

2.5 'Euphylong' (Byk Gulden Pharmaceuticals, Federal Republic of Germany)

This is a new theophylline once-daily capsule, filled with micropellets with a porous membrane. It is available in strengths of 250, 350 and 500mg.

The *in vitro* release of theophylline from 'Euphylong' is consistent, with little intercapsule variation. The dissolution is only slightly influenced by the rotation speed, and is pH independent. It is designed for administration in the evening.

The product has been extensively tested for a possible influence on the bioavailability of the drug by concomitant food intake (and by different dietary habits such as cold and hot evening meals) [Schultz et al. 1987]. Both rate and extent of absorption were identical when the preparation was taken before or 30 minutes after a cold standardised evening meal. Similar results were obtained with a hot evening meal. This indicates that time of drug intake is not important with this product (fig. 14).

The formulation was also tested by administration 30 minutes after cold and hot evening meals in a crossover study. The composition of the meal was as follows: 151g carbohydrate, 75g protein and 43g fat. A 10% decrease in AUC and a 20% decrease in C_{max} was observed when 'Euphylong' was administered after the hot meal, and t_{max} was slightly shorter (8 *vs* 10h). This observation can probably be explained by the differences in the physiological situation in the gastrointestinal tract after a hot compared with a cold meal. The differences are probably without clinical relevance.

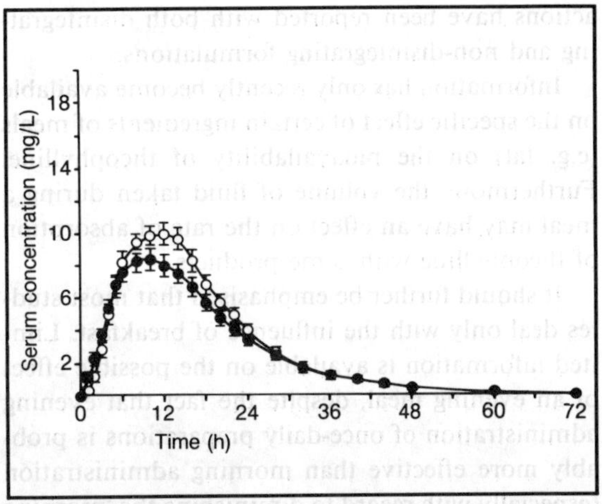

Fig. 14. Mean (± SEM) serum theophylline concentration-time curves in 12 adults after a single dose of 'Euphylong' 800mg before (●) and after (○) a hot evening meal [from Schultz et al. (1987), with permission].

2.6 Riker Once-Daily Controlled-Release Theophylline (Riker Laboratories, UK)

Riker has recently developed a bead-filled once-daily controlled-release theophylline, but it is not yet on the market. First reports on this product indicate that its absorption is not influenced by food to a significant extent (McEwen et al. 1988; Moreland et al. 1988; Pedersen & Steffensen 1987).

3. *Discussion*

Concomitant intake of food can have a substantial influence on the bioavailability of a sustained-release theophylline preparation. This phenomenon was only recently recognised, and not all brands of sustained-release theophylline preparations used in daily practice have been studied in this respect.

When theophylline (even as a solution) is taken with food, the absorption is generally delayed by about 2 to 3 hours, apparently due to delayed gastric emptying. Whether or not a further decrease (or increase) of the rate of absorption and/or the amount of absorption occurs depends predominantly on the biopharmaceutical properties of the specific sustained-release preparation. Food interactions have been reported with both disintegrating and non-disintegrating formulations.

Information has only recently become available on the specific effect of certain ingredients of meals (e.g. fat) on the bioavailability of theophylline. Furthermore, the volume of fluid taken during a meal may have an effect on the rate of absorption of theophylline with some products.

It should further be emphasised that most studies deal only with the influence of breakfast. Limited information is available on the possible effect of an evening meal, despite the fact that evening administration of once-daily preparations is probably more effective than morning administration (especially with regard to diminishing the 'morning dip'). This aspect of time of day is important because circadian rhythms in theophylline absorption have also been documented (Jonkman & Smolensky 1984; Smolensky et al. 1985). With 1 preparation ('Theo-24') it was found that the bioavailability was markedly affected by dosing time (Hiatt et al. 1986).

It appears to be very difficult to distinguish the role of food intake on day/night differences in theophylline absorption (Jonkman 1986). Moreover, the effect of posture cannot be excluded (Warren et al. 1985). Mean theophylline concentrations were significantly higher in the standing position after intake of a twice-daily sustained-release preparation.

The phenomenon of 'dose-dumping' that occurs under certain circumstances with some once-daily preparations is a matter of great concern. Because the complete daily dose is given at once, it is a particular potential danger for patients who require high doses (e.g. > 1200 mg/day). An additional problem is the fact that with 24h preparations the total daily dose is taken at once. As there are indications that theophylline obeys the rules of non-linear pharmacokinetics (Tang-Liu et al. 1982; Wagner 1985), higher doses at one time might easily result in unexpectedly high plasma concentrations. There are indications that children are more susceptible to the occurrence of 'dose-dumping' than adults.

It is difficult to predict whether food will have an effect on a specific sustained-release brand of theophylline. The manufacturers of the different brands use different methods and ingredients to obtain the sustained-release properties of their products, and these methods are usually patented. It is also difficult to predict the *in vivo* effect of food based on *in vitro* dissolution tests. If a pronounced pH-dependent release has been found *in vitro*, food can be expected to have a pronounced effect. One recent paper describes a new *in vitro* method which can probably be used to detect the effect of a high fat meal *in vivo* (Maturu et al. 1986).

The hard facts, however, will have to be defined by means of clinical studies. Probably because the clinical impact of the effect of food on bioavailability has been recognised only during the past 4 years, most registration authorities have not yet published official requirements for food-effect studies. One exception is the FDA in the United States. Since 1983, the FDA has required information on the effects of food for all prescription New Drug Applications (NDA) for controlled-release drug products submitted.

Unofficially, it has been recommended (Skelly et al. 1987) that at least 1 study be performed in order to detect a possible effect. This could be done by conducting a single-dose, three-way crossover study with the following treatments: the sustained-release formulation administered under fasting conditions; the same formulation administered concomitantly with a high fat meal; and finally, a rapidly available form of the drug administered under fasting conditions.

If no significant differences are found in the AUC and C_{max} in such a study, no further food-effect studies are necessary. But if an effect has been detected, it will need to be investigated and quantitated in more detail.

In Europe, most registration authorities have not yet published official requirements for food-effect studies.

4. Conclusion

The recent literature indicates that food can have a substantial, but variable, effect on the bioavailability of several brands of sustained-release theophylline preparations (table I).

Table I. Summary of the effects of food on various theophylline formulations

Product	Rate of absorption	Extent of absorption
Solution	–	–
12h preparations		
'Sabidal'	–	0
'Slo-Bid Gyrocaps'	––	0
'Somophyllin CRT'	–	0
'Theobid Duracap'	0	0
'Theo-Dur'	––	0
'Theo-Dur Sprinkle'	–––	–––
'Theograd'	–	+++
'Theolair SR'	–––	–
24h preparations		
'Dilatrane AP'	–	+
'Euphylong'	–	–
'Theo-24'	+++	+++
'Uniphyl'	–	++

Abbreviations: 0 = no effect; –/+ = slight decrease/increase (not clinically relevant); ––/++ = moderate decrease/increase; –––/+++ = significant decrease/increase (clinically relevant).

In light of the different influences (food interaction, circadian rhythm, posture) it is important that the patient is informed in detail about the conditions (especially time of day and time in relation to a meal) that are optimal for the product which is prescribed. In addition, the clinician should bear in mind that switching from one sustained-release theophylline product to another may be risky, and should be avoided.

References

Anderson KE, Conney AH, Kappas A. Nutrition and oxidative drug metabolism in man: relative influence of dietary lipids, carbohydrate and protein. Clinical Pharmacology and Therapeutics 26: 493-501, 1979

Anderson KE, Kappas A. Dietary influences on the metabolism of theophylline and other drugs in humans. In Jonkman et al. (Eds) Sustained release theophylline in the treatment of chronic reversible airways obstruction, pp. 83-90, Excerpta Medica, Amsterdam, 1984

Birkett DJ, Coulthard KP, Lines D, Grgurinovich N. Circadian variation in the absorption of three sustained release theophylline products in asthmatic children and the effect of food on absorption of Somophyllin® C.R.T. British Journal of Clinical Practice 38 (Suppl. 35): 17-23, 1984

Boxenbaum HG. Physiological and pharmacokinetic factors affecting performance of sustained release dosage forms. Drug Development and Industrial Pharmacy 8: 1-25, 1982

Brazier JL, Soubeyrand J, Desage M, Gillet A, Georges D. Influence de l'alimentation sur la cinétique d'une théophylline à action prolongée prise une fois par jour. Acta Therapeutica 11 (Suppl.): 35-47, 1985

Coulthard KP, Birkett DJ, Lines DR, Grgurinovich N, Grygiel JJ. Bioavailability and diurnal variation in absorption of sustained release theophylline in asthmatic children. European Journal of Clinical Pharmacology 25: 667-672, 1983

Crombeen JP, de Blaey CJ. *In vitro* testing of controlled release theophylline preparations: Theolair®, Theograd® and Theolin®. Pharmaceutisch Weekblad – Scientific Edition 5: 65-69, 1983

Delhotal-Landes B, Flouvat B, Boutin MS, Karpouzas I, Prinseau J. Influence of food on the absorption of theophylline administered in the form of sustained release tablet and microgranules. Biopharmaceutics and Drug Disposition 9: 19-29, 1988

Feldman CH, Hutchinson VE, Pippenger CE, Blumenfeld TA, Feldman BR, et al. Effect of dietary protein and carbohydrate on theophylline metabolism in children. Pediatrics 66: 956-962, 1980

Feldman CH, Hutchinson VE, Sher TH, Feldman BR, Davis WJ. Interaction between nutrition and theophylline metabolism in children. Therapeutic Drug Monitoring 4: 69-76, 1982

Flouvat B, Delhotal-Landes B, Boutin-Pannetier MS. Influence de la nourriture sur la biodisponibilité de la théophylline présentée sous une formulation à libération prolongée (Dilatrane® AP). Thérapie 41: 144-145, 1986

Golub AL, Frost RW, Betlach CJ, Gonzalez MA. Physiologic considerations in drug absorption from the gastrointestinal tract. Journal of Allergy and Clinical Immunology 78: 689-694, 1986

Green ER, Green AW, Lanc R, Slaughter R, Middleton E. Absorption characteristics of sustained release theophylline capsules administered in applesauce. Journal of Pediatrics 98: 832-834, 1981

Hendeles L, Iafrate RP, Weinberger M. A clinical and pharmacokinetic basis for the selection and use of slow release theophylline products. Clinical Pharmacokinetics 9: 95-134, 1984

Hendeles L, Massanari M, Weinberger M. Update on the pharmacodynamics and pharmacokinetics of theophylline. Chest 88 (Suppl.): 103S-111S, 1985

Hendeles L, Weinberger M, Milavetz G, Hill M, Vaughan L. Food-induced 'dose-dumping' from a once-a-day theophylline product as a cause of theophylline toxicity. Chest 87: 758-765, 1985

Hendeles L, Weinberger M. Selection of a slow release theophylline product. Journal of Allergy and Clinical Immunology 78: 743-751, 1986

Hendeles L, Weinberger M. Theophylline product and dosing interval selection for chronic asthma. Journal of Allergy and Clinical Immunology 76: 285-291, 1985

Hendeles L, Weinberger M. Theophylline: 'state of the art' review. Pharmacotherapy 3: 2-44, 1983

Hendeles L, Wubbena P, Weinberger M. Food-induced 'dose-dumping' of once-a-day theophylline. Lancet 2: 1471, 1984

Hiatt P, Scott P, Hearn D, Krames W, Smolensky M, et al. Effect of dosing time on pharmacokinetics of once daily theophylline in asthmatic children. American Review of Respiratory Diseases 133: A42, 1986

Jonkman JHG, Berg WChr, de Vries K, de Zeeuw RA, Schoenmaker R, et al. Disposition and clinical pharmacokinetics of theophylline after administration of a new sustained release tablet. European Journal of Clinical Pharmacology 21: 39-44, 1981

Jonkman JHG, Grasmeijer G, Holland A. Theophylline disposition after single-dose ingestion of a once-a-day preparation (Dilatrane AP 400mg) with and without breakfast. International Journal of Clinical Pharmacology, Therapy and Toxicology 25: 633-637, 1987

Jonkman JHG, Schoenmaker R, Grimberg N, de Zeeuw RA. A new *in vitro* dissolution test for controlled release theophylline tablets. International Journal of Pharmaceutics 8: 153-156, 1981

Jonkman JHG, Smolensky MH. Chronopharmacology of theophylline, with special reference to age. Annual Review of Chronopharmacology 1: 73-76, 1984

Jonkman JHG. The role of food intake on day-night differences in theophylline absorption. Annual Review of Chronopharmacology 3: 161-164, 1986

Jonkman JHG, van der Boon WJV, Balant LP, Le Cotonnec JY. Food reduces the rate but not the extent of the absorption of theophylline from an aqueous solution. European Journal of Clinical Pharmacology 28: 225-227, 1985

Jonkman JHG, van der Boon WJV, Balant LP, Le Cotonnec JY. No effect of food on single dose bioavailability of sustained release theophylline (Sabidal®): a comparison between Sabidal® and choline theophyllinate solution. International Journal of Pharmaceutics 25: 113-117, 1985

Jonkman JHG, van der Boon WJV, Balant LP, Schoenmaker R, Holtkamp A. Chronopharmacokinetics of theophylline after sustained release and intravenous administration to adults. European Journal of Clinical Pharmacology 25: 215-222, 1984

Juan D, Worwag EM, Schoeller DA, Kotake AN, Hughes RL, Frederiksen MC. Effects of dietary protein on theophylline pharmacokinetics and caffeine and aminopyrine breath tests. Clinical Pharmacology and Therapeutics 40: 187-194, 1986

Kappas A, Alvares AP, Anderson KE, Pantuck EJ, Pantuck CB, et al. Effect of charcoal-broiled beef on antipyrine and theophylline metabolism. Clinical Pharmacology and Therapeutics 23: 445-450, 1978

Kappas A, Anderson KE, Conney AH, Alvares AP. Influence of dietary protein and carbohydrate on antipyrine and theophylline metabolism in man. Clinical Pharmacology and Therapeutics 20: 643-653, 1976

Karim A, Burns T, Janky D, Hurwitz A. Food-induced changes in theophylline absorption from controlled release formulations, part II: importance of meal composition and dosing time relative to meal intake in assessing changes in absorption. Clinical Pharmacology and Therapeutics 38: 642-647, 1985a

Karim A, Burns T, Wearley L, Streicher J, Palmer M. Food-induced changes in theophylline absorption from controlled release formulations, part I: substantial increased and decreased absorption with Uniphyl® tablets and Theo-Dur® Sprinkle. Clinical Pharmacology and Therapeutics 38: 77-83, 1985b

Kehe CR, Ekholm BP, Chann SF, Wick KA, Rhode KA, et al. Comparative absorption of theophylline from Theolair® S.R. and two reference theophylline preparations following multiple doses with food. Current Therapeutic Research 39: 3-7, 1986

Lagas M, Jonkman JHG. Greatly enhanced bioavailability of theophylline on postprandial administration of a sustained release tablet. European Journal of Clinical Pharmacology 24: 761-767, 1983

Lagas M, Jonkman JHG. Influence of food on the rate and extent of absorption of theophylline after single dose oral administration of a controlled release tablet. International Journal of Clinical Pharmacology, Therapy and Toxicology 23: 424-426, 1985

Lagas M, Jonkman JHG. Studies on the delivery mechanisms of theophylline from a sustained release tablet. Drug Development and Industrial Pharmacy 12: 489-506, 1986

Leeder JS, Robertson C, Correia JN, Isles AF, Levison H, et al. Evaluation of serum theophylline concentrations following administration of sustained release beads in applesauce to asthmatic pre-school children. Annals of Allergy 56: 133-137, 1986

Leeds NH, Gal P, Purohit AA, Walter JB. Effect of food on the bioavailability and pattern of release of a sustained release theophylline tablet. Journal of Clinical Pharmacology 22: 196-200, 1982

Leslie S. The Contin delivery system: dosing considerations. Journal of Allergy and Clinical Immunology 78: 768-773, 1986

Maturu PK, Prasad VK, Worsley WN, Shin GK, Skelly JP. Influence of a high fat breakfast on the bioavailability of theophylline controlled release formulations: an *in vitro* demonstration of an *in vivo* observation. Journal of Pharmaceutical Sciences 79: 1205-1206, 1986

McEwen J, McMurdo MET, Moreland TA. The effect of food on the pharmacokinetics of controlled release theophylline capsules formulation following multiple dosing. Research and Clinical Forums 10: 47-54, 1988

Melander A. Influence of food on the bioavailability of drugs. Clinical Pharmacokinetics 3: 337-351, 1978

Milavetz G, Vaughan L, Weinberger M, Harris J, Mullenix T. Bioavailability of oral theophylline: single and multiple dose studies of Uniphyl®. Journal of Allergy and Clinical Immunology 77: 146, 1986

Moreland TA, McMurdo MET, McEwen J. The effect of fasting, food and antacid on the pharmacokinetics of controlled release theophylline capsules. Research and Clinical Forums 10: 43-46, 1988

Osman MA, Patel RB, Irwin DS, Welling PG. Absorption of theophylline from enteric coated and sustained release formulations in fasted and non-fasted subjects. Biopharmaceutics and Drug Disposition 4: 63-72, 1983

Pedersen S. Delay in the absorption rate of theophylline from a sustained release theophylline preparation caused by food. British Journal of Clinical Pharmacology 12: 904-905, 1981

Pedersen S, Møller-Petersen J. Erratic absorption of a slow release theophylline sprinkle product. Pediatrics 74: 534-538, 1984

Pedersen S, Møller-Petersen J. Influence of food on the absorption rate and bioavailability of a sustained release theophylline preparation. Allergy 37: 531-534, 1982

Pedersen S, Møller-Petersen J. Influence of food on the absorption of theophylline from a sustained release formulation (Somophyllin®). Clinical Allergy 15: 253-259, 1985

Pedersen S, Steffensen G. Absorption characteristics of once-a-day slow release theophylline preparation in children with asthma. Journal of Pediatrics 110: 953-959, 1987

Pedersen S, Steffensen G. Food and fasting absorption of a single dose of a sustained release theophylline sprinkle formulation in children. Allergy 41: 46-50, 1986

Rivington RN, Calcutt L, Child S, MacLeod JP, Hodder RV, et al. Comparison of morning versus evening dosing with a new once-daily oral theophylline formulation. American Journal of Medicine 79 (Suppl. 6A): 67-72, 1985

Saccar CL, Rocci Jr ML, Mansmann Jr HC. The effect of food on the *in vivo* mean absorption and dissolution times of two sustained release theophylline (SRT) preparations. Journal of Allergy and Clinical Immunology 77: 146, 1986

Schulz HU, Karlsson S, Sahner-Ahrens I, Steinijans VW, Beier W. Effect of drug intake prior to or after meals on serum theophylline concentrations: single dose studies with Euphylong®. International Journal of Clinical Pharmacology, Therapy and Toxicology 25: 222-228, 1987

Shenfield GM, Hudson BJ, Boutagy JS, Munro IA, Vandenberg RA. Effect of food and tablet division on the absorption of a sustained release preparation of theophylline. Medical Journal of Australia 140: 477-479, 1984

Sips AP, Edelbroek PM, Kulstad S, de Wolff FA, Dijkman JH. Food does not affect the bioavailability of theophylline from Theolin® Retard. European Journal of Clinical Pharmacology 26: 405-407, 1984

Skelly JP, Barr WH, Benet LZ, Doluisio JT, Goldberg AH, et al. Report of the workshop on controlled release dosage forms: issues and controversies. Pharmaceutical Research 4: 75-77, 1987

Smolensky MH, Scott PH, Barnes PJ, Jonkman JHG. The chronopharmacology and chronotherapy of asthma. Annual Review of Chronopharmacology 2: 229-273, 1985

Spector SL. Advantages and disadvantages of 24-hour theophylline. Journal of Allergy and Clinical Immunology 76: 302-311, 1985

Spector SL, Rohr AS, Rachelefsky GS, Katz RM, Siegel SC, et al. The effect of food on once daily Theo-Dur® in asthmatic subjects. Journal of Allergy and Clinical Immunology 75: 105, 1985

Spector SS. Theophylline once-a-day dosage. Chest 90: 623-625, 1986

Steffensen G, Pedersen S. Food induced changes in theophylline absorption from a once-a-day theophylline product. British Journal of Clinical Pharmacology 22: 571-577, 1986

Tang-Liu DDS, Williams RL, Riegelman S. Non-linear theophylline elimination. Clinical Pharmacology and Therapeutics 31: 358-369, 1982

Thompson PJ, Kemp MW, McAllister WAC, Turner-Warwick M. Slow release theophylline in patients with airways obstruction with particular reference to the effects of food upon serum levels. British Journal of Diseases of the Chest 77: 293-298, 1983

Thompson PJ, Skypala I, Dawson S, McAllister WAC, Turner-Warwick M. The effect of diet upon serum concentrations of theophylline. British Journal of Clinical Pharmacology 16: 267-270, 1983

Tinkelman DG, Edelman L, Decouto J, Maloch LD, Spangler DL. The effect of diet on the metabolism of long acting theophylline. Annals of Allergy 54: 280-283, 1985

Vaughan L, Milavetz G, Hill M, Weinberger M, Hendeles L. Food-induced 'dose-dumping' of Theo-24, a once-daily slow release theophylline product. Drug Intelligence and Clinical Pharmacy 18: 510, 1984

Wagner JG. Theophylline: pooled Michaelis-Menten parameters (V_{max} and K_m) and implications. Clinical Pharmacokinetics 10: 432-442, 1985

Warren JB, Cuss F, Barnes PJ. Posture and theophylline kinetics. British Journal of Clinical Pharmacology 19: 707-709, 1985

Weinberger M. Clinical and pharmacokinetic concerns of 24-hour dosing with theophylline. Annals of Allergy 56: 2-8, 1986

Welling PG. Influence of food and diet on gastrointestinal drug absorption – a review. Journal of Pharmacokinetics and Biopharmaceutics 5: 291-334, 1977

Welling PG, Lyons LL, Craig WA, Trochta GA. Influence of diet and fluid on bioavailability of theophylline. Clinical Pharmacology and Therapeutics 17: 475-480, 1975

Author's address: Dr *J.H.G. Jonkman*, Pharma Bio-Research International B.V., P.O. Box 147, NL-9400 AC Assen, The Netherlands.

Original Research Article

Clinical Pharmacokinetics 16: 180-185 (1989)
0312-5963/89/0003-0180/$03.00/0

Lack of Effect of Influenza Vaccine on the Pharmacokinetics of Antipyrine, Alprazolam, Paracetamol (Acetaminophen) and Lorazepam

Joseph M. Scavone, Gershwin T. Blyden and *David J. Greenblatt*
Division of Clinical Pharmacology, Tufts University School of Medicine and New England Medical Center, Boston, Massachusetts, USA

Summary *31 healthy male (n = 17) and female (n = 14) volunteers, aged 20 to 45 years, were divided into 4 groups and received on 3 separate occasions either: paracetamol (acetaminophen) 650mg intravenously (n = 9); alprazolam 1mg orally (n = 7); antipyrine (phenazone) 1g intravenously (n = 8); or lorazepam 2mg intravenously (n = 7). Doses were administered prior to influenza vaccine (0.5ml, intramuscularly) and at 7 and 21 days post-vaccination. The overall differences among the 3 trials in clearance of antipyrine were of borderline significance (p < 0.0611), with a trend towards reduced clearance in both of the post-vaccination trials. There were no overall differences observed in the elimination half-life of antipyrine, nor were there significant differences between trials in cumulative urinary excretion or fractional recovery of intact antipyrine, 4-hydroxyantipyrine, norantipyrine, or 3-hydroxymethyl antipyrine. For paracetamol and alprazolam, there were no significant differences among the 3 trials in any of the kinetic variables. The elimination half-life of lorazepam varied significantly among trials, but differences were small and not systematic. Lorazepam clearance did not vary significantly among trials. Thus, clearance of drugs which undergo hepatic conjugative reactions such as glucuronidation and sulphation are unlikely to be affected by the coadministration of influenza vaccine. Furthermore, not all drugs which are biotransformed by hepatic microsomal oxidation necessarily have impaired clearance due to coadministration of influenza vaccine.*

Influenza vaccination has been associated with the impaired elimination of some drugs metabolised primarily by the hepatic cytochrome P450 microsomal enzyme system (Fischer et al. 1982; Harless 1983; Kramer & McClain 1981; Kramer et al. 1984; Levine et al. 1984; Meredith et al. 1985; Renton et al. 1980; Walker et al. 1980). This effect was found to persist for up to 3 to 4 weeks after inoculation (Kramer & McClain 1981; Kramer et al. 1984). The potential clinical importance of this observation is especially obvious in chronically ill patients who frequently take drugs with low therapeutic indices. However, some studies have not confirmed the effect of influenza vaccine on drug biotransformation (Bukowskyj et al. 1984; Fischer et al. 1982; Goldstein et al. 1982; Meredith et al. 1985; San Joaquin et al. 1982; Stults & Hashisaki 1983). Thus, the actual extent and the clinical importance of impaired drug metabolism due to the influenza vaccine is not clearly established. The present study evaluates the effect of influenza vaccine on the pharmacokinetics of antipyrine (phenazone) and alprazolam, which are metabolised mainly by microsomal oxidation, and of paracetamol (acetaminophen) and lorazepam, which are metabolised mainly by conjugation.

Methods

Subjects

31 healthy male and female volunteers aged 20 to 45 years participated after giving written informed consent. All were healthy, active, ambulatory adults receiving no medication and without history of medical disease. Female subjects were not taking oral contraceptives. Screening procedures included: medical history, blood counts, laboratory screening profile (SMA-20) and urinalysis. Subjects were excluded from the study if any of these procedures revealed clinically important abnormalitics which might have made participation inappropriate or unsafe. They were also excluded if they were taking paracetamol or any benzodiazepines within 1 month of the start of the study.

Procedure

Subjects were randomly assigned to 4 groups and received either antipyrine, alprazolam, lorazepam, or paracetamol on 3 separate occasions. The influenza virus vaccine ('Trivalent', Types A and B, Wyeth Laboratories, Inc., Radnor, PA) contained the proportions and not less than the microgram amounts of haemaglutinin antigens (μg HA) representative of the following components: 15μg HA of A/Brasil/11/78 (H1N1), 15μg HA of A/Phillipines/2/82 (H3N2), and 15μg HA of B/Singapore/222/79.

At least 1 week before vaccination, each subject received either: antipyrine 1g administered intravenously by 5-minute infusion; alprazolam 1mg orally; lorazepam 2mg administered intravenously over 1 minute; or paracetamol 650mg administered intravenously by 5-minute infusion. Subjects were vaccinated with influenza vaccine (0.5ml by gluteal intramuscular injection) at least 7 days later. Seven and 21 days post-vaccination, all subjects received another single dose of the same drug. The subjects in the alprazolam group fasted overnight and ingested a single 1mg dose with 100 to 200ml of tap water. They remained fasting until 3 hours after the dose, at which time they resumed their normal diet. Subjects receiving intravenous medications had no dietary restrictions.

Venous blood samples were drawn prior to each drug administration, and at multiple points in time up to 48 hours after dosage. Samples were drawn from an indwelling butterfly cannula (kept patent by a slow infusion of physiological saline solution) for the first 8 hours, and then by separate venipuncture. All samples were collected into 'Vacutainer' heparinised tubes (Becton-Dickinson, Rutherford, NJ). Blood samples were centrifuged and the plasma was separated and stored at −20°C until the time of assay. For subjects who received antipyrine, a 48-hour urine collection commenced at the termination of the antipyrine infusion.

Analysis of Samples

Concentrations of antipyrine (Greenblatt et al. 1983) and paracetamol (Ameer et al. 1981) in plasma samples were determined by high pressure liquid chromatography (HPLC). Concentrations of intact antipyrine and its three principal metabolites (norantipyrine, 4-hydroxyantipyrine and 3-hydroxymethyl antipyrine) in all urine samples were also determined by HPLC (Blyden et al. 1986). Plasma lorazepam (Greenblatt et al. 1978) and alprazolam (Greenblatt et al. 1981) concentrations were analysed by electron-capture gas-liquid chromatography. All samples from a given subject's set of trials were extracted and analysed on the same day using the same calibration standards.

For alprazolam, the slope (β) of the terminal log-linear phase of the plasma concentration/time curves was used to calculate the apparent elimination half-life. Area under the plasma concentration-time curve (AUC) from time zero until the last detectable concentration was determined by the linear trapezoidal method. To this was added the residual area extracted to infinity, calculated as the actual final concentration divided by β, yielding the total area under the plasma concentration/time curve from time zero to infinity ($AUC_{0-\infty}$). Total

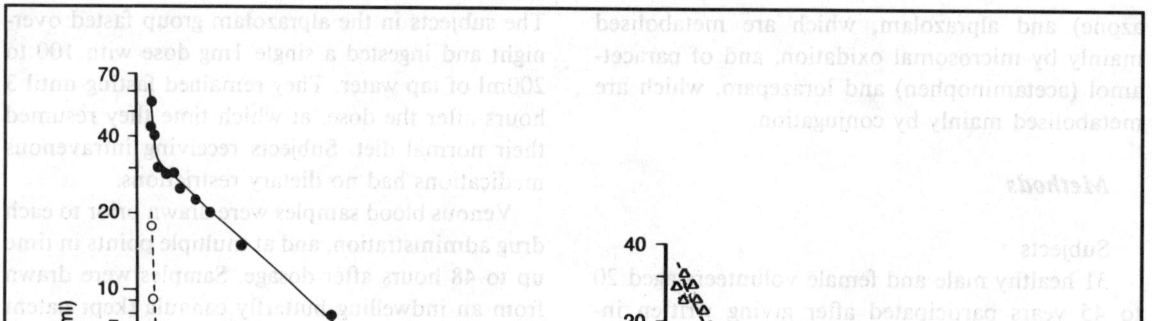

Fig. 1. Representative pre-vaccination control plasma drug concentration curves. ○ = Paracetamol (acetaminophen) 650mg IV; ● = antipyrine (phenazone) 1g IV; ▲ = alprazolam 1mg PO; △ = lorazepam 2mg IV.

oral clearance was calculated as dose divided by $AUC_{0-\infty}$ and apparent volume of distribution as clearance divided by β. Although calculated values of volume of distribution and clearance for an orally-administered medication depend on absolute bioavailability, previous studies of oral alprazolam indicate that bioavailability after oral dosage is close to 100% (Smith et al. 1984). For the other 3 drugs, data points were fitted to a linear sum of 2 or 3 exponential terms (Harmatz & Greenblatt 1987), with the choice between bi- and tri-exponential equations made on the basis of visual goodness-of-fit and on the sum of squares of weighted residual errors. The fitted function was used to calculate volume of distribution by the area method, elimination half-life, and total clearance (Greenblatt & Koch-Weser 1975).

Differences in kinetic variables among the 3 trials were analysed using analysis of variance for repeated measures (ANOVA).

Results

All 31 subjects enrolled in the study completed the 3 trials. Seven subjects (4 females and 3 males) participated in the lorazepam study, 7 subjects (1 female and 6 males) in the alprazolam trial, 8 subjects (5 females and 3 males) in the antipyrine study, and 9 subjects in the paracetamol study (4 females and 5 males).

Figure 1 shows representative plasma concentration curves from the pre-vaccination control trials.

The overall differences among the 3 trials in clearance of antipyrine were of borderline significance ($p < 0.0611$), with a trend towards reduced clearance in both of the post-vaccination trials (table I). However, Dunnett's t-test revealed no significant difference between the pre-vaccination control trial and either of the post-vaccination trials. The overall difference among the 3 trials in volume of distribution of antipyrine was of borderline significance ($p = 0.0536$), but differences between individual trials were not significant. There were no overall differences observed in the elimination half-life of antipyrine, and there were also no significant differences between trials in 48-hour cumulative urinary excretion or fractional recovery of intact antipyrine, 4-hydroxyantipyrine, norantipyrine, or 3-hydroxymethyl antipyrine (table II).

In the case of paracetamol and alprazolam, there were no significant differences among the 3 trials in any of the kinetic variables (table I). For lorazepam, elimination half-life varied significantly among trials, but differences were small and not systematic. Lorazepam clearance did not vary significantly among trials, with if anything slightly higher values after vaccination.

Discussion

The results of the study indicate that trivalent influenza vaccine may slightly impair the oxidative clearance of antipyrine but not of alprazolam. The coadministration of influenza vaccine did not affect the elimination of lorazepam and paracetamol, which are predominantly cleared by conjugative processes.

Influenza vaccine as well as natural influenza viral infections have been noted to transiently impair the clearance of some hepatically oxidised drugs (Fischer et al. 1982; Harless 1983; Kramer &

Table I. Summary of pharmacokinetic results

Parameter (units)	Mean (± SE) for trial			Value of F[a]
	Pre-vaccination control	7 days post-vaccination	21 days post-vaccination	
Antipyrine (phenazone) (n = 8)				
Vd (L)	37.3 ± 2.3	35.2 ± 2.5	34.9 ± 2.2	3.60 ($p < 0.06$)
$t_{1/2}$ (h)	9.9 ± 1.2	10.1 ± 1.0	10.1 ± 0.8	0.11 (NS)
Clearance (ml/min)	50.0 ± 7.9	43.4 ± 5.7	42.0 ± 4.7	3.43 ($p < 0.07$)
Alprazolam (n = 7)				
Vd (L)	88.4 ± 9.1	98.0 ± 10.5	94.3 ± 6.2	1.59 (NS)
$t_{1/2}$ (h)	10.9 ± 1.4	12.0 ± 2.2	11.8 ± 1.9	0.62 (NS)
Clearance (ml/min)	95.5 ± 5.0	106.6 ± 10.5	103.1 ± 6.2	0.38 (NS)
Paracetamol (acetaminophen) (n = 9)				
Vd (L)	67.6 ± 5.4	69.5 ± 7.1	68.7 ± 7.1	0.10 (NS)
$t_{1/2}$ (h)	2.2 ± 0.2	2.3 ± 0.10	2.2 ± 0.1	0.57 (NS)
Clearance (ml/min)	372.0 ± 38	352.0 ± 34	363.0 ± 43	0.33 (NS)
Lorazepam (n = 7)				
Vd (L)	113.8 ± 14.7	130.5 ± 15.2	123.1 ± 17.8	2.80 (NS)
$t_{1/2}$ (h)	14.6 ± 1.6	16.5 ± 2.1	13.7 ± 1.5	6.07 ($p < 0.025$)
Clearance (ml/min)	97.3 ± 16.8	103.4 ± 23.9	114.5 ± 22.9	1.75 (NS)

a Analysis of variance.
Abbreviations: Vd = apparent volume of distribution; $t_{1/2}$ = elimination half-life; NS = not significant; n = number of subjects.

Table II. 48-hour cumulative urinary excretion of antipyrine (phenazone) and metabolites

	Mean ± SE recovery (mg)			Value of F[a]
	Pre-vaccination control	7 days post-vaccination	21 days post-vaccination	
Antipyrine	34.2 (± 9.0)	35.7 (± 7.2)	50.4 (± 12.3)	0.70 (NS)
4-Hydroxyantipyrine	241.4 (± 21.0)	266.8 (± 31.9)	283.0 (± 35.4)	1.20 (NS)
Norantipyrine	133.8 (± 11.6)	171.5 (± 20.5)	166.8 (± 23.8)	1.11 (NS)
3-Hydroxymethylantipyrine	97.8 (± 10.4)	104.3 (± 13.4)	122.6 (± 16.1)	3.11 (NS)

a Analysis of variance.
Abbreviation: NS = not significant.

McClain 1981; Kramer et al. 1984; Levine et al. 1984; Meredith et al. 1985; Renton et al. 1980; Walker et al. 1980). This effect was found to persist for up to 3 to 4 weeks after vaccination (Kramer & McClain 1981; Kramer et al. 1984). However, it is not clearly established which patients will be affected, when they will be affected, and for how long the influenza vaccine will affect drug clearance if such effect occurs.

Therapeutic Implications

The present study indicates that clearance of drugs which undergo hepatic conjugative reactions such as glucuronidation and sulphation are unlikely to be affected by the coadministration of influenza vaccine. Furthermore, not all drugs which are biotransformed by hepatic microsomal oxidation necessarily have impaired clearance due to coadministration of influenza vaccine.

Acknowledgements

This study was supported in part by grants MH-34223 and AG-10016 from the United States Department of Public Health.

We are grateful for the assistance of Ann Locniskar, Rita Matlis, Barbara W. LeDuc, Jerold S. Harmatz, Richard I. Shader, and the staff of the Clinical Study Unit, New England Medical Center Hospital (supported by grant RR-00054 from the United States Public Health Service).

References

Ameer B, Greenblatt DJ, Divoll M, Abernethy DR, Shargel L. High performance liquid chromatography determination of acetaminophen in plasma: single dose pharmacokinetic studies. Journal of Chromatography – Biomedical Applications 226: 224-230, 1981

Blyden GT, LeDuc BW, Greenblatt DJ. Large theophylline requirements due to high theophylline clearance: verification by the antipyrine test. Pharmacology 32: 226-231, 1986

Bukowskyj M, Mont PW, Wigle R, Nakatsu K. Theophylline clearance. Lack of effect of influenza vaccine and ascorbic acid. American Review of Respiratory Disease 129: 672-675, 1984

Fischer RG, Booth BH, Mitchell DQ, Kibbe AM. Influence of trivalent influenza vaccine on serum theophylline levels. Canadian Medical Association Journal 126: 1312-1314, 1982

Goldstein RS, Cheung OT, Seguin R, Lobley G, Johnson AC. Decreased elimination of theophylline after influenza vaccination. Canadian Medical Association Journal 126: 470, 1982

Greenblatt DJ, Abernethy DR, Divoll M. Kinetics of low dose intravenous antipyrine: use of liquid chromatography. International Journal of Clinical Pharmacology 21: 51-55, 1983

Greenblatt DJ, Divoll M, Moschitto LJ, Shader RI. Electron-capture gas chromatographic analysis of the triazolobenzodiazepines alprazolam and triazolam. Journal of Chromatography – Biomedical Applications 225: 202-207, 1981

Greenblatt DJ, Franke K, Shader RI. Analysis of lorazepam and its glucuronide metabolite by electron-capture gas-liquid chromatography: use in pharmacokinetic studies of lorazepam. Journal of Chromatography – Biomedical Applications 146: 311-320, 1978

Greenblatt DJ, Koch-Weser J. Clinical pharmacokinetics. New England Journal of Medicine 293: 702-705, 964-970, 1975

Harless GR. Note on interactions involving theophylline kinetics. Drug Intelligence and Clinical Pharmacy 17: 132-133, 1983

Harmatz JS, Greenblatt DJ. A SIMPLEX procedure for fitting nonlinear pharmacokinetic models. Computers in Biology and Medicine 17: 199-208, 1987

Kramer P, McClain CJ. Depression of aminopyrine metabolism by influenza vaccination. New England Journal of Medicine 305: 1262-1264, 1981

Kramer P, Tsuru M, Cook CE, McClain CJ, Holtzman JL. Effect of influenza vaccine on warfarin anticoagulation. Clinical Pharmacology and Therapeutics 35: 416-418, 1984

Levine M, Jones MW, Gribble M. Increased serum phenytoin concentration following influenza vaccine. Clinical Pharmacy 3: 505-509, 1984

Meredith CG, Christian CD, Johnson RF, Troxell R, Davis GL, et al. Effects of influenza virus vaccine on hepatic drug metabolism. Clinical Pharmacology and Therapeutics 37: 396-401, 1985

Renton KW, Gray JD, Hall RI. Decreased elimination of theophylline after influenza vaccination. Canadian Medical Association Journal 123: 288-290, 1980

San Joaquin VH, Reyes S, Marks MI. Influenza vaccination in asthmatic children on maintenance theophylline therapy. Clinical Pediatrics 21: 724-726, 1982

Smith RB, Kroboth PD, Vanderlugt JT, Phillips JP, Juhl RP. Pharmacokinetics and pharmacodynamics of alprazolam after oral and IV administration. Psychopharmacology 84: 452-456, 1984

Stults BM, Hashisaki PA. Influenza vaccination and theophylline pharmacokinetics in patients with chronic obstructive lung disease. Western Journal of Medicine 139: 651-654, 1983

Walker S, Schreiber L, Middelkamp JN. Serum theophylline levels after influenza vaccination. Canadian Medical Association Journal 125: 243-244, 1980

Authors' address: Dr *David J. Greenblatt*, Division of Clinical Pharmacology, Tufts-New England Medical Center, Box 1007, 171 Harrison Avenue, Boston MA 02111 (USA).

Clinical Pharmacokinetics 16: 186-191 (1989)
0312-5963/89/0003-0186/$03.00/0

Tianeptine and its Main Metabolite
Pharmacokinetics in Chronic Alcoholism and Cirrhosis

R.J. Royer, M.J. Royer-Morrot, F. Paille, D. Barrucand, J. Schmitt, R. Defrance and *C. Salvadori*

Service de Pharmacologie Clinique et Toxicologie, Hôpital Central, Nancy; Service de Médecine Interne, Hôpital Fournier, Nancy; and Institut de Recherches Internationales Servier, Neuilly sur Seine, France

Summary

The effect of chronic alcoholism (with or without associated moderate cirrhosis) on the disposition of the antidepressant tianeptine, which is devoid of substantial first-pass metabolism, was examined in 21 patients and 11 age-matched controls.

Pharmacokinetic parameters for tianeptine and its C_5 acid analogue metabolite (MC_5 metabolite) were estimated by non-compartmental analysis.

The area under the curve (AUC) for tianeptine, following a 12.5mg single oral dose, was decreased by 31% in chronic alcoholics and increased by only 14% in cirrhotics, compared to controls. These changes did not attain statistical significance. The trend of changes in the AUC for the MC_5 metabolite was similar to that observed for the parent drug. No statistical difference was found in the terminal half-life for both tianeptine and its MC_5 metabolite between patients and controls. On the basis of this study, it appears unnecessary to modify the proposed dosage regimen used in clinical trials (tianeptine sodium salt 12.5mg 3 times daily) in chronic alcoholics with or without associated moderate cirrhosis.

The influence of liver disease on the kinetics of a drug may not be generally predictable, with the exception that the oral availability of drugs with a high hepatic extraction ratio is increased (Blaschke & Rubin 1979; Klotz et al. 1979; Williams & Mamelok 1980).

Little information is currently available on the pharmacokinetics of tricyclic antidepressants in patients who abuse alcohol and/or present with cirrhosis. Nevertheless, first-pass metabolism is extensive with tricyclic antidepressants (Molnar & Gupta 1980), and a small change in this process can greatly affect the amount of the drug reaching the tissues and thus alter drug effect.

The pharmacokinetics of tianeptine, an antidepressant with an original serotoninergic neurochemical action (Kato & Weitsch 1988; Mennini et al. 1987), has been studied in healthy young subjects (Salvadori et al., unpublished data); in these individuals this drug is rapidly [time to peak plasma drug concentration (t_{max}) close to 1h] and completely absorbed when given orally, with an absolute bioavailability on average of about 99%. The drug is extensively metabolised and the renal clearance of unchanged tianeptine is about 0.024 L/h. Tianeptine is converted to metabolites mainly by β-oxidation of the side chain (Campbell & Taylor 1981), its C_5 acid analogue being the most abundant: 32% of total radioactivity after an oral dose of ^{14}C-tianeptine (12.5mg; 50 μCi) is converted to metabolites at plasmatic level, and 22% to MC_5 metabolite [7-(3-chloro-6,11-dihydro-5,5 dioxo-6-

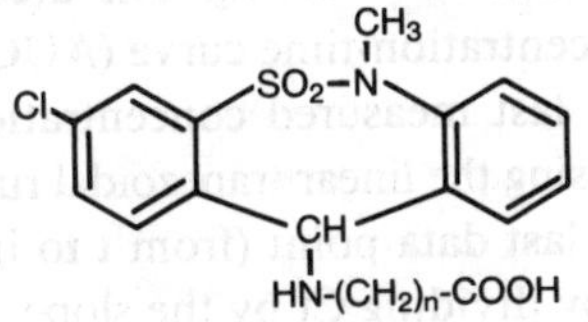

n = 6 Tianeptine

n = 4 MC_5 metabolite

Fig. 1. Structure of tianeptine and its principal metabolite MC_5.

methyldibenzo (c,f) (1,2) thiazepin-11-ylamino) pentanoic acid] (fig. 1).

A previous study in healthy young adults has shown that the MC_5 metabolite reaches peak plasma concentration later than tianeptine (t_{max} = 1h and 2.2h for tianeptine and MC_5 metabolite, respectively). The plasma metabolite concentrations are lower than those of the parent drug, but decline with a longer terminal half-life ($t_{½}$): 7.2 *vs* 2.5h on average.

Since tianeptine shows an antidepressant activity equal to that of amitriptyline in depressed chronic alcoholics (Lôo et al. 1988), it seemed logical to study tianeptine pharmacokinetics in such patients. Thus, the present study was performed to determine the pharmacokinetic profile of a single oral dose of tianeptine in chronic alcoholics with or without moderate liver cirrhosis, and to compare it with the profile in non-alcoholic patients.

Methods

Clinical aspects of this study were conducted in departments of Médecine Interne (Professor Barrucand, Fournier Hospital, and Professor Schmitt, Central Hospital, Nancy). The protocol was approved by the local ethical committee.

After giving informed consent, 32 inpatients were enrolled in the study. All subjects were examined before the first day of the study, including a complete medical history, physical examination and complete serum biochemical profile. All patients were without abnormal cardiovascular or renal function. Other medication was discontinued the day before and during the sampling period. The patients were divided into 3 groups (table I).

Group 1 (n = 10; age range 30 to 62 years) included patients having combined depression and alcoholism defined by the criteria of DSM III (American Psychiatric Association 1980) and consisting of either 'alcohol abuse' or 'alcohol dependence'. Lack of liver cirrhosis was confirmed by liver biopsy and prothrombin time > 70%.

Group 2 (n = 11; age range 36 to 59 years) included patients with alcoholic cirrhosis confirmed by liver biopsy or previous icteroascitic decompensation. Cirrhosis was inactive and laboratory data were only slightly abnormal.

Group 3 (n = 11; age range 31 to 74 years) included non-alcoholic patients with normal liver function confirmed by clinical and laboratory findings.

Table I. Summary of pre-trial evaluation of patients in the study

Patients	Sex M/F	Age (y)	Bodyweight (kg)	Bilirubin (μmol/L)	ALT (IU/L)	Albumin (g/L)	PT (%)	γ-GT (IU/L)
Group 1 (n = 10)								
Mean ± SD	10/0	42.7 ± 11.7	64.8 ± 7.5	11.81 ± 4.79	31.9 ± 13.5	39.91 ± 3.76	92.0 ± 11.1	130.5 ± 204.1
Group 2 (n = 11)								
Mean ± SD	9/2	45.7 ± 8.4	65.9 ± 9.5	19.91 ± 11.77	46.9 ± 37.9	36.56 ± 5.24	75.8 ± 15.6	192.5 ± 147.7
Group 3 (n = 11)								
Mean ± SD	7/4	48.4 ± 12.9	62.0 ± 12.9	11.50 ± 6.76	10.6 ± 7.9	39.95 ± 2.39	91.0 ± 10.0	20.0 ± 31.0

Abbreviations: ALT = alanine aminotransferase; PT = prothrombin time; γ-GT = γ-glutamyl transferase

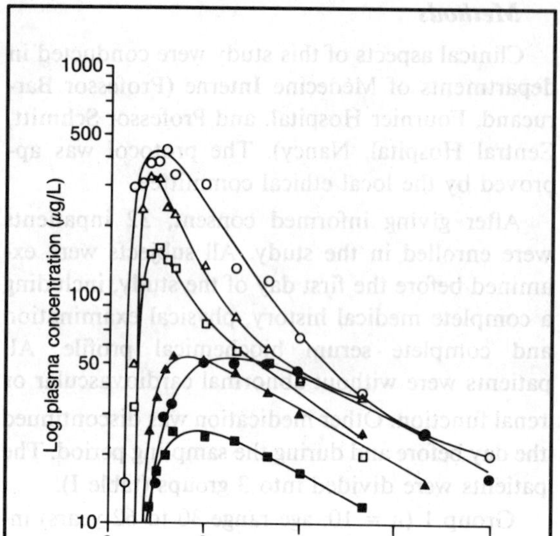

Fig. 2. Plasma concentration *versus* time profiles of tianeptine (open symbols) and MC_5 metabolite (black symbols) in three patients: □, ■ = chronic alcoholic; ○, ● = cirrhotic; △, ▲ = control.

An oral dose of tianeptine 12.5mg (tablet form) was administered at 8a.m. following an overnight fast. Venous blood (6ml on dry heparin) was drawn before and at 0.5, 0.75, 1, 1.25, 1.5, 1.75, 2, 3, 4, 5, 6, 8, 10, 12, 18 and 24 hours after drug intake. Fasting conditions were maintained for 4 hours after administration. The blood was centrifuged and plasma was separated and frozen at −20°C until assayed. Tianeptine and its MC_5 metabolite plasma concentrations were determined by high performance liquid chromatography (HPLC) using the method described by Nicot et al. (1986).

Pharmacokinetic parameters were estimated from plasma concentrations by non-compartmental analysis. Peak plasma concentration (C_{max}) and t_{max} were determined directly from the plasma concentrations *versus* time profile for tianeptine. The elimination rate constant λ_z was determined from the terminal log-linear phase by linear least squares regression.

The terminal phase elimination half-life was calculated from $t_{½} = \ln 2/\lambda_z$. The area under the plasma concentration-time curve (AUC) from zero time to the last measured concentration [Ct] was calculated using the linear trapezoidal rule. The area beyond the last data point (from t to infinity) was estimated by dividing Ct by the slope λ_z. The total area under the curve is the sum of these two areas.

MC_5 metabolite parameters, marked with the (m) qualifier, were calculated in the same way.

Using the value of λ_z and AUC for tianeptine, the following parameters were calculated: apparent oral clearance CL/f = D/AUC and apparent volume of distribution $V/f = D/AUC \cdot \lambda_z$ where f was the absolute bioavailability and D the administered dose.

Differences in the parameters of drug disposition between the 3 groups were analysed using a one-way analysis of variance. Values of $p < 0.05$ were considered statistically significant. In such cases, analysis of variance was continued by a Newman Keuls test for comparison of treatments in pairs.

Results

Figure 2 shows representative log plasma concentration time profiles of tianeptine and its MC_5 metabolite in a chronic alcoholic patient, a cirrhotic patient and a control subject. The kinetic parameters of tianeptine for each group of patients are shown in table II.

C_{max} and t_{max} were comparable in the 3 groups, whereas there was a decreased AUC in the chronic alcoholic group. The mean AUC was 488 ± 135 µg/L • h for this group, smaller than the mean AUC for the cirrhotic group (AUC = 803 ± 340 µg/L • h; $p < 0.05$) and for the control group (AUC = 703 ± 315 µg/L • h). The difference with this last group did not reach significance. Apparent oral clearance was increased in the chronic alcoholic group compared with the 2 other groups. No statistical difference was found in the V/f and the $t_{½\lambda z}$ between the 3 groups but $t_{½}$ appeared slightly shorter in the chronic alcoholic group (2.3 ± 0.9h) compared to

Table II. Pharmacokinetic data for tianeptine in chronic alcoholic, cirrhotic and control patients (mean ± SD)

Parameter (units)	Chronic alcoholics	Cirrhotics	Controls	Analysis of variance
C_{max} (μg/L)	165 ± 30	222 ± 96	211 ± 73	NS
t_{max} (h)	1.62 ± 0.26	1.66 ± 0.53	1.94 ± 0.85	NS
AUC (μg/L · h)	488 ± 135[a]	803 ± 340[a]	703 ± 315	$p < 0.05$
CL/f (L/h)	26.0 ± 6.6	17.9 ± 9.1	20.4 ± 9.3	NS
V/f (L/kg)	1.28 ± 0.50	1.20 ± 0.80	1.16 ± 0.29	NS
$t_{½λz}$ (h)	2.3 ± 0.9	3.3 ± 2.1	3.3 ± 1.7	NS

a Newman Keuls test.

Abbreviations: C_{max} = peak plasma drug concentration; t_{max} = time to C_{max}; AUC = area under the plasma concentration-time curve; CL/f = apparent oral clearance; V/f = apparent volume of distribution; $t_{½λz}$ = terminal phase elimination half-life; NS = not significant.

the cirrhotic group (3.3 ± 2.1h) and the control group (3.3 ± 1.7h).

The MC_5 metabolite kinetic parameters are shown in table III. The trend and extent of changes in the parameters for the MC_5 metabolite were similar to those observed for the parent drug. Administration of tianeptine resulted in a significant decrease of plasma MC_5 concentrations in the chronic alcoholic group.

The AUC(m) was 208 ± 70 μg/L·h in this group and 363 ± 115 and 390 ± 147 μg/L·h in cirrhotic and control groups, respectively. The mean ratio AUC(m)/AUC was comparable in the 3 groups (0.41 ± 0.13, 0.41 ± 0.16 and 0.54 ± 0.16 in chronic alcoholic, cirrhotic and control groups, respectively).

The $t_{½λz}$ of the MC_5 metabolite was slightly longer than that of tianeptine, with mean values between 3 and 4 hours for the 3 groups.

Discussion

Liver disease in humans results in a variety of pathophysiological changes which may have important effects on drug elimination. Hepatocyte function, hepatic blood flow, protein binding or biliary secretion may be affected. To interpret the effect of liver disease on drug disposition, it is important to assess the severity of the disease because, as shown by Zilly et al. (1978), significant differences exist between patients with compensated and decompensated cirrhosis. Pronounced changes may develop between the early stage of compensated liver cirrhosis and the decompensated stage with ascites, hypoalbuminaemia, portocaval shunting and accumulation of endogenous substances. Nevertheless, moderate cirrhosis may affect drug disposition, as shown by Neal et al. (1979) for analgesics.

Table III. Pharmacokinetic data of the MC_5 metabolite of tianeptine in chronic alcoholic, cirrhotic and control subjects (mean ± SD)

Parameter (units)	Chronic alcoholics	Cirrhotics	Controls	Analysis of variance
C_{max}(m) (μg/L)	45 ± 22	59 ± 24	61 ± 22	NS
t_{max}(m) (h)	2.54 ± 0.82	2.60 ± 0.68	3.06 ± 1.43	NS
AUC(m) (μ/L · h)	208 ± 70[a,b]	363 ± 115[a]	390 ± 147[b]	$p < 0.05$
AUC(m)/AUC	0.41 ± 0.13	0.41 ± 0.16	0.54 ± 0.16	NS
$t_{½λz}$(m)	3.0 ± 2.0	3.9 ± 1.2	4.0 ± 1.3	NS

a,b Newman Keuls test.

Abbreviations: (m) = metabolite; for other abbreviations see table II.

The pharmacokinetic parameters for tianeptine and its MC_5 metabolite in healthy young adults were previously reported (Salvadori et al. 1988) and showed that tianeptine was rapidly absorbed following oral administration (mean t_{max} = 0.938 ± 0.466h). Our present results showed that following the same oral dose, plasma concentrations of tianeptine rose more slowly to a lower C_{max} in all the patients studied than in healthy young subjects. This finding could be attributed to a lower absorption rate of the oral drug in the patients. Absorption rate was affected in every patient group, with and without liver disease, but the effect was more pronounced in chronic alcoholics. In this group, both the C_{max} and AUC for tianeptine were lower than those observed in control subjects. A study in chronic alcoholics given intravenous tianeptine would be necessary to show whether these results were due to an increase in volume of distribution, a decrease in bioavailability or an increased biotransformation. Nevertheless, the third hypothesis appeared unlikely because plasma MC_5 metabolite concentrations were not increased in these patients; the AUC(m)/AUC ratio was not statistically different between chronic alcoholics, cirrhotics and control subjects.

No important change was observed in the pharmacokinetic parameters of tianeptine and MC_5 metabolite in cirrhotics. Mean tianeptine AUC was slightly higher than in control subjects but this increase did not attain a statistical significance; this is not surprising for a drug which normally does not undergo substantial first-pass metabolism and which has a bioavailability close to 100% in healthy young subjects. This characteristic differentiates tianeptine from most of the tricyclic antidepressants (Molnar & Gupta 1980) and also non-tricyclics such as zimeldine (Heel et al. 1982) and mianserin (Brogden et al. 1978).

The lack of substantial first-pass effect implies that the normal liver has a low intrinsic tianeptine metabolism capacity and that the extraction ratio is lower than 0.3. This would place tianeptine in the protein binding-limited hepatic clearance class (Blaschke 1977). Tianeptine is highly bound (around 94%) to plasma proteins, mainly albumin, the binding involving 2 classes of binding-sites, of which one is saturable with a low affinity for tianeptine (affinity constant approximately 38,000 mol/L) [Tillement & Zini, personal communication]. Thus, in theory, the consequences of reduced protein binding in hypoalbuminaemic states could substantially alter tianeptine pharmacokinetics. However, in the present study no change in albuminaemia was observed between cirrhotic and control subjects, and thus a rise in free drug concentration would be unlikely in those patients with moderate liver cirrhosis.

Therapeutic Implications

No statistically significant decrease in tianeptine clearance was observed in chronic alcoholics with or without associated moderate cirrhosis compared to controls; therefore steady-state plasma tianeptine concentrations would not be expected to change in such patients. Thus, it would appear unnecessary to modify the proposed dosage regimen used in clinical trials (tianeptine sodium salt 12.5mg three times daily) in these patients.

References

American Psychiatric Association. Diagnostic and statistical manual of mental disorders, 3rd ed., American Psychiatric Association, Washington D.C., 1980

Blaschke TF. Protein binding and kinetics of drugs in liver disease. Clinical Pharmacokinetics 2: 32-44, 1977

Blaschke TF, Rubin PC. Hepatic first-pass metabolism in liver disease. Clinical Pharmacokinetics 4: 423-432, 1979

Brogden RN, Heel RC, Speight TM, Avery GS. Mianserin: a review of its pharmacological properties and therapeutic efficacy in depressive illness. Drugs 16: 273-301, 1978

Campbell DB, Taylor AR. A species comparison of the pharmacokinetics and metabolism of ^{14}C-tianeptine. In Struwe & Jansson (Eds). Biological psychiatry, Proceedings of the Third World Congress of Biological Psychiatry, June 28-July 3, 1981, Stockholm, Sweden, pp 585-588, Elsevier, North Holland, 1981

Heel RC, Morley PA, Brogden RN, Carmine AA, Speight TM, et al. Zimeldine: a review of its pharmacological properties and therapeutic efficacy in depressive illness. Drugs 24: 169-206, 1982

Kato G, Weitsch AF. Neurochemical profile of tianeptine, a new antidepressant drug. Clinical Neuropharmacology 11 (Suppl. 2): S43-S50, 1980

Klotz U, Fischer C, Muller-Seydlitz P, Schultz J, Muller WA. Alterations in the disposition of differently cleared drugs in patients with cirrhosis. Clinical Pharmacology and Therapeutics 26 (2): 221-227, 1979

Lôo H, Malka R, Defrance R, Barrucand D, Benard JY, et al. Tianeptine and amitriptyline: controlled double-blind trial in depressed alcoholic patients. Neuropsychobiology 19: 79-85, 1988

Mennini T, Mocaer E, Garattini S. Tianeptine, a selective enhancer of serotonin uptake in rat brain. Naunyn-Schmiedeberg's Archives of Pharmacology 336: 478-482, 1987
Molnar G, Gupta RN. Plasma levels and tricyclic antidepressant therapy: part 2. Pharmacokinetic, clinical and toxicological aspects. Biopharmaceutics and Drug Disposition 1: 283-305, 1980
Neal EA, Meffin PJ, Gregory PB, Blaschke TF. Enhanced bioavailability and decreased clearance of analgesics in patients with cirrhosis. Gastroenterology 77: 96-102, 1979
Nicot G, Lachatre G, Gonnet C, Mallon J, Mocaer E. Paired-ion extraction and high performance liquid chromatographic determination of tianeptine and its metabolites in human plasma, urine and tissues. Journal of Chromatography – Biomedical Applications 381 (1): 115-126, 1986
Williams RL, Mamelok RD. Hepatic disease and drug pharmacokinetics. Clinical Pharmacokinetics 5: 528-547, 1980
Zilly W, Breimer DD, Richter E. Hexobarbital disposition in compensated and decompensated cirrhosis of the liver. Clinical Pharmacology and Therapeutics 23 (5): 525-534, 1978

Authors' address: Mrs *Catherine Salvadori*, Institut de Recherches Internationales Servier, 27, rue du Pont, 92202 Neuilly sur Seine Cédex (France).

Information for Authors

Manuscript Preparation: Articles are published in English. Submit 2 copies of the complete manuscript, including title page, text pages, references, tables, legends, footnotes and figures. Only typed copy, double-spaced on 1 side of preferably A4 (206mm × 294mm) typewriter paper with liberal margins is acceptable. Articles in the current issue of the Journal should be consulted for the general layout of the paper.

Subdivision of Articles: Manuscripts should be prepared and paginated in the following manner:

a) Title page
b) Summary
c) Text pages
  i) Original articles
    Introduction
    Methods
    Results
    Discussion
    Therapeutic Implications
  ii) Review articles
    Outline will be provided
d) Acknowledgements
e) List of references
f) Address for correspondence
g) Tables
h) Figures and legends
i) Footnotes

Title Page: There should be a separate title page with title, authors and institutions where the work was done, indicating the city, and a condensed running title of not more than 50 letters including spaces.
The name and address of author to whom correspondence should be addressed should appear separately at the end of the references.

Summary: For *original articles,* the summary should not exceed 150 words. It should be factual, not descriptive, and should present the reason for the study, the main findings (giving specific data if possible), and the principal conclusions. For *review articles,* the summary should be about 5% of the length of the article and should highlight the salient points discussed.

Results/Discussion/Implications (for Original Articles): Description of the experimental results should be succinct, but of sufficient detail to allow the experiment to be repeated by others. Conclusions and theoretical considerations must not appear in the results section, nor is a recapitulation of the results acceptable for the discussion section. Where relevant, a concise statement of the implications of the experimental results, particularly in the clinical use of drug(s), should appear as a separate section.

References: In the text, reference to published work is cited by author (alphabetically) and year — viz. (Hart 1986, 1987; Lind et al. 1980; Mariner & Jamieson 1976) . . . (Tipping 1982b; Wilson & Payne 1984b,c,d).
The list of references must be arranged alphabetically by first author's name (and initials if more than one author of the same name) or by second or third, etc. authors if more than one author of the same name and initials. If the sequence of the authors' names and initials is identical, the references should be arranged chronologically by year of publication. Only the first 5 authors are required.
Sample references are listed below. *Note:* titles of journals are *not* to be abbreviated. Supply inclusive pagination for all articles.

Journal article: Ashby J, Piddock LJV, Wise R. An investigation of the hydrophobicity of the quinolones. Journal of Antimicrobial Chemotherapy 16: 805-810, 1985

Silke B, Verma SP, Frais MA, Reynolds G, Jackson N, et al. Haemodynamic analysis of the effects of nicardipine and metoprolol alone and in combination in coronary artery disease. European Heart Journal 6: 930-938, 1985a

Silke B, Verma SP, Hussain M, Jackson NC, Hafizullah M, et al. Comparative haemodynamic effects of nicardipine and verapamil in coronary artery disease. Herz 10: 112-119, 1985b

Journal abstract: Sando H, Katagiri H, Okada M, Shoda R, Arai Y, et al. The effect of nifedipine and nicardipine on glucose tolerance, insulin and C-peptide. Abstract no. 262. Diabetes 32 (Suppl. 1): 6A, 1983

Book: Hart AH. Pharmacokinetics and metabolism of the benzamides. In Platts et al. (Eds) The benzamides: pharmacology and clinical aspects, Vol. 35, pp. 143-162, Raven Press, New York, 1986

Clinical Pharmacokinetics 16: 193-214 (1989)
0312-5963/89/0004-0193/$11.00/0

Clinical Pharmacokinetic Properties of the Macrolide Antibiotics
Effects of Age and Various Pathophysiological States (Part I)[1]

Piero Periti, Teresita Mazzei, Enrico Mini and *Andrea Novelli*

Department of Preclinical and Clinical Pharmacology, University of Florence, Florence, Italy

Contents

Summary 193
1. Analytical Methods 195
 1.1 Microbiological Assays 195
 1.2 Chemical Assays 196
2. Erythromycin 196
3. Oleandomycin 206
4. Spiramycin 206
5. Josamycin 207
6. Midecamycin 211
7. Miocamycin 211
8. Rosaramicin 214

Summary

The pharmacokinetic aspects in humans of macrolide antibiotics that are currently or soon to be on the market (i.e. erythromycin, oleandomycin, spiramycin, josamycin, midecamycin, miocamycin, rosaramycin, roxithromycin and azithromycin) are reviewed.

Macrolide antibiotics are basic compounds, poorly soluble in water, which are mostly absorbed in the alkaline intestinal environment. They are acid unstable, but the newer semisynthetic derivatives (i.e. roxithromycin and azithromycin) are characterised by increased stability under acidic conditions. Macrolides are highly liposoluble and consequently penetrate well into tissue, especially bronchial secretions, prostatic tissue, middle ear exudates and bone tissues, as evidenced by tissue/serum concentration ratios greater than 1. They do not penetrate well into the CSF. Macrolides undergo extensive biotransformation in the liver. With a few exceptions (e.g. miocamycin), the metabolites of these drugs are characterised by little or no antimicrobial activity.

Plasma protein binding is variable from one compound to another. At therapeutic concentrations, protein-bound erythromycin accounts for 80 to 90% of the total drug present in the blood, and the fraction is 95% for roxithromycin. The lowest values of protein-bound fraction are observed for midecamycin and josamycin (about 15%), and intermediate values are reported for spiramycin and miocamycin. However, the clinical relevance of this parameter is not clearly established.

1 A complete reference list will appear in Part II of this article in the following issue of the Journal.

Plasma half-life ($t_{1/2}$) values vary for the macrolides described: erythromycin, oleandomycin, josamycin and miocamycin have a $t_{1/2}$ ranging from 1 to 2 hours; spiramycin, erythromycin stearate, the mercaptosuccinate salt of propionyl erythromycin and rosaramicin have an intermediate $t_{1/2}$ (about 7, 6.5, 5 and 4.5 hours, respectively); the newer semisynthetic compounds roxithromycin and azithromycin are characterised by high $t_{1/2}$ values (i.e. 11 and 41 hours, respectively).

Under normal conditions, the major route of elimination is the liver. Renal elimination also takes place but it contributes to total clearance only to a small degree, as evidenced by low renal clearance values. The degree of modification of macrolide pharmacokinetics by renal insufficiency or hepatic disease is usually not considered clinically relevant, and no recommendation for dose modification is necessary in these patients.

The pharmacokinetics of macrolides are modified in elderly patients. Accordingly, their use must be accompanied by a closer than usual clinical monitoring of the older patient.

Clinically the newer semisynthetic macrolides, such as roxithromycin, possess an antibacterial spectrum at least equivalent to that of erythromycin, and superior pharmacokinetic properties (i.e. longer elimination half-life, higher tissue penetration) over erythromycin and other macrolides, allowing longer intervals between doses.

Macrolides are antibiotics composed of a macrocyclic lactone nucleus containing 12 to 16 atoms substituted by sugars via glycosidic bonds (Bryskier et al. 1986). The group was discovered in the early 1950s and chemically it is possible to distinguish 3 groups of representative products of the class in relation to the number of lactone atoms. 14-membered macrolides include the classical erythromycins A, B, C and D, oleandomycin, and more recent compounds such as albocycline, megalomycin, lankamycin and roxithromycin. 16-membered macrolides include the traditional spiramycin, tylosin, josamycin, rosaramicin, midecamycin, rokitamycin, miocamycin and kitasamycin. Azithromycin is a new 15-membered-ring macrolide.

Macrolide antibiotics were originally isolated from various *Streptomyces* species and can be synthesised by condensation of acetate, propionate or butyrate units. However, total synthesis is no longer the most economical way of obtaining new macrolides.

Semisynthetic modification of the natural macrolide structure represents the third useful possibility aimed at improving the antimicrobial activity and pharmacokinetic characteristics of the parent compounds (Steigbigel 1985).

Despite a certain disparity in the chemical structure, macrolide antibiotics constitute a homogeneous class of antimicrobial drugs characterised by similar antibacterial spectrum, mechanisms of action and resistance, but by relatively different pharmacokinetic properties.

Macrolides reversibly bind to the P site of the 50s ribosomal subunit and inhibit RNA-dependent protein synthesis by stimulating the dissociation of peptidyl *t*-RNA from ribosomes (Kucers & Bennet 1987). Amphenicols and lincosamides compete with macrolides for binding to the P site and therefore exert antagonistic activity (Steigbigel 1985).

Macrolides are weak bases and their activity is increased in alkaline pH, probably because of the better penetration of non-ionised drug through the bacterial cell wall (Chow 1984). Depending on drug concentration, microbial species, phase of growth and inoculum density, macrolides are bacteriostatic or bactericidal (Brittain 1987).

In the last 35 years, macrolides have been widely used in the treatment of infections caused by susceptible Gram-positive organisms; in addition they have become standard therapy for infections caused by *Mycoplasma pneumoniae, Legionella* species, ampicillin-resistant *Haemophilus influenzae, Bordetella pertussis* and *Campylobacter* species. Erythromycin is useful in the eradication of *Corynebacterium diphtheriae* from the nasopharynx and together with the other macrolides it is accepted for the treatment of acne, soft tissue and skin infections, otitis media, bronchitis and sexually

Table I. *In vitro* antimicrobial activity of erythromycin (modified from Steigbigel 1985)

Organism	Minimum inhibitory concentration (mg/L)	
	range	median
Gram-positive bacteria		
S. aureus	0.005->100	0.4
S. epidermidis	0.2->100	0.6
S. pyogenes	0.005-0.2[a]	0.04
S. pneumoniae	0.001-0.2[a]	0.05
S. viridans	0.02-3.1[a]	0.06
S. faecalis	0.1->100	1.5
Clostridium perfringens	0.1-6[a]	0.8
Corynebacterium diphtheriae	0.006-3.1[a]	0.02
Listeria monocytogenes	0.1-0.3	0.2
Gram-negative bacteria		
N. gonorrhoeae	0.005-0.4[a]	0.1
N. meningitidis	0.1-1.6	0.4
H. influenzae	0.1-6	3.1
Bordetella pertussis	0.02-1.6	0.3
Legionella pneumophila	0.06-0.5	0.1
Campylobacter jejuni	0.05->50	0.2
Bacteroides fragilis	0.1->100	≥0.25
Miscellaneous		
Mycoplasma pneumoniae	0.001-0.02	0.005
Chlamydia trachomatis	0.1-0.5	0.1

a Occasional clinical isolates are more resistant.

transmitted diseases, particularly those caused by *Chlamydia* species (Auckenthaler et al. 1987; Griffith & Black 1970; Kucers & Bennet 1987).

MIC values of erythromycin against sensitive bacterial species are shown in table I. Macrolides described in this review have the same broad spectrum as erythromycin and in general similar potency (Katsumi et al. 1981; Saito et al. 1973; Shadomy et al. 1976), with the exception of spiramycin which displays higher MIC values (Kernbaum 1982). Somewhat superior activity against specific bacterial strains has been described for roxithromycin (Bryskier et al. 1986).

Since 1977, macrolides have recaptured clinical interest through the development of semisynthetic molecules with improved pharmacokinetics (Bryskier et al. 1986; McDonald 1986). Macrolide antibiotics are normally administered orally and are readily absorbed from the intestinal tract, if not inactivated by stomach acids; they are characterised by their high lipid solubility and good tissue penetration.

Macrolides enter pleural and ascitic fluids, middle ear exudates, and the sputum. Under normal conditions they do not enter the cerebrospinal fluid but may do so when the meninges are inflamed. These antibiotics also achieve high intracellular concentrations, and this property may contribute to their proven clinical efficacy (Brittain 1987; McDonald 1986; Prokesch & Hand 1982).

The metabolism of macrolides has not been studied extensively; substantial conversion to less active derivatives has, however, been demonstrated for most molecules. Macrolide antibiotics are excreted in both the urine and bile. Percentages excreted vary, depending on the mode of administration, being higher after intravenous than after oral route dosing (Auckenthaler et al. 1987; Garrod et al. 1981; Wiley 1983).

Macrolides bind to serum proteins but this pharmacokinetic factor does not influence clinical efficacy: it appears to affect their *in vitro* antibacterial activity only slightly (McDonald 1986; Nilsen 1987).

1. Analytical Methods

Macrolide concentrations in biological fluids and tissues may be determined either by microbiological assays or by chemical methods.

1.1 Microbiological Assays

The bioassay, based on the agar well diffusion technique (radial agar diffusion assay), can be performed with minimal equipment and very low cost for reagents (Grove & Randall 1955; Sabath & Anhalt 1980), and it is commonly used for determination of macrolide levels, generally employing *Micrococcus luteus* ATCC 9341 (Mini et al. 1987; Tserng & Wagner 1976) or less frequently *Bacillus subtilis* ATCC 6633 (Bégué et al. 1987; Lin et al. 1980) as the test organism. However, because of their polyfunctional structure and amphipathic characteristics, macrolide antibiotics may be good substrates for drug-metabolising enzyme systems in mammals, including humans. Therefore, in addition to its sensitivity limitations, the microbiological assay, measuring not only the parent drug but also partially or totally biologically active metabolites, may produce results which are not specific enough, and not fully usable in therapeutic drug monitoring or pharmacokinetic studies. Moreover, the controversy over the relative effectiveness of different erythromycin prodrugs may also be due to the difficulty of establishing the actual amount of the active form in blood samples. For example, when samples containing erythromycin propionate (a microbiologically inactive ester which may represent the major circulating form following administration of erythromycin estolate) are measured by microbiological assay, a large but unknown amount of the ester is hydrolysed to erythromycin during the assay, thus invalidating the result (Tserng & Wagner 1976).

1.2 Chemical Assays

Among chemical assay methods, high performance liquid chromatography (HPLC) serves an important role in determining macrolide serum and urine concentrations. This technique usually requires extraction procedures, and in some cases complex and expensive equipment (Tsuji 1978). Nevertheless, HPLC methods seem preferable to bioassay because of their specificity, sensitivity and accuracy (Stubbs et al. 1985). Macrolides may be detected by different HPLC techniques using fluorimetric (Tremblay et al. 1985; Tsuji 1978), ultraviolet (Lin et al. 1980; Stubbs et al. 1985) or electrochemical detection (Chen & Chiou 1983; Saint-Salvi et al. 1987; Shepard 1987).

Injection of plasma directly into the HPLC system without pretreatment of the sample, using column switching for sample clean-up, has been described for josamycin (Raeder et al. 1985) and spiramycin (Dow et al. 1985). Finally, liquid scintillation spectrometry (LSS), using ^{14}C-radiolabelled compounds, has been employed both in animals and man in order to evaluate the metabolism and faecal excretion of some macrolides (Lee et al. 1956; Lin et al. 1984a,b, 1986; McLean et al. 1988).

2. *Erythromycin*

Erythromycin is only slightly soluble in water, and is a weak base with a pKa of 8.8. It is a bitter crystalline compound, readily inactivated in an acid medium (Brittain 1987). The active form of the drug is erythromycin base and originally the drug was only available in this form, but subsequently a number of modifications were made to improve oral absorption, eliminate the bitter taste or make it suitable for intravenous use.

Erythromycin base is now marketed in acid-resistant enteric-coated form to retard gastric inactivation and consequently improve absorption. Other approaches were also taken in an attempt to overcome the problems of oral bioavailability of erythromycin by converting the base to acid-stable palatable salt (stearate), ester (ethylsuccinate and propionate) or salt of an ester, such as dodecyl sulphate (estolate) or mercaptosuccinate (RV11) of the propionyl ester (fig. 1). These salts and esters are more acid-resistant than the parent compound (Chow 1984; Periti et al. 1986a,b).

Two relatively water-soluble salts of erythromycin, gluceptate and lactobionate, are available for intravenous injection (Brittain 1987; McDonald 1986).

2.1 Fundamental Pharmacokinetic Properties

The pharmacokinetics of erythromycin have been extensively reviewed in the past 10 years (Auckenthaler et al. 1987; Bergogne-Bérézin 1985; Chow 1984; Kucers & Bennet 1987; McDonald 1986; Nilsen 1987; Osono & Umezawa 1985; Wilson & Van Boxtel 1978; Washington & Wilson 1985).

2.1.1 Absorption and Bioavailability

Unfortunately, many of the available pharmacokinetic data concerning erythromycin are derived using microbiological assays that do not dis-

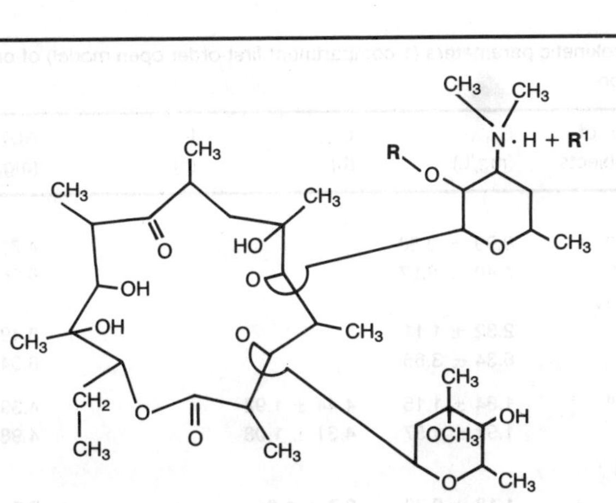

	R	R^1	
Erythromycin	H		(base)
Propionyl erythromycin	$(CH_2)_2CO$		(ester)
Erythromycin ethylsuccinate	$(CH_2)_2OOC(CH_2)_2COO$		(ester)
Erythromycin stearate	H	$C_{17}H_{35}COO$	(salt)
Erythromycin estolate	$(CH_2)_2CO$	$C_{12}H_{25}OSO_3$	(salt of an ester)
Propionil erythromycin mercaptosuccinate	$(CH_2)_2CO$	COOH-CH-SH / COOH-CH_2	(salt of an ester)

Fig. 1. Chemical structure of erythromycin A and its ester and salt derivatives for oral use.

tinguish between the parent drug and its metabolites or the free drug and its protein-bound or unhydrolysed ester forms. Comparisons of erythromycin bioavailability data among the different formulations and the clinical significance of antibiotic concentrations measured are, therefore, particularly difficult to evaluate.

Erythromycin Base

The only form of erythromycin known to be biologically active *in vivo* is the free base; when given orally, however, erythromycin base is inactivated by gastric acid, resulting in decreased gastrointestinal absorption and erratic bioavailability. Erythromycin base is absorbed intact. In fact, volunteers given oral preparations showed considerable intersubject variability, and patients with pernicious anaemia and achlorhydria regularly exhibited higher blood concentrations than healthy subjects (Griffith & Black 1970; Josselyn & Sylvester 1953; McDonald et al. 1977; Rutland et al. 1979).

The time course and total amount of absorption are affected by the nature of the coating applied to erythromycin base (i.e. pellets in capsules and film, or tablets) and, for some preparations, by food intake. Excellent bioavailability has been demonstrated for enteric-coated erythromycin base in both fasting and non-fasting states on single- and multiple-dose regimens (Griffith & Black 1970). Available pharmacokinetic data for these formulations are reported in table II.

Table II. Mean (± SD) pharmacokinetic parameters (1-compartment first-order open model) of oral erythromycin base in adults with normal hepatic and renal function

Oral dosage[a]	No. of subjects	C_{max} (mg/L)	t_{max} (h)	$t_{1/2}$ (h)	AUC (mg/L · h)	Reference
Enteric-coated tablets						
250/1/F	24[b]	0.99 ± 0.68			4.70 ± 2.25	Hovi & Heikinheimo
	–[b]	1.40 ± 0.87			6.25 ± 3.40	(1985)
Enteric-coated pellets (capsules)						
250/1/F	–[c]	2.32 ± 1.11			8.49 ± 4.30	Hovi & Heikinheimo
250/1/NF	–[c]	6.34 ± 3.65			6.34 ± 3.65	(1985)
500/1/before breakfast	16[d]	1.84 ± 1.15	4.44 ± 1.92		4.39 ± 2.98	Rutland et al.
500/1/after breakfast	–[d]	1.91 ± 1.57	4.31 ± 1.08		4.98 ± 3.17	(1979)
250 qid/5/F	10					McDonald et al.
1st dose		1.18 ± 0.73	2.7 ± 1.3		2.9 ± 1.8	(1977)
5th dose		2.59 ± 0.76	2.1 ± 0.3		7.9 ± 2.2	
250 qid/10/F	24					Yakatan et al.
1st dose		0.60 ± 0.20	3.48 ± 0.94		1.67 ± 0.56	(1985)
2nd dose		0.79 ± 0.41	4.02 ± 0.91		2.25 ± 0.67	
9th dose		1.19 ± 0.25	3.38 ± 0.82		4.81 ± 1.19	
10th dose		0.92 ± 0.27	3.92 ± 0.97		4.81 ± 1.19	
250 qid/13/F	8					Josefsson et al.
1st dose		1.4 ± 0.9	2.3 ± 0.5	1.4 ± 0.6	5.8 ± 2.2	(1982)
5th dose		3.2 ± 1.1	2.2 ± 0.3	1.7 ± 0.2	11.9 ± 2.2	
13th dose		3.5 ± 1.2	2.1 ± 0.2	2.1 ± 0.3	15.3 ± 5.1	
500 bid/13/F	8					Yakatan et al.
1st dose		3.2 ± 1.5	2.5 ± 0.5	1.9 ± 0.8	14.2 ± 4.9	(1985)
3rd dose		3.7 ± 2.1	1.7 ± 0.5	1.9 ± 0.5	16.4 ± 7.6	
13th dose		3.0 ± 2.0	1.9 ± 0.4	2.8 ± 2.7[e]	14.3 ± 9.0	

a Dose (mg)/no. of doses/schedule.
b Trials conducted in same subjects.
c Trials conducted in same subjects.
d Trials conducted in same subjects.
e If an atypical $t_{1/2}$ value of 8.8 hours for 1 subject is excluded, the mean $t_{1/2}$ is 1.9 hours on day 7.
Abbreviations: C_{max} = peak plasma concentration; t_{max} = time to C_{max}; $t_{1/2}$ = elimination half-life; AUC = area under the plasma concentration-time curve from zero to infinity; F = fasting; NF = non-fasting; qid = 4 times daily; bid = twice daily.

Absorption of film-coated erythromycin base tends to be erratic, and administration under fasting conditions is required (Brittain 1987). Although erratic absorption of the enteric-coated tablets has been reported (Disanto et al. 1980; Disanto & Chodos 1981; Yakatan et al. 1980), other preparations, such as enteric-coated pellets in capsule, provide excellent bioavailability in the fasting and non-fasting states with both single- and multiple-dose regimens (Fraser 1980; Gribble & Chow 1982; Hovi & Heikinheimo 1985; Josefsson et al. 1982, 1983a,b; McDonald et al. 1977; Rutland et al. 1979; Yakatan et al. 1985).

Ingestion of a pelletised, encapsulated enteric-coated form of erythromycin base achieves peak serum concentrations (C_{max}) of 1 to 2 mg/L after a single 250 or 500mg dose, and food does not appear to affect the bioavailability of the preparation. The pelletised preparation displays a better and more regular absorption than the enteric-coated tablet of erythromycin base (Hovi & Heikinheimo 1985). However, the enteric-coated tablet or pellets in the capsule are protected from the acidic environment of the stomach and do not release erythromycin base for absorption until the more alkaline environment of the intestine is reached.

When erythromycin base was given orally to fasting subjects as multiple 250 or 500mg doses, steady-state conditions appear to have been reached on day 2 with C_{ss} between 3.2 and 3.7 mg/L, and the mean time before the serum peaks occurred (t_{max}) was about 2 hours (Josefsson et al. 1982). In other comparative studies using erythromycin tablets with or without coating the mean C_{max} values were lower, varying from 0.5 to 2 mg/L with t_{max} between 3 and 8 hours depending on formulation type and timing of treatment in relation to meals (Disanto et al. 1980; Disanto & Chodos 1981; Hovi & Heikinheimo 1985; Yakatan et al. 1980). Low C_{max} values (0.6 to 1.2 mg/L) and t_{max} values of more than 3 hours were reported by Yakatan et al. (1985) even after ingestion of enteric-coated pellets in a capsule.

Erythromycin Stearate

Erythromycin stearate is less readily destroyed in the stomach than the base and dissociates in the duodenum, liberating the active form which is absorbed at this site. Relative pharmacokinetic parameters are shown in table III. Peak serum concentrations after oral administration of commercial preparations of this erythromycin salt were low after a single dose, but considerably higher after multiple doses (McDonald et al. 1977). However, serum concentrations achieved using the drug in the form of capsules or film-coated tablets are lower than the mean values obtained with the erythromycin base preparations (Josefsson et al. 1982). Multiple fasting 250mg doses produce peak serum concentrations ranging from 0.8 to 1.5 mg/L. A single fasting dose of 500mg resulted in a peak serum concentration of 1.81 mg/L at 6 hours, while the same dose ingested immediately after a meal achieved 1.1 mg/L at 1.5 hours (Josefsson et al. 1983a,b).

A high loading dose of oral erythromycin stearate has been recommended for antibiotic prophylaxis of endocarditis in susceptible dental patients who are allergic to penicillin. Shanson et al. (1983) compared 3 high single doses in a crossover study measuring serum erythromycin concentrations. Erythromycin stearate 500mg tablets were administered in doses of 1.0, 1.5 or 2.0g, 1 hour after a light breakfast. For all 3 doses there were considerable variations between individuals in the antibiotic concentrations obtained, but the differences between mean peak levels were significant. The serum concentrations of 3.5 mg/L achieved after the 1.5g single dose given 1 to 1.5 hours before a dental procedure should give effective bactericidal cover against *Streptococcus viridans* released into the bloodstream. Formulation factors are known to affect the bioavailability of erythromycin stearate tablets (Chow 1984; Disanto et al. 1980; McDonald 1986; Posti & Salonen 1983; Steigbigel 1985; Welling & Tse 1982; Wilson & Van Boxtel 1978; Yakatan et al. 1979, 1980, 1985). The value of comparative bioavailability studies of marketed synonym drug products is demonstrated by a recent pharmacokinetic study in humans performed with 3 erythromycin stearate formulations, 2 in the form of conventional tablets and the third coated with an acid-resistant film (Venho et al. 1987). Despite delays in absorption, the highest erythromycin plasma C_{max} values were obtained with the acid-resistant film-coated product. The 2 erythromycin stearate tablet formulations without a film coating had a significantly lower bioavailability. A significant difference in bioavailability existed also between these 2 non-film-coated products: one of them in fact disintegrated slowly, exposing the drug to the gastric acid in the fasted stomach for a longer time (Venho et al. 1987).

Food seems to play a significant role in the bioavailability of erythromycin stearate, as some formulations are best absorbed when taken immediately before meals (Disanto & Chodos 1981; Malmborg 1979; Rutland et al. 1979; Welling & Tse 1982).

Erythromycin Esters

Unlike the free base and salt forms of erythromycin, the esters are less water soluble and more resistant to acid-catalysed degradation: conse-

Table III. Mean (± SD) pharmacokinetic parameters (1-compartment first-order open model) of oral erythromycin stearate in adults with normal hepatic and renal function (microbiological assay)

Oral dosage[a]	No. of subjects	C_{max} (mg/L)	t_{max} (h)	AUC (mg/L · h)	Reference
Tablet					
500/1/F	12	1.81 ± 1.2	6	4.9 ± 2.9	Josefsson et al. (1983a)
500/1/immediately after food	18	1.1 ± 1.0	1.5	3.8 ± 3.5	Josefsson et al. (1983b)
1000/1/1h after breakfast	9[b]	1.5 ± 1.3	2		Shanson et al. (1983)
1500/1/1h after breakfast	–[b]	3.5 ± 2.2	1.5		
2000/1/1h after breakfast	–[b]	4.9 ± 2.6	1.5		
500/1/F (product B)	12[c]	1.93 ± 0.72	1.6 ± 0.8	7.22 ± 2.61	Venho et al. (1987)
500/1/F (product C)	–[c]	1.01 ± 0.65	2.1 ± 0.9	3.61 ± 2.41	
500/1/before breakfast	16[d]	2.09 ± 1.06	3.34 ± 0.27	4.99 ± 2.41	Rutland et al. (1979)
500/1/after breakfast	–[d]	0.37 ± 0.40	2.28 ± 0.93	1.04 ± 1.57	
Film-coated tablet					
500/1/F (product A)	12[c]	2.31 ± 0.78	2.3 ± 0.8	8.48 ± 2.38	Venho et al. (1987)
250 qid/10/fast≥2h	12				Disanto & Chodos (1981)
1st dose		0.62	3		
2nd dose		0.30	2	3.05[e]	
9th dose		1.45	3		
10th dose		0.80	3	9.28[f]	
250 qid/12/immediately after meals	21				
4th dose		0.40	2	6.88[g]	
12th dose		0.50	2	8.93[h]	
Capsule					
250 qid/5/1h before meals	10				McDonald et al (1977)
1st dose		0.41 ± 0.34	2.1 ± 0.6	1.0 ± 0.3	
5th dose		1.38 ± 0.87	2.1 ± 0.6	4.1 ± 2.6	

a Erythromycin base-equivalent dose/mg/schedule.
b Trials conducted in same subjects.
c Trials conducted in same subjects.
d Trials conducted in same subjects.
e 0-12 hours.
f 48-60 hours.
g 0-24 hours.
h 48-72 hours.
Abbreviations: see table II.

quently, they can be administered in the form of capsules and suspension.

Erythromycin ethylsuccinate ester is well absorbed from the gastrointestinal tract as esterified molecule, and hydrolysed to the base in the blood. Absorption is, however, delayed by food. The main pharmacokinetic studies of erythromycin ethylsuccinate are summarised in table IV. Under fasting conditions, peak serum concentrations (2.7 mg/L) occurred 1.3 hours after an 800mg single dose, with an area under the concentration-time curve (AUC) of 7.48 mg/L · h · C_{max} and AUC values were significantly higher than those observed with the same dose administered immediately after food, and the absorption process was faster (shorter t_{max}). Likewise, the C_{max} was significantly greater and t_{max} less than the values for the erythromycin ester administered either immediately or 1 hour after food (Thompson et al. 1980).

High peak serum erythromycin concentrations are obtained after administration of a single dose of 3g ethylsuccinate granules 1 hour after a light breakfast: at 1 hour the C_{max} was 2.8 mg/L (Shanson et al. 1984). The same authors demonstrated significantly higher serum drug concentrations following a single oral dose of erythromycin stearate 1.5g compared with a 3g dose of the ethylsuccinate ester (Shanson et al. 1983) [table III]. The mean C_{max} of total erythromycin derived from multiple dose administration of the ethylsuccinate ester tablets equivalent to 400mg base was in the range of 0.48 to 0.74 mg/L between the first and the tenth of 6-hourly doses in 24 fasting subjects (Yakatan et al. 1985). This study demonstrates that there are no absorption advantages to the ethylsuccinate ester over the acid-labile erythromycin base when assay methods capable of measuring the microbiologically active base in the presence of the ester are used (tables II and IV). In fact, the enteric-coated pellets of erythromycin base deliver more drug at steady-state than does the immediate-release erythromycin ethylsuccinate product. These differences are magnified even further by the fact that the ethylsuccinate product contains 1.6 times as much erythromycin as the enteric-coated pellets of the base product. Plasma concentrations for erythromycin ethylsuccinate comprise equal proportions of ester and free base (Welling & Tse 1982).

Erythromycin estolate, the dodecyl sulphate salt of the propionyl ester, is more acid-stable than the ethylsuccinate, and is absorbed from the gastrointestinal tract more completely and mainly as the ester. It is subsequently hydrolysed back to free base for about 20 to 35% of the total drug present in the blood. Pharmacokinetic parameters of erythromycin estolate are reported in table V. High serum concentrations are obtained rapidly and remain elevated for a prolonged period. The peak serum level obtained after erythromycin estolate as base plus ester is about 3 to 4 times higher than that achieved with a single dose of the base, the stearate or the ethylsuccinate ester. Food does not appreciably alter the absorption of estolate: its effects vary depending on the commercial preparations used (Disanto et al. 1980; Malmborg 1979; Welling & Tse 1982; Yakatan et al. 1980). The es-

Table IV. Mean (± SD) pharmacokinetic parameters (1-compartment, first-order open model) of oral erythromycin ethylsuccinate (microbiological assay)

Oral dosage[a]	No. of subjects	C_{max} (mg/L)	t_{max} (h)	AUC (mg/L · h)	Reference
Film-coated tablet	18				
800/1/immediately before food		2.71 ± 1.34	1.28 ± 0.79	7.48 ± 3.98	Thompson et al. (1980)
800/1/immediately after food		1.54 ± 1.05	2.39 ± 0.93	4.86 ± 3.28	
800/1/1h after food		1.72 ± 0.89	2.97 ± 0.81	5.51 ± 3.06	
Granules	11				
3000/1/1h after breakfast		2.8 ± 1.4	1		Shanson et al. (1984)
Tablet (conventional)	24				
400 qid/10/F					
1st dose		0.48 ± 0.27	1.50 ± 0.88	1.22 ± 0.68	Yakatan et al. (1985)
2nd dose		0.64 ± 0.29	1.50 ± 0.72	1.76 ± 0.81	
9th dose		0.57 ± 0.23	1.17 ± 0.48	2.19 ± 0.77	
10th dose		0.74 ± 0.41	1.40 ± 0.68	2.16 ± 1.00	

a Erythromycin base-equivalent dose (mg)/no. of doses/schedule.
Abbreviations: see table II.

ters of erythromycin give rise to circulating levels of both the esterified form of the drug, and also free base resulting from hydrolysis: plasma concentrations of erythromycin estolate comprise approximately 80% ester and 20% free base (table V). The actual levels of base are similar to those achieved by other oral preparations taken in the fasting state. Although the estolate form of erythromycin is better absorbed from the gastrointestinal tract, the serum concentrations may be spuriously high because only a percentage of the propionyl ester is hydrolysed to active erythromycin base *in vivo*. Moreover, the erythromycin estolate has the disadvantage of potential hepatotoxicity at therapeutic doses (Kucers & Bennet 1987).

Excellent bioavailability has been demonstrated recently for the propionyl erythromycin mercaptosuccinate: this new ester salt in the form of enterosoluble tablets on single- and multiple-dose regimens of 1g resulted in peak serum concentrations of 5.6 to 6.3 mg/L at 1.6 hours (Periti et al. 1986b). However, it is still not clear precisely how much of this erythromycin salt is hydrolysed *in vivo*.

Erythromycin glucoheptonate (gluceptate) and lactobionate are suitable for intravenous administration; intramuscular injection is also possible but causes pain at the injection site, and the dose should not exceed 100mg. Following a single intravenous injection of 250mg of gluceptate the peak serum concentration in adults is between 3.5 and 10.7 mg/L (Garrod et al. 1981). Pharmacokinetic parameters describing the disposition of erythromycin after intravenous administration of lactobionate in various single doses are given in table VI. A peak plasma concentration of approximately 10 mg/L

Table V. Mean (± SD) pharmacokinetic parameters (1-compartment, first-order open model) of oral erythromycin estolate

Oral dosage[a]	No. of subjects	C_{max} (mg/L)	t_{max} (h)	AUC (mg/L · h)	Assay	Reference
Tablet (conventional)						
250/1/4h fast before treatment	8	base 0.39 ± 0.22	3.63 ± 1.69	1.85 ± 1.06[b]		
		base+ester 1.66 ± 1.12	2.5			
250 qid/5/4h fast before and 2h fast after treatment	24					
1st dose		base 0.39 ± 0.18	3	1.34[c]	Micro	Yakatan et al. (1980)
		base+ester 2.50 ± 1.10	3			
5th dose		base 1.13 ± 0.37	3	7.37[b]		
		base+ester 4.35 ± 1.21	3			
Capsule						
250 qid/12/fast ≥ 2h	16	base 0.73	4.5		Fluorometric	Disanto et al. (1980)
		base+ester 3.0	3			
2nd dose		base 1.27	3	6.76[b]		
		base+ester 4.75	4.5			
9th dose		base 1.36	4.5	11.68[b]		
		base+ester 4.85	3			
12th dose		base 1.38	3			
		base+ester 4.60	3			

a Erythromycin base-equivalent dose (mg)/no. of doses/schedule.
b 0-12 hours.
c 0-6 hours.
Abbreviations: micro = microbiological assay; also see table II.

Table VI. Mean (±SD) pharmacokinetic parameters (2-compartment open model) of intravenous erythromycin lactobionate (microbiological assay)

IV dosage[a]	No. of subjects	Vd_{ss} (L)	$t_{1/2}$ (h)	CL (L/h)	CL_R (L/h)	A_{ur} (%)	AUC (mg/L · h)	Reference
250/1/F (3 min)	24	44.4 ± 11.4	1.5 ± 0.3	26.3 ± 7.5	3.4 ± 2.4	12		Austin et al. (1980)
125/1/F (15 min)	5	33.0 ± 4.5	1.3 ± 0.1	28.1 ± 5.9	1.5 ± 0.4	5.6 ± 2.3	4.6 ± 0.9	
250/1 (15 min)	5	40.4 ± 25.1	1.3 ± 0.2	28.9 ± 14.4	1.3 ± 0.8	4.8 ± 1.2	10.5 ± 3.0	
500/1 (15 min)	4	70.3 ± 11.4	2.4 ± 0.4	25.3 ± 4.3	2.7 ± 0.5	16.3 ± 2.3	19.4 ± 3.3	
900/1 (15 min)	3	76.7 ± 26.6	2.4 ± 0.4	26.3 ± 11.8	4.4 ± 3.6	17.1 ± 11.0	41.0 ± 23.1	

a Erythromycin base-equivalent dose (mg)/ no. of doses/schedule (duration of infusion time).

Abbreviations: Vd_{ss} = volume of distribution at steady-state; CL = total body clearance; CL_R = renal clearance; A_{ur} = amount of drug excreted in urine (percentage of administered dose); also see table II.

was present immediately after the 250mg dose infused over 3 minutes; a 500mg dose produced peak serum levels of 11.5 to 30.0 mg/L (Garrod et al. 1981).

Incremental doses of erythromycin lactobionate between 125 and 900mg were administered by 15-minute infusions to assess the linearity of the kinetics. Erythromycin kinetics were described by a 2-compartment model with little intersubject variation. Mean peak serum concentrations varied from about 8 to 35 mg/L with some evidence of non-linear pharmacokinetics as a function of dose (Austin et al. 1980).

Erythromycin base or lactobionate, administered rectally as a suppository, demonstrated satisfactory absorption and therapeutic plasma concentrations for 6 hours after a dose similar to that used orally (Bosco 1973; Pozzi et al. 1982).

2.1.2 Distribution

Erythromycin appears to be distributed throughout the total body water. The volume of distribution at steady-state (Vd_{ss}) reaches about 45L in adult subjects (McDonald 1986; Spitzy & Hitzenberger 1958; Wilson & Boxtel 1978).

Erythromycin is highly bound to plasma proteins: the binding ranges from 65 to 90% of total drug concentration, depending on the method used. In contrast to acidic drugs, for which serum albumin is the major binding protein, erythromycin is primarily bound to α_2-globulin (Bergan et al. 1987; Chow 1984; Dette et al. 1981, 1982; Wilson & Boxtel 1978). Erythromycin binding to serum proteins is reversible, and varies as a function of serum protein levels. As shown by equilibrium dialysis, at concentrations achieved with therapeutic doses, erythromycin binding is not linearly related to total drug concentration: the amount of the bound drug fraction decreases with increasing total concentration. Total binding can be divided into 2 components: specific binding, which is saturable with increasing erythromycin concentrations, and nonspecific binding, which does not reach a plateau and increases linearly with increasing antibiotic concentrations. The affinity of specific erythromycin binding is rather high and follows hyperbolic saturation kinetics (Dette et al. 1982). Protein binding has only a minor impact on erythromycin penetration into extravascular tissue sites; distinct lymph drug concentrations are observed with a low peak and a protracted disposition, with nearly horizontal concentration curves. The explanation for the slow decrease of lymph levels is the interaction of erythromycin with the lattice of the α_2-globulin fibrillae within the intracellular space, like the stationary phase of a chromatographic system (Bergan et al. 1987). The relation between serum protein binding and erythromycin tissue penetration, indicated as a percentage of the lymph/serum AUC ratio, corresponds well in humans to a penetration ratio of 35% for a serum protein binding of 70% according to a regression line among various chemical classes of antibacterial agents (Bergan et al. 1987).

Erythromycin is usually well distributed to various tissues and fluids. In general, animal studies indicate that tissue concentrations are higher than those in serum, and persist longer. In humans the ratios of tissue or body fluid to contemporaneous serum concentrations vary from 0.1 for saliva, cord serum and cerebrospinal fluid with meningitis to values of more than 1 for bronchial secretions, lung tissues, breast milk and bile; for other body tissues and fluids the values are intermediate (reviewed by Bergogne-Bérézin 1986; Steigbigel 1985; Wilson & Van Boxtel 1978). These data are reported in detail in table VII.

An interesting aspect of erythromycin is its ability to penetrate phagocytes as measured by microscope-autoradiography with ^{3}H-labelled drug. Compared with extracellular fluid, the intracellular concentration of erythromycin is 9 to 23 times higher in alveolar macrophages, and 4 to 24 times higher in polymorphonuclear leucocytes (Carlier et al. 1987; Dette & Knothe 1986; Miller et al. 1984; Pocidalo et al. 1985; Vosbeck et al. 1984).

^{14}N-CH_3-erythromycin is massively concentrated by alveolar macrophages obtained by bronchoalveolar lavage from smokers with associated pulmonary abnormalities (Hand et al. 1985). The base is highly concentrated by human-derived tissue culture cells of normal bronchus, kidney, liver, lung and skin and by cancer cells derived from breast, liver and lung; intracellular concentrations 4 to 12 times that of the extracellular milieu are obtained in both early-passage and transformed cells (Martin et al. 1985).

2.1.3 Metabolism and Elimination

Erythromycin is concentrated by the liver and excreted into the bile as active drug in high concentrations ranging from 5 to 250 mg/L: 10 mg/L in subjects receiving the propionyl ester, and 64 mg/L in those receiving the base. Only about 1.5% of the dose of the base and 0.2% of the estolate appears in the bile in the first 8 hours, the bile : serum concentration ratio being approximately 4 for the propionyl ester, and 30 for the base (Garrod et al. 1981); much of the rest is presumably demethylated or otherwise degraded. Erythromycin is *N*-demethylated in the liver microsomal system; indeed, a large proportion of absorbed drug cannot be accounted for by urinary or biliary excretion or by tissue binding. The distribution of *N*-demethylated erythromycin is apparently similar to the parent drug (Wilson & Boxtel 1978). The substantial bowel intraluminal concentrations seen reflect both this biliary excretion and residual unabsorbed drug. In patients with biliary obstruction, bile concentrations and therefore stool concentrations are correspondingly lower (Brittain 1987). An enterohepatic recirculation may also contribute to the high concentrations of erythromycin in faecal samples (Chelvan et al. 1979; Hammond & Griffith 1961; Sabath et al. 1968; Twiss et al. 1956).

Up to 4.5% of an oral dose and 15% of a parenteral dose of erythromycin are recoverable in the urine: urine concentrations after oral doses are often high but quite variable (Garrod et al. 1981; Nicholas 1977), and only a minor fraction of the dose can be accounted for in this way. Urine concentrations from 1 g/day of propionyl erythromycin have been reported to be 13 to 46 mg/L, and from similar doses of erythromycin base 11 to 24 mg/L; peak concentrations of 7.4 to 15.2 mg/L 3 to 4 hours after a dose of 250mg of the estolate have been found. Clearance data suggest an active transfer and net tubular reabsorption of erythromycin.

The elimination half-life ($t_{1/2}$) of erythromycin base in adult patients with normal renal and hepatic function varies between 1.9 and 2.1 hours following multiple oral drug administration of 500mg twice daily or 250mg four times daily (Yakatan et al. 1985; Josefsson et al. 1982). Longer $t_{1/2}$ values have been reported for the stearate salt (6.6 hours: Ducci et al. 1981) and for the propionyl ester in the form of the mercaptosuccinate salt (about 5 hours: Periti et al. 1986b). Garrod et al. (1981) reported a $t_{1/2}$ of 1 to 2 hours for erythromycin glucoheptonate. Austin et al. (1980), studying the pharmacokinetics of incremental doses of erythromycin lactobionate between 125 and 900mg, administered by a 15-minute infusion, found the pharmacokinetics to be non-linear: as doses increase so too do $t_{1/2}$ and Vd_{ss}. Reasons for this ap-

Table VII. Mean (±SD) or range of erythromycin concentrations in body tissues and fluids (different formulations)

Body tissue or fluid	Dose (mg)	Route	C_{max}[a]	C_{max}/C_s	Reference
Lymph	500 bid	PO	0.93 ± 0.24	0.25-0.35	Bergan et al. (1982, 1987)
Suction blister fluid	1000	PO	0.34	0.43-0.77	Vaillant et al. (1987)
			3.3 ± 0.5		Periti et al. (1986a)
Skin-window	500	PO	0.41	0.6	Magliulo et al. (1979)
Saliva	500 bid	PO/IV	0.84 ± 0.09	0.2-0.3	Ducci et al. (1981)
			0.35±0.15; 0.1		Heimdahl & Nord (1981)
					Austin et al. (1980)
Bronchial secretions	1000 bid	PO	1.05 ± 0.49	0.25-0.45	Bergogne-Bérézin (1985)
			0.6-3.8		Kosmidis & Marosis (1985)
Healthy lung	270/500-1000	PO/IV	6.6 ± 2.2	1.1-3.2	Wolmer et al. (1982)
			4.2-5.9		Walstad & Hellum (1984)
			6.35 ± 3.18 -		Brun et al. (1981)
			4.23 ± 2.16		
Pleural fluid	500 bid	PO	1.0-7.4	0.7	Nicholas (1977)
Middle ear exudate	250-500 tid	PO	0.8-4.2	0.6-1.0	Bass et al. (1971)
					Sundberg et al. (1979)
Maxillary sinus mucosa	500 tid	PO	<0.1-5.4	0.8	Paavolainen et al. (1977)
Nasal mucosa	500 bid	PO	1.96 ± 1.56	0.74	Periti et al. (1986b)
Adenoids	600 bid	PO	0.9-1.4	1.1	Sundberg et al. (1981)
Tonsil	100 bid	PO	3.39 ± 0.28	0.3-1.2	Falchi et al. (1985)
Breast milk	500 bid	PO	30	5.0	Wilson & Van Boxtel (1978)
Bile					
(unobstructed)	1000	IV	81	28.0-30.0	Chelvan et al. (1979)
(T-tube drainage)	200-400 qid	PO	5.0-90.0	2.0-10.0	Twiss et al. (1956)
(unobstructed)	200-400 qid	PO	35.0-250.0	25.0-250.0	
(T-tube drainage)	500	PO	10.0-64.0	4.0-30.0	Hammond & Griffith (1961)
Semen	500 bid	PO	0.2-0.9	0.3	Armstrong et al. (1968)
Prostatic fluid	1000	IV	0.35	0.4	Chow (1984)
Cord serum	600-1000	PO	0.04-0.6	0.1	Wilson & Van Boxtel (1978)
Amniotic fluid	500	PO/IV	0.23-0.36	0.05	Philipson et al. (1973)
Fetal tissues	500	PO/IV	0.08-0.35[b]	0.01-0.7	Philipson et al. (1973)
Uterine tissue	1000	IV	4.5-17.6	1.5-3.0	Segui et al. (1987)
Lymph node	1000 bid	PO	1.51±1.07 -	1.1-1.5	Brun et al. (1981)
			4.77±2.85		

a Tissue (mg/kg) or fluid (mg/L).
b Mean values of different tissues.

Abbreviations: PO = oral administration; IV = intravenous administration; tid = 3 times daily; C_s = serum concentration; also see table II.

parent non-linearity may be related to changes in plasma protein binding over the concentration range of the antibiotic: certainly plasma protein binding of erythromycin is high and in the range where its effects are important (Gordon et al. 1973).

2.2 Effects of Age and Various Pathophysiological States on Kinetics

There is a dearth of adequate information on age-specific pharmacokinetics for erythromycin in children or in the elderly (Coyne et al. 1978; Nilsen 1987; Patamasucon et al. 1981; Washington & Wilson 1985).

Renal impairment has only a minor impact on the pharmacokinetics of erythromycin (Disse et al. 1986; Kunin 1967), while alcoholic liver disease increases the elimination half-life from 2.0 to 3.2 hours (Hall et al. 1982). No adjustment of the dose of erythromycin in these categories of patients is necessary (Nilsen 1987).

2.2.1 Renal Disease

Erythromycin is not removed by peritoneal dialysis or haemodialysis (Steigbigel 1985).

Renal clearance of erythromycin has been found to be significantly correlated to the creatinine clearance. Total recovery in urine did not exceed 7.5%. As expected from the small fraction excreted via the kidneys, the elimination half-life and total clearance of erythromycin did not depend on renal function (Disse et al. 1986).

In patients with complete renal failure receiving large doses of the drug (i.e. ⩾ 4 g/day), however, erythromycin may accumulate, and many toxic effects have been seen in this setting: an increase in the interval between doses to 8 or 12 hours might be prudent under these circumstances (Brittain 1987).

2.2.2 Liver Disease

Comparative serum concentration/time data from subjects with normal liver function and alcoholic liver disease after a single oral dose of erythromycin base show a shorter lag time and an earlier time to peak concentration in patients (Kroboth et al. 1982).

Patients with biliary obstruction or severe hepatocellular disease may benefit from a reduced dosing schedule to lessen the change in drug accumulation: if large doses of erythromycin are administered to such patients, serum drug concentration monitoring may be necessary (Kucers & Bennet 1987).

3. Oleandomycin

Oleandomycin phosphate can be given by oral route or slow intravenous infusion. Oleandomycin is also available in an oral preparation as the triacetyl ester, troleandomycin.

The mean peak concentration is about 0.8 mg/L after an oral dose of oleandomycin 500mg, whereas an identical dose of triacetyloleandomycin produced a C_{max} of 2.0 mg/L (De Louvois 1982). The serum half-life of oleandomycin has been reported to be about 1 hour (Duthu 1985). Oleandomycin is significantly excreted in bile, reaching levels 10 to 15 times greater than serum concentrations (De Louvois 1982). The drug is well distributed in tissues, achieving elevated concentrations which persist for prolonged periods in various organs or body fluids including middle-ear exudate, tissue secretions, adenoids, bronchial secretions and skin window fluids (Bergogne-Bérézin 1985; Magliulo et al. 1979).

4. Spiramycin

Spiramycin is well absorbed from the gastrointestinal tract, and the simultaneous administration of food does not affect its bioavailability (Kamme et al. 1978; Welling 1980). Serum concentrations during treatment with 2 to 3 g/day ranged from 0.5 to 3.7 mg/L, with peaks of 7.2 and 8 mg/L and $t_{1/2}$ of about 2 hours (Bergogne-Bérézin et al. 1978; Chabbert 1955; Gaillot & Lemar 1981; Hudson et al. 1956; Macfarlane et al. 1968; Taranger et al. 1972).

Spiramycin penetrates well into tissues such as lung, prostate and muscle, and into body fluids, persisting for prolonged periods at these sites. Kamme et al. (1978) demonstrated that it is secreted in saliva with peaks that are 1.3 to 4.8 times higher than serum concentrations. According to Macfarlane et al. (1968), tissue concentrations of spiramycin are at maximum after 7 days of treatment. Spiramycin showed good and rapid penetration into bronchial secretions with levels varying from 2 to 7.3 mg/L (Bergogne-Bérézin et al. 1978; Lamy et al. 1977).

Spiramycin does not enter the cerebrospinal fluid, even in the case of meningitis (Kernbaum 1982). Protein binding is about 30%.

Renal clearance of spiramycin is less than 10% (Videau 1978), but biliary excretion is significant, with bile concentrations 15 to 40 times higher than serum concentrations (Gaillot and Lemar 1981). The serum $t_{1/2}$ has been estimated at between 4 and 8 hours (Gaillot & Lemar 1981; Kamme et al. 1978).

Only recently have the pharmacokinetics of spiramycin after single and multiple intravenous administration of a 500mg dose (1-hour infusion) been investigated in healthy volunteers by Le Roux et al. (1985). After a single dose the C_{max} was 2.50 mg/L and the $t_{1/2}$ 5.16 hours. At the end of 6 days of treatment with 500mg three times daily the mean steady-state concentration was 2.91 mg/L, and the trough level was 0.51 mg/L.

5. Josamycin

5.1 Fundamental Pharmacokinetic Properties

5.1.1 Absorption and Bioavailability

Table VIII summarises the most important pharmacokinetic parameters in adults with normal hepatic and renal function. Josamycin is administered only by oral route and is well absorbed from the gastrointestinal tract.

A single dose of 400mg produces peak concentrations of 0.33 mg/L within 0.77 hours (Shiiki & Sakamoto 1987), and single doses of 500mg provide peak concentrations of 0.61 to 0.71 mg/L within 1 hour (Strausbaugh et al. 1976). According to Fourtillan et al. (1983) the administration of a single dose of 1000mg does not cause an increase in plasma peak concentrations (mean values of 0.21 mg/L in 6 healthy subjects). However, in our experience a higher mean peak concentration of 2.4 mg/L occurred within 1 hour of the administration of a similar dose in 10 healthy volunteers (Nicoletti et al. 1983a). In a previous study, Fourtillan et al. (1982) also reported a C_{max} as high as 2.41 mg/L in 5 healthy adults after the same dose. The mean values of AUC are similar in both studies: 4.4 mg/L • h (Nicoletti et al. 1983) and 4.9 mg/L • h (Fourtillan et al. 1982). Strausbaugh et al. (1976) obtained a peak concentration of 5.06 mg/L within 1 hour after a loading dose of 1500mg followed by 500mg four times daily over 10 days in 4 healthy subjects.

The absorption of josamycin free base is delayed by food, as reflected by the t_{max} which was 0.72 hours in fasting and 1.95 hours in non-fasting subjects (Ikeda et al. 1985). The same authors demonstrated that the bioavailability of josamycin propionate was 3 times higher after food.

Increases in C_{max} with multiple-dose regimens of 500mg three times daily, 500mg four times daily and 1000mg three times daily over 3 days were obtained by Strausbaugh et al. (1976) and Fourtillan et al. (1983). A comparative study of josamycin and erythromycin pharmacokinetics was conducted by Strausbaugh et al. (1976) in 21 healthy volunteers and demonstrated that the 2 drugs, in comparable doses, produced similar plasma concentrations.

5.1.2 Distribution

The ability of josamycin to penetrate and accumulate in various tissues and body fluids has been well documented and data from the literature have been summarised in table IX. Josamycin showed good penetration into bronchial secretions after both single and repeated doses of 500mg and 1000mg (Bergogne-Bérézin et al. 1985; Fraschini et al. 1982). The mean sputum concentrations ranged from 0.45 to 1.00 mg/L with sputum : serum concentration ratios varying from 0.2 to 0.3 (Fraschini et al. 1982). Lower concentrations were achieved in bronchial aspirates (0.26 to 0.52 mg/L) with a bronchial aspirate : serum ratio ranging from 0.2 to 0.4 (Bergogne-Bérézin et al. 1985).

The mean concentrations of josamycin in pulmonary tissue after multiple doses varied from 0.9

Table VIII. Mean (± SD) pharmacokinetic parameters of oral josamycin in adults with normal hepatic and renal function

Oral dosage[a]	No. of subjects	C_{max} (mg/L)	t_{max} (h)	$t_{1/2}$ (h)	AUC (mg/L · h)	A_{ur} (%)	Assay	References
400/1	12	0.33	0.77	1.51	0.91		Micro	Shiiki & Sakamoto (1987)
1000/1	10	2.4 ± 0.9		0.9 ± 0.1	4.4 ± 1.6		Micro	Nicoletti et al. (1983a)
1000/1	5	2.41	0.75	2.0	4.9[b]		HPLC	Fourtillan et al. (1982)
1000/1							Micro	Ikeda et al. (1985)
F		3.78	0.72		7.92	3.19[c]		
NF		1.95	1.95		10.8	4.49[c]		
1000/1								
F		0.87	1.57		3.27	1.64[c]		
NF		2.11	1.86		9.84	4.39[c]		
1000 tid/1[d]	6	0.21 ± 0.07[e]	1.0		0.91		HPLC	Fourtillan et al. (1983)
1000 tid/7[d]	6	2.28 ± 0.49[e]	1.1	5.8 ± 0.8				
500 tid/1	21	0.71	1	1.48			Micro	Strausbaugh et al. (1976)
500 tid/7	21	1.64	1	1.53				
500 qid/1	20	0.61	1	1.56				
500 qid/1	20	2.31	1	1.34				
500 qid/1[f,g]	4	5.06	1			8.35		
1500 followed by 500 qid/37[f,g]	4	2.61	1			16.46		

a Dose (mg)/no. of doses/schedule.
b 0-8g.
c 0-6 hours.
d Josamycin base.
e Standard error.
f Following a loading dose of 1500mg.
g Josamycin propionate.

Abbreviations: HPLC = high performance liquid chromatography; micro = microbiological assay; A_{ur} = amount of drug excreted in urine (percentage of administered dose); tid = 3 times daily; also see table II.

to 3.68 mg/kg (Fraschini et al. 1982; Wildfeuer et al. 1985).

In 20 adult patients undergoing tonsillectomy, administration of josamycin base 500mg in a single dose produced a mean tonsillar concentration of 13.65 mg/kg with a tissue : serum ratio of 7.54. After administration of the same dose of josamycin propionate in 30 paediatric patients, the mean tonsillar levels were higher at 21.24 mg/kg (Carlone et al. 1982). Josamycin also demonstrated good penetration into middle-ear fluid, sinus secretions and adenoids (Bergogne-Bérézin 1985). Carlone et al. (1982) also investigated the distribution of multiple doses of josamycin in eye fluids: in 50 patients undergoing cataract extraction the mean concentrations were: aqueous humour 0.4 mg/L, subretinal fluid 6 mg/L and tears 2.3 mg/L. In their earlier study, Strausbaugh et al. (1976) reported similar tear concentrations after 10 days of treatment.

The distribution of multiple doses of josamycin into long bones and the jaw bone was studied by Fraschini et al. (1982) and found to be respectively 83% and 39% of blood concentration. The saliva concentrations varied from 0.15 mg/L after a single dose of 400mg (Shiiki & Sakamoto 1987) to 1.03 mg/L after multiple doses (Strausbaugh et al. 1976). Higher concentrations were reached in prostatic tissue in 12 male subjects undergoing prostatectomy for prostatic hypertrophy: the mean level at the fourth 500mg dose was 5.0 mg/kg (Fagioli et al. 1982).

The penetration of josamycin into extracellular fluid was quite good and the fluid : serum ratio varied, with various regimens and methods, from 0.24 to 0.73 (Magliulo et al. 1982; Nicoletti et al. 1983a).

The intracellular accumulation of ^{14}C-labelled josamycin has been investigated by Wildfeuer et al. (1985). The ratio of the cellular to the extracellular concentration (C : E) of josamycin demonstrated a significant accumulation of the drug by polymorphonuclear leucocytes and monocytes *in vitro* (C : E = 20.8 and 20.7 respectively, after 45 minutes of incubation at 37°C).

Josamycin binding to plasma proteins is 15% (Yamanouchi Ltd, data on file, 1984).

5.1.3 Metabolism and Elimination

Josamycin is metabolised in the liver and excreted mainly in the bile (Mitsuhashi 1971). Less than 20% of the drug is excreted via the urine in an active form (Ikeda et al. 1985; Strausbaugh et al. 1976). The metabolic pathway of josamycin in humans leads to 4 metabolites (Fourtillan et al. 1982). Metabolite I, the major derivative hydroxylated at C-15, is measurable in plasma and the 3 others are detectable only in urine samples. The antimicrobial activity of metabolite I is reduced from that of the parent compound.

Most authors reported a serum half-life following a single dose of josamycin ranging between 0.9 and 2 hours (Nicoletti et al. 1983a; Shiiki and Sakamoto 1987; Strausbaugh et al. 1976). However, Fourtillan et al. (1982), using an HPLC assay method for measurement of plasma josamycin concentrations, reported a terminal half-life of 12.7 hours for unmetabolised josamycin and 1.3 hours for its main metabolite.

5.2 Effects of Age and Various Pathological States on Kinetics

The pharmacokinetics of a single dose of josamycin 1250mg have been studied by Bergan et al. (1972) in 5 patients with parenchymal liver disease in comparison with 14 healthy subjects. The C_{max} values were significantly higher in healthy subjects than in patients (6.87 *vs* 1.66 mg/L), but no differences were demonstrated in serum half-lives. In 2 patients with biliary occlusion in the same study the elimination of josamycin was markedly slower and the $t_{1/2}$ values were undetermined within the period of observation (Bergan et al. 1972).

Josamycin pharmacokinetics were impaired in one study conducted by Okolicsanyi et al. (1985) in patients with liver cirrhosis and Gilbert's syndrome. Plasma josamycin concentrations, in fact, after both single and multiple 1000mg doses, were higher in patients than in normal subjects. The half-life was also significantly higher in cirrhotics (5.36 *vs* 1.05 hours), and the author suggests that a dosage adjustment is indicated when dealing with these patients (Okolicsanyi et al. 1985).

The pharmacokinetics of josamycin in the elderly have been studied by Ghanassia et al. (1985). Comparison of the main pharmacokinetic parameters between aged and young subjects after a single dose of 1000mg showed a significant increase in the half-life in aged subjects (3.4 ± 0.67 hours). The authors suggested lower doses and longer intervals between doses.

6. Midecamycin

Few data are available concerning the pharmacokinetic properties of midecamycin in humans. Saito et al. (1973) observed in 5 healthy male volunteers a mean peak serum concentration of 0.8 mg/L 1 hour after oral administration of 600mg, serum levels of 0.2 mg/L or less after 4 to 6 hours, urine concentrations ranging from 21 to 100 mg/L 2 to 4 hours after administration and a urinary recovery after 6 hours of 3.3% on average. When administered at an oral dosage of 1000 to 1200mg, midecamycin proved to be rapidly absorbed by the gastrointestinal tract with peak serum concentrations occurring within 1 to 2 hours and ranging from 1.27 to 1.9 mg/L (Clauzel et al. 1981; Iwasawa 1973). Midecamycin undergoes liver metabolisation and a major metabolite formed by direct

Table IX. Mean (± SD) concentration of oral josamycin in body tissues and fluids (microbiological assay)

Body tissue/ fluid	Oral dosage[a]	No. of subjects [Time to sample (h)]	C_s (mg/L)	C_t (mg/kg or mg/L)	C_t/C_s ratio	Reference
Respiratory tract						
Bronchial aspirates	1000/1	5 [1]	1.74 ± 0.76	0.52 ± 0.23	0.30	Bergogne-Bérézin (1985)
	1000/1	5 [2]	1.24 ± 1.85	0.35 ± 0.18	0.28	
	1000/1	5 [4]	0.55 ± 0.29	0.27 ± 0.11	0.48	
Sputum	500/1	10 [1]	1.36	0.45	0.33	Fraschini et al. (1982)
	500 qid/25	10 [1]	1.75	0.53	0.30	
	1000/1	10 [1]	3.30	0.75	0.23	
	1000 bid/13	10 [1]	3.80	1.00	0.26	
Healthy lung	500 qid/25	8 [3.20-4.20]	0.7	0.9	1.28	Fraschini et al. (1982)
Pathological lung				1.3	1.85	
Lung	100 bid[b]	12 [2.28 ± 0.36]	1.29 ± 1.10	3.68 ± 4.6	2.85	Wildfeuer et al. (1985)
Tonsil	500/1[c]	30 [1]	0.76 ± 0.22	21.24 ± 6.5	27.94	Carlone et al. (1982)
	500/1[d]	20 [1]	1.81 ± 0.6	13.65 ± 2.7	7.54	
Middle ear exudate						Bergogne-Bérézin (1985)
acute otitis media	1000 bid[b]	10 [3]	0.55 ± 0.33	1.24 ± 1.87	2.25	
chronic otitis media	1000 bid[b]	5 [3]	1.95 ± 1.69	0.97 ± 0.74	0.49	
serous middle ear effusion	1000 bid[b]	4 [3]	0.45 ± 0.30	1.88 ± 3.46	4.17	
Sinus secretions	1000 bid[b]	8 [3]	0.91 ± 0.66	2.80 ± 1.47	3.07	
Adenoids	1000 bid[b]	6 [3]	0.45 ± 0.34	1.60 ± 1.52	3.55	
Eye fluids						
Aqueous humour	500 every 4h/ 6 followed by one 1g dose	50	2.8 ± 0.21	0.4 ± 0.03	0.14	Carlone et al. (1982)
Sub-retinal fluid	500 every 4h/ 6 followed by one 1g dose	50	2.8 ± 0.21	6.0 ± 1.05	2.0	
Tears	500 every 4h/ 6 followed by one 1g dose	50	2.8 ± 0.21	2.3 ± 0.36	0.82	
Tears	500 qid/37[e]	4		2.62 ± 0.72		Strausbaugh et al. (1976)
Bone						
Long bones	500 qid/25	7 [1.45-3.55]	1.2	(spongy) 1.0	0.83	Fraschini et al. (1982)
				(compact) 1.0	0.83	
Jaw bone tissue	500 qid/9	22 [2.00-2.45]	1.47 ± 0.36	0.57 ± 0.26	0.39	

Table IX. Contd

Body tissue/ fluid	Oral dosage[a]	No. of subjects [Time to sample (h)]	C_s (mg/L)	C_t (mg/kg or mg/L)	C_t/C_s ratio	Reference
Miscellanea						
Healthy gums	500 qid/9	22 [2.00-2.45]	1.47 ± 0.36	0.43 ± 0.21	0.29	Fraschini et al. (1982)
Pathological gums				0.50 ± 0.15	0.34	
Saliva	400/1	12 [1]	0.34 ± 0.08[f]	0.15 ± 0.04[f]	0.44	Shiiki & Sakamoto (1987)
Saliva	500 qid/39[e]	4		1.03 ± 0.43		Strausbaugh et al. (1976)
Sweat	500 qid/37[e]	4		0.95 ± 0.30		
Prostate	500 tid/4	12 [1.86 ± 0.45]		5.00 ± 1.00		Fagioli et al. (1982)
Extracellular fluids						
Window chamber fluid	500/1	6 [2]	0.60 ± 0.16	0.26 ± 0.10	0.43[g]	Magliulo et al. (1982)
	1000/1	3 [4]	1.26 ± 0.60	0.93 ± 0.23	0.73[g]	
	1000 tid/9	3 [4]	2.50 ± 1.22	0.76 ± 0.15	0.30[g]	
Suction blister fluid	500/1	6 [4]		0.32 ± 0.06		
	1000/1	3 [4]		1.46 ± 0.10		
Suction blister fluid	1000/1	10 [1]	2.4 ± 0.9	0.58 ± 0.15	0.24[g]	Nicoletti et al. (1983a)

a Dose (mg)/no. of doses/schedule.
b Repeated dose, not specified.
c Josamycin propionate in paediatric patients.
d Josamycin base in adult patients.
e Following a loading dose of 1500mg.
f Standard error.
g AUC_{fluid}/AUC_{serum} (%).
Abbreviations: qid = 4 times daily; tid = 3 times daily; C_s = serum concentration; C_t = tissue or fluid concentration.

14-hydroxylation, with reduced activity (almost 50%) compared with the parent drug, is detected in human urine (Inouye & Niida 1981). Pharmacokinetic studies performed in rats demonstrate that midecamycin has a wide tissue distribution, reaching concentrations in main organs higher than those in the blood (Inovye & Niida 1981; Shomura & Umemura 1973). However, early observations in humans with oral doses of midecamycin 1000mg demonstrated a mean concentration of 0.3 mg/kg in palatine tonsil compared to an average plasma level of 1.9 mg/L, with a tissue : plasma ratio of 0.16. The compound was detectable only in traces, or not at all, in maxillary sinus mucosa (Iwasawa 1973).

Nevertheless, relatively high concentrations of the antibiotic were observed in bronchial secretions 4 hours after single or multiple oral administration of 1200mg with an average bronchial secretion : plasma ratio of 0.86 (Clauzel et al. 1981), thus confirming a good diffusion and tropism for the respiratory tract (table X).

7. *Miocamycin*

Miocamycin, a semisynthetic derivative of midecamycin bearing 2 acetyl groups at C-9 and C-3″, is rapidly and almost completely absorbed by the gastrointestinal tract (Fukaya et al. 1981, 1985). After oral administration of miocamycin 400mg Sawae et al. (1987) found a mean peak serum concentration of 1.65 mg/L; with a dose of 600mg

Table X. Mean (± SD) or range of pharmacokinetic parameters of oral miocamycin and rosaramicin in adults with normal hepatic and renal function

Dosage (mg)	No. of subjects	C_{max} (mg/L)	t_{max} (h)	$t_{½}$ (h)	CL (L/h)	Vd (L)	A_{ur} (%)	Assay	References
Miocamycin									
400	5	1.65	1	0.61 ± 0.17			0.9[d]	Micro	Sawae et al. (1987)
600	11	2.7-3	0.66	0.83			4-5	Micro	Fraschini et al. (1985)
600[a]	30	1.31	1	0.78				Micro	Fukaya et al. (1985)
600[b]	30	1.36	0.66	0.86					
800[c]	6	2.7	0.72	1			<0.5		
800[c]	6	1.7	1.28				<0.5	Micro	Sanders et al. (1985)
800[c,d]	12	1.3	0.75	0.73			0.225		
800[c,e]	12	1.9	0.75	1.52			0.4		
Rosaramicin									
250	10	0.165-0.485	2	4.4	26.63	238.7 ± 114.8		HPLC	Stoehr et al. (1985)
500[f]	12	0.448	1.5				0.4	HPLC	Lin et al. (1980)
500[c]	12	0.418 ± 0.111	1.58 ± 0.62	4.53 ± 1.19			6		Lin et al. (1984a)
500[a]	12	0.486 ± 0.125	1.83 ± 0.8	4.82 ± 1.25				HPLC	
500[g]	8	0.73 ± 0.24	0.94±0.12	5.01±1.08			6.98± 3.65	LSS	
500[h]	12			3.28±0.37	56.32± 8.69	264.6± 39.9		HPLC	

a Tablets.
b Dry syrup.
c Oral solution.
d 1st dose.
e 12th dose.
f Intravenous administration.
g ^{14}C-Rosaramicin oral solution.
h 1h infusion.

Abbreviations: Vd = apparent volume of distribution; A_{ur} = amount of drug excreted in urine (percentage of dose administered); LSS = liquid scintillation spectrometry; HPLC = high performance liquid chromatography; micro = microbiological assay; also see table II.

(tablets or dry syrup) peak serum concentrations, obtained within 40 to 60 minutes, range from 1.31 to 3 mg/L on average (Fraschini et al. 1985; Fukaya et al. 1985) [table XI]. Absorption of the compound, unlike that of various erythromycin salts, appears not to be influenced by the presence of food in the stomach: Fukaya et al. (1981) reported mean peak serum levels of 2.38 and 1.83 mg/L after oral administration of miocamycin 600mg in fasting and non-fasting subjects, respectively. Sanders et al. (1985) found, however, that the absorption of an oral suspension of 800mg of the antibiotic in 100ml water was actually delayed in non-fasting subjects.

Protein binding is about 47%, and seems to be independent of the dosage regimen (Fukaya et al. 1981). The elimination half-life of miocamycin ranges from 0.61 to 1.49 hours, being shorter with lower dosage, and the compound is usually detectable in blood 6 hours after administration (Fraschini et al. 1985; Fukaya et al. 1981, 1985; Sanders et al. 1985; Sawae et al. 1987). Miocamycin is excreted as unchanged drug, as fully active metabolites and as metabolites with reduced biological activity (almost half that of the parent compound) through hydroxylation in the C-14 position of the lactonic ring or deacetylation in C-4″ of the mycarose molecule (Fukaya et al. 1981; Inouye & Niida 1981). Biliary excretion represents the main elimination route of miocamycin and its derivatives (Fukaya et al. 1981; Inouye & Niida 1981).

Renal excretion of unchanged drug and active metabolites is usually low and ranges from 0.3 to 5%, according to different studies (Fraschini et al. 1985; Fukaya et al. 1981, 1985; Sanders et al. 1985; Sawae et al. 1987), with urinary concentrations of 10 to 20 mg/L in the 4-hour period following administration of miocamycin 600mg (Fukaya et al. 1985). Similar pharmacokinetic parameters were observed in children after an oral dose of 10 or 20 mg/kg, with mean peak serum concentrations of 0.76 mg/L and 1.01 mg/L, respectively, occurring 1 hour after administration (Nishimura 1983). Miocamycin demonstrates rapid diffusion in the extravascular compartment, with tissue concentrations always higher than those in serum in the 6 hours after a single or multiple dose of 600mg (Fraschini et al. 1985; Nicoletti et al. 1983b). During the 1- to 2-hour period following administration, lung and palatine tonsil concentrations ranged from 2.4 to 4 mg/kg, being 1.5 to 3 times higher than corresponding plasma levels, while in larynx and nasal mucosa miocamycin concentrations at 2 hours post administration were 1.0 mg/kg and 1.4 mg/kg, respectively. After the sixth oral dose of 600mg every 8 hours, miocamycin achieved prostatic concentrations 2-fold higher than plasma levels (Fraschini et al. 1985; Nicoletti et al. 1983b;

Table XI. Mean (±SD) or ranges of concentrations of midecamycin, miocamycin and rosaramicin in body tissues and fluids

Body tissue/ fluid	Oral dosage (mg)	No. of subjects	Time to sample (h)	C_s (mg/L)	C_t (mg/kg or mg/L)	C_t/C_s ratio	Assay	References
Midecamycin								
Palatine tonsils	1000	3	1	1.9	0.3	0.16	Micro	Iwasawa (1973)
Bronchial secretion	1200	10	4	0.52 ± 0.26[a]	0.56 ± 0.27[a]	1.08	Micro	Clauzel et al. (1981)
					0.47 ± 0.33[b]			
					0.37 ± 0.36[a]			
Miocamycin								
Bronchial secretion[d]	600	6	2	0.81 ± 0.33	5.16 ± 4.93	6.37	Micro	Fioretti et al. (1984)
Sputum		6	4	0.32 ± 0.05	1.82 ± 1.92	5.69		
	600	6	1	0.54 ± 0.18	1.45 ± 1.88	2.69		
		6	3	0.6-1.1	0.68 ± 0.84	1.0		
		6	6	0.26 ± 0.18	0.40 ± 0.13	1.5		
Sputum	600	11 (F)	0.66	2.7-3.0	1	0.35	Micro	Fraschini et al. (1985)
Bronchial secretion	600 bid[e]	11 (F)	1.5-2		2.4-1.7			
Rosaramicin								
Breast milk	250	10	2-4	0.165-0.485[f]	0.0278-0.0447	0.12	HPLC	Stoehr et al. (1985)

a 1st day.
b 3rd day.
c 10th day.
d Obtained by means of bronchoaspiration.
e 14th day.
f Occurred at the first sampling time.

Abbreviations: HPLC = high performance liquid chromatography; micro = microbiological assay; bid = twice daily. C_s = serum concentration; C_t tissue or fluid concentration; F = fasting.

Periti, personal communication; Pignanelli et al. 1984). Moreover, miocamycin was detected in bronchial secretion and sputum at concentrations ranging from 0.68 to 5.16 mg/L within 2 to 4 hours after administration (Fioretti et al. 1984; Fraschini et al. 1985; Nicoletti et al. 1983b) [table X]. In lactating women receiving treatment with an oral dose of miocamycin 400mg every 8 hours, the antibiotic was excreted in breast milk at concentrations ranging from 0.4 to 1.7 mg/L (Nicoletti et al. 1983b).

8. Rosaramicin

Rosaramicin is rapidly absorbed after oral administration as tablet or solution, with absorption and disposition kinetics independent of the form of the dose (Lin et al. 1984a). There are few published data describing the pharmacokinetics and metabolism of this drug in humans, partly because after oral or intravenous administration of 250 to 500mg blood concentrations are generally low, and often below the lower limit of sensitivity of bioassay (Baumueller et al. 1977; Lin et al. 1980).

For this reason, rosaramicin concentrations in serum and body fluids are assayed by HPLC or by liquid scintillation spectrometry using a radiolabelled compound (Lin et al. 1980, 1984a,b; Stoehr et al. 1985). Stoehr et al. (1985) observed peak serum concentrations ranging from 0.165 to 0.485 mg/L 2 hours after an oral dose of 250mg in 10 fasting healthy lactating women (table XI). The mean serum concentration of rosaramicin at the end of a 1-hour infusion of 500mg was almost 4 mg/L. The disposition kinetics are biexponential, with a rapid distribution phase and a slow elimination half-life (3.28 hours). With the same dosage either in oral solution or in tablets a mean peak serum concentration of 0.418 to 0.486 mg/L was achieved within 1.58 to 1.83 hours from administration with a mean bioavailability of 32% and 39%, respectively, while after oral dosing with ^{14}C-rosaramicin a mean peak serum concentration of 0.73 mg/L was observed within 56 minutes (Lin et al. 1984a). With the oral route the elimination half-life ranges from 4.4 to 5.01 hours, with a cumulative urinary recovery of 6 to 7% (Lin et al. 1984a; Stoehr et al. 1985). Rosaramicin undergoes extensive hepatic metabolism and at least 4 metabolites are present in urine. Only 20-*bis*-ureido-rosaramicin has been identified, and it may be considered as the major metabolite (Lin et al. 1984a,b). This metabolite, obtained by conjugation with urea, is formed in the body and represents a novel transformation pathway. Although rosaramicin, like erythromycin, has a dimethylamine group, the *N*-demethylated metabolite has not yet been recognised (Lin et al. 1984b). The amount of unchanged drug excreted by the kidney is only 7 to 9% and the compound is primarily excreted into the faeces via the biliary tract (Lin et al. 1984a). In dogs the macrolide was highly concentrated in urethral and vaginal secretions (Hoyme et al. 1978). Nevertheless, in lactating women the compound was only minimally excreted in breast milk and peak milk concentration averaged only 10% of peak serum level (Stoehr et al. 1985). However, Baumueller et al. (1977) obtained high prostatic concentrations after multiple oral doses of rosaramicin 250mg in patients with benign prostatic hyperplasia; these levels were higher than those observed after the same dosage of erythromycin gluceptate.

(Part II of this article, including references, will appear in the following issue of Clinical Pharmacokinetics)

Authors' address: Professor *P. Periti*, Department of Preclinical and Clinical Pharmacology, University of Florence, Viale Morgagni, 65, 50134 Florence (Italy).

Clinical Pharmacokinetics 16: 215-237 (1989)
0312-5963/89/0004-0215/$11.50/0

Clinical Pharmacology of 5-Fluorouracil

Robert B. Diasio and *Barry E. Harris*

Division of Clinical Pharmacology, University of Alabama at Birmingham, Birmingham, Alabama, USA

Contents

Summary ... 215
1. Physicochemical Properties ... 216
2. Cellular Pharmacology ... 217
   2.1 Cellular Entry ... 217
   2.2 Catabolism ... 218
   2.3 Anabolism ... 219
   2.4 Resistance ... 224
3. Assay Methods for Drug and Metabolites ... 225
   3.1 Assays in Biological Fluids ... 225
   3.2 Pharmacodynamic Assays ... 226
4. Clinical Pharmacokinetics ... 226
   4.1 Routes of Administration and Absorption ... 226
   4.2 Distribution ... 230
   4.3 Elimination ... 230
5. Effect of Pathophysiological State on Pharmacokinetics ... 230
6. Pharmacokinetic Interactions with Other Drugs ... 231
   6.1 Interactions with Other Chemotherapy Drugs ... 231
   6.2 Interactions with Non-Chemotherapy Drugs ... 232
7. Implications of Pharmacokinetics for Clinical Use ... 232

Summary

5-Fluorouracil, first introduced as a rationally synthesised anticancer agent 30 years ago, continues to be widely used in the management of several common malignancies including cancer of the colon, breast and skin. This drug, an analogue of the naturally occurring pyrimidine uracil, is metabolised via the same metabolic pathways as uracil. Although several potential sites of antitumour activity have been identified, the precise mechanism of action and the extent to which each of these sites contributes to tumour or host cell toxicity remains unclear.

Several assay methods are available to quantify 5-fluorouracil in serum, plasma and other biological fluids. Unfortunately, there is no evidence that plasma drug concentrations can predict antitumour effect or host cell toxicity. The recent development of clinically useful pharmacodynamic assays provides an attractive alternative to plasma drug concentrations, since these assays allow the detection of active metabolites of 5-fluorouracil in biopsied tumour or normal tissue.

5-Fluorouracil is poorly absorbed after oral administration, with erratic bioavailability. The parenteral preparation is the major dosage form, used intravenously (bolus or continuous infusion). Recently, studies have demonstrated the pharmacokinetic rationale and

clinical feasibility of hepatic arterial infusion and intraperitoneal administration of 5-fluorouracil. In addition, 5-fluorouracil continues to be used in topical preparations for the treatment of malignant skin cancers.

Following parenteral administration of 5-fluorouracil, there is rapid distribution of the drug and rapid elimination with an apparent terminal half-life of approximately 8 to 20 minutes. The rapid elimination is primarily due to swift catabolism of 5-fluorouracil in the liver.

As with all drugs, caution should be used in administering 5-fluorouracil in various pathophysiological states. In general, however, there are no set recommendations for dose adjustment in the presence of renal or hepatic dysfunction. Drug interactions continue to be described with other antineoplastic drugs, as well as with other classes of agents.

Although it was introduced over 30 years ago, 5-fluorouracil continues to be one of the most widely used anticancer drugs. It is used in the treatment of a number of different malignancies, either alone or in combination with other drugs. It has been shown to have palliative activity in the management of cancer of the breast, gastrointestinal tract (particularly cancer of the colon) and ovary, and to be curative in the treatment of non-invasive basal cell carcinomas (DeVita et al. 1985).

Over the past 30 years, much has been learned about the biochemical and clinical pharmacology of fluoropyrimidines. However, despite extensive studies on the metabolism of 5-fluorouracil, there remain many large gaps in our current knowledge. In particular, the relative importance of the various intracellular targets has not been fully elucidated at a biochemical level. Furthermore, although many assays for 5-fluorouracil have been available and many pharmacokinetic studies have been conducted since the introduction of the drug, the best method or schedule of administration is still unclear. Several routes of administration are currently used, including intravenous bolus, continuous infusion (over several days) and, more recently, 'protracted' infusion via an ambulatory pump for 1 to 2 weeks or longer. The pharmacological rationale for using many of these regimens and the means of drug delivery has not been rigorously assessed. Lastly, as 5-fluorouracil continues to be widely used clinically, the list of drug interactions continues to increase. This includes other chemotherapeutic drugs that can 'biochemically modulate' the antitumour efficacy or toxicity of 5-fluorouracil (e.g. methotrexate, folinic acid), as well as drugs from other classes (e.g. allopurinol, cimetidine) which can also affect the availability of active drug. The purpose of this article is to review our current understanding of the clinical pharmacology of this important anticancer drug.

1. Physicochemical Properties

5-Fluorouracil is one of only a few clinically useful antineoplastic drugs that have been rationally designed on the basis of knowledge of tumour biochemistry. Experimental studies had demonstrated that certain tumours (rat hepatomas) utilised exogenous uracil more avidly than healthy tissues (Rutman et al. 1954). The uracil was necessary for sustaining nucleic acid synthesis required for tumour growth. This led to the hypothesis that if a pyrimidine analogue could be synthesised with physicochemical properties similar to uracil, it might interfere with nucleic acid synthesis and slow tumour growth (Heidelberger 1975). In attempting to design a uracil analogue that would interfere with tumour cell growth, consideration was given to fluorine. Earlier studies had shown that by substituting fluorine for a hydrogen, a relatively non-toxic molecule (e.g. acetate) could be converted into one with increased toxicity (e.g. fluoroacetate) [Liebecq & Peters 1949]. In addition, the van der Waal's radius of the fluorine atom (1.35Å) was similar to that of hydrogen (1.2Å), thus minimising alteration of the molecular conformation (fig. 1) and increasing the likelihood that such a molecule could be metabolised by the same enzymes that metabolised uracil. The hydrogen at the '5' position appeared particularly attractive for substitution since most mammalian cells obtain the thymidine-5′-triphosphate (dTTP) needed for DNA synthesis from 2′-deoxyuridine-5′-monophosphate (dUMP) by replacing the hydrogen on the '5' carbon with a methyl group to form thymidine-5′-monophosphate (dTMP). Lastly, it was hypothesised (Heidelberger 1975) that the carbon-fluorine bond would be more stable with less chemical reactivity, thereby preventing substitution of the methyl group at the '5' position of the uracil analogue [i.e. 5-fluoro-2′-deoxyuridine-5′-monophosphate (FdUMP)].

5-Fluorouracil was originally synthesised by Duschinsky from acyclic precursors (Duschinsky et al. 1957). This method is still utilised in the commercial synthesis of the drug. An alternative method of synthesis using direct fluorination of uracil by trifluoromethyl hypofluorite has also been described (Robins & Naik 1971).

5-Fluorouracil is more acidic than its natural pyrimidine analogue and is also more soluble in aqueous solutions. It is stable in solution at physiological pH for weeks. On exposure to ultraviolet irradiation, it forms an alkali-labile, acid-stable compound that has been identified as 5-fluoro-5-hydroxy-5,6-dihydrouracil (Lozeron et al. 1964). There is no evidence for dimer formation.

2. *Cellular Pharmacology*

Unmetabolised 5-fluorouracil is essentially harmless to mammalian host and tumour cells. Upon administration, the drug is subject to 1 of 2 opposing metabolic fates (fig. 2). Inactivation and elimination are accomplished by avid catabolism, which inactivates more than 80% of administered 5-fluorouracil, and urinary excretion which eliminates 5 to 20% of the unmetabolised drug. However, the cytotoxicity of 5-fluorouracil in host and tumour cells only occurs following anabolism to nucleotides in actively proliferating cells. The availability of 5-fluorouracil for anabolism is determined by the extent of its catabolism, suggesting that detailed knowledge of the balance between catabolism and anabolism is essential to understand the biological effects of the drug (Myers 1981).

2.1 Cellular Entry

Early studies utilising Ehrlich ascites cells (Jacquez 1962) and normal human leucocytes (Kessel & Hall 1967) suggested that 5-fluorouracil and the naturally occurring pyrimidines uracil and thymine made use of a simple diffusion process to enter cells achieving a rapid equilibrium between intracellular and extracellular compartments. These early studies were limited technically in that fluxes could not be assessed over very short intervals. Subsequent studies (Wohlhueter et al. 1980) using rapid sampling techniques in several established cell lines suggested that both 5-fluorouracil and uracil enter the cell via a carrier-mediated transport process which appeared to be saturable and non-concentrative. Concentrations that resulted in 'half saturation' were very high, such that entry of either agent at pharmacological or physiological concentrations was first-order. At low extracellular con-

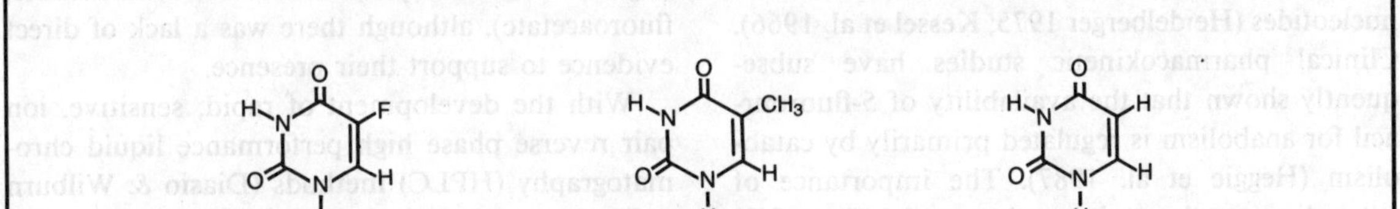

Fig. 1. Chemical structures of 5-fluorouracil, thymine and uracil.

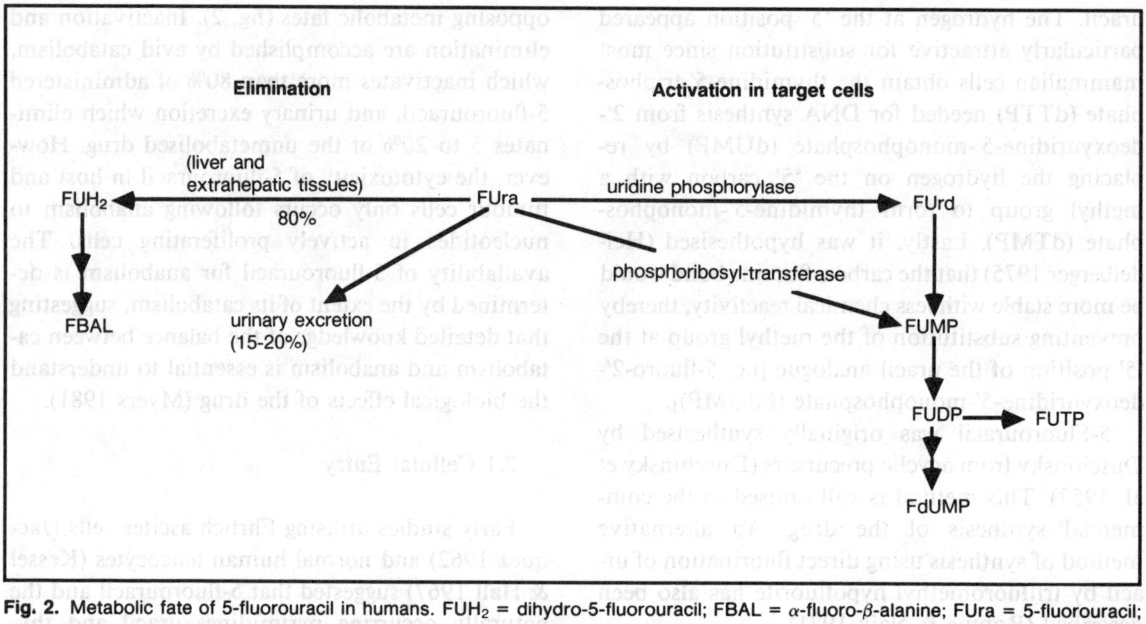

Fig. 2. Metabolic fate of 5-fluorouracil in humans. FUH_2 = dihydro-5-fluorouracil; FBAL = α-fluoro-β-alanine; FUra = 5-fluorouracil; FUrd = 5-fluorouridine; FUMP = 5-fluorouridine-5′-monophosphate; FUDP = 5-fluorouridine-5′-diphosphate; FUTP = 5-fluorouridine-5′-triphosphate; FdUMP = 5-fluoro-2′-deoxyuridine-5′-monophosphate.

centrations of 5-fluorouracil or uracil, the transport was not rate-limiting to the intracellular metabolism of either pyrimidine.

2.2 Catabolism

Until recently, most studies of the metabolism of 5-fluorouracil have focused almost exclusively on anabolism, due to the fact that earlier cellular studies with the drug had emphasised the importance of anabolism with the demonstration that antitumour activity and host cell toxicity were dependent on initial conversion of 5-fluorouracil to nucleotides (Heidelberger 1975; Kessel et al. 1966). Clinical pharmacokinetic studies have subsequently shown that the availability of 5-fluorouracil for anabolism is regulated primarily by catabolism (Heggie et al. 1987). The importance of catabolism in determining the availability of 5-fluorouracil for anabolism (with resultant antitumour activity and host toxicity) has been further demonstrated by clinical studies in which the drug was coadministered with other pyrimidines, such as thymine or uracil, resulting in increased availability of 5-fluorouracil and, in turn, increased antitumour activity and host toxicity (Au et al. 1982).

Until the early 1980s our knowledge of 5-fluorouracil catabolism was limited to the studies of Heidelberger and his associates done 20 years earlier (Chadhuri et al. 1959; Mukherjee & Heidelberger 1960). These studies utilised time-consuming, open column low pressure chromatography under conditions that could lead to decomposition of some of the pH-labile catabolites. Several metabolites were alleged to be formed (e.g. fluoroguanidopropionic acid, fluorocitrate, fluoroacetate), although there was a lack of direct evidence to support their presence.

With the development of rapid, sensitive, ion pair reverse phase high performance liquid chromatography (HPLC) methods (Diasio & Wilburn 1979; Sommadossi et al. 1982), it is now possible to resolve virtually all of the catabolites as well as 5-fluorouracil and its anabolites. This method has been used in conjunction with radiolabelled drug where the label (tritium) is at the ‘6’ position on the pyrimidine ring, thus enabling resolution by HPLC and quantification of the radioactivity in each resolved peak. We have used this approach with isolated rat hepatocytes (Sommadossi et al. 1982, 1985a,b), isolated perfused rat liver (Sweeny et al. 1988a) and clinical pharmacokinetic studies (Diasio et al. 1988; Heggie et al. 1987). These studies have helped to clarify the catabolism of 5-fluorouracil with several new findings: (1) the initial catabolite of 5-fluorouracil, dihydrofluorouracil (FUH_2), is not as transient (Sommadossi et al. 1982) as earlier studies (Chaudhuri et al. 1959; Mukherjee & Heidelberger 1960) had suggested and follows Michaelis-Menten kinetics (Mentre et al. 1984); (2) FUH_2 itself demonstrates potential toxicity in some tumour lines (Diasio et al. 1985); (3) there is no evidence of fluoroguanidopropionic acid, fluorocitrate or fluoroacetate in either the animal or human studies; (4) 5-fluoroureidopropionic acid (FUPA) and α-fluoro-β-alanine (FBAL) are the 2 other metabolites found in both cellular and clinical studies; and (5) novel metabolites which are conjugates of FBAL and the naturally occurring bile acids (cholic acid and chenodeoxycholic acid) have been isolated from human bile (Sweeny et al. 1987, 1988b). The FBAL-chenodeoxycholate conjugate has been shown to produce cholestasis in the isolated perfused rat liver (Sweeny et al. 1988a). This conjugate may have a role in the biliary toxicity that typically occurs with prolonged hepatic arterial infusion of fluoropyrimidine drugs, particularly fluorodeoxyuridine (FdUrd).

Figure 3 summarises our current understanding of the catabolic pathway of 5-fluorouracil metabolism in man. The enzymes in the catabolic pathway have not been well characterised (Wasternak 1980). The initial enzyme dihydropyrimidine dehydrogenase (DPD) is responsible for reducing the double bond in the pyrimidine ring. Although DPD is the best studied enzyme in the catabolic pathway, there are no data on the human enzyme. It is thought to be the rate-limiting enzyme in the pathway (Shiotani & Weber 1981) and to be reversible. The product of DPD, FUH_2, is unstable in aqueous solution and can break down spontaneously. The enzyme responsible for further catabolising FUH_2 to FUPA is dihydropyrimidinase (Maguire & Dudley 1978; Sanno et al. 1970). FUPA appears to be a transient intracellular catabolite (Sommadossi et al. 1982) and is thought to be converted to FBAL by β-ureidopropionase (Sanno et al. 1970).

FBAL represents the major urinary catabolite in man (> 95%). We have recently shown that FBAL can also be conjugated with bile acids in place of taurine and glycine and that FBAL-bile acid conjugates are the major biliary metabolites of 5-fluorouracil in cancer patients (Sweeny et al. 1987). The enzyme that is responsible for formation of these conjugates is thought to be an *n*-acyl CoA transferase (Vessey 1979). In addition to the catabolic pathway, metabolism of 5-fluorouracil in the liver may also lead to the formation of an inactive glucuronide conjugate (Sommadossi et al. 1985a). In our studies we have not found any evidence of 5-fluorouracil anabolism in either rat or human hepatocytes.

2.3 Anabolism

As with catabolism, the presence of the fluorine does not interfere with the anabolism of 5-fluorouracil via the pyrimidine pathway. The anabolic pathways of 5-fluorouracil are essentially the same pathways used by the *de novo* pyrimidine uracil (fig. 4). There are 3 pathways by which 5-fluorouracil may be anabolised to form cytotoxic nucleotides. The first utilises uridine phosphorylase and uridine kinase for conversion to the ribonucleotide 5-fluorouridine-5′-monophosphate (FUMP). The second is the direct conversion of 5-fluorouracil to FUMP by orotidine-5′-monophosphate phosphoribosyltransferase. The third, which is quantitatively less important, uses thymidine phosphorylase and thymidine kinase for conversion of 5-fluorouracil to the deoxyribosylnucleotide FdUMP. This pathway is more important when FdUrd is administered as a drug.

Due to the addition of the charged phosphate group, nucleotides are retained in the cell (in contrast to the base and nucleosides which can diffuse

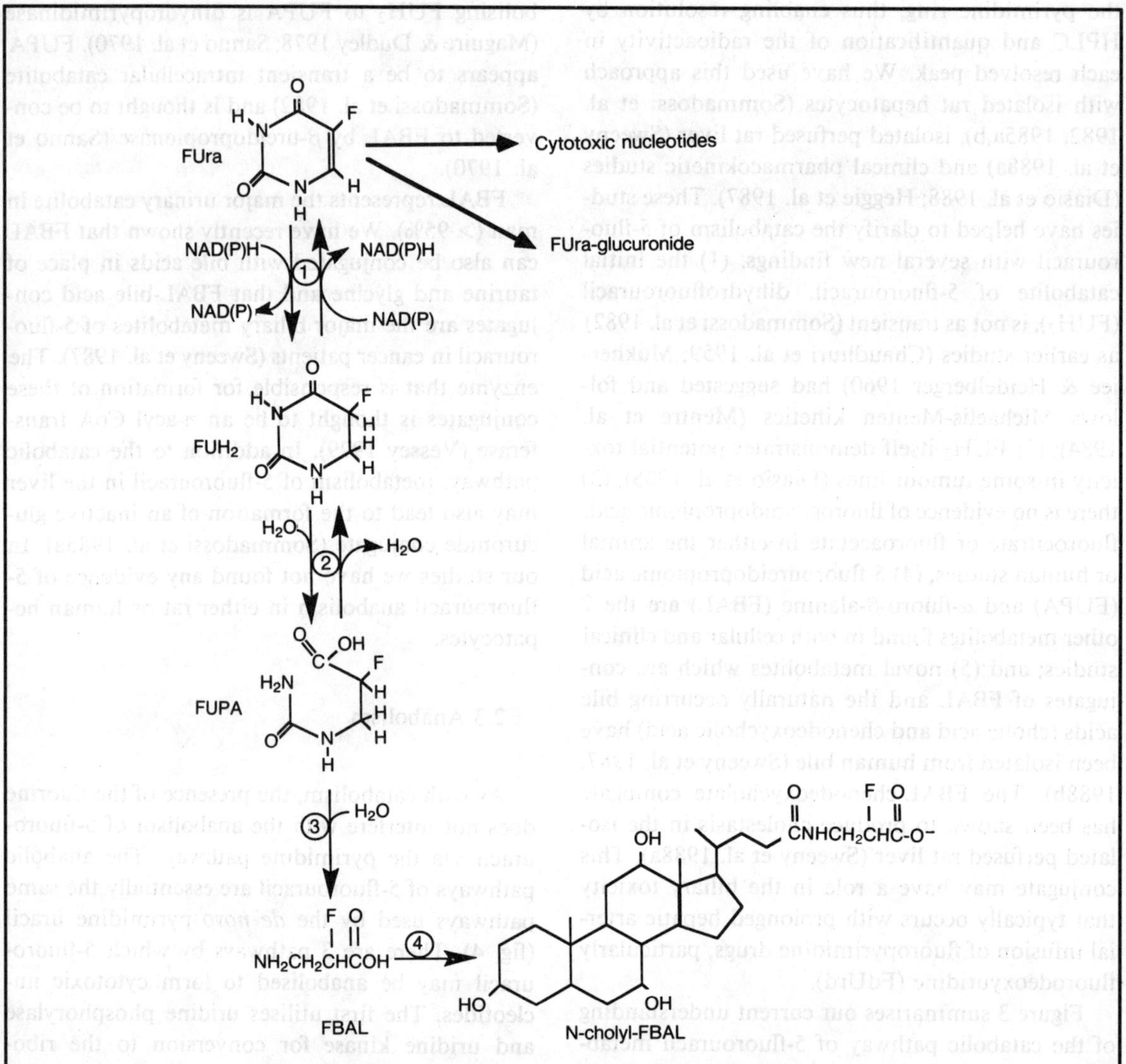

Fig. 3. Catabolism of 5-fluorouracil in humans. 1, dihydropyrimidine dehydrogenase (DPD); 2, dihydropyrimidinase; 3, β-ureidopropionase; 4, *n*-acyl CoA transferase. FUPA = 5-fluoroureidopropionic acid; for other abbreviations, see fig. 2.

back out of the cell), allowing interconversions to other nucleotides. Thus, FUMP may be metabolised to 5-fluorouridine-5′-diphosphate (FUDP) which can then be converted either to 5-fluorouridine-5′-triphosphate (FUTP) or to the deoxyribosylnucleotide 5-fluoro-2′-deoxyuridine-5′-diphosphate (FdUDP) by ribonucleotide reductase. FdUDP can then be converted to 5-fluoro-2′-deoxyuridine-5′-triphosphate (FdUTP) or FdUMP.

Of critical importance, but still not completely clear after 30 years of research, is the question of which nucleotide is ultimately responsible for cellular cytotoxicity. Thus, the relative importance of the following remains unclear: (1) formation of

FdUMP with inhibition of thymidylate synthase activity; (2) formation of FUTP, which may substitute for uridine triphosphate (UTP) in RNA and result in RNA dysfunction; (3) formation of FdUTP, which may substitute for dTTP and be incorporated and subsequently excised from DNA, resulting in damage in newly synthesised DNA; and (4) effect of 5-fluorouracil on cell membranes, with an alteration in membrane structure possibly related to a decrease in glycoprotein biosynthesis and a decrease in fucose incorporation. Of particular interest are the questions: first, does 5-fluorouracil result in a cytocidal effect or a transient effect on cell proliferation; secondly, does 5-fluorouracil have different mechanisms of cytotoxicity in tumour versus host cells; and thirdly, does more than 1 mechanism contribute to the cytotoxicity of 5-fluorouracil.

2.3.1 Inhibition of Thymidylate Synthase

Inhibition of thymidylate synthase by FdUMP is by far the best studied and best understood site of action for 5-fluorouracil. As noted earlier, most mammalian cells use thymidylate synthase to make the dTMP needed for DNA synthesis from dUMP, obtaining the methyl group for the '5' position of the pyrimidine ring from 5,10-methylene tetrahydrofolate (fig. 5). Because FdUMP has a greater affinity for thymidylate synthase than the natural substrate dUMP, it can prevent the formation of dTMP. Subsequent inhibition of DNA synthesis combined with continued RNA and protein synthesis produces an imbalance that is incompatible with cell survival. To produce this effect, FdUMP must form a ternary covalent complex with 5,10-methylene tetrahydrofolate and thymidylate synthase (Danenberg & Danenberg 1978; Santi & McHenry 1972; Santi et al. 1974). This complex is shown in figure 5.

The reaction catalysed by thymidylate synthase is a sequence of 2 different chemical reactions. The first reaction involves the transfer of a methylene group from 5,10-methylene tetrahydrofolate to the '5' position of the pyrimidine ring. This occurs in a similar fashion with either dUMP or FdUMP, but the ternary complex that is formed with FdUMP does not proceed past this point. The second reaction involves a reduction of the methylene group to a methyl group by the removal of a proton from the '5' carbon, forming an intermediate

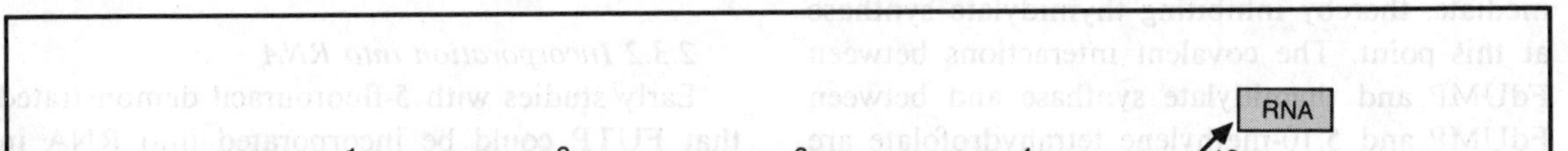

Fig. 4. The anabolic metabolism of 5-fluorouracil in humans. 1, uridine (thymidine) phosphorylase; 2, uridine kinase; 3, (deoxy)uridine monophosphate kinase; 4, (deoxy)uridine diphosphate kinase; 5, orotidine monophosphate phosphoribosyltransferase; 6, ribonucleotide reductase; 7, thymidine kinase; 8, thymidylate synthase; 9, deoxyuridine triphosphate diphosphohydrolase; 10, thymidine monophosphate kinase; 11, thymidine diphosphate kinase; 12, RNA polymerase; 13, DNA polymerase α. FdUrd = 5-fluoro-2′-deoxyuridine; FdUDP = 5-fluoro-2′-deoxyuridine-5′-diphosphate; FdUTP = 5-fluoro-2′-deoxyuridine-5′-triphosphate; dUMP = 2′-deoxyuridine-5′-monophosphate; dTMP = thymidine-5′-monophosphate; dTDP = thymidine-5′-diphosphate; dTTP = thymidine-5′-triphosphate; for other abbreviations, see fig. 2.

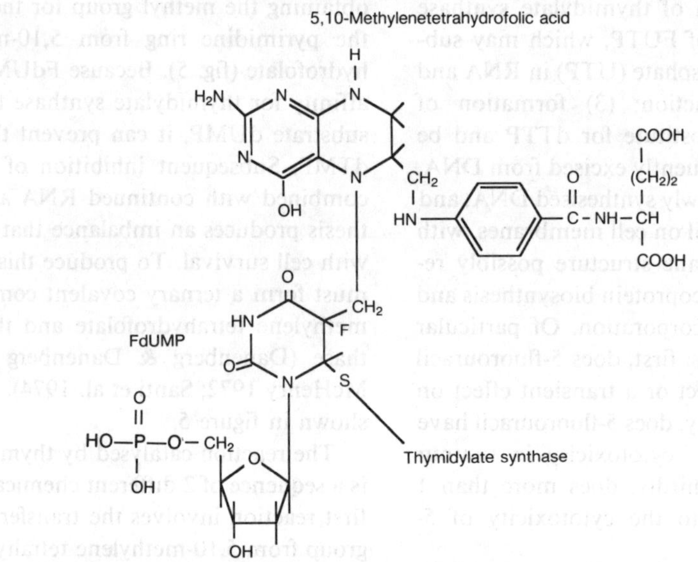

Fig. 5. Ternary complex of N^5,N^{10}-methylene tetrahydrofolate, 5-fluoro-2′-deoxyuridine monophosphate (FdUMP), and thymidylate synthase.

which may act as a hydride acceptor in the reduction reaction (Danenberg & Lockshin 1981). The presence of a fluorine on the '5' carbon of the pyrimidine ring prevents the formation of this intermediate, thereby inhibiting thymidylate synthase at this point. The covalent interactions between FdUMP and thymidylate synthase and between FdUMP and 5,10-methylene tetrahydrofolate are chemically stable, but reversible (Santi et al. 1974). The dissociation of the ternary complex formed with FdUMP results in free active enzyme (Danenberg 1984).

The importance has been demonstrated of having adequate intracellular concentrations of reduced folates to interact with thymidylate synthase and FdUMP to form a stable ternary complex (Ullman et al. 1978). As the concentration of reduced cofactor increases, the dissociation of FdUMP from the ternary complex is inhibited (Danenberg & Danenberg 1978), which in turn has led to the recognition that the antitumour effectiveness of 5-fluorouracil could be improved by coadministering a reduced folate such as folinic acid. This has been shown both in cellular (Evans et al. 1981; Hakala 1984) and, more recently, in clinical studies (DeLap 1988; Grem et al. 1987). The interaction of 5-fluorouracil and folinic acid is described in more detail in section 6.1.

2.3.2 Incorporation into RNA

Early studies with 5-fluorouracil demonstrated that FUTP could be incorporated into RNA in place of UTP (Mandel 1969). It has since been shown that 5-fluorouracil is incorporated into each of the species of RNA including ribosomal (Cohen & Glazer 1985; Herrick & Kufe 1984), messenger (Armstrong et al. 1986a; Dolnick & Pink 1983) and transfer (Ramberg et al. 1978) as well as other small molecular weight species (Armstrong et al. 1986b). What remains unclear is the specific functional damage that may result following incorporation of 5-fluorouracil into any of these RNA species and the subsequent relation of this incorporation to fluoropyrimidine cytotoxicity.

Generally, cellular toxicity that is not reversed by thymidine (which may bypass the block at thymidylate synthase, providing dTTP for DNA synthesis) is referred to as RNA-mediated cytotoxicity. Characterisation of the effects of 5-fluorouracil on RNA and/or RNA processing may be especially important when it is given in combination with other antineoplastic agents. Cadman et al. (1979) demonstrated that the combination of methotrexate and 5-fluorouracil enhanced cytotoxicity, and that this increased toxicity correlated specifically with the incorporation of 5-fluorouracil into RNA. However, some investigators (Houghton & Houghton 1980) have had difficulty correlating tumour response with the level of incorporation of the drug in total cellular RNA. Subsequent studies on 5-fluorouracil incorporation into RNA have begun to focus on specific RNA species (Herrick & Kufe 1982; Major et al. 1982) and have suggested that incorporation into distinct species of RNA may be more closely related to cellular toxicity than to total incorporation. This was clearly demonstrated by the studies of Major et al. (1982) who found that the combination of 5-fluorouracil with several other antineoplastic agents produced enhanced 5-fluorouracil cytotoxicity that only weakly correlated with the level of the drug in total cellular RNA but showed a highly significant correlation with newly synthesised RNA.

Recent studies with various other drugs that can 'biochemically modulate' the metabolism of 5-fluorouracil and its incorporation into RNA have led to renewed interest in the importance of specific RNA targets as a mechanism of action for the drug, but the precise contribution to toxicity remains unclear.

2.3.3 Incorporation into DNA

It is now recognised that both 5-fluorouracil and uracil can be incorporated into DNA (Ingraham et al. 1982). Following anabolism of 5-fluorouracil to FdUTP (Caradonna & Cheng 1980), FdUTP can substitute as a substrate for DNA polymerase (Cheng & Nakayama 1983), and be incorporated into DNA in place of dTTP. The presence of dUTPase (fig. 6) decreases the dUTP and FdUTP pool, further lessening the likelihood of incorporation of these deoxyribosylnucleotides into DNA (Ingraham et al. 1980, 1982).

Inhibition of thymidylate synthase by FdUMP may actually predispose the cell to incorporate both FdUTP and dUTP into DNA. The dTTP pools would be expected to decrease while dUMP (and in turn dUTP) pools would be expected to increase, as has been shown to occur when thymidylate synthase is inhibited by FdUMP (Myers et al. 1975). Furthermore, as the FdUMP pool expands there is greater likelihood that the FdUTP pool will expand. Thus, in the presence of decreased dTTP pools, both FdUTP and dUTP pools increase (Schuetz et al. 1984). Since both FdUTP and dUTP are substrates for DNA polymerase (Cheng & Nakayama 1983; Tanaka et al. 1981), they can be incorporated into DNA (fig. 6). This has been shown to occur in a number of cells, including human cells (Kufe et al. 1981; Major et al. 1982). Once 5-fluorouracil or uracil is incorporated into DNA, uracil glycosylase, a DNA repair enzyme, may remove the incorporated uracil or 5-fluorouracil (Caradonna & Cheng 1980; Lindahl et al. 1977; Schuetz et al. 1988). An apyrimidine endonuclease (Lindahl 1979) may then break the sugar-phosphate backbone which can subsequently be repaired with the correct pyrimidine base. However, it should be emphasised that if sufficient 5-fluorouracil and/or uracil is incorporated into DNA, the repair process may actually produce damage to the DNA structure (Schuetz et al. 1988).

The significance of the incorporation of 5-fluorouracil into DNA in terms of cellular toxicity remains unclear. Although some studies suggest that the extent of its incorporation into DNA cannot account for the observed cytotoxicity in mammalian tumour cells (Danenberg et al. 1981; Parker et al. 1987), other reports suggest a possible correlation of incorporation into DNA with cell survival in host (Schuetz et al. 1984) and tumour cells (Kufe et al. 1983). In studies from our laboratory we have shown that DNA repair does occur following incorporation of 5-fluorouracil into DNA (Schuetz et al. 1988). In the presence of sufficient damage, the DNA may not be able to repair itself effectively, which may lead to DNA fragmentation (Lonn & Lonn 1984, 1986; Schuetz et al. 1986). In a study with murine bone marrow cells, we demonstrated that 5-fluorouracil resulted in a time-dependent

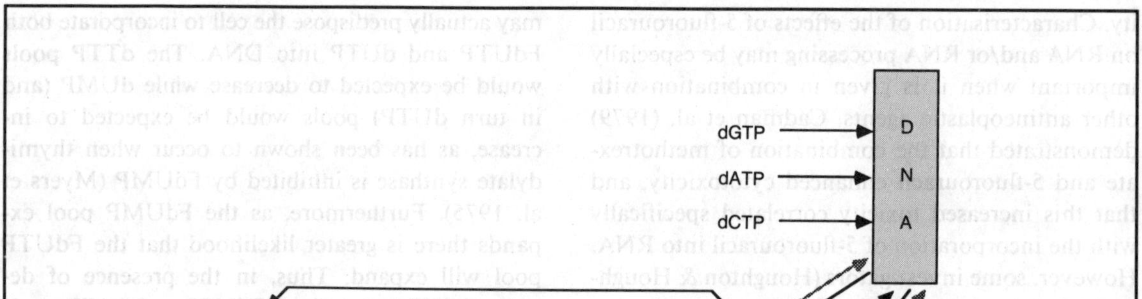

Fig. 6. Effect of 5-fluorouracil on DNA synthesis. dUMP = 2′-deoxyuridine-5′-monophosphate; dTMP = thymidine-5′-monophosphate; FdUMP = 5-fluoro-2′-deoxyuridine-5′-monophosphate; dTDP = thymidine-5′-disphosphate; dUDP = 2′-deoxyuridine-5′-diphosphate; FdUDP = 5-fluoro-2′-deoxyuridine-5′-diphosphate; dTTP = thymidine-5′-triphosphate; dUTP = 2′-deoxyuridine-5′-triphosphate; FdUTP = 5-fluoro-2′-deoxyuridine-5′-triphosphate.

fragmentation of DNA with a concomitant time-dependent excision of the drug from DNA. This suggests an association between excision of 5-fluorouracil from DNA and changes in the secondary structure of newly synthesised DNA (Schuetz et al. 1986). The excision of the drug from nascent DNA chains may prevent further elongation of DNA (Schuetz & Diasio 1985).

2.3.4 Interaction with Cellular Membranes

5-Fluorouracil has also been noted to result in membrane effects that may have a role in the cytotoxicity produced: it can alter membrane function with changes in transmembrane potential and surface charge (Walliser & Redmann 1978), and can also change membrane structure with impairment of glycoprotein synthesis (Kessel 1980). The latter author has demonstrated that these structural changes may be associated with an increase in cell volume, making these cells more susceptible to lysis. The relative importance of these membrane effects has not been well studied and their contribution to toxicity remains unclear.

2.4 Resistance

As with other anticancer drugs, there are various mechanisms of both innate (*de novo*) and acquired resistance which may be exhibited by tumour cells in response to 5-fluorouracil. Resistance may develop at any of the various steps, from entry into the cell to interaction with the intracellular target responsible for toxicity in the particular cell. A recent review details many of the studies of 5-fluorouracil resistance in both *in vivo* and cellular (human and animal) trials (Houghton & Houghton 1984). Unfortunately, the studies of resistance in man are in the minority.

Theoretically, it is possible that the 5-fluorouracil transport mechanism may be altered either *de novo* or through some acquired mechanism. To our knowledge, such a mechanism has not been reported. It is interesting that 5-fluorouracil differs from many of the diverse anticancer drugs that have been associated with so-called 'pleotropic' or 'multiple drug mechanisms' where resistance has been shown to be due to accelerated pumping or efflux of the drug from the cell (Beck 1987). Most of the drugs exhibiting this resistance pattern have chemical structures that are foreign, in contrast to the 'natural appearing' structure of the antimetabolite 5-fluorouracil.

Another poorly characterised but potentially important mechanism of resistance to the drug involves its catabolism. The initial step in 5-fluorouracil catabolism (by DPD) regulates the amount of the drug that is available for anabolism. It is possible that some cells may be more resistant to 5-fluorouracil because they can degrade it faster and more efficiently, due to increased levels of DPD. Further studies on the catabolism in sensitive and resistant cell lines are needed to determine its importance in either innate or acquired resistance.

There is much more data available on resistance to 5-fluorouracil resulting from a deficiency or alteration of anabolic enzymes which convert it to the necessary nucleotide precursors. Such alterations may lead to a decrease in the production of active metabolites, resulting in a decrease in cell lethality. Resistance has been attributed to defects at several steps in the anabolic pathway, including conversion of the parent compound to its nucleosides (Goldberg et al. 1966; Reichard et al. 1959), conversion of the nucleosides to nucleotides (Reichard et al. 1959, 1962; Skold 1963) and conversion of 5-fluorouracil to FUMP (Ardalan et al. 1978), as well as other anabolic conversions to nucleotides which interact with intracellular targets.

Although alteration of cellular metabolism (see above) is probably the predominant mechanism of 5-fluorouracil resistance, another potential site is at the level of the various intracellular targets. Thymidylate synthase may be altered, resulting in complete inhibition by FdUMP (Heidelberger et al. 1960a,b); or it may be present in excess, as occurs with gene amplification (Berger et al. 1985; Clark et al. 1987), resulting in resistance because thymidylate is still produced. It is also possible that cells resistant to 5-fluorouracil may have an altered form of the target enzyme which allows the enzyme to better discriminate between its natural substrate dUMP and its fluorinated analogue, FdUMP (Houghton & Houghton 1984). Other plausible target-directed mechanisms of resistance may include tolerance to the incorporation of fluorinated analogues into cellular RNA and/or DNA.

Lastly, resistance can occur from an alteration in the turnover of enzymes, nucleic acids or the natural nucleotide precursors (e.g. dUMP). This has been shown particularly with dUMP accumulation (Myers et al. 1975).

With better understanding of the mechanisms of resistance to 5-fluorouracil, there have been a number of pharmacological approaches to overcome this resistance that have used various pyrimidines or purines to 'biochemically modulate' metabolism of the drug. These schemes are described more fully in section 6.

3. Assay Methods for Drug and Metabolites

3.1 Assays in Biological Fluids

Over the years a number of assays have been developed to measure 5-fluorouracil in various biological fluids. Initial assays utilised microbiological procedures (Clarkson et al. 1964) which were cumbersome and time-consuming, and lacked sensitivity. Thin layer (Ikenaka et al. 1979) and open column low pressure chromatographic techniques (Chaudhuri et al. 1959; Mukherjee & Heidelberger 1960) were shown to be useful (particularly when used with radiolabelled drug) for separating 5-fluorouracil from its metabolites, but were also limited by similar problems. The development of gas chromatographic and subsequently gas chromatographic-mass spectrometric (GC-MS) methods (Aubert et al. 1981, 1982; Lakings et al. 1978) permitted shorter analysis time and more sensitivity. These assays proved to be useful particularly in clinical pharmacokinetic studies.

The assay used most often today in both cellular and clinical pharmacokinetic studies is HPLC. Most of the current methods use reverse phase columns. Several different sample preparation techniques, including organic extraction and ion exchange resins, are used together with the HPLC and permit determination of. 5-fluorouracil in the nanogram range (6.5 to 50 ng/ml), approaching the sensitivity available with GC-MS (Aubert et al. 1981; Buckpitt & Boyd 1980; Christophidis et al. 1979). Thus HPLC methods are useful for measuring 5-fluorouracil concentrations in the range observed in patients receiving the drug via continuous infusion. Reverse phase HPLC has also proven useful in both cellular (Sommadossi et al. 1982) and clinical (Heggie et al. 1987) metabolism studies, which used ion pair reagents together with reverse phase to resolve 5-fluorouracil from its anabolites and catabolites.

3.2 Pharmacodynamic Assays

A major limitation in the assay of 5-fluorouracil in plasma (serum) has been the lack of any demonstrable predictive value for either antitumour effect or host cell toxicity. Recently, several pharmacodynamic tests have been developed using serial needle biopsies in the clinical setting. These assays permit the quantification of FdUMP, dUMP, free and total thymidylate synthase, tetrahydrofolate and methylene tetrahydrofolate (Moran et al. 1979; Spears & Gustavsson 1988). Spears and his associates (1988a) have suggested that these pharmacodynamic parameters may be useful in predicting patient response to 5-fluorouracil, with statistically significant correlations between short and long term inhibition of thymidylate synthase activity and patient response, and between inhibition of this activity and survival.

The identification of intratumour mechanisms of resistance to thymidylate synthase developed during administration of 5-fluorouracil can thus be readily made in the clinic. Such a capability may help determine early in a patient's course of treatment whether doses should be increased, decreased, or omitted altogether, and may also suggest plausible alterations in the course of therapy such as the addition of a biochemical modulator (e.g. folinic acid) to improve thymidylate synthase inhibition by increasing FdUMP concentrations, decreasing dUMP concentrations or increasing reduced cofactor levels (Spears et al. 1988b).

4. Clinical Pharmacokinetics

There have been numerous studies examining the pharmacokinetics of 5-fluorouracil and other fluoropyrimidines in humans. With the development of the newer analytic techniques (particularly GC-MS and, more recently, HPLC) there has been a better understanding and more general agreement on the disposition and initial kinetics of the drug following intravenous bolus administration. However, pharmacokinetic studies following continuous and protracted infusion have been more difficult because plasma (serum) concentrations are often at or below the limits of sensitivity of the assay; and until recently such studies have paid little attention to the metabolites of 5-fluorouracil, particularly its catabolites.

4.1 Routes of Administration and Absorption

4.1.1 Oral Administration

Oral administration of 5-fluorouracil has been used much less frequently in the last several years, largely due to the findings from several pharmacokinetic studies that there is significant variation in the bioavailability (0 to 80%) of the drug when administered via this route (Christophidis et al. 1978; Cohen et al. 1974). Variation occurs in peak concentrations and the time to reach peak, both in studies of different patients and in repeat studies of the same patient.

The basis for this apparently erratic bioavailability is not completely understood. It would appear that, since 5-fluorouracil has a pKa of 8.1, pH conditions in the upper gastrointestinal tract would favour absorption. The possible role of catabolism of the drug within the gastrointestinal mucosa has not been fully assessed. The initial enzyme in catabolism, DPD, is known to be present in this tissue (Naguib 1985), so that it is possible that this may contribute to the observed variations in bioavailability.

4.1.2 Intravenous Bolus Administration

Most of the published studies on the pharmacokinetics of 5-fluorouracil have focused on intravenous bolus administration, which continues to be the most common route. The drug is usually given at a dosage of 10 to 15 mg/kg every week or daily for 5 days once a month. Table I summarises the pharmacokinetic data from several reported studies. In these studies the elimination half-life ($t_{1/2\beta}$) varied from 8 to 22 minutes, with the volume of distribution (Vd) varying between 14 and 54L and plasma clearance (CL) between 48 and 114 L/h. A recent study using radiolabelled drug examined the disposition of 5-fluorouracil and its metabolites in plasma, urine and bile of patients given [^{3}H-6]-5-fluorouracil in a typical dose (500 mg/m^2) by intravenous bolus (Heggie et al. 1987). This study utilised ion pair reversed phase HPLC to separate the drug from its metabolites, thereby permitting individual measurement of both. Figure 7 shows a typical profile of plasma concentrations of 5-fluorouracil and its catabolites observed over 24 hours following an intravenous bolus dose. This study demonstrates that 5-fluorouracil has a $t_{1/2\beta}$, Vd and CL similar to those reported by previous studies (table I). In addition, it shows that the $t_{1/2\beta}$ of the catabolites FUH_2, FUPA, and FBAL is much longer than that of the parent compound, with values of 1, 4 and 33 hours, respectively.

4.1.3 Continuous Infusion

For many years it has been recognised that if 5-fluorouracil is given by infusion rather than by bolus, the type and severity of the side effects and toxicity will change. It was also recognised that a larger amount of drug could be given and tolerated when administered by infusion, which made this method theoretically appealing. In the past, most infusions were by gravity and thus often poorly controlled. More recently, with the advent of sophisticated pumps with flow control devices and alarms, continuous delivery of drug by infusion has been more realistic. In addition, with the development of battery-operated ambulatory microprocessor pumps, it has been possible to explore 'protracted' infusions of 5-fluorouracil (Lokich et al. 1983) continuing for 2 weeks or more.

Despite interest in the administration of 5-

Table I. Pharmacokinetic parameters of 5-fluorouracil in humans

Reference	Dose	No. of patients	$t_{1/2\beta}$ (min)	C_{ss} (μmol/L)	Vd (L)	CL_p (L/h)
IV bolus						
Sitar et al. (1977)	11 mg/kg	16	20		54	114
Christophidis et al. (1978)	11 mg/kg	12	19		25	48
MacMillan et al. (1978)	11 mg/kg	8	11		18	78
Cano et al. (1979)	750-1000mg	9	12			48
Finch et al. (1979)	500mg	11	8		13	60
Fraile et al. (1980)	500-900 mg/m^2	3	9		17	102
McDermott et al. (1982)	10 mg/kg	12	22			
Heggie et al. (1987)	500 mg/m^2	10	13		14	60
Schaaf et al. (1987)	15 mg/kg	6	12			90
Continuous infusion						
Clarkson et al. (1964)	10 mg/kg/day	2		0.8		240
Garrrett et al. (1977)	175 mg/kg/day	3		15.0		216
Ensminger et al. (1978)	134 mg/kg/day	8		71.0		54
Hillcoat et al. (1978)	30 mg/kg/day	28		1.6		420
Spicer et al. (1988)	300-500 mg/m^2/day	25		11.2		

Abbreviations: $t_{1/2\beta}$ = apparent terminal half-life; C_{ss} = plasma drug concentration at steady-state; Vd = apparent volume of distribution; CL_p = clearance of drug from plasma; IV = intravenous administration.

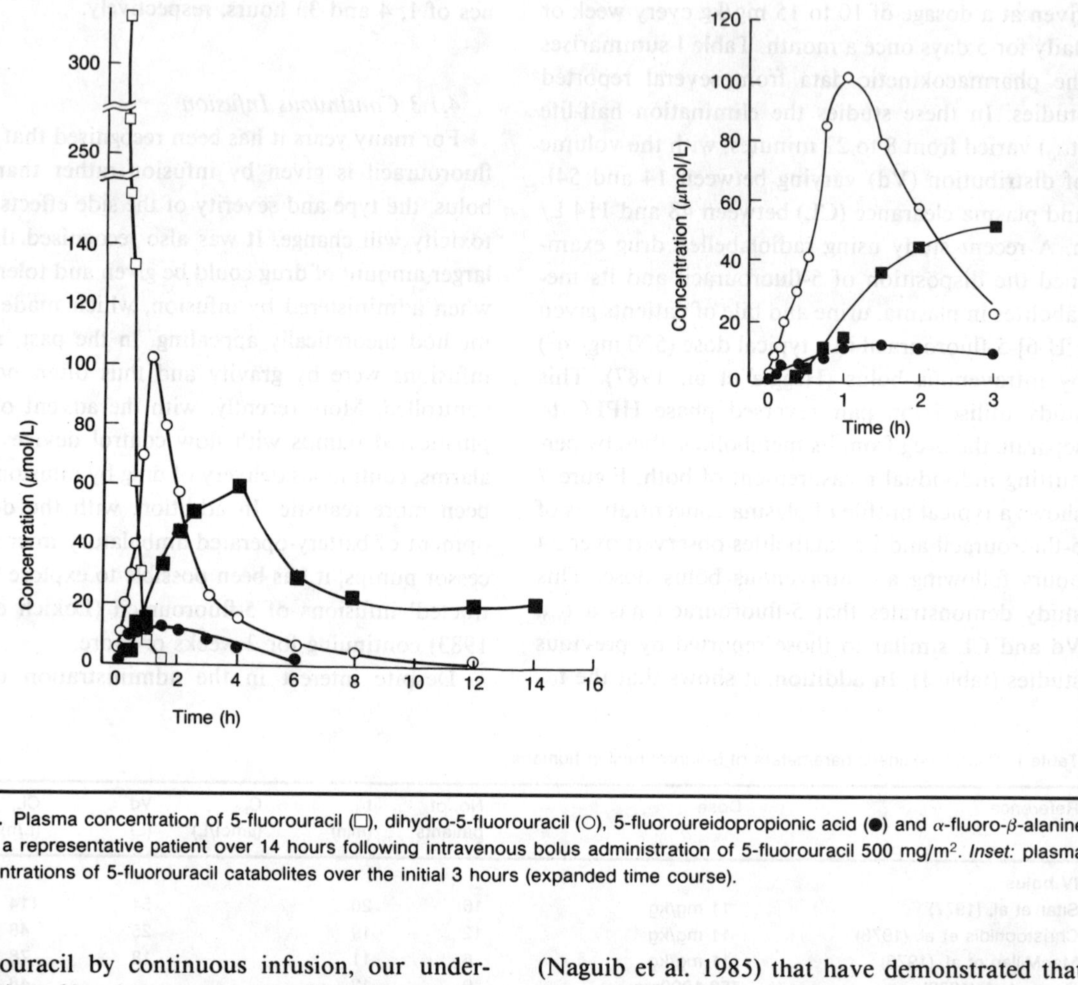

Fig. 7. Plasma concentration of 5-fluorouracil (□), dihydro-5-fluorouracil (○), 5-fluoroureidopropionic acid (●) and α-fluoro-β-alanine (■) in a representative patient over 14 hours following intravenous bolus administration of 5-fluorouracil 500 mg/m². *Inset:* plasma concentrations of 5-fluorouracil catabolites over the initial 3 hours (expanded time course).

fluorouracil by continuous infusion, our understanding of its pharmacokinetics when given by this route is limited. One problem is that 5-fluorouracil concentrations with continuous or protracted infusions are very low, near the limits of sensitivity of most of the assays. Table I lists the pharmacokinetic data obtained from several representative studies. Steady-state concentrations typically ranged between 0.8 and 71.0 μmol/L, with clearance values between 54 and 420 L/h. As noted by Myers (1981), clearance values often approach cardiac output. This implies that degradation of 5-fluorouracil must be occurring in organs besides the liver, a conclusion which is supported by recent studies (Naguib et al. 1985) that have demonstrated that dihydropyrimidine dehydrogenase is present in many tissues (e.g. pancreas, lung, intestinal mucosa and lymphocytes) in addition to the liver.

One interesting recent observation is that when plasma concentrations were measured at various times over 24 hours in patients receiving 5-fluorouracil by continuous infusion via a pump, there was marked variation in the values obtained at the various times, demonstrating that there is a circadian variation (3- to 25-fold) in the plasma concentrations of 5-fluorouracil (Petit et al. 1988). The clinical importance of the observed diurnal variation in plasma 5-fluorouracil concentration is currently being evaluated in our own laboratory. Several recent studies have suggested that the basis for this observation may be a circadian variation in the level of DPD in patients (Harris et al. 1988a; Tuchman et al. 1988). Additional support for the importance of circadian variation in DPD has been shown in studies in rat liver (Harris et al. 1988b). Studies are presently in progress in our laboratory to determine the relationship between DPD activity and plasma concentrations of 5-fluorouracil following administration by continuous infusion. With the development of the computerised ambulatory pumps, it is now possible to alter the rate of drug delivery throughout the day (Roemeling & Hrushesky 1987). By monitoring those critical metabolic enzymes (e.g. DPD) which display a circadian pattern, it should be possible to rationally alter the drug delivery to maximise therapeutic effect.

4.1.4 Hepatic Arterial Infusion

Regional infusion of chemotherapy has many theoretical advantages over systemic chemotherapy. Infusion of 5-fluorouracil or its derivatives into the liver via the hepatic artery or the portal vein is pharmacologically attractive, since many of the tumours that metastasise to the liver are relatively sensitive to this drug (e.g. adenocarcinoma from the gastrointestinal tract). Because 5-fluorouracil is rapidly cleared and degraded by the liver, hepatic arterial infusion results in low systemic drug concentrations, approximately 60% of that observed following peripheral intravenous infusion (Ensminger et al. 1978). This in turn may protect bone marrow and gastrointestinal mucosa from drug-induced cytotoxicity.

The pharmacological basis for hepatic arterial infusion of fluoropyrimidine drugs has been demonstrated by Ensminger & Gyves (1983). Both 5-fluorouracil and FdUrd are efficiently extracted by the liver with extraction ratios of 0.22 to 0.45 and 0.69 to 0.92, respectively (Ensminger et al. 1978). Using this route of administration, the apparent terminal half-life of both drugs was shown to be 10 minutes or less (Ensminger & Gyves 1983). It is therefore attractive to infuse drug continuously into the liver in an attempt to increase the concentration/time profile and hopefully achieve maximal antitumour effect. Several clinical studies have demonstrated the clinical efficacy of hepatic arterial infusion, even in patients previously unresponsive to 5-fluorouracil, with response rates greater than 50% (Balch & Levin 1987; Ensminger et al. 1978; Hohn et al. 1986). Unfortunately, this approach is not without toxic effect. The major toxicities observed have been hepatic. While it was initially thought to be hepatocellular, recent studies have demonstrated that this toxicity is mainly cholestatic (Hohn et al. 1985; Kemeny et al. 1985, 1986). Recent studies have shown that a novel conjugate can be detected in the bile of patients given radiolabelled 5-fluorouracil that is formed from the FBAL catabolite and bile acids (Sweeny et al. 1987, 1988b). These conjugates have recently been shown to produce cholestasis in the isolated perfused rat liver (Sweeny et al. 1988a). Their role in biliary toxicity in humans is currently being evaluated.

Less clear is how efficiently the fluoropyrimidines are converted into active metabolites in tumours located within the liver. Future studies are needed to address these pharmacodynamic questions.

4.1.5 Intraperitoneal Administration

Intraperitoneal administration is another type of regional therapy approach that enables delivery of high concentrations of drug to the peritoneal area for varying periods of time (Dedrick et al. 1978). As with hepatic arterial administration, this approach is attractive for tumours that are potentially sensitive to 5-fluorouracil, such as gastrointestinal tumours and ovarian cancer (Myers 1984). Moreover, as the peritoneal cavity drains into the portal venous system, the remaining 5-fluorouracil is catabolised in the liver, reducing systemic blood drug concentrations and diminishing the occurrence of systemic toxicities such as bone marrow depression or gastrointestinal mucositis. Several studies have described in detail the pharmacokinetics of intraperitoneal administration of 5-fluorouracil (Collins et al. 1980; Gyves 1985; Myers 1984). In the study of Gyves using a continuous 5-day intraperitoneal infusion of 5-fluorouracil, it was shown that it was possible to maintain a 2 to 3 log greater concentration of 5-fluorouracil in the peritoneal cavity than in the systemic circulation.

4.1.6 Topical Administration

5-Fluorouracil has been used as a topical agent in the treatment of several premalignant and malignant skin diseases. It is usually administered by application directly to the skin lesions as a 1% or 5% cream or solution, twice daily for 14 to 21 days. This therapy has been demonstrated to be useful in the treatment of the premalignant lesion actinic keratosis (Stoll 1979), and suggested to be potentially curative in basal cell carcinoma (Haynes et al. 1985). The disposition of 5-fluorouracil administered topically has not been fully examined; however, there appears to be minimal absorption of the drug into the systemic circulation.

4.2 Distribution

In earlier animal studies (Chadwick & Chang 1976) 5-fluorouracil was shown to distribute readily to all tissues examined, including most notably bone marrow, small intestine, kidney, liver and spleen. In clinical studies 5-fluorouracil has been demonstrated to distribute freely throughout the body, penetrating the extracellular space, cerebrospinal fluid, ascites and pleural effusions (Chabner 1982). The Vd with intravenous bolus administration has been estimated to be 0.1 to 0.4 L/kg (Christophidis et al. 1978; Fraile et al. 1980). This figure represents a volume of distribution that is just slightly in excess of extracellular fluid space.

4.3 Elimination

4.3.1 Routes of Elimination

As shown in figure 2, 5-fluorouracil is eliminated by 1 of 2 pathways – catabolism by the liver and other tissues, and urinary excretion – with the former representing the major route of elimination. Following an intravenous bolus dose of 9 to 16 mg/kg, 5-fluorouracil reaches a peak plasma concentration of 0.4 to 1.0 mmol/L (Christophidis et al. 1978). Plasma clearance is monoexponential (Fraile et al. 1980) with a $t_{1/2\beta}$ of 8 to 20 minutes. Using a highly sensitive assay, a terminal phase has also been reported with a $t_{1/2\gamma}$ of 20 hours (Finn & Sadee 1975).

Recent pharmacokinetic studies (Heggie et al. 1987) utilising radiolabelled 5-fluorouracil with HPLC analysis of drug and metabolite concentrations in plasma and urine have shown that less than 10% of the administered drug is excreted intact. In the presence of certain rare metabolic abnormalities such as the recently described inherited syndrome of DPD deficiency (Diasio et al. 1988), the pharmacokinetics can be markedly altered and the amount of 5-fluorouracil excreted via the kidneys becomes significant, with more than 89% of administered drug being excreted in the urine.

The study of Heggie et al. (1987) with radiolabelled drug also demonstrated that trace amounts of unchanged 5-fluorouracil are eliminated via the biliary route.

4.3.2 Metabolism

Metabolism of 5-fluorouracil in humans is mainly via reductive catabolism (by DPD) in the liver and other tissues, which accounts for the elimination of more than 80% of an administered dose (Heggie et al. 1987). The liver represents the primary site of catabolic elimination of systemic 5-fluorouracil. However, on the basis of a hepatic extraction of 50% (Ensminger et al. 1978) and hepatic blood flow of 1 to 1.5 L/min, hepatic clearance falls significantly short of the observed total body clearance values for 5-fluorouracil (Myers 1981). This suggests that extrahepatic tissues and urinary excretion may also contribute to the elimination of the drug.

5. Effect of Pathophysiological State on Pharmacokinetics

Cancer patients often have concomitant diseases. Because renal and hepatic disease can alter the pharmacokinetics of chemotherapy agents (Powis 1982), the practitioner must consider its effect in the case of 5-fluorouracil.

Although there is a lack of published data on

the effect of renal dysfunction on the pharmacokinetics and toxicity of 5-fluorouracil, a reduction of dose in patients with renal dysfunction is usually not recommended.

The liver is the primary site of 5-fluorouracil catabolism; hence it might be expected that the dose would need to be reduced in the presence of hepatic dysfunction. However, only a few studies have addressed the effect of hepatic dysfunction on 5-fluorouracil pharmacokinetics and toxicity. Bioavailability of the drug did not appear to vary with alterations in standard liver function tests or presence of metastatic tumour (Christophidis et al. 1978). There are reports of prolonged plasma concentrations of 5-fluorouracil in patients with liver disease (Ensminger et al. 1978; MacMillan et al. 1978; Mukherjee et al. 1965). Although there are no specific guidelines for reducing the dose in the presence of hepatic dysfunction, several authors have recommended caution in the administration of 5-fluorouracil to patients with hepatic dysfunction (Bender et al. 1978; Carter 1977; Powis 1982).

6. Pharmacokinetic Interactions with Other Drugs

Because cancer patients are often treated with multiple drug therapy (including not only other chemotherapy agents but also non-chemotherapy drugs as well), one must be alert for possible interactions that may either increase or decrease tumour and/or host toxicity.

6.1 Interactions with Other Chemotherapy Drugs

Perhaps the interaction that has stimulated the most interest is that of 5-fluorouracil with methotrexate. These drugs are routinely used together in the treatment of adjuvant and metastatic breast cancer, and occasionally in head and neck cancer. The possible role of methotrexate in 'biochemically modulating' the metabolism of 5-fluorouracil has led to consideration of the use of a combination of the 2 drugs in other tumours (e.g. gastrointestinal tumours) where methotrexate itself has no significant activity as a single agent. Interest in possible interactions between these 2 drugs arose from experimental studies that suggested that the sequence of administration was important. Administration of 5-fluorouracil followed by methotrexate led to an antagonistic interaction (Bowen et al. 1978; Tattersall et al. 1973), while a reversal of the order led to a synergistic interaction (Bertino et al. 1977). The biochemical basis for the synergistic interaction between methotrexate and 5-fluorouracil given in sequence has been suggested to be due to increased uptake of the latter drug, increased incorporation of it into RNA, and increased formation of FdUMP. The modulation of 5-fluorouracil metabolism was suggested to be secondary to an increase in the availability of 5-phosphoribose-1-pyrophosphate (PRPP) pools following methotrexate pretreatment (Cadman et al. 1979). Unfortunately, *in vivo* studies in animal models (Mulder et al. 1981) have shown that the effect is not beneficial, with no differential selectivity between tumour and normal cells. Similarly, no clinical studies have demonstrated a significant response or survival advantage to sequential administration of methotrexate and 5-fluorouracil (Cano et al. 1981).

Recently there has been increased interest in the use of folinic acid with 5-fluorouracil, following on the observation that inhibition of thymidylate synthase requires the presence of reduced folate for maximal effect (Ullman et al. 1978). Studies with tumour lines *in vitro* have confirmed this effect (Hakala 1984), and several clinical studies have shown evidence that there may be some increased therapeutic benefit from providing a source of reduced folate (DeLap 1988; Petrelli et al. 1988).

Another approach has been to utilise other pyrimidines, such as thymidine or uridine, to biochemically modulate the metabolism and activity of 5-fluorouracil. There was interest in this approach because it had been thought that the metabolism of 5-fluorouracil could be shifted towards either incorporation into RNA or inhibition of thymidylate synthase activity. Clinical studies with 5-fluorouracil and thymidine demonstrated toxicity (Au et al. 1982; Martin et al. 1978) thought to be due mainly to competition for the same catabolic pathway (probably at the DPD step), resulting in increased and possibly prolonged concentrations of 5-fluorouracil. Uridine has similar effects, although these are not so pronounced as those of thymidine (Groeningen et al. 1986).

A similar approach has been to utilise drugs which interfere with pyrimidine biosynthesis. Many of these were evaluated as single agents themselves in Phase 1 or Phase 2 trials. Combinations have included 5-fluorouracil with inhibitors of *de novo* pyrimidine biosynthesis such as pyrazofurin and 6-azuridine, inhibitors of orotidylate decarboxylase (Chabner 1982) and PALA, an inhibitor of aspartate transcarbamylase (Erlichman et al. 1982). To date none of these combinations has demonstrated much success, but interest in this approach continues.

There have also been attempts to use purine analogues to 'modulate' 5-fluorouracil metabolism and the resultant toxicity. The drug that has been used most frequently is allopurinol, a purine analogue which (following conversion to its nucleotide) can inhibit OMP decarboxylase, leading to an accumulation of orotic acid. This in turn can compete with 5-fluorouracil for OMP phosphoribosyltransferase. Since many host tissues utilise this enzyme to anabolise 5-fluorouracil, in contrast to many tumours which do not, it may be possible to selectively reduce host toxicity. Several investigators have shown potential increased therapeutic effect with this combination in humans (Fox et al. 1979; Howell et al. 1981). However, the therapeutic advantage of this combination remains to be demonstrated.

Misonidazole is a radiosensitiser of hypoxic cells which has been shown to enhance the antitumour activity of several chemotherapy drugs (McNally 1982; Millar 1982). The pharmacokinetic rationale for using 5-fluorouracil and misonidazole together has been examined (McDermott et al. 1983) with demonstration that the clearance of the former was significantly reduced. The reduced clearance was associated with an earlier onset of the non-linear phase of 5-fluorouracil pharmacokinetics and an increased $t_{1/2\beta}$. Several clinical studies have demonstrated that the combination results in a reduction of the therapeutic index of 5-fluorouracil, with increased toxicity but no improvement in therapeutic benefit (Bardkji et al. 1986; Spooner et al. 1982).

6.2 Interactions with Non-Chemotherapy Drugs

The clinician must always be aware that other drugs besides chemotherapy agents may also interfere with the pharmacokinetics of 5-fluorouracil. Phenobarbitone and prednisone are known to alter the pharmacokinetics of several other drugs, and are often used in cancer patients; however, studies with these drugs failed to detect any pharmacokinetic effects on 5-fluorouracil (Ambre & Fischer 1971). The potential interaction of cimetidine and 5-fluorouracil has been examined (particularly with oral administration of the latter) to determine whether the bioavailability and pharmacokinetics of 5-fluorouracil could be altered (Harvey et al. 1984). Pretreatment with a single dose or daily treatment (1000mg) for 1 week had no effect on 5-fluorouracil pharmacokinetics. Pretreatment daily (1000mg) for 4 weeks led to increased peak plasma concentrations of 5-fluorouracil with an increased AUC. The total body clearance of 5-fluorouracil was decreased, but its $t_{1/2\beta}$ was not altered. The basis for the interaction of cimetidine and 5-fluorouracil is not understood but has been suggested by these authors to be possibly due to an effect on liver blood flow or inhibition of drug metabolism. They suggest care be taken when the drugs are administered concomitantly.

7. *Implications of Pharmacokinetics for Clinical Use*

The major impact of pharmacokinetic studies of 5-fluorouracil is in providing a basis for selecting a specific route of administration. Thus several of the studies with oral drug have shown that the bioavailability of 5-fluorouracil varies markedly between individuals, and even within the same individual on repeat dosing. Oral administration cannot be recommended although some clinical investigators have demonstrated that 5-fluorouracil is relatively well tolerated by the oral route and responses have been seen. In contrast to oral administration, pharmacokinetic studies have shown that there is a good rationale for the administration of 5-fluorouracil and its derivatives via both the intraperitoneal and hepatic arterial routes, which offer optimal drug delivery to the tumour bed while at the same time permitting sufficient degradation of the drug in the liver to decrease systemic toxicity.

Unfortunately, pharmacokinetic studies, and specifically measurements of concentrations of 5-fluorouracil in the blood following intravenous bolus or continuous (including protracted) infusions, have not proven useful in predicting tumour response or host cell (bone marrow, gastrointestinal mucosa) toxicity. With the development of the newer pharmacodynamic assays which can measure 5-fluorouracil metabolites or their effect on intracellular targets (e.g. FdUMP, inhibition of thymidylate synthase activity, FUTP incorporated into RNA), it may be possible to correlate these parameters with toxicity in both tumour and host cell.

References

Ambre JJ, Fischer LJ. The effect of prednisone and other factors on the catabolism of 5-fluorouracil in rats. Journal of Laboratory and Clinical Medicine 78: 343-353, 1971

Ardalan B, Buscaglia MD, Schein PS. Tumor 5-fluorodeoxyuridylate concentrations as a determinant of 5-fluorouracil response. Biochemical Pharmacology 27: 2009-2013, 1978

Armstrong RD, Lewis M, Stern SG, Cadman EC. Acute effect of 5-fluorouracil on cytoplasmic and nuclear dihydrofolate reductase messenger RNA metabolism. Journal of Biological Chemistry 261: 7366-7371, 1986a

Armstrong RD, Takimoto CH, Cadman EC. Fluoropyrimidine-mediated changes in small nuclear RNA. Journal of Biological Chemistry 261: 21-24, 1986b

Au JL, Rustum YM, Ledesma EJ, Mittelman A, Greaven PJ. Clinical pharmacological studies of concurrent infusion of 5-fluorouracil and thymidine in treatment of colorectal carcinoma. Cancer Research 42: 2930-2937, 1982

Aubert C, Luccioni C, Coassolo P, Sommadossi JP, Cano JP. Comparative determination of 5-fluorouracil in plasma using GC/MS and HPLC. Arzneimittel-Forschung 31: 2048-2053, 1981

Aubert C, Sommadossi JP, Coassolo P, Cano JP, Rigault JP. Quantitative analysis of 5-fluorouracil and 5,6-dihydrofluorouracil in plasma by gas chromatography mass spectrometry. Biomedical Mass Spectrometry 9: 336-339, 1982

Balch CM, Levin B. Regional and systemic chemotherapy for colorectal metastases to the liver. World Journal of Surgery 11: 521-526, 1987

Bardkji Z, Jolivet J, Langelier Y, Besner JG, Ayoub J. 5-Fluorouracil-metronidazole combination therapy in metastatic colorectal cancer. Cancer Chemotherapy and Pharmacology 18: 140-144, 1986

Beck WT. The cell biology of multiple drug resistance. Biochemical Pharmacology 36: 2879-2887, 1987

Bender RA, Zwelling LA, Doroshow JH, Myers CE, Chabner BA, et al. Antineoplastic drugs: clinical pharmacology and therapeutic use. Drugs 16: 46-87, 1978

Berger SH, Jenh CH, Johnson LF, Berger FG. Thymidylate synthase overproduction and gene amplification in fluorodeoxyuridine-resistant human cells. Molecular Pharmacology 28: 461-467, 1985

Bertino JR, Sawicki WL, Linquist CA, et al. Schedule-dependent antitumor effects of methotrexate and 5-fluorouracil. Cancer Research 37: 327-328, 1977

Bowen D, White JC, Goldman ID. A basis for fluoropyrimidine-induced antagonism to methotrexate in Ehrlich ascites tumor cells *in vitro*. Cancer Research 38: 219-222, 1978

Buckpitt AR, Boyd MR. A sensitive method for determination of 5-fluorouracil and 5-fluoro-2′-deoxyuridine in human plasma by high-pressure liquid chromatography. Analytical Biochemistry 106: 432-437, 1980

Cadman E, Hermer R, Davis L. Enhanced 5-fluorouracil nucleotide formation after methotrexate administration: explanation for drug synergism. Science 205: 1135-1137, 1979

Cano JP, Aubert C, Rigault JP, Gilli R, Coassolo P, et al. Advantages and limitations of pharmacokinetic studies in the rationalization of anticancer therapy: methotrexate and 5-FU. Cancer Treatment Reports 65: 33-42, 1981

Cano JP, Rigault JP, Aubert C, Carcassione Y, Seitze JF. Determination of 5-fluorouracil in plasma by GC/MS using an internal standard. Applications to pharmacokinetics. Bulletin du Cancer 66: 67-74, 1979

Caradonna SJ, Cheng YC. The role of deoxyuridine triphosphate nucleotidohydrolase, uracil-DNA glycosylase, and DNA polymerase α in the metabolism of FUdR in human tumor cells. Molecular Pharmacology 18: 513-520, 1980

Carter SK (Ed.). Chemotherapy of cancer, Wiley, New York, 1977

Chabner BA. Pyrimidine antagonists. In Chabner BA (Ed.) Pharmacologic principles of cancer treatment, pp. 183-212, WB Saunders Co., Philadelphia, 1982

Chadwick M, Chang C. Comparative physiologic dispositions of 5-fluoro-2′-deoxyuridine and 5-fluorouracil in mice bearing solid L1210 lymphocytic leukemia. Cancer Treatment Reports 60: 845-855, 1976

Chaudhuri NK, Mukherjee KL, Heidelberger C. Studies on fluorinated pyrimidines. VII. The degradative pathway. Biochemical Pharmacology 1: 328-341, 1959

Cheng YC, Nakayama K. Effects of 5-fluoro-2′-deoxyuridine on DNA metabolism in HeLa cells. Molecular Pharmacology 23: 171-174, 1983

Christophidis N, Mihaly G, Vajda F, Louis W. Comparison of liquid- and gas-liquid chromatographic assays of 5-fluorouracil in plasma. Clinical Chemistry 25: 83-86, 1979

Christophidis N, Vajda FJE, Lucas I, Drummer O, Moon WJ, et al. Fluorouracil therapy in patients with carcinoma of the large bowel: a pharmacokinetic comparison of various rates and routes of administration. Clinical Pharmacokinetics 3: 330-336, 1978

Clark JL, Berger SH, Mittelman A, Berger FG. Thymidylate synthase gene amplification in a colon tumor resistant to fluoropyrimidine chemotherapy. Cancer Treatment Reports 71: 261-265, 1987

Clarkson B, O'Connor A, Winston L, Hutchison D. The physiological disposition of 5-fluorouracil and 5-fluorodeoxyuri-

dine in man. Clinical Pharmacology and Therapeutics 5: 581-610, 1964
Cohen JL, Irwin LE, Marshall GJ, Darvey H, Bateman JR. Clinical pharmacology of oral and intravenous 5-fluorouracil (NSC-19893). Cancer Chemotherapy Reports 58: 723-731, 1974
Cohen MB, Glazer RI. Cytotoxicity and the inhibition of ribosomal RNA processing in human colon carcinoma cells. Molecular Pharmacology 27: 308-313, 1985
Collins JM, Dedrick RL, King FG, Speyer JL, Myers CE. Nonlinear pharmacokinetic models for 5-fluorouracil in man: intravenous and intraperitoneal routes. Clinical Pharmacology and Therapeutics 28: 235-246, 1980
Danenberg PV. The role of reduced folates in the enhanced binding of FdUMP to dTMP synthetase. In Bruckner & Rustum (Eds) The current status of 5-fluorouracil-leucovorin calcium combination, pp. 5-11, John Wiley & Sons, New York, 1984
Danenberg PV, Danenberg KD. Effect of 5,10-methylenetetrahydrofolate on the dissociation of 5-fluoro-2′-deoxyuridylate from thymidylate synthetase: evidence for an ordered mechanism. Biochemistry 17: 4018-4024, 1978
Danenberg PV, Heidelberger C, Mulkins MA, Peterson AR. The incorporation of 5-fluoro-2-deoxyuridine into DNA of mammalian tumor cells. Biochemical and Biophysical Research Communications 102: 654-658, 1981
Danenberg PV, Lockshin A. Fluorinated pyrimidines as tight-binding inhibitors of thymidylate synthase. Pharmacological Therapeutics 13: 69-90, 1981
Dedrick R, Myers C, Bungay P, et al. Pharmacokinetic rationale for peritoneal drug administration in the treatment of ovarian cancer. Cancer Treatment Reports 62: 1-11, 1978
DeLap RJ. The effect of leucovorin on the therapeutic index of fluorouracil in cancer patients. Yale Journal of Biology and Medicine 61: 23-34, 1988
DeVita VT, Hellman S, Rosenberg SA (Eds). Cancer, principles and practice of oncology, 2nd ed., JB Lippincott Company, Philadelphia, 1985
Diasio RB, Beavers TL, Carpenter JT. Familial deficiency of dihydropyrimidine dehydrogenase: biochemical basis for familial pyrimidinemia and severe 5-fluorouracil-induced toxicity. Journal of Clinical Investigation 81: 47-51, 1988
Diasio RB, Schuetz JD, Wallace HJ, Sommadossi JP. Dihydrofluorouracil, a fluorouracil catabolite with antitumor activity in murine and human cell. Cancer Research 45: 4900-4903, 1985
Diasio RB, Wilburn ME. Effect of column temperature on resolution of fluoropyrimidines by reverse phase high performance liquid chromatography. Journal of Chromatographic Science 17: 565-567, 1979
Dolnick BJ, Pink JJ. 5-Fluorouracil modulation of dihydrofolate reductase RNA levels in methotrexate-resistant KB cells. Journal of Biological Chemistry 258: 13299-13306, 1983
Duschinsky R, Pleven E, Heidelberger C. The synthesis of 5-fluoropyrimidines. Journal of the American Chemical Society 79: 4559-4560, 1957
Ensminger WD, Gyves JW. Clinical pharmacology of hepatic arterial chemotherapy. Seminars in Oncology 10: 176-182, 1983
Ensminger WD, Rosowsky A, Raso V, Levin DC, Glode M, et al. A clinical-pharmacological evaluation of hepatic arterial infusions of 5-fluoro-2′-deoxyuridine and 5-fluorouracil. Cancer Research 38: 3784-3792, 1978
Erlichman C, Donehower RC, Speyer JL, Klecker R, Chabner BA. Phase I-phase II trial of N-phosphonacetyl-L-aspartic acid given by intravenous infusion and 5-fluorouracil given by bolus injection. Journal of the National Cancer Institute 68: 227-231, 1982
Evans RM, Laskin JD, Hakala MT. Effect of excess folates and deoxyinosine on the activity and site of actions of 5-fluorouracil. Cancer Research 41: 3288-3295, 1981
Finch RE, Bending MR, Lant AF. Plasma levels of 5-fluorouracil after oral and intravenous administration in cancer patients. British Journal of Clinical Pharmacology 7: 613-617, 1979
Finn C, Sadee W. Determination of 5-fluorouracil (NSC-19893) plasma levels in rats and man by isotope dilution-mass fragmentography. Cancer Chemotherapy Reports 59: 279-286, 1975
Fox RM, Woods RL, Tattersall MHN. Allopurinol modulation of high dose fluorouracil toxicity. Cancer Treatment Reports 6: 143-147, 1979
Fraile RJ, Baker LH, Buroker TR, Horwitz J, Vaitkevicius VK. Pharmacokinetics of 5-fluorouracil administered orally, by rapid intravenous and by slow infusion. Cancer Research 40: 2223-2228, 1980
Garrett ER, Hurst GH, Green JR. Kinetics and mechanisms of drug action on microorganisms. XXIII. Microbial kinetic assay for fluorouracil in biological fluids and its application to human pharmacokinetics. Journal of Pharmaceutical Sciences 66: 1422-1429, 1977
Goldberg AR, Machledt JH Jr, Pardee AB. On the action of fluorouracil on leukemia cells. Cancer Research 26: 1611-1615, 1966
Grem J, Hoth D, Hamilton JM. Overview of current status and future direction of clinical trials with 5-fluorouracil in combination with folinic acid. Cancer Treatment Reports 12: 1249-1264, 1987
Groeningen CJV, Leyva A, Kraal I, Peters GJ, Pinedo HM. Clinical and pharmacokinetic studies of prolonged administration of high-dose uridine intended for rescue from 5-FU toxicity. Cancer Treatment Reports 70: 745-750, 1986
Gyves J. Pharmacology of intraperitoneal infusion 5-fluorouracil and mitomycin-C. Seminars in Oncology 12: 29-32, 1985
Hakala MT. Basis for the effect of leucovorin on the activity and site of action of 5-fluorouracil in human cells. In Bruckner & Rustum (Eds) The current status of 5-fluorouracil-leucovorin calcium combination, pp. 33-39, John Wiley & Sons, New York, 1984
Harris BE, Song R, He Y, Diasio RB. Circadian periodicity of dihydropyrimidine dehydrogenase (DPD) activity in humans: possible relevance to toxicity from fluoropyrimidine (FP) drugs with implications for FP infusion by programmable pumps. Proceedings of the American Society of Clinical Oncology 7: 77, 1988a
Harris BE, Song R, He Y, Soong SJ, Diasio RB. Circadian rhythm of rat liver dihydropyrimidine dehydrogenase: possible relevance to fluoropyrimidine chemotherapy. Biochemical Pharmacology 37: 4759-4762, 1988b
Harvey VJ, Slevin ML, Dilloway MR, Clark PI, Johnston A, et al. The influence of cimetidine on the pharmacokinetics of 5-fluorouracil. British Journal of Clinical Pharmacology 18: 421-430, 1984
Haynes HA, Mead KW, Goldwyn RM. Cancers of the skin. In DeVita et al. (Eds) Cancer, principles and practice of oncology, 2nd ed., pp. 1343-1369, J.B. Lippincott Co., Philadelphia, 1985
Heggie GD, Sommadossi JP, Cross DS, Huster WJ, Diasio RB. Metabolism of 5-fluorouracil in cancer patients with quantitation of fluorouracil catabolites in plasma, urine, and bile over time. Cancer Research 47: 2203-2206, 1987
Heidelberger C. Fluorinated pyrimidines and their nucleosides. In Sartorelli & Johns (Eds) Antineoplastic and immunosuppressive agents, part II, pp. 193-231, Springer-Verlag, New York, 1975
Heidelberger C, Ghobar A, Baker RK, Mukherjee KL. Studies on fluorinated pyrimidines. X. *In vivo* studies on tumor resistance. Cancer Research 20: 897-902, 1960a
Heidelberger C, Kaldor G, Mukherjee KL, Danenberg PV. Studies on fluorinated pyrimidines. XI. *In vitro* studies on tumor resistance. Cancer Research 20: 905-909, 1960b
Herrick D, Kufe DW. Lethality associated with incorporation of 5-fluorouracil into preribosomal RNA. Molecular Pharmacology 21: 468-473, 1982
Herrick D, Kufe DW. Lethality associated with incorporation of

5-fluorouracil into preribosomal RNA. Molecular Pharmacology 26: 135-140, 1984
Hillcoat BL, McCulloch PB, Figueredo AT, Ehsan MH, Rosenfeld JM. Clinical response and plasma levels of 5-fluorouracil in patients with colonic cancer treated by drug infusion. British Journal of Cancer 38: 719-724, 1978
Hohn D, Melnick J, Stagg R, Altman D, Friedman M, et al. Biliary sclerosis in patients receiving hepatic arterial infusions and floxuridine. Journal of Clinical Oncology 3: 98-102, 1985
Hohn DC, Rayner AA, Economou JS, Ignoffo RJ, et al. Toxicities and complications of implanted pump hepatic arterial infusions and intravenous floxuridine infusion. Cancer 57: 465-470, 1986
Houghton JA, Houghton PJ. On the mechanism of cytotoxicity of fluorinated pyrimidines in four human colon adenocarcinoma xenografts maintained in immune-deprived mice. Cancer 45: 1159-1167, 1980
Houghton JA, Houghton PJ. 5-Halogenated pyrimidines and their nucleosides. In Fox & Fox (Eds) Antitumor drug resistance, pp. 515-549, Springer-Verlag, New York, 1984
Howell SB, Wung WE, Taetle R, et al. Modulation of 5-fluorouracil toxicity by allopurinol in man. Cancer 48: 1281-1289, 1981
Ikenaka K, Shirasaka T, Kitano S, Fujii S. Effect of uracil on metabolism of 5-fluorouracil *in vitro.* Gann 70: 353-359, 1979
Ingraham HA, Tseng BY, Goulian M. Mechanism for exclusion of 5-fluorouracil from DNA. Cancer Research 40: 998-1001, 1980
Ingraham HA, Tseng BY, Goulian M. Nucleotide levels and incorporation of 5-fluorouracil and uracil into DNA of cells treated with 5-fluorodeoxyuridine. Molecular Pharmacology 21: 211-216, 1982
Jacquez JA. Permeability of Ehrlich cells to uracil, thymine, and fluorouracil. Proceedings of the Society of Experimental Biology and Medicine 109: 132-135, 1962
Kemeny MM, Goldberg DA, Browning S, Metter GE, Miner PJ, et al. Experience with continuous regional chemotherapy and hepatic resection as treatment of hepatic metastases from colorectal primaries. Cancer 55: 1265-1270, 1985
Kessel D. Cell surface alterations associated with exposure of leukemia L1210 cells to fluorouracil. Cancer Research 40: 322-324, 1980
Kessel D, Hall TC. Studies on drug transport by normal human leukocytes. Biochemical Pharmacology 16: 2395-2403, 1967
Kessel D, Hall TC, Wodinsky I. Nucleotide formation as a determinant of 5-fluorouracil response in mouse leukemias. Science 154: 911-913, 1966
Kufe DW, Major PP, Egan EM, Loh E. 5-Fluoro-2′-deoxyuridine incorporation in L1210 DNA. Journal of Biological Chemistry 256: 8885-8888, 1981
Kufe DW, Scott P, Fram R, Major P. Biological effect of 5-fluoro-2′-deoxyuridine incorporation in L1210 deoxyribonucleic acid. Biochemical Pharmacology 32: 1337-1340, 1983
Lakings DB, Adamson RH, Diasio RB. Quantitative analysis of 5-fluorouracil in human serum by selected ion monitoring gas chromatography-mass spectrometry. Journal of Chromatography – Biomedical Applications 146: 512-517, 1978
Liebecq C, Peters RA. The toxicity of fluoroacetate and the tricarboxylic acid cycle. Biochimica Biophysica Acta 3: 215-230, 1949
Lindahl T. DNA glycosylases, endonucleases for apurinic/apyrimidinic sites, and base excision repair. In Cohen WE (Ed.) Progress in nucleic acid research molecular biology, Vol. 22, pp. 135-192, Academic Press, New York, 1979
Lindahl T, Ljunquist S, Siegert N, Nyberg B, Sperens B. DNA N-glycosidases: Properties of uracil-DNA glycosidase from Escherichia coli. Journal of Biological Chemistry 252: 3286-3294, 1977
Lokich J, Fine N, Perri J, Bothe A. Protracted ambulatory venous infusion of 5-fluorouracil. American Journal of Clinical Oncology Cancer Clinical Trials 6: 103-107, 1983
Lonn U, Lonn S. Interaction between 5-fluorouracil and DNA of human colon adenocarcinoma. Cancer Research 44: 3414-3418, 1984
Lonn U, Lonn S. DNA lesions in human neoplastic cells and cytotoxicity of 5-fluoropyrimidines. Cancer Research 46: 3866-3870, 1986
Lozeron HA, Gordon MP, Gabriel T, Tautz W, Duschinsky R. The photochemistry of 5-fluorouracil. Biochemistry 3: 1844-1850, 1964
MacMillan WE, Wolberg WH, Welling PG. Pharmacokinetics of 5-fluorouracil in humans. Cancer Research 38: 3479-3482, 1978
Maguire JH, Dudley KH. Partial purification and characterization of dihydropyrimidinase from calf and rat liver. Drug Metabolism and Disposition 6: 601-610, 1978
Major PP, Egan E, Herrick D, Kufe DW. 5-Fluorouracil incorporation in DNA of human breast carcinoma cells. Cancer Research 42: 3005-3009, 1982
Mandel HG. The incorporation of 5-fluorouracil into RNA and its molecular consequences. Progress in Molecular and Subcellular Biology 1: 82-135, 1969
Martin DS, Nayak P, Sawyer RC, Stolfi RL, Young CW, et al. Enhancement of 5-fluorouracil chemotherapy with emphasis on the use of excess thymidine. Cancer Bulletin 30: 219-224, 1978
McDermott BJ, Van den Berg HW, Martin WMC, Murphy RF. Pharmacokinetic rationale for the interaction of 5-fluorouracil and misonidazole in humans. British Journal of Cancer 48: 705-710, 1983
McDermott BJ, Van den Berg HW, Murphy RF. Nonlinear pharmacokinetics for the elimination of 5-fluorouracil after intravenous administration in cancer patients. Cancer Chemotherapy and Pharmacology 9: 173-178, 1982
McNally NJ. Enhancement of chemotherapy agents. International Journal of Radiation Oncology Biology & Physics 8: 593-598, 1982
Mentre F, Steimer JL, Sommadossi JP, Diasio RB, Cano JP. A mathematical model of the kinetics of 5-fluorouracil and its catabolites in freshly isolated rat hepatocytes. Biochemical Pharmacology 33: 2727-2732, 1984
Millar BC. Hypoxic cell radiosensitizers as potential adjuvants to conventional chemotherapy for the treatment of cancer. Biochemical Pharmacology 31: 2439-2445, 1982
Moran RG, Spears CPO, Heidelberger C. Biochemical determinants to tumor sensitivity to 5-fluorouracil: ultrasensitive methods for the determination of 5-fluoro-2′-deoxyuridylate, 2′-deoxyuridylate, and thymidylate synthetase. Proceedings of the National Academy of Science 76: 1456-1460, 1979
Mukherjee KL, Boohar J, Wentland D, Ansfield FJ, Heidelberger C. Studies on fluorinated pyrimidines. XVI. Metabolism of 5-fluorouracil-2-^{14}C and 5-fluoro-2′-deoxyuridine-2-^{14}C in cancer patients. Cancer Research 23: 49-66, 1965
Mukherjee KL, Heidelberger C. Studies on fluorinated pyrimidines. IX. The degradation of 5-fluorouracil-6-C^{14}. Journal of Biological Chemistry 235: 433-437, 1960
Mulder JH, Smink T, van Putten LM. 5-Fluorouracil and methotrexate combination chemotherapy: the effect of drug scheduling. European Journal of Cancer and Clinical Oncology 17: 831-837, 1981
Myers CE. The pharmacology of the fluoropyrimidines. Pharmacological Reviews 33: 1-15, 1981
Myers CE. The use of intraperitoneal chemotherapy in the treatment of ovarian cancer. Seminars in Oncology 11: 275-284, 1984
Myers CE, Young RC, Chabner BA. Biochemical determinants of 5-fluorouracil response *in vivo.* The role of deoxyuridylate pool expansion. Journal of Clinical Investigation 56: 1231-1238, 1975

Naguib FMN, el Kouni MH, Cha S. Enzymes of uracil catabolism in normal and neoplastic human tissue. Cancer Research 45: 5404-5412, 1985
Parker WB, Kennedy KA, Klubes P. Dissociation of 5-fluorouracil into DNA and its cytotoxicity in murine T-lymphoma (S-49) cells. Cancer Research 47: 979-982, 1987
Petit E, Milano G, Levi F, et al. Circadian rhythm-varying plasma concentration of 5-fluorouracil during a five-day continuous venous infusion at a constant rate in cancer patients. Cancer Research 48: 1676-1679, 1988
Petrelli N, Stablein D, Bruckner H, et al. A prospective randomized phase III trial of 5-fluorouracil (5FU) versus 5FU + high dose leucovorin (HDCF) versus 5FU + low dose leucovorin (LDCF) in patients (PTS) with metastatic colorectal adenocarcinoma. Proceedings of the American Society of Clinical Oncology 7: 94, 1988
Powis G. Effect of human renal and hepatic disease on the pharmacokinetics of anticancer drugs. Cancer Treatment Reviews 9: 85-124, 1982
Ramberg ES, Ishaq M, Rulf S, Moeller B, Horowitz J. Inhibition of transfer RNA function by replacement of uridine and uridine-derived nucleosides with 5-fluorouridine. Biochemistry 17: 3978-3985, 1978
Riechard P, Skold O, Klein G. Possible enzymic mechanism for the development of resistance against fluorouracil in ascites tumors. Nature 183: 939-941, 1959
Reichard P, Skold O, Klein G, Revesz L, Magnusson P-H. Studies on resistance against fluorouracil. I. Enzymes of the uracil pathway during development of resistance. Cancer Research 22: 235-243, 1962
Robins MJ, Naik SR. Nucleic acid related compounds III. A focile synthesis of 5-fluorouracil bases and nucleosides by direct fluorination. Journal of the American Chemical Society 93: 5277-5278, 1971
Roemeling RV, Hrushesky WJM. Circadian pattern of continuous FUDR infusion reduces toxicities. Progress in Clinical and Biological Research 227B: 357-373, 1987
Rutman RJ, Cantarow A, Paschkis KE. Studies in 2-acetylaminofluorene carcinogenesis III. The utilization of uracil-2-^{14}C by preneoplastic rat liver and rat hepatoma. Cancer Research 14: 119-134, 1954
Sanno Y, Holzer M, Schimple RT. Studies of a mutation affecting pyrimidine degradation in inbred mice. Journal of Biological Chemistry 245: 5658-5676, 1970
Santi DV, McHenry CS. 5-Fluoro-2′-deoxyuridylate: covalent complex with thymidylate synthetase. Proceedings of the National Academy of Sciences, USA 69: 1855-1857, 1972
Santi DV, McHenry CS, Sommer H. Mechanism of interaction of thymidylate synthetase with 5-fluorodeoxyuridylate. Biochemistry 13: 471-481, 1974
Schaaf LJ, Dobbs BR, Edwards IR, Perrier DG. Nonlinear pharmacokinetic characteristics of 5-fluorouracil (5-FU) in colorectal cancer patients. European Journal of Clinical Pharmacology 32: 411-418, 1987
Schuetz JD, Collins JM, Wallace HJ, Diasio RB. Alteration of the secondary structure of newly synthesized DNA from murine bone marrow cells by 5-fluorouracil. Cancer Research 46: 119-123, 1986
Schuetz JD, Diasio RB. The effect of 5-fluorouracil on DNA chain elongation in intact bone marrow cells. Biochemical and Biophysical Research Communications 133: 361-367, 1985
Schuetz JD, Wallace HJ, Diasio RB. 5-Fluorouracil incorporation into DNA of CF-1 mouse bone marrow cells as a possible mechanism of toxicity. Cancer Research 44: 1358-1363, 1984
Schuetz JD, Wallace HJ, Diasio RB. DNA repair following incorporation of 5-fluorouracil into DNA of mouse bone marrow cells. Cancer Chemotherapy and Pharmacology 21: 208-210, 1988
Shiotani T, Weber G. Purification and properties of dihydrothymine dehydrogenase from rat liver. Journal of Biological Chemistry 256: 219-224, 1981
Sitar DS, Shaw DHJ, Thirwell MP, Ruedy JR. Disposition of 5-fluorouracil after intravenous bolus doses of a commercial formulation to cancer patients. Cancer Research 37: 3981-3984, 1977
Skold O. Studies on resistance against 5-fluorouracil. IV. Evidence for an altered uridine kinase in resistant cells. Biochimica et Biophysica Acta 76: 160-162, 1963
Sommadossi JP, Cross DS, Gewirtz DA, Goldman ID, Diasio RB. Evidence from rat hepatocytes of an unrecognized pathway of 5-fluorouracil metabolism with the formation of a glucuronide derivative. Cancer Research 45: 2450-2455, 1985a
Sommadossi JP, Gewirtz DA, Cross DS, Goldman ID, Diasio RB. Modulation of 5-fluorouracil catabolism in freshly isolated rat hepatocytes by thymine or uracil: therapeutic implications. Cancer Research 45: 116-121, 1985b
Sommadossi JP, Gewirtz DA, Diasio RB, Aubert C, Cano JP, et al. Rapid catabolism of 5-fluorouracil in freshly isolated rat hepatocytes as analyzed by high performance liquid chromatography. Journal of Biological Chemistry 357: 8171-8176, 1982
Spears CP, Gustavsson BG. Methods for thymidylate synthase pharmacodynamics: serial biopsy, free and total TS, FdUMP and dUMP, and H_4PteGlu and CH_2-H_4PteGlu assays. In Rustum et al. (Eds) The expanding role of folates and fluoropyrimidines in cancer chemotherapy, Plenum Press, New York, 1988
Spears CP, Gustavsson BG, Berne M, Frosing R, Hayes AA. Mechanisms of innate resistance to thymidylate synthase inhibition after 5-fluorouracil. Cancer Research, in press, 1988a
Spears CP, Gustavsson BG, Karlsson G, Frosing R. Fluorouracil/leucovorin pharmacodynamics: determination by serial biopsy. Proceedings of the American Association for Cancer Research 29: 186, 1988b
Spicer DV, Ardalan B, Daniels JB, Silbermann H, Johnson K. Reevaluation of the maximum tolerated dose of continuous venous infusion of 5-fluorouracil with pharmacokinetics. Cancer Research 48: 459-461, 1988
Spooner D, Bugden RD, Peckham MJ, Wist EA. The combination of 5-fluorouracil with misonidazole in patients with advanced colorectal cancer. International Journal of Radiation Oncology Biology and Physics 8: 387-389, 1982
Stoll HL. Topical chemotherapy. In Helm F (Ed.) Cancer dermatology, pp. 435-448, Lea & Febiger, Philadelphia, 1979
Sweeny DJ, Barnes S, Diasio RB. Production of cholestasis by 2-fluoro-β-alanine-chenodeoxycholic acid: possible role of this metabolite in the cholestasis associated with hepatic arterial infusion of fluoropyrimidines. Proceedings of the American Association for Cancer Research 29: 486, 1988a
Sweeny DJ, Barnes S, Heggie GD, Diasio RB. Metabolism of 5-fluorouracil to a N-cholyl-2-fluoro-β-alanine conjugate: a novel role for bile acids in drug conjugation. Proceedings of the National Academy of Sciences, USA 84: 5439-5443, 1987
Sweeny DJ, Martin M, Diasio RB. N-chenodeoxycholyl-2-fluoro-β-alanine: a biliary metabolite of 5-fluorouracil in man. Drug Metabolism and Disposition 16: 892-894, 1988b
Tanaka M, Yoshida S, Saneyoshi M, Yamaguchi T. Utilization of 5-fluoro-2′-deoxyuridine triphosphate and 5-fluoro-2′-deoxycytidine triphosphate in DNA synthesis by DNA polymerase α and β from calf thymus. Cancer Research 41: 4132-4135, 1981
Tattersall MHN, Jackson RG, Connors TA, Harrap KR. Combination chemotherapy: The interaction of methotrexate and 5-fluorouracil. European Journal of Cancer 9: 733-739, 1973
Tuchman M, Roemeling RV, Lanning RM, Sothern RB, Hrushesky WJM. Sources of variability of dihydropyrimidine dehydrogenase activity in human blood mononuclear cells. Annual Review of Chronopharmacology, in press, 1988
Ullman B, Lee M, Martin DW Jr, et al. Cytotoxicity of 5-fluoro-2′-deoxyuridine: requirement for reduced folate cofactors and

antagonism by methotrexate. Proceedings of the National Academy of Sciences, USA 75: 980-983, 1978

Vessey DA. The co-purification and common identity of cholyl CoA:glycine- and CoA:taurine-n-acyltransferase activities from bovine liver. Journal of Biological Chemistry 254: 2059-2063, 1979

Walliser S, Redmann K. Effect of 5-fluorouracil and thymidine on the transmembrane potential and zeta potential of HeLa cells. Cancer Research 38: 3555-3559, 1978

Wasternak C. Degradation of pyrimidines and pyrimidine analogs – pathways and mutual influences. Pharmacology Therapeutics 8: 629-651, 1980

Wohlhueter RM, McIvar RS, Plageman PGW. Facilitated transport of uracil and 5-fluorouracil, and permeation of orotic acid into cultured mammalian cells. Journal of Cellular Physiology 104: 309-319, 1980

Authors' address: Dr *Robert B. Diasio*, Box 600 Volker Hall, Division of Clinical Pharmacology, Comprehensive Cancer Center, University of Alabama at Birmingham, Birmingham, AL 35294 (USA).

Clinical Pharmacokinetics 16: 238-253 (1989)
0312-5963/89/0004-0238/$08.00/0

Clinical Pharmacokinetic Considerations in the Control of Oral Anticoagulant Therapy

H.G.M. Shetty, A.G. Fennerty and *P.A. Routledge*

Department of Pharmacology and Therapeutics, University of Wales College of Medicine, Health Park, Cardiff, Wales

Contents

Summary 238
1. Pharmacokinetics of Warfarin 239
 1.1 Absorption 239
 1.2 Distribution 239
 1.3 Metabolism 240
2. Pharmacokinetic Causes of Altered Response to Warfarin Therapy 240
 2.1 Absorption 240
 2.2 Distribution 241
 2.3 Metabolism 243
 2.4 Excretion 245
3. Pharmacodynamic Factors 245
 3.1 Genetic Factors 245
 3.2 Vitamin K Excess or Deficiency 245
 3.3 Variations in the Levels of Vitamin K-Dependent Clotting Factors 248
4. Clinical Pharmacokinetic Considerations 248
 4.1 Investigation of Patients with Abnormal Response to Warfarin 248
 4.2 Initiation and Cessation of Warfarin Therapy 249
 4.3 Prediction of Warfarin Dosage 250
 4.4 Treatment of Warfarin Overdosage 250
5. Conclusion 251

Summary *Aspects of the pharmacokinetics of warfarin that are clinically relevant are reviewed here. Since warfarin is normally completely absorbed, resistance to treatment due to impaired absorption is unusual, even in severe short bowel syndrome. Warfarin is highly albumin-bound; thus, hypoalbuminaemic states result in an increased free fraction of the drug and a decreased half-life but, as might be expected, there is no evidence of altered response at steady-state. Warfarin is completely metabolised by the liver to hydroxywarfarins and warfarin alcohols, and although the latter have some biological activity they do not contribute significantly to the drug effect. No information is available concerning the metabolism of warfarin in chronic liver disease, but there is evidence of increased sensitivity due to impaired vitamin K-dependent clotting factor synthesis. Impaired renal function does not appear to alter the effect of warfarin. Lowered response to the drug may be secondary to poor compliance, kinetic resistance or pharmacodynamic resistance. These factors can be identified using algorithms based on population values for plasma warfarin concentrations and clearances at steady-state.*

The pharmacokinetics and pharmacodynamics of warfarin indicate that several days' overlap with heparin on initiation of warfarin, and gradual (rather than sudden) discontinuation of warfarin, might theoretically be necesssary. However, those studies which have been performed have indicated that a long overlap and gradual discontinuation are not associated with greater safety or efficacy of the drug.

Because of the long elimination half-life of warfarin and the short elimination half-life of vitamin K, many days' treatment with phytomenadione may be required after warfarin overdose. The elimination half-life and therefore the duration of therapy may be reduced by regular oral cholestyramine, although the means by which the latter enhances warfarin elimination is still unknown.

Of the various oral anticoagulants, warfarin is the most widely used drug world-wide and probably the most extensively investigated. Warfarin has a very narrow therapeutic index and, therefore, for a safe, rational anticoagulant therapy, an understanding of various factors that influence an individual's response to the drug is essential.

In this review we discuss the normal pharmacokinetics of warfarin; the various clinical settings which alter its pharmacokinetics; the investigation of a patient with abnormal response to warfarin; the advantages or potential risks involved in the different ways of initiating and discontinuing warfarin therapy; how to predict the warfarin dosage; and, finally, how to treat warfarin overdosage.

1. *Pharmacokinetics of Warfarin*

1.1 Absorption

The sodium salt of warfarin is non-polar below a pH of 5.1 and is absorbed completely from the stomach and proximal small intestine (Deykin 1970). When administered orally in tablet form, warfarin is 100% bioavailable and a comparison of area under the curve after oral and intravenous administration indicates that 'first-pass' metabolism does not occur (Andreasen & Vesell 1974). Food slightly decreases the rate but not the extent of absorption (Melander 1978); unchanged warfarin has not been recovered from stool (Aggeler & O'Reilly 1966). Using high performance liquid chromatography, peak plasma concentrations have been observed between 0.3 and 4 hours, but 1 study reports a secondary peak between 1 and 8 hours (Stirling et al. 1982).

1.2 Distribution

Warfarin is highly protein bound, binding almost entirely to albumin (O'Reilly 1973). It appears to have 1 to 3 primary binding sites per molecule of albumin in humans at physiological pH. The measured affinity constant varies between 0.75 × 10^5 mol/L and 2.5 × 10^5 mol/L depending on the method used (Bachman & Shapiro 1977). Equilibrium dialysis techniques have shown that S(−) and R(+) warfarin have similar protein binding characteristics at 27°C (O'Reilly 1971b), but at 37°C S(−) warfarin is more significantly albumin bound than the R(+) enantiomer (Sellers & Koch-Weser 1975). Because elimination occurs only from the central compartment, warfarin kinetics can be adequately described by a 1-compartment open model (Wagner 1975). The apparent volume of distribution (Vd) of warfarin ranges between 7.6 L/70kg (Slattery et al. 1979) and 13.9 L/70kg (Toon et al. 1986). The volumes of distribution of the R(+) and S(−) enantiomers are similar to each other and to that of the racemate (Banfield et al. 1983; Breckenridge et al. 1974; Hignite et al. 1980).

The uptake of warfarin by erythrocytes is less than 1% in humans (O'Reilly et al. 1963). Warfarin therapy during pregnancy is associated with increased incidence of fetal abnormalities (Hall 1976), indicating that it does cross the placental barrier; but although traces of warfarin are secreted into the breast milk, no measurable anticoagulant effect occurs in infants breast-fed by mothers receiving the drug (Orme et al. 1977).

1.3 Metabolism

Warfarin is eliminated almost entirely by metabolism, with only small traces of unmetabolised warfarin appearing in urine (Banfield et al. 1983). Plasma clearance of warfarin is about 0.2 L/h/70kg (Andreasen & Vesell 1974) and hepatic extraction is small.

Warfarin is metabolised by the cytochrome P450 system in the endoplasmic reticulum of the liver parenchyma (Brodie 1964). After administration of racemic warfarin 4 metabolites are found: 7-hydroxywarfarin, 6-hydroxywarfarin, and 2 diastereoisomeric warfarin alcohols (Lewis & Trager 1971). Of these, 7-hydroxywarfarin is the first metabolite detected in human urine (O'Reilly et al. 1962).

The terminal half-life ($t_{1/2}$) of warfarin is about 35 hours. Steady-state is reached in about a week, and relatively little fluctuation in plasma concentration occurs during the daily dosing interval (Holford 1986).

The clearance of R(+) warfarin is approximately half that of S(−) warfarin when administered as the racemate; hence the half-life of the R(+) enantiomer is longer than that of the S(−) enantiomer, because the Vd of the enantiomers appears to be the same (Holford 1986). S(−) warfarin is predominantly oxidised to 7-hydroxywarfarin, with a smaller proportion oxidised to 6-hydroxywarfarin (Lewis et al. 1974) or reduced to (S,S) warfarin alcohol and (S,R) alcohol; R(+) warfarin is primarily reduced to (R,S) warfarin alcohol with traces of (R,R) alcohol. S(−) warfarin, and some R(+) warfarin, is oxidised to 6-hydroxywarfarin (Lewis et al. 1974).

All 4 configurations of warfarin alcohols lower vitamin K-dependent clotting factors in man. They do not appear to be metabolised but are excreted completely in urine. The rates of clearance of (S,S), (S,R) and (R,R) warfarin alcohols are rapid, ranging from 4.1 to 6.3% per hour. However, the (R,S) enantiomer is eliminated even more slowly than the parent compound, at about 2% per hour (Lewis et al. 1973). The potency of the alcohols is markedly lower than that of the parent compound, and at concentrations found during warfarin therapy their effect on anticoagulation is likely to be negligible.

2. *Pharmacokinetic Causes of Altered Response to Warfarin Therapy*

A 20-fold or even greater interindividual variation in the warfarin dose required to achieve an equivalent anticoagulant effect has been noted during long term therapy (Routledge et al. 1979b). Several factors that have been identified as determinants of response to a given dose of warfarin in an individual patient are considered in the following discussion.

2.1 Absorption

As warfarin is completely absorbed from the stomach and proximal small intestine, resistance to treatment due to impaired absorption is ex-

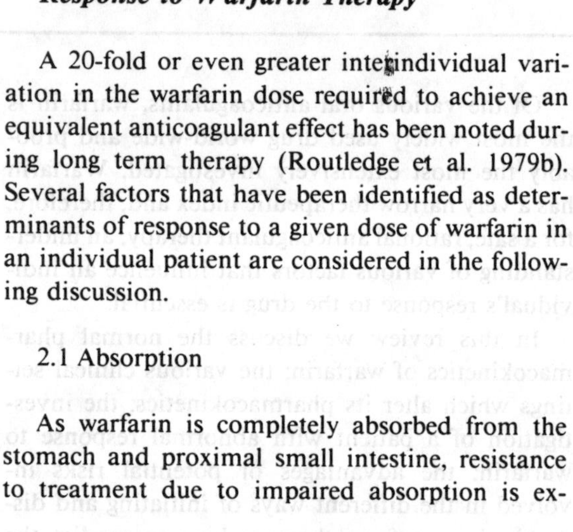

Fig. 1. Relationship between the free fraction of warfarin and total plasma warfarin clearance in a patient with idiopathic hypoalbuminaemia (■) and patients with normal albumin concentrations (○) [± SD]. (Data from Piroli et al. 1981.)

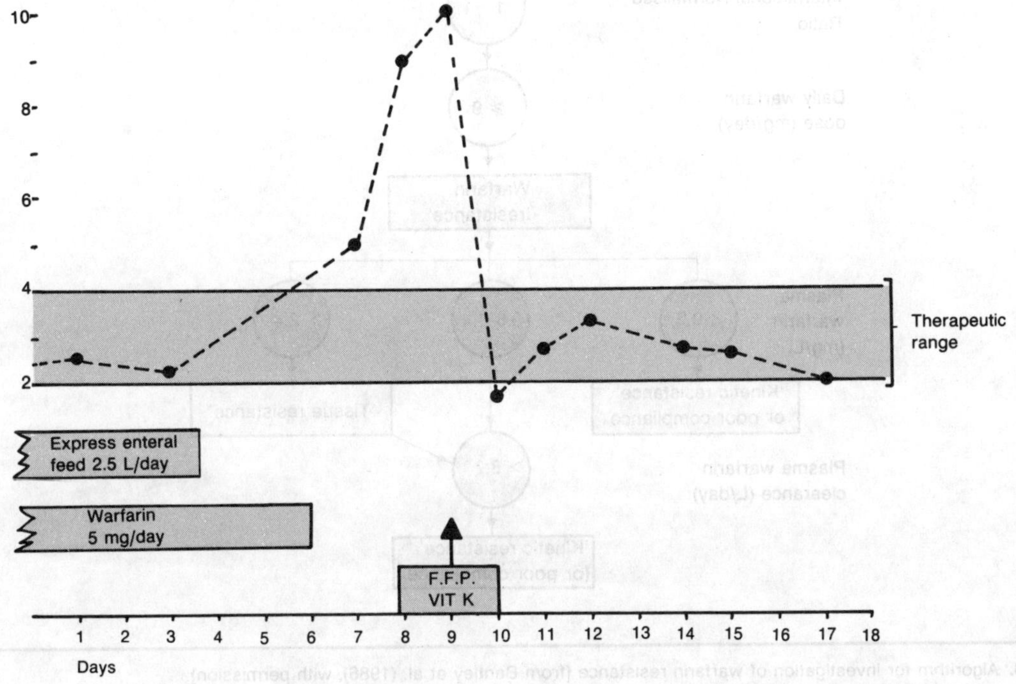

Fig. 2. The effect of discontinuation of enteral feeds on the International Normalised Ratio of an 81-year-old female receiving warfarin 5mg daily after venous thromboembolism. 'Express' enteral feed contains phytomenadione 225 μg/L.

tremely unusual. Even in a patient who was left with only 30cm of jejunum following ileal resection, less than 0.05 μg/ml of unchanged warfarin was recovered from the stool (Kearns & O'Reilly 1986). Selective malabsorption of warfarin has been reported in a patient with articular form of Danlos syndrome in the absence of clinical and biochemical evidence of malabsorption syndrome (Lefrere et al. 1986). Intravenous administration of warfarin resulted in therapeutic prolongation of prothrombin time within 24 hours, and the $t_{1/2}$ of warfarin was found to be 29 hours, suggesting normal metabolism. The dose of intravenous warfarin required to produce therapeutic effect was 37.5mg, however, indicating that there is also a relative pharmacodynamic resistance whose mechanism is unclear.

Cholestyramine binds to both the warfarin molecules and vitamin K in the gut and results in resistance to warfarin therapy, possibly by impairing absorption (Robinson et al. 1971). If the 2 drugs are to be given together, separation of doses by 3 to 6 hours may reduce the effects of interaction to some extent (see section 4.4).

2.2 Distribution

In view of the fact that warfarin is highly albumin bound it is important to consider its disposition in hypoalbuminaemic patients, the effect

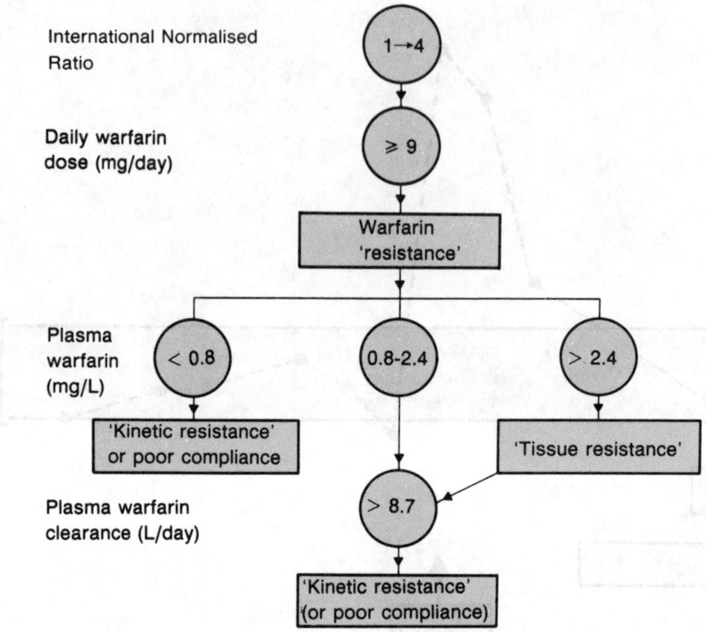

Fig. 3. Algorithm for investigation of warfarin resistance [from Bentley et al. (1986), with permission].

of drugs which compete for the binding sites and the effect of disease states which impair protein binding.

A study of warfarin disposition in a patient with idiopathic hypoalbuminaemia showed that in this condition there is an increase in the free fraction of warfarin in the plasma (fig. 1), with increased rate of clearance and decreased plasma half-life of the drug. The Vd of warfarin was found to be normal. The numbers of warfarin binding sites per albumin molecule and the affinity of the sites in the patient were of the same order as those in controls, indicating that the reduced warfarin protein binding in the patient was due to the hypoalbuminaemia rather than a qualitative abnormality of albumin (Piroli et al. 1981).

The distribution of warfarin in patients with chronic liver disease is unknown.

In patients with nephrotic syndrome and hypoalbuminaemia a 2-fold increase in the free fraction and a 3-fold increase in clearance of warfarin was found when compared with controls. There was no change in Vd (Ganeval et al. 1986) and no major change in anticoagulant response. Patients with chronic renal disease given a large single dose of warfarin had a significantly increased Vd, indicating decreased protein binding (Aggeler & O'Reilly 1966). There is evidence that the decreased protein binding of warfarin in uraemic serum may be partly due to the presence of endogenous binding inhibitors (Sjoholm et al. 1976). This phenomenon could cause a transient increase in sensitivity, since the free plasma warfarin concentration for a given dose of drug will initially be higher. However, free plasma warfarin would be similar to that in healthy individuals at steady-state, and therefore long term warfarin sensitivity should not occur.

Drugs which displace warfarin from its albumin

binding sites could theoretically increase sensitivity to the drug initially, but this effect would be transient and its true significance has probably been overestimated. Drug interactions with warfarin have been reviewed elsewhere (Serlin & Breckenridge 1983) and are not discussed in detail in this review.

2.3 Metabolism

As warfarin is almost entirely metabolised in the liver, impaired hepatic function might be expected to increase sensitivity to the drug. The synthesis of clotting factors is decreased in the presence of liver disease (Gallus et al. 1972) which also causes a predisposition to increased pharmacodynamic sensitivity.

Increased sensitivity to dicoumarol, without significant pharmacokinetic changes, has been observed in patients with macronodular cirrhosis (Brodie et al. 1959). However, no data are available about the metabolism of warfarin in patients with chronic liver disease.

Warfarin clearance and protein binding are unaltered in patients with acute viral hepatitis during or after the acute episode (Williams et al. 1976), but increased sensitivity to anticoagulant therapy, probably secondary to impaired protein synthesis, occurs in viral hepatitis as indicated by histological abnormalities of rough endoplasmic reticulum in the hepatocytes (Schaffner 1970).

Phytomenadione sometimes reverts prothrombin time to normal in some patients with liver disease, suggesting a decreased sensitivity to or avail-

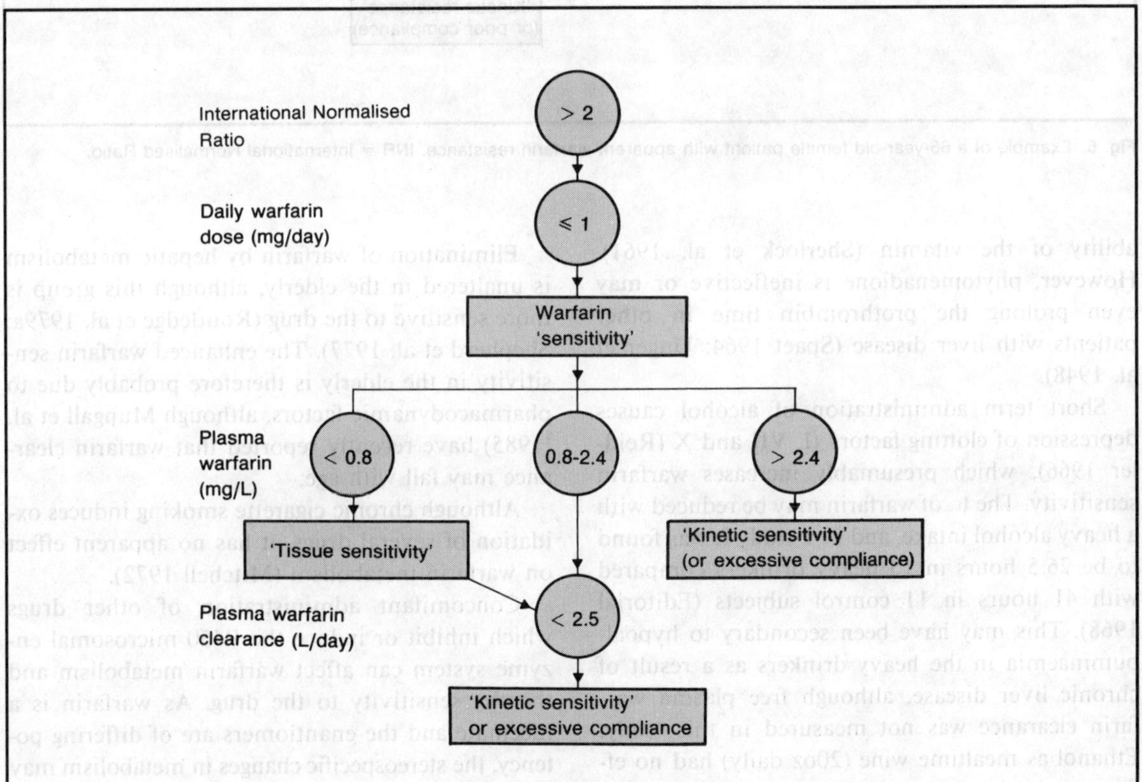

Fig. 4. Algorithm to investigate warfarin sensitivity [from Bentley et al. (1986), with permission].

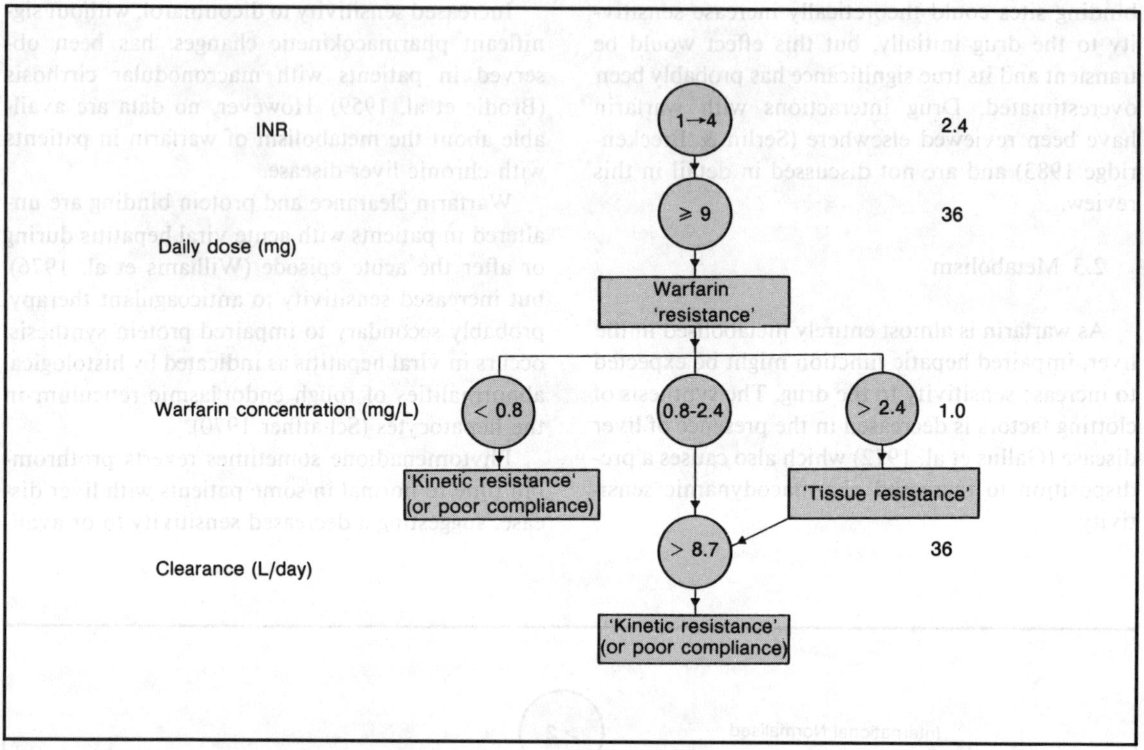

Fig. 5. Example of a 66-year-old female patient with apparent warfarin resistance. INR = International Normalised Ratio.

ability of the vitamin (Sherlock et al. 1961). However, phytomenadione is ineffective or may even prolong the prothrombin time in other patients with liver disease (Spaet 1964; Unger et al. 1948).

Short term administration of alcohol causes depression of clotting factors II, VII and X (Reidler 1966), which presumably increases warfarin sensitivity. The $t_{1/2}$ of warfarin may be reduced with a heavy alcohol intake, and in 1 study it was found to be 26.5 hours in 15 heavy drinkers compared with 41 hours in 11 control subjects (Editorial 1968). This may have been secondary to hypoalbuminaemia in the heavy drinkers as a result of chronic liver disease, although free plasma warfarin clearance was not measured in this study. Ethanol as mealtime wine (20oz daily) had no effect on the hypoprothrombinaemia of long term warfarin administration (O'Reilly 1981).

Elimination of warfarin by hepatic metabolism is unaltered in the elderly, although this group is more sensitive to the drug (Routledge et al. 1979a; Shepherd et al. 1977). The enhanced warfarin sensitivity in the elderly is therefore probably due to pharmacodynamic factors, although Mungall et al. (1985) have recently reported that warfarin clearance may fall with age.

Although chronic cigarette smoking induces oxidation of several drugs, it has no apparent effect on warfarin metabolism (Mitchell 1972).

Concomitant administration of other drugs which inhibit or induce the P450 microsomal enzyme system can affect warfarin metabolism and thereby sensitivity to the drug. As warfarin is a racemate and the enantiomers are of differing potency, the stereospecific changes in metabolism may cause differences in anticoagulant action not necessarily reflected in changes in pharmacokinetic parameters of the racemate. Examples of drugs causing stereoselective inhibition of warfarin metabolism are: cimetidine, which selectively inhibits the metabolism of the R(+) enantiomer (Choonara et al. 1986), and phenylbutazone (Lewis et al. 1974) and sulphonamides (O'Reilly 1980), both of which inhibit the metabolism of the S(−) enantiomer. The effects of concomitantly administered drugs on warfarin metabolism are reviewed elsewhere (Serlin & Breckenridge 1983).

2.4 Excretion

Since warfarin is almost totally cleared by hepatic metabolism, and since the renally excreted metabolites have only a very low anticoagulant effect, impaired renal function is unlikely to alter significantly its pharmacokinetics or effect. Although patients with chronic renal disease had a markedly increased Vd, the degree of depression of prothrombin complex activity after a single dose of warfarin did not appear to be significantly different (Aggeler & O'Reilly 1966). Similarly, age-related reduction in renal function has no effect on warfarin sensitivity (Davies & Shock 1950).

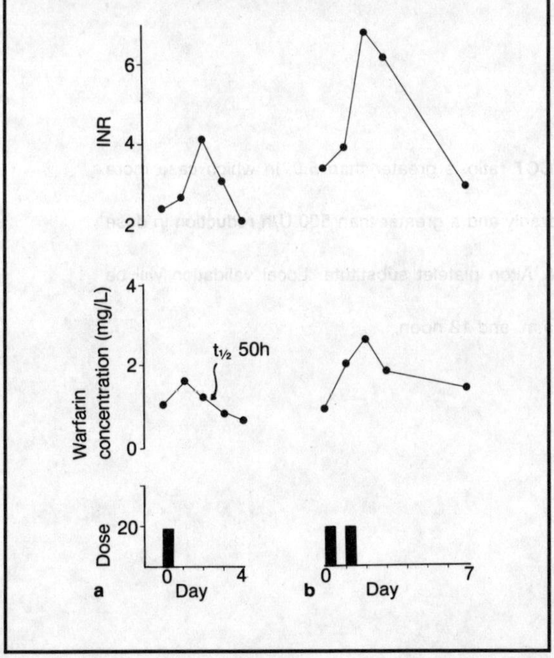

Fig. 6. Effect of warfarin administered intravenously **(a)** and in solution **(b)** on International Normalised Ratio in the patient described in fig. 5.

3. Pharmacodynamic Factors

3.1 Genetic Factors

A study of 14 identical and 14 fraternal twins indicated that the variance of half-lives was much greater in the latter than in the former group (Vesell & Page 1968), and the authors concluded that hereditary factors could account for almost all the variations observed in half-lives (La Du 1969). Since idential twins also share common environmental conditions, however, these studies do not rule out the importance of the latter factor.

Warfarin resistance inhcrited as an autosomal dominant trait has been described (O'Reilly et al. 1964). The pharmacokinetics of warfarin in such patients are normal, and the requirement for vitamin K is markedly increased (O'Reilly 1971a).

3.2 Vitamin K Excess or Deficiency

Dietary deficiency of vitamin K is a rare cause of warfarin sensitivity (Douglas 1962). Diseases of the small bowel which hinder the delivery of bile to the small intestine can cause deficiency of this fat-soluble vitamin and result in increased warfarin sensitivity. Broad spectrum oral antibiotics (e.g. neomycin) which may deplete the intestinal bacterial source of vitamin K have little effect on anticoagulant therapy in general, unless there is already an associated dietary deficiency of vitamin K. Certain cephalosporins [e.g. cefoperazone and latamoxef (moxalactam)] which have a methylthiotetrazole side chain, however, have a warfarin-like effect themselves and may augment the anticoagulant effects of warfarin (Uotila & Suttie 1983). α-Tocopherol in large doses antagonises the action of vitamin K (Corrigan 1982).

Warfarin resistance has been encountered with surreptitious intake of excessive vitamin K in the

ANTICOAGULANT SCHEME

General guidelines

Day 1 - Day 5 (inclusive)		Check baseline kaolin cephalin clotting time (KCCT) and INR before therapy. Heparin infusion. Give loading dose of 5000 units followed by heparin infusion of 1400 units/hour. Check KCCT after 4-6 hours of infusion and daily thereafter, adjusting infusion rate to keep KCCT 1.5-2.5 × control.
Day 3	(5 p.m.)	Induction dose of warfarin 10mg.
Day 4	(9-10 a.m.)	Send blood for KCCT and INR.
	(5 p.m.)	Warfarin as per day 4 INR (see table).
Day 5	(9-10 a.m.)	Send blood for KCCT and INR.
	(5 p.m.)	Warfarin as per day 5 INR (see table).
Day 6	(9-10 a.m.)	Send blood for day 6 INR. Suggested maintenance dose of warfarin will depend on this result.
	(5 p.m.)	Warfarin as per day 6 INR (this is projected maintenance dose).
Day 7 onwards		INR taken as usual and warfarin dose adjusted accordingly.

Heparin schedule

Loading dose – 5000U over 5 minutes.
Infusion – Start at 1400 U/hour (e.g. 8400U in 100ml over 6 hours).
Check KCCT after 6 hours.
Adjust dose according to the ratio of KCCT to control (KCCT ratio) as follows:

KCCT ratio	*Change in heparin infusion rate*
> 7	See note 2 below.
> 5.0	Reduce 500 U/h.
4.1-5.0	Reduce 300 U/h.
3.1-4.0	Reduce 100 U/h.
2.6-3.0	Reduce 50 U/h.
1.5-2.5	No change.
1.2-1.4	Increase 200 U/h.
< 1.2	Increase 400 U/h.

1. Wait 10 hours before next KCCT estimation, unless KCCT ratio is greater than 5.0, in which case more frequent estimation (e.g. 4-hourly) is advised.
2. If KCCT > 7, the infusion should be discontinued temporarily and a greater than 500 U/h reduction in dose made.
3. These guidelines were drawn up using 'Diagen' Bell & Alton platelet substitute. Local validation will be necessary.
4. If possible, measure KCCT in the mornings between 9 a.m. and 12 noon.

Fig. 7. A scheme to adjust heparin and warfarin therapy and to predict the dose of warfarin for anticoagulation [from Fennerty et al. (1984, 1986), with permission].

Warfarin schedule

Day	KCCT (9-10 a.m.)	Heparin dose	INR (BCR) (9-10 a.m.)	Warfarin dose given at 5 p.m.
1	1.5-2.5 × control	as per KCCT	–	nil
2	1.5-2.5 × control	as per KCCT	–	nil
3	1.5-2.5 × control	as per KCCT	< 1.4	10mg
4	1.5-2.5 × control	as per KCCT	< 1.8	10mg
			1.8	1mg
			> 1.8	0.5mg
5	1.5-2.5 × control	as per KCCT	< 2.0	10mg
			2-2.1	5mg
			2.2-2.3	4.5mg
			2.4-2.5	4mg
			2.6-2.7	3.5mg
			2.8-2.9	3mg
			3.0-3.1	2.5mg
			3.2-3.3	2mg
			3.4	1.5mg
			3.5	1mg
			3.6-4.0	0.5mg
			> 4.0	0mg
		STOP HEPARIN		
6				Predicted maintenance dose
			< 1.4	> 8mg
			1.4	8mg
			1.5	7.5mg
			1.6-1.7	7mg
			1.8	6.5mg
			1.9	6mg
			2-2.1	5.5mg
			2.2-2.3	5mg
			2.4-2.6	4.5mg
			2.7-3.0	4mg
			3.1-3.5	3.5mg
			3.6-4.0	3mg
			4.1-4.5	Miss out next day's dose then give 2mg
			> 4.5	Miss out 2 days' doses then give 1mg

Notes:

1. KCCT should be within or below therapeutic range (1.5-2.5 times control). If KCCT is above this range, the heparin effect on INR is neutralised with protamine (0.4 μg/ml plasma) added to the sample by the haematologist.
2. If heparin therapy is not being given, commence the schedule at Day 3.
3. Special care should be taken with patients with heart failure, liver disease or immediately post-operative since their sensitivity to warfarin may vary with time.
4. If INR on day 6 is less than 2.0, heparin can be recommended until the INR is within the desired range.
5. If the INR on day 3 is 1.4 or greater, the initial dose of warfarin should be reduced and the schedule is no longer relevant.

form of health food (O'Reilly & Rytand 1980) or a weight-reducing diet (Qureshi et al. 1981). Large quantities of phytomenadione administered with enteral feeds have also been associated with increased resistance to warfarin (Watson et al. 1984), and an example of this interaction is shown in figure 2.

3.3 Variations in the Levels of Vitamin K-Dependent Clotting Factors

The synthesis of vitamin K-dependent clotting factors is decreased in the presence of liver disease (Gallus et al. 1972), and administration of warfarin to such patients results in greater hypoprothrombinaemia than in healthy subjects.

Factor VII level may be slightly diminished in uraemia but there is no clear evidence of an associated increase in warfarin sensitivity (Cheney & Bonnim 1962).

The rates of decay of vitamin K-dependent factos have been noted to be increased up to 3-fold in hyperthyroid patients given a standard dose of coumarin anticoagulant compared with those in healthy controls, and they are decreased in hypothyroid patients (Loeliger et al. 1964). In hyperthyroid patients, the factor II activity is lower and partial thromboplastin time with kaolin (PTT-K) is shorter than in those in the euthyroid state. Warfarin produces a greater fall in factors II and VIII, and a greater increase in prothrombin ratio and PTT-K, in the hyperthyroid state than in the euthyroid state (Kellett et al. 1986).

Pregnancy is associated with elevation of factors VII (Loeliger & Koller 1952), VIII (Kasper et al. 1964), IX (Ratnoff & Holland 1959) and X (Pechet & Alexander 1961). There is often a 2-fold increase in factors VIII, IX and X and the level of circulating fibrinogen is also elevated (Plass & Matthew 1926). The levels of factors II and V are unaffected (Alexander et al. 1956). No data are available on warfarin requirements in pregnancy because of its contraindications in this condition (Hall 1976) but some degree of warfarin resistance might be expected.

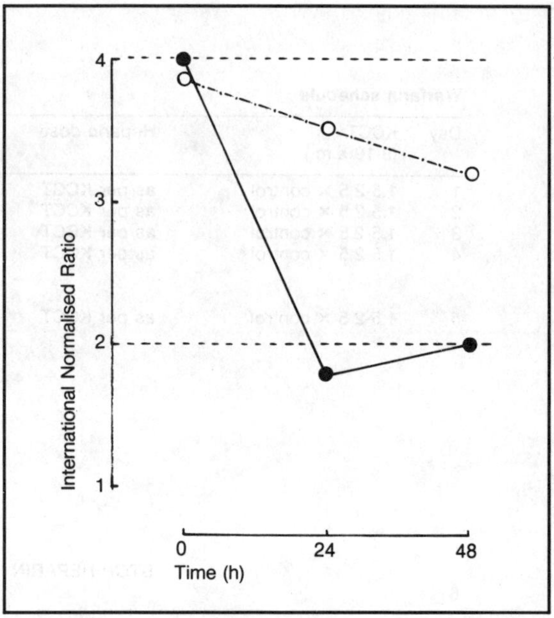

Fig. 8. Effect of discontinuing warfarin (○) or administration of phytomenadione (1mg IV) [●] on the International Normalised Ratio in patients receiving warfarin. Calculated from the data of Andersen and Godal (1975).

4. Clinical Pharmacokinetic Considerations

4.1 Investigation of Patients with Abnormal Response to Warfarin

Patients who require very large, very small or markedly varying doses of warfarin are not uncommonly encountered in clinical practice. An abnormal response to warfarin therapy may be secondary to poor compliance, kinetic resistance, tissue resistance, tissue sensitivity or kinetic sensitivity. The value of estimating plasma warfarin clearance and plasma warfarin concentrations in such patients has recently been highlighted (Bentley et al. 1986). By using algorithms (figs 3 and 4) which correlate plasma warfarin concentration and plasma warfarin clearance with the patient's International Normalised Ratio (INR), it is possible to correctly identify the cause of abnormal warfarin responsiveness and thereby modify correctable factors.

To cite an example (fig. 5), a 66-year-old female

patient who required warfarin 36 mg/day was found to have a plasma warfarin concentration of 1 mg/L and plasma warfarin clearance of 36 L/day, indicating either kinetic resistance or poor compliance. When she was given similar doses of intravenous warfarin and subsequently oral warfarin solution she rapidly became excessively anticoagulated, confirming that the cause of apparent warfarin resistance was indeed at least in part due to poor compliance (fig. 6).

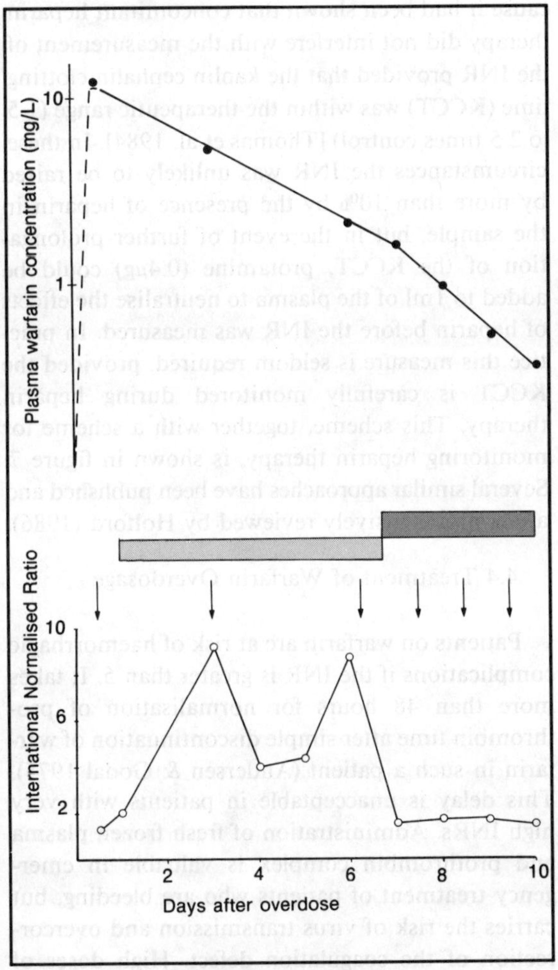

Fig. 9. Effect of cholestyramine on the elimination of warfarin in a patient after overdose. The elimination half-life fell from 53 to 33 hours. ▭ = Oral phytomenadione 10 mg/day; ▩ = oral cholestyramine 4g 4 times daily; ↓ = parenteral phytomenadione 10mg (first 2 doses intramuscular, remainder intravenous). From Renowden et al (1985), with permission.

4.2 Initiation and Cessation of Warfarin Therapy

It is a common clinical practice to initiate anticoagulation with heparin and overlap the first 2 to 3 days of warfarin therapy with heparin therapy. When a patient is started on warfarin, vitamin K-dependent factor VII level falls much faster than factors II, IX and X (O'Reilly & Aggeler 1968). Thus, while the prothrombin time, which is particularly sensitive to factor VII levels, may be in the therapeutic range early in therapy, there may still be high levels of factors II, IX and X, with the patient remaining at risk of further thromboembolism. It is suggested, therefore, that patients should continue heparin for 2 to 4 days despite a therapeutic INR, while factors II, IX and X fall (Coon & Willis 1972). As yet, however, there is no evidence that the delay in reduction of factors II, IX and X is clinically important, or whether a prolonged overlap of heparin and warfarin is necessary. Indeed, the only study to examine this showed that when warfarin was started almost immediately after heparin in patients with venous thromboembolism, there was no increased risk of recurrence compared with those patients in whom 7 days of heparin therapy preceded warfarin administration (Gallus et al. 1986).

Whether warfarin should be discontinued abruptly or tailed off gradually has been a matter for considerable debate. The concept of rebound hypercoagulable state on abrupt cessation of warfarin was derived from studies which found an increased incidence of rethrombosis in patients after warfarin was stopped abruptly compared with patients who had not been treated with anticoagulants or in whom warfarin had been tailed off (Carter et al. 1958; Lieberman & Lindner 1965). Other studies were unable to detect a difference in recurrence rates regardless of how the therapy was discontinued (Michaels & Beamish 1967; Sharland 1966; van Clere 1966). These studies included many patients with arterial thrombosis, and were poorly controlled. The diagnostic end points were unclear and the confidence limits unacceptably wide.

It has been demonstrated that factor VIII is elevated in patients on long term oral anticoagulants and that it remains elevated for 1 to 2 weeks after discontinuation of treatment (Poller & Thomson 1964). There is also a true rebound increase in factor VII on cessation of anticoagulation therapy (Poller & Thomson 1964). Theoretically, therefore, there is a risk of thrombosis once the vitamin K-dependent factors return to normal levels after cessation of anticoagulant therapy. This hypercoagulable state could be ameliorated by slowly tailing off the oral anticoagulant therapy over a period of 4 weeks (Poller & Thomson 1965). There has been only 1 randomised study looking at the effects of the rate of warfarin cessation on the recurrence of thrombosis in patients with venous thromboembolic disease. No significant difference was found in the recurrence rates of venous thrombosis in patients who stopped the treatment abruptly compared with those in whom the treatment was tailed off (O'Sullivan 1972). The number of patients in this study was too small to provide a definitive answer to the problem, and as yet there is no firm clinical evidence to indicate how rapidly warfarin therapy should be discontinued.

4.3 Prediction of Warfarin Dosage

The pharmacokinetic and pharmacodynamic variability in response to oral anticoagulants results in wide variability in dose, which of course gives the greatest problems on initiation of treatment. It seemed reasonable to assume, however, that this variability would lead to altered response so that, if patients were given a fixed induction dose, the most sensitive individuals initially would require the smallest maintenance dose of warfarin, and vice versa. This approach was validated using thrombotest reagent to measure prothrombin time (Routledge et al. 1977) but the major problem with this approach was that one-third of patients were excessively anticoagulated initially, and a further third were under-anticoagulated. Using a semi-empirical approach, we therefore designed a variable dose induction scheme which allowed tailoring of the initial loading doses depending on the INR in the first 3 days of warfarin treatment (Fennerty et al. 1984). This prevented the excessive anticoagulation seen with the fixed loading dose technique, but still allowed prediction of the warfarin dose using the INR on the fourth day of warfarin treatment. This scheme was only possible because it had been shown that concomitant heparin therapy did not interfere with the measurement of the INR provided that the kaolin cephalin clotting time (KCCT) was within the therapeutic range (1.5 to 2.5 times control) [Thomas et al. 1984]. In these circumstances the INR was unlikely to be raised by more than 10% by the presence of heparin in the sample, but in the event of further prolongation of the KCCT, protamine (0.4μg) could be added to 1ml of the plasma to neutralise the effects of heparin before the INR was measured. In practice this measure is seldom required, provided the KCCT is carefully monitored during heparin therapy. This scheme, together with a scheme for monitoring heparin therapy, is shown in figure 7. Several similar approaches have been published and are comprehensively reviewed by Holford (1986).

4.4 Treatment of Warfarin Overdosage

Patients on warfarin are at risk of haemorrhagic complications if the INR is greater than 5. It takes more than 48 hours for normalisation of prothrombin time after simple discontinuation of warfarin in such a patient (Andersen & Godal 1975). This delay is unacceptable in patients with very high INRs. Administration of fresh frozen plasma and prothrombin complex is valuable in emergency treatment of patients who are bleeding, but carries the risk of virus transmission and overcorrection of the coagulation defect. High doses of phytomenadione, although effective in reversing the coagulation defect within 24 hours, may result in refractoriness to anticoagulation for up to a week. Administration of very low doses (1mg) of phytomenadione overcomes this problem (Andersen

& Godal 1975) [fig. 8]. In major overdose, cholestyramine increases the clearance of warfarin (Jahnchen et al. 1978) and helps to reduce the period for which regular doses of intravenous phytomenadione are required (Renowden et al. 1985) [fig. 9]. This may be due to an interruption of enterohepatic recycling of the drug, since the high protein binding of the drug makes it unlikely that warfarin can be 'dialysed' from the splanchnic circulation back into the gut lumen to bind to cholestyramine.

5. Conclusion

Although warfarin was initially felt to be only useful as a rodenticide, its successful use as an anticoagulant in a president of the United States (Link 1959) encouraged its use in humans and it is now the most popular oral anticoagulant in clinical practice. Although its long half-life makes it useful for once-daily dosing, its narrow therapeutic ratio means that it must be prescribed only for those in whom the benefits outweigh the risks. A knowledge of warfarin's pharmacokinetics can help in its optimal use and in understanding the reasons for poor or excessive response.

References

Aggeler PM, O'Reilly RA. Pharmacological basis of oral anticoagulant therapy. Thrombosis et Diathesis Haemorrhagica 21 (Suppl.): 227-256, 1966

Alexander B, Meyers L, Kenny J, Goldstein R, Gurewich V, et al. Blood coagulation in pregnancy. Proconvertin and prothrombin and hypercoagulable state. New England Journal of Medicine 254: 358-363, 1956

Andersen P, Godal HC. Predictable reduction in anticoagulant activity of warfarin by small amounts of vitamin K. Acta Medica Scandinavica 198: 269-270, 1975

Andreasen P, Vesell E. Comparison of plasma levels of antipyrine, tolbutamide and warfarin after oral and intravenous administration. Clinical Pharmacology and Therapeutics 16: 1059-1065, 1974

Bachman K, Shapiro R. Protein binding of coumarin anticoagulants in disease states. Clinical Pharmacokinetics 2: 110-126, 1977

Banfield C, O'Reilly R, Chan E, Rowland M. Phenylbutazone-warfarin interaction in man: further stereochemical and metabolic considerations. British Journal of Clinical Pharmacology 16: 669-675, 1983

Bentley DP, Backhouse G, Hutchings A, Haddon RL, Spragg B, et al. Investigation of patients with abnormal response to warfarin. British Journal of Clinical Pharmacology 22: 37-41, 1986

Breckenridge AM, Orme M, Wesseling H, Lewis RJ, Gibbons R. Pharmacokinetics and pharmacodynamics of the enantiomers of warfarin in man. Clinical Pharmacology and Therapeutics 15: 424-430, 1974

Brodie BB. Of mice, microsomes and man. Pharmacologist 6: 12-26, 1964

Brodie BB, Burns JJ, Weiner M. Metabolism of drugs in subjects with Laennec's cirrhosis. Medicina Experimentalis 1: 290-292, 1959

Carter SA, McDevitt E, Gatje BW, Wright IS. Analysis of factors affecting the recurrence of thromboembolism off and on anticoagulant therapy. American Journal of Medicine 25: 43-51, 1958

Cheney K, Bonnin JW. Haemorrhage, platelet dysfunction and other coagulation defects in uraemia. British Journal of Haematology 8: 215-222, 1962

Choonara I, Cholerton S, Haynes B, Breckenridge A, Park BK. Stereoselective interaction between R enantiomer of warfarin and cimetidine. British Journal of Clinical Pharmacology 21: 271-277, 1986

Coon WW, Willis III PW. Thromboembolic complications during anticoagulant therapy. Archives of Surgery 105: 209-212, 1972

Corrigan Jr JJ. The effect of vitamin E on warfarin induced vitamin K deficiency. Annals of the New York Academy of Sciences 393: 361-368, 1982

Davies DF, Shock NW. Age changes in glomerular filtration rate, effective renal plasma flow and the tubular excretory capacity in adult males. Journal of Clinical Investigation 29: 496-507, 1950

Deykin D. Warfarin therapy. New England Journal of Medicine 283: 691-694, 801-803, 1970

Douglas AS. Anticoagulant therapy, p.394, FA Davies, Philadelphia, 1962

Editorial. Heavy drinking accelerates drugs' breakdown in liver. Journal of the American Medical Association 206: 1709, 1968

Fennerty A, Dolben J, Thomas P, et al. Flexible induction dose regimen for warfarin and prediction of maintenance dose. British Medical Journal 288: 1268-1270, 1984

Fennerty AG, Renowden S, Scolding N, Bentley DP, Campbell IA, et al. Guidelines to control heparin treatment. British Medical Journal 292: 579-580, 1986

Gallus A, Jackaman J, Tillett J, Mills W, Wytherley A. Safety and efficacy of warfarin started early after submassive venous thrombosis or pulmonary embolism. Lancet 2: 1293-1296, 1986

Gallus AS, Lucas CR, Hirsch V. Coagulation studies in patients with acute infectious hepatitis. British Journal of Haematology 22: 761-771, 1972

Ganeval D, Fischer AM, Barre J, Pertuiset N, Dautzenberg MD, Pharmacokinetics of warfarin in the nephrotic syndrome and effect on vitamin K-dependent clotting factors. Clinical Nephrology 25(2): 75-80, 1986

Hall JG. Warfarin and foetal abnormality. Lancet 1: 1127, 1976

Hignite C, Uetrecht J, Tschariz C, Azarnoff D. Kinetics of R and S warfarin enantiomers. Clinical Pharmacology and Therapeutics 28: 99-105, 1980

Holford NHG. Clinical pharmacokinetics and pharmacodynamics of warfarin: understanding the dose-effect relationship. Clinical Pharmacokinetics 11: 483-504, 1986

Jahnchen E, Meinertz HJ, Gifrich F, Kersting F, Groth U. Enhanced elimination of warfarin during treatment with cholestyramine. British Journal of Clinical Pharmacology 5: 437-440, 1978

Kasper CK, Hoag MS, Aggeler PM, Stone S. Blood clotting factors in pregnancy: factor VIII concentrations in normal and AHF-deficient women. Obstetrics and Gynecology 24: 242-247, 1964

Kearns Jr PR, O'Reilly RA. Bioavailability of warfarin in a patient with severe short bowel syndrome. Journal of Parenteral and Enteral Nutrition 10 (1): 100-101, 1986

Kellett HA, Sawers JSA, Boulton FE, Cholerton S, Park BK, et al. Problems of anticoagulation with warfarin in hyperthyroidism. Quarterly Journal of Medicine. New Series 58 (225): 43-51, 1986

La Du Jr BN. Pharmacogenetics. Medical Clinics of North America 53: 839-855, 1969

Lefrere J, Guyon F, Horellou M, Conard J, Samama M. Selective malabsorption of anticoagulants. Journal of the American Medical Association 256(5): 595, 1986

Lewis RJ, Trager WF. The metabolic fate of warfarin: studies on the metabolites in plasma. Annals of the New York Academy of Sciences 179: 205-212, 1971

Lewis RJ, Trager WF, Chan KK, Breckenridge A, Orme M, et al. Warfarin – stereochemical aspects of its metabolism and the interaction with phenylbutazone. Journal of Clinical Investigation 53: 1607-1617, 1974

Lewis RJ, Trager WF, Robinson AJ, Chan KK. Warfarin metabolites: the anticoagulant activity and pharmacology of warfarin alcohols. Journal of Laboratory and Clinical Medicine 81: 925-931, 1973

Lieberman LS, Lindner M. Effective termination of anticoagulation in coronary artery disease. Circulation 32 (Suppl. 2): II-138, 1965

Link KP. The discovery of dicoumarol and its sequels. Circulation 19: 97-107, 1959

Loeliger EA, Koller F. Behaviour of factor VII and prothrombin in late pregnancy and in the newborn. Acta Haematologica 7: 157-161, 1952

Loeliger EA, van der Esch B, Mattern MJ, Hemkev HC. Biological disappearance rate of prothrombin, factors VII, IX and X from plasma in hypothyroidism, hyperthyroidism and during fever. Thrombosis et Diathesis Haemorrhagica 10: 267-277, 1964

Melander A. Influence of food on the bioavailability of drugs. Clinical Pharmacokinetics 3: 337-351, 1978

Michaels L, Beamish RE. Relapses of thromboembolic disease after discontinued anticoagulant therapy. A comparison of the incidence after abrupt and after gradual termination of treatment. American Journal of Cardiology 20: 670-673, 1967

Mitchell AA. Smoking and warfarin dosage. New England Journal of Medicine 287: 1153-1154, 1972

Mungall DR, Ludden TM, Marshall J, Hawkins DW, Talbert RL, et al. Population pharmacokinetics of racemic warfarin in adult patients. Journal of Pharmacokinetics and Biopharmaceutics 13 (3): 213-227, 1985

O'Reilly RA. Vitamin K in hereditary resistance to oral anticoagulant drugs. American Journal of Physiology 221: 1327-1330, 1971a

O'Reilly RA. Interaction of several coumarin compounds with human and canine plasma albumin. Molecular Pharmacology 7: 209-218, 1971b

O'Reilly RA. The binding of sodium warfarin to plasma albumin and its displacement by phenylbutazone. Annals of the New York Academy of Sciences 226: 293-308, 1973

O'Reilly RA. Stereoselective interaction of trimethoprim sulfamethoxazole and the separated enantiomorphs of racemic warfarin in man. New England Journal of Medicine 302: 33-35, 1980

O'Reilly RA. Lack of effect of fortified wine ingested during fasting and anticoagulant therapy. Archives of Internal Medicine 141: 458, 1981

O'Reilly RA, Aggeler PM. Studies on couramin anticoagulant drugs: initiation of warfarin therapy without a loading dose. Circulation 38: 169-177, 1968

O'Reilly RA, Aggeler PM, Hoag MS, Leong L. Studies on the coumarin anticoagulant drugs: assay of warfarin and its biological application. Thrombosis et Diathesis Haemorrhagica 8: 89-95, 1962

O'Reilly RA, Aggeler PM, Hoag MS, Leong LS, Kropatkin ML. Hereditary transmission of exceptional resistance to coumarin anticoagulant drugs: the first reported kindred. New England Journal of Medicine 271: 809-815, 1964

O'Reilly RA, Aggeler PM, Leong LS. Studies on the coumarin anticoagulant drugs: the pharmacodynamics of warfarin in man. Journal of Clinical Investigation 42: 1542-1551, 1963

O'Reilly RA, Rytand DA. 'Resistance' to warfarin due to unrecognised vitamin K supplementation. New England Journal of Medicine 303(3): 160-161, 1980

Orme ML, Lewis PJ, de Swiet M, Serlin MJ, Sibeon R, et al. May mothers given warfarin breast-feed their infants? British Medical Journal 1: 1564-1565, 1977

O'Sullivan EF. Duration of anticoagulant therapy in venous thromboembolism. Medical Journal of Australia 2: 1104-1107, 1972

Pechet L, Alexander B. Increased clotting factors in pregnancy. New England Journal of Medicine 265: 1093-1097, 1961

Piroli RJ, Passananti GT, Shively CA, Vesell ES. Antipyrine and warfarin disposition in a patient with idiopathic hypoalbuminaemia. Clinical Pharmacology and Therapeutics 30(6): 810-816, 1981

Plass ED, Matthew CW. Plasma protein fractions in normal pregnancy, labour, and puerperium. American Journal of Obstetrics and Gynecology 12: 346-358, 1926

Poller L, Thomson J. Evidence for 'rebound' hypercoagulability after stopping anticoagulants. Lancet 2: 62-64, 1964

Poller L, Thomson JM. Reduction of 'rebound' hypercoagulability by gradual withdrawal ('tailing off') of oral anticoagulants. British Medical Journal: 1475-1476, 1965

Qureshi GD, Reinders TP, Swint JJ, et al. Acquired warfarin resistance and weight-reducing diet. Archives of Internal Medicine 141: 507-509, 1981

Ratnoff OD, Holland TR. Coagulation components in normal and abnormal pregnancies. Annals of the New York Academy of Sciences 75: 626-633, 1959

Reidler G. Einfluss des Alkohols auf die antikoagulantien Therapie. Thrombosis et Diathesis Haemorrhagica 16: 613, 1966

Renowden S, Westmoreland D, White JP, Routledge PA. Oral cholestyramine increases elimination of warfarin after overdose. British Medical Journal 291: 513-515, 1985

Robinson DS, Benjamin DM, McCormack JJ. Interaction of warfarin and non systemic gastrointestinal drugs. Clinical-Pharmacology and Therapeutics 12: 492-495, 1971

Routledge PA, Bell SM, Davies DM, Cavanagh JS, Rawlins MD. Predicting patients' warfarin requirements. Lancet 2: 854-855, 1977

Routledge PA, Chapman DH, Davies DM, Rawlins MD. Pharmacokinetics and pharmacodynamics of warfarin at steady state. British Journal of Clinical Pharmacology 8: 243-247, 1979a

Routledge PA, Chapman PH, Davies DM, Rawlins MD. Factors affecting warfarin requirements – a prospective population study. European Journal of Clinical Pharmacology 15: 319-322, 1979b

Schaffner F. The structural basis of altered hepatic function in viral hepatitis. American Journal of Medicine 49: 658-668, 1970

Sellers E, Koch-Weser J. Interaction of warfarin stereoisomers with human albumin. Pharmacology Research Communications 7: 331-336, 1975

Serlin MJ, Breckenridge AM. Drug interactions with warfarin. Drugs 25: 610-620, 1983

Sharland DE. Effect of cessation of anticoagulant therapy on the course of ischaemic heart disease. British Medical Journal 2: 292, 1966

Shepherd AMM, Hewick DS, Moreland TA, Stevenson IH. Age as a determinant of sensitivity to warfarin. British Journal of Clinical Pharmacology 4: 315-320, 1977

Sherlock S, Barber KM, Bell JL, Watt PJ. Anticoagulants and the

liver. In Pickering GW (Ed.) Symposium on anticoagulant therapy, p. 14-36, Harvey and Blythe Ltd., London, 1961
Sjoholm I, Kober A, Odar-Cederlof I, Borga O. Protein binding of drugs in uraemic and normal serum: the role of endogenous binding inhibitors. Biochemical Pharmacology 25: 1205-1213, 1976
Slattery JT, Levy G, Jain A, McMahon FG. Effect of naproxen on the kinetics of elimination and anticoagulant activity of a single dose of warfarin. Clinical Pharmacology and Therapeutics 25: 51-60, 1979
Spaet TH. Clinical implications of acquired blood coagulation abnormalities. Blood 23: 839-842, 1964
Stirling Y, Howarth DJ, Stockley R, Bland R, Towler CM, et al. Comparison of the bioavailability and anticoagulant activities of two warfarin formulations. British Journal of Haematology 51: 37-45, 1982
Thomas P, Fennerty A, Backhouse G, Bentley DP, Campbell IA, et al. Monitoring oral anticoagulants during heparin therapy. British Medical Journal 288: 191, 1984
Toon S, Hopkins KJ, Garstang FM, Digret B, Rowland M. The warfarin-cimetidine interaction: stereochemical considerations. British Journal of Clinical Pharmacology 21: 245-246, 1986
Unger PM, Weiner M, Shapiro S. Vitamin K tolerance test. American Journal of Clinical Pathology 18: 835-851, 1948
Uotila L, Suttie JW. Inhibition of vitamin K-dependent carboxylase *in vitro* by cefamandole and its structured analogues. Journal of Infectious Diseases 148: 571, 1983
Van Clere RB. Letting go of the bear's tail. Experience with discontinuation of long-term anticoagulation therapy. Journal of the American Medical Association 196(13): 140-142, 1966
Vesell ES, Page JG. Genetic control of dicoumarol levels in man. Journal of Clinical Investigation 47: 2657-2663, 1968
Wagner J. Dosage regimen calculations. In Fundamentals of Clinical Pharmacokinetics, p. 129-172, Drug Intelligence, Hamilton, Ill, 1975
Watson AJM, Pegg M, Green JRB. Enteral feeds may antagonise warfarin. British Medical Journal 288: 557, 1984
Williams R, Schary W, Blaschke T, Meffin P, Melmon K, et al. Influence of viral hepatitis on disposition and pharmacological effect of warfarin. Clinical Pharmacology and Therapeutics 20: 90-97, 1976

Authors' address: Dr *P.A. Routledge*, Department of Pharmacology and Therapeutics, University College of Medicine, Heath Park, Cardiff CF4 4XN (Wales).

Original Research Article

Clinical Pharmacokinetics 16: 254-260 (1989)
0312-5963/89/0004-0254/$03.50/0

Phenytoin Dosage Predictions in Paediatric Patients

Geoffrey J. Yuen, Patricia T. Latimer, Louis C. Littlefield and *Ray W. Mackey*

School of Pharmacy, University of Maryland, Baltimore, Maryland, College of Pharmacy, Oregon State University, Corvallis, Oregon, College of Pharmacy, University of Texas, Austin, Texas, and Department of Pediatrics, University of Texas Health Science Center, San Antonio, Texas, USA

Summary

Phenytoin dosing in paediatric patients is complicated both by alterations in patient requirements due to growth and maturation changes and by the capacity-limited characteristics of phenytoin metabolism. This study examines 2 pharmacokinetic methods to adjust phenytoin dosage based on a single dosing-rate/steady-state serum phenytoin concentration pair. A Bayesian forecaster and a fixed parameter [rate of metabolism (V_{max})] method were examined with previously published sets of a priori *parameter estimates. The fixed V_{max} method was utilised with the parameter derived from native Japanese (method 1), US Caucasian (method 2) and European (method 3) patients. The Bayesian forecaster used* a priori *parameter estimates obtained from native Japanese (method 4) and European (method 5) patients. Each method was examined retrospectively in 34 paediatric patients with a total of 48 predictions possible. Measures of absolute predictability, bias (mean error, % dose) and precision (root mean squared error, % dose), were −3.58/12.2, −1.51/12.2, 4.06/9.96, −4.38/13.2, and −3.10/11.5, for methods 1, 2, 3, 4 and 5, respectively. There was no significant difference among the 5 methods. However, the Bayesian algorithm tended to be more robust over a broad range of situations, providing predictions in all cases. The fixed V_{max} methods could not provide predictions in every case. Finally, all methods had a significant number of overpredictions of dosage. Poorer results were observed when prediction of steady-state serum concentrations were performed, partly due to the retrospective nature of the study. We conclude that close monitoring of patients, regardless of the method chosen to adjust dosage, is recommended.*

Phenytoin is an anticonvulsant agent introduced in 1938 by Merritt and Putman. Despite the long clinical experience, many problems still arise in attempting to determine the appropriate dose for a particular patient. Phenytoin has a narrow therapeutic range of 10 to 20 mg/L, to which the majority of patients respond without undue side effects (Lund 1974). Phenytoin also exhibits capacity-limited metabolism which is consistent with Michaelis-Menten saturable enzyme kinetics (Arnold & Gerber 1969; Gerber & Wagner 1972; Lund et al. 1974; Perucca et al. 1978). Clinically, this is important, since small dosage changes may produce large, non-proportional changes in steady-state serum concentrations. To aid clinicians in making dosage adjustments, a number of methods have been proposed using one or more serum phenytoin concentrations (Ludden et al. 1977; Martin et al. 1977; Mullen 1978; Rambeck et al. 1979; Richens & Dunlop 1975; Vozeh et al. 1981). While these methods have proven useful in adult populations, their use in paediatric patients has not been investigated extensively.

Paediatric patients treated for chronic diseases present some unique problems. Frequent dosage adjustments must take place over time due to changes in physiology, body size and, presumably, metabolism. Most dosing methods for phenytoin require 2 or more dose/steady-state concentration pairs. Dodson (1982) has shown relatively good predictability with a correlation coefficient of 0.83 (predicted versus observed serum concentrations) employing techniques utilising the multiple-dose and steady-state concentration pairs. Despite this success, these multiple data point methods may be less applicable in paediatric patients, in whom growth and maturation may occur rapidly over a short period of time. Methods which can use 1 dose/steady-state concentration pair provide a more rapid prediction and will thus help to remove the problem of body changes during the predictive period.

The purpose of this study is to examine the applicability of 2 methods utilising a single dose/steady-state concentration pair to predict subsequent phenytoin dosages in paediatric seizure patients.

Methods

Drug monitoring profiles of 52 patients were compiled prospectively as part of routine clinical pharmacy consultations from patients at the Pediatric Seizure Disorder Clinic at the Brady Green Community Health Center in San Antonio, Texas. These profiles were then retrospectively reviewed to determine if the data were suitable for inclusion in the present study. Patients were included in the study if they were from 0.5 to 16 years old inclusive, had stable steady-state serum phenytoin concentrations at least 4 weeks after a dosage change with a difference of less than 20% on 2 different occasions, and demonstrated no more than 1kg change in bodyweight during the predictive period. Patients could not be receiving any concurrent medication which is known to displace phenytoin from protein binding sites; however, those with concurrent medications which have enzyme induction or inhibition properties were allowed into the study if the dosages of these medications remained constant during the predictive period. A total of 34 patients fitted the above criteria. During the study 27 patients received other medications, primarily other anticonvulsants.

Table I. Values for maximal metabolic rate (V_{max}) [mg/kg/day]

	Age (y)			
	0.5-3	4-6	7-9	10-13
Ethnic group				
Japanese	13.80	11.20	9.50	8.00
US Caucasian	13.95	10.93	10.00	8.25

Serum phenytoin concentration at steady-state can be described by the following adaptation of the Michaelis-Menten equation:

$$D = V_{max} \times C_{p,ss}/(K_m + C_{p,ss}) \qquad \text{(Eq. 1)}$$

where D is the daily dose of phenytoin acid; V_{max} is the maximal metabolic rate; K_m is the serum concentration at half the maximal metabolic rate; and $C_{p,ss}$ is the steady-state serum concentration. The following methods used the most recent phenytoin dose/steady-state concentration pair to predict the subsequent dose for a given steady-state serum concentration using equation 1.

Methods 1, 2 and 3

The first 3 methods utilise the method proposed by Chiba and co-workers (1980) and described by equation 2.

$$D\ (p) = \frac{V_{max} \times C_{p,ss}\ (d)}{C_{p,ss}\ (o) \times (V_{max}/D(o)-1) + C_{p,ss}\ (d)} \qquad \text{(Eq. 2)}$$

where (p) = predicted, (o) = observed and (d) = desired.

This method assumes that V_{max} is constant and K_m varies within the population. V_{max} is set to an age-adjusted population mean value (see table I). The V_{max} values used were derived from Japanese

Table II. Bayesian parameter values

Parameter	European	Japanese
K_m > 15y, mg/L	5.7	3.8
< 15y, mg/L	3.2	2.2
V_{max}, %CV	20.0	11.0
K_m, %CV	50.0	56.0
Dose, %CV	8.60	12.0
V_{max}, mg/day	415 $(Wt/70kg)^{0.6}$	

Abbreviations: K_m = serum drug concentration at half the maximal metabolic rate; V_{max} = maximal metabolic rate; CV = coefficient of variation.

paediatric patients (method 1; Chiba et al. 1980), US Caucasian patients (method 2; Bauer & Blouin 1983) and European patients (method 3; Grasela et al. 1983). Preliminary studies suggested that the V_{max} values derived from European patients in the last study may be similar to the current study population (see table II).

Methods 4 and 5

Methods 4 and 5 utilise the general Bayesian method proposed for drug dosage by Sheiner and Beal (1982). This method minimises the following function in the case of phenytoin:

$$(V_{max} - \hat{V}_{max})^2/Var_{V_{max}} + (K_m - \hat{K}_m)^2/Var_{K_m} \sum_{i=1}^{n} (D_i - \hat{D}_i)^2/Var_D \quad \text{(Eq. 3)}$$

$\hat{V}_{max}$ and $\hat{K}_m$ are the population mean values. V_{max} and Km are the individual parameter estimates to which the expression is to be minimised. $\hat{D}_i$ is the predicted dose for the *i*th observed $C_{p,ss}$/dosage pair; D_i is the actual dosage associated with the *i*th pair; n is the total number of $C_{p,ss}$/dosage pairs. $Var_{V_{max}}$ and Var_{K_m} are the interindividual standard deviations for V_{max} and K_m, respectively; Var_D is the combined residual error which includes intraindividual variability (i.e. day-to-day variability in absorption, metabolism, model misspecification error, etc.).

The function assumes that parameters are normally distributed and uncorrelated as to pairs, and that intersubject deviations and intrasubject residual errors are uncorrelated. Table 2 lists the population mean values used in methods and 4 and 5. Method 4 utilised Japanese-derived parameters, while for method 5 the parameters used were derived from patients in Germany and Britain (Grasela et al. 1983).

The Bayesian estimation procedure was implemented on an IBM-compatible computer using the ADAPT software package (D'Argenio & Schmitzky 1979). This particular implementation was specifically designed for the present study (doses and serum concentration at steady-state).

Absolute predictability for each method was assessed using measures of bias [mean error (ME)] and precision [root mean squared error (RMSE)] expressed as the percentage of the actual dose received (Sheiner & Beal 1981). The percentage of 'poor' predictions, i.e. those that yielded errors greater than 10% of acutal doses and cases where no prediction was possible, was tabulated for each method.

The Friedman test, a non-parametric test for analysis of variance which minimises the assumptions regarding the statistical distribution of the prediction errors, was used to compare the absolute predictability of the different dosing methods. χ-Square analysis was performed on the tabulated data of poor predictions (Steel & Torrie 1980). Finally, steady-state serum concentration predictions, based on the estimated parameter values from each method, were made for each subsequent dose administered.

Table III. Absolute predictability of all cases. Figures in parentheses indicate the 95% confidence intervals.

Method	No. of patients	Bias (ME, % dose)	Precision (RMSE, % dose)
1	45	−3.58 (−8.78, 1.61)	11.2 (9.06, 13.0)
2	47	−1.51 (−8.07, 5.05)	12.2 (9.40, 14.4)
3	43	4.53 (1.58, 7.48)	10.5 (8.31, 12.4)
4	46	−4.38 (−11.2, 2.52)	13.2 (8.75, 16.4)
5	48	−3.10 (−8.38, 2.17)	11.5 (8.58, 13.8)

Abbreviations: ME = mean error; RMSE = root mean squared error.

Table IV. Absolute predictability of matched cases (n = 43). Friedman χ^2 = 3.44, p = 0.48

Method	Bias (ME, % dose)	Precision (RMSE, % dose)
1	−3.16 (−8.60, 2.34)	11.2 (8.76, 13.1)
2	−1.45 (−7.14, 4.23)	11.0 (7.02, 13.8)
3	4.53 (1.58, 7.48)	10.5 (8.31, 12.4)
4	−5.34 (−9.62, −1.06)	10.8 (2.82, 15.0)
5	−4.22 (−9.20, 0.74)	11.0 (7.16, 13.8)

Abbreviations: ME = mean error; RMSE = root mean squared error.

Results

The measures of absolute predictability for all predicted doses are shown in table III. Method 2 was the least biased, with an ME of −1.51% of the dose. Method 3 was the most precise, with an RMSE of 10.5% of the dose, but only 43 out of 48 predictions could be performed. Method 5 was the next most precise with an RMSE of 11.5% of the dose. Only the Bayesian algorithm (methods 4 and 5) could provide predictions in all cases.

Predictions common to all methods were compared (table IV). A total of 43 predictions were possible. Again, method 2 was the least biased, with an ME of −1.45% of the dose. All the methods tended to have the same precision, with an RMSE of around 11%. In the matched predictions there were no statistically significant differences between the methods (Friedman χ^2 = 3.44; p = 0.48).

Table V compares the number of 'poor' predictions for each method. These included both dosing error greater than 10% and cases where no prediction was possible. The number of 'poor' predictions ranged from 33.3 to 45.8%. In general, most of the 'poor' predictions were underpredictions, but each method had a number of overpredictions ranging from 8.3% (method 4) to 20.8% (method 3) of the total. In a comparison of the methods on the basis of 'good' *vs* 'poor' predictions, method 5 had significantly fewer 'poor' predictions than method 3 (p = 0.02) or method 2 (p = 0.04). All other comparisons showed no significant differences.

The prediction error versus observed steady-state concentration for each method is shown in figure 1. The number of possible steady-state serum concentration predictions was less than the number of predicted doses. In some cases the administered dose was greater than the estimated V_{max} values, and therefore no predictions were possible. The numbers of possible predictions were 36, 43, 37, 36 and 41, of a total possible of 43, for methods 1 to 5, respectively.

Discussion

The maturation process is a significant confounding factor in predicting drug dosages using pharmacokinetic data, particularly for drugs which take a long time to reach steady-state. Several studies have noted age- or weight-related changes in phenytoin pharmacokinetics in paediatric patients. Bach and co-workers (1981) have demonstrated that free phenytoin clearance is correlated to both age and a corresponding decrease in liver volume in the elderly. This change in the ratio of liver size to body size and drug metabolism can occur during periods of growth seen in childhood, thereby altering dosage requirements. Phenytoin is unique, since it has a relatively narrow therapeutic index

Table V. 'Poor' predictions

Method	Error > +10%	Error > −10%	No prediction	%[a]
1	4	15	3	45.8
2	7	13	1	43.8
3	10	2	5	35.4
4	4	16	2	45.8
5	5	11	0	33.3

a Percentage of total possible predictions.

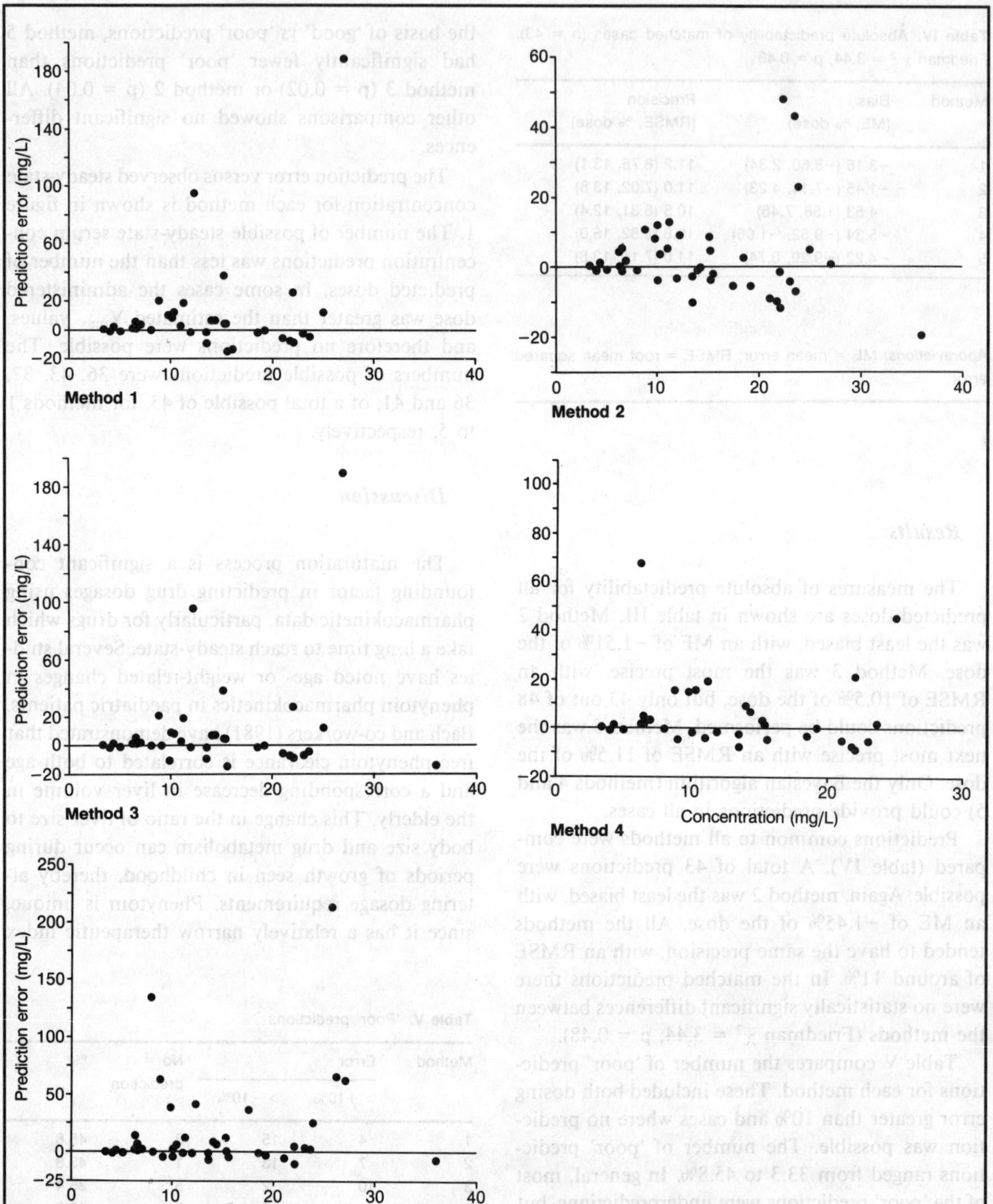

Fig. 1. Prediction error *versus* observed steady-state phenytoin concentration for each method.

and the time to reach steady-state is dependent both on the individual and the dose. Computer simulations have shown that the time to reach steady-state may be as long as 50 days or more in some cases (Tozer & Winter 1980). During the time required to obtain at least 2 steady-state serum concentrations on different doses, significant age- and/or weight-related changes in the rate of metabolism of phenytoin may occur. This is likely to confound the predictability of previous serum concentrations.

The present study examined 2 general methods using a single dosing rate/steady-state concentration pair to predict future phenytoin dosage methods in paediatric patients. Different sets of ethnic groups and age/weight-adjusted *a priori* parameter estimates were employed in each method. The results of the tests of absolute predictability were similar to the predictability of methods reported in a retrospective study performed in adults (Yuen et al. 1983). The Bayesian algorithm, regardless of population parameters, tended to be more robust than the fixed V_{max} methods. In all cases the Bayesian algorithm could provide reasonable predicted doses, but there were certain cases where the fixed V_{max} method could not provide a prediction since the actual administered dose was greater than the population V_{max} value.

Although the general Bayesian-dosing method can allow for utilisation of more than 1 dose/steady-state concentration pair, no such predictions were performed. This is in part due to the small number of predictions which would be possible for our population, given the constraints we defined to screen the patient charts. Previous studies in adults suggest that more data would slightly improve the predictions of subsequent doses (Yuen et al. 1983); however, the maturation process in paediatric patients may preclude the collection of large amounts of data during a constant 'physiological state'.

Despite the relatively 'good' predictability of the techniques examined, it is still somewhat disconcerting that there is a sizable number of predictions with an error of more than 10%. While this is trivial for most other drugs, such an error can become significant in the case of phenytoin because of the Michaelis-Menten characteristics of the drug (Mawer et al. 1974). The majority of 'poor' predictions for all methods were underpredictions, thus minimising the risk of potentially toxic dosages; a small number of patients would have received overdosages. The lack of predictability in these cases may be a problem inherent in using retrospective, more poorly controlled, data. Dodson (1982) has demonstrated excellent predictability using a multiple data point method with a correlation coefficient of 0.896 in a prospective manner. It is likely that in a more controlled setting an improvement in predictability may be seen.

The results of analysis of predictions of steady-state concentrations for a given dose were discouraging. In some cases large overpredictions of attained steady-state concentrations were observed. In other cases predictions could not be performed, since the administered dose was above the predicted V_{max} value, and hence steady-state would theoretically never be reached. However, one should not conclude that the methods are invalid; rather, this is an inherent problem of a retrospective study where there is no control over the dose that is actually administered.

This study examined only dosages predicted from steady-state information. Two studies have examined the Bayesian algorithm utilising non-steady-state data in adults receiving phenytoin (Crowley et al. 1987; Ludden et al. 1986) with excellent results. Such an algorithm can be developed using a number of pharmacokinetic packages, including the ADAPT software package for paediatric patients, using appropriate population parameters. Further study utilising such an algorithm may prove useful for early estimation of paediatric patients' maintenance dosage requirements.

Therapeutic Implications

The Bayesian method appears to be a reasonable approach to phenytoin dosage; however, the selection of appropriate population parameters is important in the success of this technique. Whichever technique is chosen to calculate phenytoin dosage in paediatric patients, the pharmacokinetic approaches described above or a more conservative empirical stepwise approach as proposed by Koren (1983), some individuals may still receive an inappropriate regimen. It is therefore important to monitor serum phenytoin concentrations and the clinical status at appropriate intervals after dosage alterations.

References

Arnold K, Gerber N. The rate of decline of diphenylhydantoin in human plasma. Clinical Pharmacology and Therapeutics 11: 121-134, 1969

Bach B, Hansen JM, Kampmann JP, Rasmussen SN, Skovsted L. Disposition of antipyrine and phenytoin correlated with age and liver volume in man. Clinical Pharmacokinetics 6: 389-396, 1981

Bauer LA, Blouin RA. Phenytoin Michaelis-Menten pharmacokinetics in Caucasian paediatric patients. Clinical Pharmacokinetics 8: 545-549, 1983

Chiba K, Ishizaki T, Miura H, Minagawa K. Michaelis-Menten pharmacokinetics of diphenylhydantoin and application in the pediatric age patient. Journal of Paediatrics 96: 479-481, 1980

Crowley JJ, Koup JR, Cusack BJ, Ludden TM, Vestal RE. Evaluation of a proposed method for phenytoin maintenance dose prediction following an intravenous loading dose. European Journal of Clinical Pharmacology 32: 141-148, 1987

D'Argenio D, Schumitzky A. A user's guide to the ADAPT programs. Technical Report, Laboratory of Applied Pharmacokinetics, University of Southern California, 1979

Dodson WE, Nonlinear kinetics of phenytoin in children. Neurology 32: 42-48, 1982

Gerber N, Wagner J. Explanation of dose-dependent decline of diphenylhydantoin plasma levels by fitting to the integrated form of the Michaelis-Menten equation. Research Communications in Chemical Pathology 3: 455-466, 1972

Grasela TH, Sheiner LB, Rambeck B, Boenigk HE, Dunlop A, et al. Steady-state pharmacokinetics of phenytoin from routinely collected patient data. Clinical Pharmacokinetics 8: 355-363, 1983

Koren G. Predicting phenytoin serum concentrations. Neurology 33: 1251, 1983

Ludden TM, Allen JP, Valutsky WA, Vicuna AV, Nappi JM, et al. Individualization of phenytoin dosage regimens. Clinical Pharmacology and Therapeutics 21: 287-293, 1977

Ludden TM, Beal SL, Peck CC, Godley PJ. Interpretation of phenytoin concentration-time data using Bayesian regression analysis: an initial evaluation. Clinical Pharmacy 5: 580-585, 1986

Lund L. Anticonvulsant effect of diphenylhydantoin relative to plasma levels. Archives of Neurology 31: 289-294, 1974

Lund L, Alvan G, Berlin A, Alexanderson B. Pharmacokinetics of single and multiple doses of phenytoin in man. European Journal of Clinical Pharmacology 7: 81-86, 1974

Martin E, Tozer T, Sheiner L, Riegelman S. The clinical pharmacokinetics of phenytoin. Journal of Pharmacokinetics and Biopharmaceutics 5: 579-596, 1977

Mawer GE, Mullen PW, Rodgers M, Robins AJ, Lucas SB. Phenytoin dose adjustment in epileptic patients. British Journal of Clinical Pharmacology 1: 163-168, 1974

Mullen PW. Optimal phenytoin therapy: a new technique for individualizing dosage. Clinical Pharmacology and Therapeutics 23: 228-232, 1978

Perucca E, Makki K, Richens A. Is phenytoin metabolism dose dependent by enzyme saturation or by feedback inhibition? Clinical Pharmacology and Therapeutics 24: 46-51, 1978

Rambeck B, Boenigk H, Dunlop A, Wadsworth J, Richens A. Predicting phenytoin dose: a revised nomogram. Therapeutic Drug Monitoring 3: 325-333, 1979

Richens A, Dunlop A. Serum phenytoin levels in management of epilepsy. Lancet 2: 247-248, 1975

Sheiner LB, Beal SL. Some suggestions for measuring predictive performance. Journal of Pharmacokinetics and Biopharmaceutics 9: 503-512, 1981

Sheiner LB, Beal SL. Bayesian individualization of pharmacokinetics: simple implementation and comparison with non-Bayesian methods. Journal of Pharmaceutical Sciences 71: 1344-1348, 1982

Steel RGD, Torrie JH. Principles and procedures of statistics: a biometrical approach, 2nd edition, pp. 444-446, 495-520, McGraw-Hill Book Company, New York, 1980

Tozer TN, Winter ME. Phenytoin. In Evans et al. (Eds) Applied pharmacokinetics: principles of therapeutic drug monitoring, pp. 275-314, Applied Therapeutics Inc., San Francisco, 1980

Vozeh S, Muir KT, Sheiner LB, Follath F. Predicting individual phenytoin dosage. Journal of Pharmacokinetics and Biopharmaceutics 9: 131-147, 1981

Yuen GJ, Taylor JW, Ludden TM, Murphy MJ. Predicting phenytoin dosages using Bayesian feedback: a comparison with other methods. Therapeutic Drug Monitoring 5: 437-441, 1983

Author's address: Dr *Geoffrey J. Yuen*, School of Pharmacy, University of Maryland, 20 North Pine Street, Baltimore, MD 21201 (USA).

Clinical Pharmacokinetics 16: 261-282 (1989)
0312-5963/89/0005-0261/$11.00/0

Clinical Pharmacokinetic Properties of the Macrolide Antibiotics
Effects of Age and Various Pathophysiological States (Part II)[1]

Piero Periti, Teresita Mazzei, Enrico Mini and *Andrea Novelli*
Department of Preclinical and Clinical Pharmacology, University of Florence, Florence, Italy

Contents

9. Roxithromycin 261
9.1 Pharmacokinetics 261
9.2 Influence of Age on Pharmacokinetics 269
9.3 Influence of Various Pathophysiological States on Pharmacokinetics 271
10. Azithromycin 273
11. Pharmacokinetic Drug Interactions 273
12. Conclusions 273

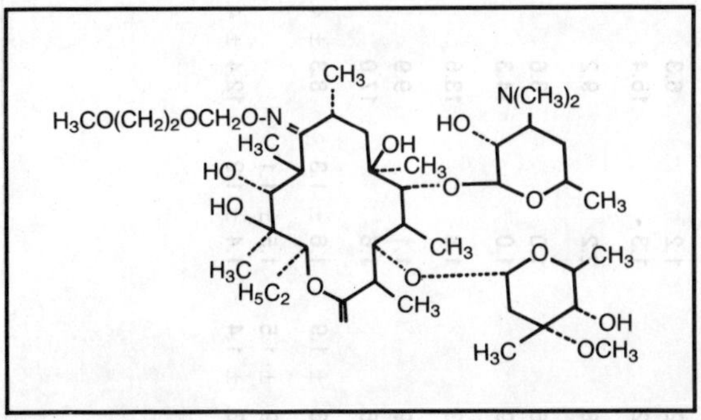

Fig. 2. Chemical structure of roxithromycin.

9. Roxithromycin

Roxithromycin (fig. 2) is a semisynthetic macrolide derived from erythromycin A by oximation of the keto group at position 9 of the aglycone nucleus. Its antibacterial spectrum of activity *in vitro* is similar to that of erythromycin (Barlam & Neu 1984; Jones et al. 1983; Rolston et al. 1986; Young et al. 1989). It is more stable in acidic medium than the parent compound as a consequence of the prevention of internal ketalisation of the glycone by the oxime function, and has improved pharmacokinetic properties and efficacy in experimental infections *in vivo* (Bryskier et al. 1986).

9.1 Pharmacokinetics

The pharmacokinetics and metabolism of roxithromycin have been extensively reviewed by Bégué et al. (1987), Bergogne-Bérézin (1987), Nilsen (1987), Periti and Mazzei (1987) and Puri and Lassman (1987). Some relevant pharmacokinetic parameters in healthy subjects are listed in table XII.

---

1 Part I of this article appeared in the previous issue of the Journal.

Table XII. Mean (± SD) pharmacokinetic parameters of oral roxithromycin in adults with normal hepatic and renal function

Oral dosage[a]		No. of subjects	C_{max} (mg/L)	t_{max} (h)	$t_{1/2}$ (h)	CL_R (L/h)	AUC (mg/L · h)	A_{ur} (%)	Assay	Reference
150/1		4	3.20 ± 0.66	3.3 ± 0.4	13.3 ± 2.7		37.4 + 6.6	7.4 ± 1.7[b]	R/C	McLean et al. (1988)
150/1		21	6.8 ± 1.2	1.9 ± 1.2	8.4 ± 4.2	0.40 ± 0.06	70.8 ± 20.0[c]	11.5 ± 4.3[c]	Micro	Puri & Lassman (1987)
300/1			9.1 ± 1.7	1.9 ± 1.3	10.5 ± 5.2	0.43 ± 0.12	113.6 ± 23.8[c]	10.4 ± 3.3[c]		
450/1			10.8 ± 1.4	1.6 ± 1.0	10.3 ± 2.6	0.58 ± 0.22	148.7 ± 31.8[c]	11.8 ± 4.5[c]		
150/1		12	7.90 ± 2.29	1.9 ± 1.8	10.5 ± 4.5	0.25 ± 0.11[d]	81 ± 34.6[e]	11.6 ± 6.9[e]	HPLC	Tremblay et al. (1988a)
300/1			10.82 ± 2.29	1.5 ± 0.9	11.9 ± 1.7	0.34 ± 0.19[d]	132 ± 59.9[e]	12.6 ± 4.5[e]		
450/1			12.24 ± 2.7	1.4 ± 0.8	13.8 ± 3.4	0.42 ± 0.14[d]	170 ± 69.3[e]	10.7 ± 3.6[e]		
50/1		10	2.5	2.8	5.9		25.7	14.3[e]	Micro	Puri et al. (1986)
50 bid/21	day 1		3.2	1.6	6.6		29.8			
	day 11		4.4	2.0	10.7		65.5	9.1[g]		
100/1			4.8	1.9	5.8		45.0	10.7[e]		
100 bid/21	day 1		5.7	1.5	6.0		51.7			
	day 11		7.9	1.8	12.7		147.5	10.0[f]		
200/1			8.9	2.2	7.4		96.4	11.4[e]		
200 bid/21	day 1		9.2	1.2	6.3		92.7			
	day 11		11.2	1.3	15.4		190.2	8.3[f]		
300/1			11.8	2.2	9.2		153.9	10.6[e]		
300 bid/21	day 1		13.6	1.0	6.6		137.7			
	day 11		13.9	1.0	14.3		268.8	9.0[f]		
400/1			16.3	1.8	13.6		227.2	10.5[e]		
400 qd/11	day 1		17.9	1.1	9.9		342.1			
	day 11		16.6	1.6	17.0		310.6	10.2[f]		
150/1		40	6.6 ± 1.9	1.6 ± 1.3	8.3 ± 4.3	0.33 ± 0.14	43.3 ± 12.6[g]	8.4 ± 1.9[e]	Micro	Puri & Lassman (1987)
150 bid/22	day 1		7.9 ± 1.5	1.5 ± 1.1			50.5 ± 10.3[g]			
	day 11		9.3 ± 1.4	1.4 ± 1.2	12.4 ± 4.9		70.8 ± 14.4[g]	6.4 ± 1.5[f]		

300/1		9.7 ± 2.0	1.3 ± 1.3	10.9 ± 6.5	0.40 ± 0.14	66.3 ± 11.89	8.1 ± 2.2[e]		
300 qd/11 day 1		10.4 ± 1.9	0.9 ± 0.4			68.9 ± 12.49			
day 11		10.9 ± 1.4	1.2 ± 0.8	13.0 ± 6.8		77.4 ± 11.09	7.5 ± 2.0[f]		
150/1	10	6.61 ± 1.9	1.75 ± 1.71	15.5 ± 4.3		79.3 ± 27.9	6.34 ± 1.61[c]	HPLC	Kees et al. (1988)
300/1	8	7.0 ± 2.63	2.8 ± 0.65	14.1 ± 11.99		91.4 ± 31.89[c]		Micro	Segre et al. (1988)

a Dose (mg)/no. of doses/schedules.
b 0-168 hours.
c 0-48 hours.
d 0-8 hours.
e 0-72 hours.
f 0-336 hours.
g 0-12 hours.
Abbreviations: R/C = radiometric/chromatographic; HPLC = high performance liquid chromatography; micro = microbiological assay; bid = twice daily; qd = every day; A_{ur} = amount of drug excreted in urine (percentage of dose administered); also see table II.

9.1.1 Absorption and Disposition Kinetics

Roxithromycin is well absorbed from the gastrointestinal tract. In the study of McLean et al. (1988) a 150mg oral dose containing 30.7 μCi of ^{14}C-roxithromycin produced peak plasma concentrations of 3.2 mg/L within about 3 hours.

Puri and Lassman (1987), comparing single doses of 150, 300 and 450mg of roxithromycin, have shown that peak plasma concentrations increased in a dose-dependent manner, but t_{max} was not affected. The AUC also increased but dose proportionality was not observed. Tremblay et al. (1988a) have also obtained similar data within the same dose interval using an HPLC assay method. In contrast, in an earlier study by Puri et al. (1986) with a very limited number of adult subjects (10) receiving single oral doses (50, 100, 200, 300 or 400mg) of roxithromycin or placebo, a dose-related increase in C_{max} and AUC was observed.

Micronisation does not significantly improve absorption characteristics, while enteric coating results in even slower absorption (5.3 *versus* 1.6 hours) [Tremblay et al. 1985].

The comparative pharmacokinetics of roxithromycin and erythromycin were studied by Kees et al. (1988) in 10 subjects receiving a single dose of roxithromycin 150mg or erythromycin 500mg according to a crossover design with a 1-week interval. The peak plasma concentrations obtained with roxithromycin were 3.75-fold higher than those following erythromycin (6.61 *vs* 1.78 mg/L). Similarly, normalised AUCs were 38 times greater for roxithromycin, indicating superior bioavailability and/or a lower clearance of the latter (529 *vs* 13.9 mg/L • h/g). Segre et al. (1988), comparing the pharmacokinetics of single doses of roxithromycin 300mg and erythromycin 500mg in fasting conditions, found higher peak plasma concentrations (7.0 *vs* 2.1 mg/L) and higher AUCs (91.4 *vs* 7.0 mg/L • h) for roxithromycin.

With multiple dosing regimens of roxithromycin 150mg twice daily or 300mg every day given over 11 days, dose-related increases in C_{max} and AUC on day 1 of multiple dosing were seen. No clinically meaningful differences were seen at day 11. During multiple dosing, steady-state concentrations were reached by day 4. The trough plasma concentrations of roxithromycin at steady-state (days 4 to 11) ranged from 3.22 to 3.69 mg/L with 150mg twice daily, and from 2.2 to 2.22 mg/L with 300mg every day. Similar results, in a limited number of patients (10) receiving 50, 100, 200 or 300mg twice daily or 400mg once daily for 10 days and a final dose on day 11, have been observed by Puri et al. (1986).

Administration of roxithromycin 15 minutes after a standard breakfast resulted in a significant delay in the t_{max} (1.8 *vs* 4.5 hours) and in a 21% reduction of AUC (147.1 *vs* 111.3 mg/L) [Lassman et al. 1986]. Tremblay et al. (1986) confirmed the reduction of roxithromycin bioavailability when drug administration followed food, while showing that it was not affected when the drug was administered before the meal. This is not considered clinically important, however, since the plasma concentrations in both cases were above the MICs necessary for antibacterial activity. Administration of roxithromycin with milk resulted in significantly higher C_{max} and AUC, but these differences are not clinically relevant.

Segre et al. (1988) studied the influence of food on the availability of roxithromycin *vs* erythromycin stearate. Results of comparative pharmacokinetic analysis in fasting conditions have been reported above in this section. After a standard meal, C_{max} and AUC of roxithromycin were higher than those of erythromycin. The erythromycin absorption rate was higher, however (higher k_{12} and lower t_{max}). The meal had no effect on the rate of absorption of erythromycin but delayed the absorption of roxithromycin (k_{12}). The relative bioavailability of this compound (AUC) was essentially unaffected (91.4 *vs* 89.2 mg/L • h) as were the peak concentrations and the elimination half-life.

9.1.2 Distribution

Data on roxithromycin distribution to various tissues have been summarised in table XIII.

In respiratory tract: The mean concentrations of roxithromycin in pulmonary tissue after a 300mg loading dose followed by 3 doses of 150mg at 12-hour intervals were 5.64 and 3.70 mg/kg at 6 and 12 hours after the last dose, respectively, whereas in serum the levels were 6.26 and 5.85 mg/L at the same times. The ratio of lung tissue : serum concentrations was about 1 at both 6 and 12 hours (Tremblay et al. 1988b). In another group of subjects, after 7 doses of 150mg at 12-hour intervals, the pulmonary concentrations of roxithromycin were 2.1, 2.1 and 3.2 mg/kg at 3, 6 and 10 hours, respectively. The tissue/serum concentration ratio was about 0.3 at all times (Mini et al. 1987).

Roxithromycin showed good penetration into bronchial secretions. In patients with superinfected chronic bronchitis, sputum concentrations were consistently higher than those in serum (sputum : serum concentration ratios ranging from 1.20 to 1.63). Stable levels ranging from 4.52 to 5.27 mg/L from 2 to 8 hours were followed by a slow decrease (2.9 mg/L at 24 hours) [Rimoldi et al. 1988]. In another group of patients roxithromycin concentrations were measured in bronchial aspirates after 4 days of treatment (150mg twice daily). Peak bronchial concentrations were 3.1 mg/L at 4 hours after the last dose and decreased slowly (2.4 mg/L at 12 hours). The bronchial aspirate : serum concentration ratio ranged from 0.83 to 1.02 as a function of sampling time (Rimoldi et al. 1988). The concentrations of roxithromycin were also determined in cells and fluid lining the epithelial surface of the lower respiratory tract. These were obtained by fibreoptic bronchoscopy with bronchoalveolar lavage in patients given ten 300mg doses at 12 hour intervals. At 2 hours after the last dose, the mean concentration in epithelial lining fluid was 2.0 mg/L, that is 17% of the simultaneous mean plasma concentrations (11.4 mg/L). Concentrations of roxithromycin in cells recovered by bronchoalveolar lavage (21 mg/L) were 2 and 10 times higher than in plasma and epithelial lining fluid, respectively (Chastre et al. 1987).

In tonsillar tissue: The mean concentrations of roxithromycin in tonsillar tissue taken during surgery after a 5 mg/kg loading dose followed by 1 and 2 doses of 2.5 mg/kg at 12 hour intervals were 2.63 and 1.65 mg/kg of tissue, respectively, at 6 and 12 hours after the last dose (Bégué et al. 1988). Similar results were obtained by Kafetzis et al.

(1988b) in children undergoing surgery at 1 to 12 hours after a single oral dose (3.0 mg/kg) or after 4 doses (3.0 mg/kg twice daily). The mean values of roxithromycin concentrations in tonsils were 6.10 mg/kg for a single dose and 4.63 mg/kg for multiple doses. Levels in tonsils were approximately the same as simultaneous serum concentrations. Lower mean concentrations of roxithromycin in tonsillar tissue are reported in adult subjects receiving either a single 300mg dose 3 to 4 hours prior to surgery or a 300mg loading dose followed by three 150mg doses at 12-hour intervals, the last one 1 to 4 hours prior to surgery (0.9 and 1.8 mg/L, respectively) [Galioto et al. 1987].

In adenoids: Roxithromycin concentrations in adenoids were very high, with median values of 10.25 mg/kg (range 1.96 to 62.74 mg/kg) following administration of a single 3 mg/kg dose, and 13.30 mg/kg (range 3.92 to 59.91 mg/kg) following multiple administration of the same dose. These were higher than the concurrent plasma concentrations (Kafetzis et al. 1988b).

In the middle ear: The diffusion of roxithromycin into the middle ear exudate of children suffering from otitis media was studied by Bégué et al. (1987). Ten children aged from 1 to 10 years, undergoing surgery for insertion of a tube through the tympanic membrane, were included in the trial. They received a loading dose of roxithromycin 5 to 6 mg/kg, followed by 1 dose of 2.5 mg/kg. Blood and middle ear fluid samples were taken 12 hours after the last administration and concentrations averaged 0.87 mg/L, about double those in plasma at the same time.

In the sinus: In sinus mucosa samples taken at sinoscopy in 15 patients with chronic sinusitis receiving five 150mg doses twice daily following a 300mg loading dose, mean tissue concentrations were 4.15 mg/kg at 4 hours after the last dose, and declined slowly to 3.54 mg/kg at 12 hours. Tissue : serum concentration ratios varied between 0.54 and 2.83 at 4 and 12 hours, respectively (Dewever 1988).

In reproductive tissues: Concentrations of roxithromycin were also measured in myometrial, endometrial and ovarian tissues and oviduct in 15 women undergoing total hysterectomy; measurements were made at various times after 3 doses of 150mg, preceded by a 300mg loading dose. High mean tissue drug concentrations of about 2 mg/kg were found in all samples taken, independent of time (De Grandi et al. 1988).

In a group of male patients undergoing surgery for a prostatic disease, after the same regimen of roxithromycin administration, the mean concentrations in prostatic tissue after the last dose were 2.16, 2.81 and 2.35 mg/kg at 2, 6 and 12 hours, respectively. At 12 hours, tissue concentrations approximated those in plasma (2.79 mg/L) [Botto et al. 1988].

Placental transfer: The placental transfer of roxithromycin was evaluated by Bergogne-Bérézin et al. (1987) in 23 pregnant women undergoing caesarean section, using the same dose schedules as above. The penetration of roxithromycin into the fetal compartment was slow and progressive: maximum concentrations in amniotic fluid were reached at 12 hours (1.25 mg/L); concentrations in fetal cord blood paralleled those in maternal blood, and peak was achieved 4 hours after the last dose (0.58 mg/L). On the whole placental transfer of roxithromycin was good, with a ratio of fluid/serum concentrations of about 0.3 to 0.4.

In other tissues/fluids: Roxithromycin distribution was determined in other tissues and fluids. After a loading dose of 300mg followed by 6 doses of 150mg at 12-hour intervals, roxithromycin was undetectable in saliva, while in contrast it reached a mean concentration of 4.25 mg/L in tears 12 hours after the last dose; this was higher than that found in plasma (2.18 mg/L) [Acar et al. 1988]. In synovial fluid collected from 40 arthritic patients, roxithromycin reached concentrations as high as those in simultaneous serum samples, with a maximum value of 3.89 mg/L 4 hours after a loading dose of 300mg and repeated 150mg doses administered every 12 hours (Meirovich et al. 1988). The penetration of roxithromycin into cerebrospinal fluid is poor: no detectable concentrations were observed in patients with normal meninges receiving 2 doses of roxithromycin (150mg at 12-hour intervals) [Puri & Lassman 1987].

Table XIII. Mean (± SD) or median (range in parentheses) oral roxithromycin concentrations in body tissues and fluids

Body tissue/ fluid	Oral dosage[a]	No. of subjects [time to sample (h)]	Cs (mg/L)	Ct (mg/kg or mg/L)	Ct/Cs ratio	Assay	Reference
Respiratory tract							
Lung	150 bid/3[b]	11 [6]	6.26 ± 2.33	5.64 ± 1.76	0.9	HPLC	Tremblay et al. (1988b)
		12 [12]	5.85 ± 1.90	3.70 ± 1.69	0.63		
	150 bid/7	4 [3]	7.4 ± 3.0	2.1 ± 2.2	0.28	Micro	Mini et al. (1987)
		4 [6]	10.6 ± 4.4	2.1 ± 1.6	0.20		
		3 [10]	10.3 ± 5.2	3.2 ± 0.7	0.31		
Sputum	150/1	10 [0-2]		4.52 ± 1.87	1.33	Micro	Rimoldi et al. (1988)
		[10-24]		2.90 ± 1.2	1.63		
Bronchial secretion	150 bid/8	4 [12]	3.0 ± 1.48	2.4 ± 0.74	0.84		
Epithelial lung fluid	150 bid/10	8 [2]	11.4 ± 5.7	2.0 ± 1.7	0.18	HPLC	Chastre et al. (1987)
BAL cells				21.0 ± 10.0	1.84		
Tonsils	2.5 per kg/2-3[c]	11[d] [6]	1.93 ± 1.39	2.70 ± 1.76/	1.4	Micro	Bégué et al. (1988)
		12[d] [12]	1.30 ± 0.52	2.55 ± 1.09[e]	1.32[e]		
				2.50 ± 1.00/	1.15		
				1.80 ± 1.21[e]	1.38[e]		
	3.0 per kg/1	6[d] [1]	4.9 ± 1.2	4.94		Micro	Kafetzis et al. (1988b)
		5 [2]	6.6 ± 1.55	(1.35-15.02)			
		3 [4]	4.71 ± 1.36				
		7 [6]	2.71 ± 0.44				
		4 [12]	1.60 ± 0.22				
	3.0 per kg (repeated doses)	3[d] [1]	8.0 ± 1.7	3.51			
		3 [2]	5.9 ± 2.1	(0.86-12.85)			
		3 [4]	5.6 ± 1.9				
		4 [6]	4.6 ± 1.9				
		5 [12]	1.78 ± 0.53				
	300/1	13 [3.3 ± 0.36]	6.7 ± 3.7	0.9 ± 0.8	0.19 ± 0.24	Micro	Galioto et al. (1987)
	150 bid/3[b]	16 [2.33 ± 1.02]	8.7 ± 6.4	1.8 ± 1.9	0.25 ± 0.17		
Adenoids	3.0 per kg/1	6[d] [1]	4.9 ± 1.2	10.25		Micro	Kafetzis et al. (1988b)
		5 [2]	6.6 ± 1.55	(1.96 ± 62.74)			
		3 [4]	4.71 ± 1.36				
		7 [6]	2.71 ± 0.44				
		4 [12]	1.60 ± 0.22				
	3.0 per kg (repeated doses)	3[d] [1]	8.0 ± 1.7	13.30			
		3 [2]	5.9 ± 2.1	(3.92 ± 59.91)			
		3 [4]	5.6 ± 1.9				
		4 [6]	4.6 ± 1.9				
		5 [12]	1.78 ± 0.53				
Glue[f]	2.5 per kg (repeated doses)	10 [12]	0.58 ± 0.06	0.93 ± 0.26	1.60	Micro	Bégué et al. (1987)
				0.81 ± 0.26[g]	1.40		
Sinus mucosa	150 bid/3[b]	5 [4]	7.64 ± 2.38	4.15 ± 2.81	0.54	HPLC	Dewever et al. (1988)
		5 [8]	2.92 ± 2.99	3.12 ± 2.91	1.07		
		5 [12]	1.25 ± 0.61	3.54 ± 2.36	2.83		
Genital tract							
Ovary	150 bid/3[b]	15 [4]			0.33	Micro	De Grandi et al. (1988)
Oviduct		[12]			0.31		
Myometrium		[12]			0.21		
Endometrium					0.29		

Table XIII. Contd

Body tissue/ fluid	Oral dosage[a]	No. of subjects [time to sample (h)]	Cs (mg/L)	Ct (mg/kg or mg/L)	Ct/Cs ratio	Assay	Reference
Prostate	150 bid/3	8 [2]	5.3 ± 3.11	2.16 ± 1.16	0.41	Micro	Botto et al. (1988)
		9 [6]	4.86 ± 1.56	2.81 ± 2.04	0.58		
		8 [12]	2.79 ± 0.59	2.35 ± 1.61	0.84		
Amniotic fluid	150 bid/3[b]	9 [4]	1.59 ± 0.38	0.54 ± 0.45	0.34	Micro	Bergogne-Bérézin et al. (1987b)
		8 [8]	1.36 ± 0.84	1.15 ± 1.34	0.85		
		6 [12]	1.04 ± 0.98	1.21 ± 0.60	1.0		
Cord fluid	150 bid/3[b]	9 [4]	1.59 ± 0.38	0.58 ± 0.50	0.36		
		8 [8]	1.36 ± 0.84	0.21 ± 0.31	0.15		
		6 [12]	1.04 ± 0.98	0.27 ± 0.6	0.26		
Extracellular fluids							
Skin blister fluid	150/1	7 [2]	6.2 ± 2.0	1.47 ± 0.4	0.37	Micro	Mini et al. (1987)
		[8]	3.4 ± 1.1	1.53 ± 0.4			
		[24]	1.9 ± 0.7	1.2 ± 0.3			
	150 bid/5	6 [2]	7.2 ± 1.4	3.5 ± 1.6	0.85	Micro	Wise et al. (1987)
		[6]	4.0 ± 1.1	3.8 ± 1.0			
		[26]	1.3 ± 0.4	1.4 ± 0.3			
	150 bid/7	6			0.63	Micro	Concia et al. (1988)
Synovial fluid	150 bid (repeated doses)	40 [4]	4.61 ± 0.42	3.89 ± 0.39	0.84	Micro	Meirovich et al. (1988)
		[12]	2.79 ± 0.60	1.93 ± 0.60	0.69		
Tears	150 bid/6[b]	6 [1]	5.25 ± 1.86	4.32 ± 1.2	0.82	Micro	Acar et al. (1988)
		[12]	2.18 ± 0.78	4.25 ± 1.35	1.95		
Saliva	150 bid/6[b]	[1]	5.25 ± 1.86	< 0.05			
		[12]	2.18 ± 0.78	< 0.05			

a Dose (mg)/no. of doses.
b Following a 300mg loading dose.
c Following a loading dose of 5-6 mg/kg.
d Children.
e Left/right tonsil.
f Serous effusion in chronic serous otitis.
g Left/right ear.
Abbreviations: BAL = bronchoalveolar lavage; HPLC = high performance liquid chromatography; micro = microbiological assay; bid = twice daily.

The diffusion of roxithromycin in skin blister fluid, a model representative of inflamed interstitial fluid (Bergan 1981), has been studied following single or multiple doses. Penetration into suction blister fluid was good following a single 150mg dose (Mini et al. 1987), with a mean penetration index, as defined by the ratio of blister fluid AUC and plasma AUC, of 36.8%. The mean peak concentrations of roxithromycin reached 2.0 mg/L in blister fluid at 6.6 hours, which indicates a slow and progressive diffusion when compared to serum kinetics (C_{max} 8.6 mg/L; t_{max} 1.2 hours). A higher penetration index has been observed by Wise et al. (1987) and Concia et al. (1988), respectively, in chemically induced and suction blister fluid following 5 and 7 doses of 150mg administered twice daily (85 and 63%, respectively).

Intracellular and subcellular distribution: Intracellular accumulation and subcellular distribution of ^{14}C-labelled roxithromycin, in comparison with that of ^{14}C-labelled erythromycin, has been investigated in polymorphonuclear neutrophils and macrophages of human and animal origin in a variety of phagocytic cells, including the J774 macrophage cell line, mouse peritoneal macrophages, human alveolar macrophages from both smokers and non-smokers, and polymorphonuclear neutrophils from hypersideraemic patients, human volunteers and bovine blood (Carlier et al. 1987).

Roxithromycin was consistently found to accumulate more than erythromycin, reaching intracellular/extracellular concentration ratios between 14 (in polymorphonuclear neutrophils) and 190 (in alveolar macrophages from smokers), compared with a mean erythromycin ratio of 8. The accumulation was reversible when cells were placed in an antibiotic-free medium. Some 50 to 70% of intracellular roxithromycin was associated to lysosomes in macrophages and 30% to azurophil granules in polymorphonuclear leucocytes.

A comparative study by Carlone et al. (1987) demonstrated that penetration of both radiolabelled roxithromycin and erythromycin in mouse resident or phagocytosis-stimulated peritoneal macrophages is excellent, always achieving cellular concentrations higher than those of the surrounding medium (i.e., ratios between 2 and 8 at a 2 mg/L concentration of the two macrolides). At 10 to 20 mg/L erythromycin intracellular levels were, however, only slightly higher than those observed extracellularly. In both resident and stimulated macrophages, roxithromycin achieved higher intracellular concentrations than erythromycin.

Hand et al. (1987) examined the entry of radiolabelled roxithromycin into human polymorphonuclear leucocytes in comparison with other antibiotics (i.e. imipenem, cefotaxime, trimethoprim and metronidazole). On the basis of the ratio of intracellular/extracellular concentrations, roxithromycin was more avidly concentrated by polymorphonuclear leucocytes than any other antibiotic tested. Uptake of roxithromycin into phagocytes was an active process and displayed saturation kinetics characteristic of a carrier-mediated membrane transport system.

Villa et al. (1988) have studied the uptake and the subcellular distribution of roxithromycin as compared to erythromycin base in rat hepatocytes. On the basis of the intracellular/extracellular concentration ratio they have shown that roxithromycin is taken up and accumulated more than erythromycin base; both macrolides have a similar subcellular distribution, being concentrated mainly in cytosol and lysosomes. Roxithromycin, however, is less concentrated in microsomes and in fact is less demethylated than erythromycin base.

9.1.3 Protein Binding

Roxithromycin is preferentially bound to α_1-acid glycoprotein. The binding is strong, specific and saturable. Protein binding is in fact about 96% at 0.84 to 3.3 mg/L of roxithromycin, and decreases with concentrations of 4.2 mg/L and higher (Zini et al. 1988). Furthermore, the serum free fraction of roxithromycin increases with a decrease in the concentration of α_1-acid glycoprotein (Andrews et al. 1987).

9.1.4 Elimination

Following oral administration of a dose of roxithromycin 150mg containing ^{14}C-radiolabelled drug, 74.2% of the drug was recovered. Most of it was eliminated unchanged, predominantly by faecal excretion (53.4%), followed by pulmonary (13.4%) and urinary (7.4%) excretion.

Three metabolites were identified in the urine: descladinose roxithromycin and mono- and didemethylated roxithromycin. The profile in faeces was similar to urine, with two further unidentified minor metabolites. In the plasma, only unmetabolised roxithromycin was detected.

McLean et al. (1988) reported an elimination half-life of about 13 hours following oral administration of ^{14}C-radiolabelled roxithromycin 150mg. Puri and Lassman (1987) and Tremblay et al. (1988a), studying the pharmacokinetics of single 150, 300 and 450mg doses, showed that the elimination half-life of the drug was not affected by dose variations, but the amount of drug excreted in the urine increased as a function of dose. These data, along with the above reported dose-dependent increase of plasma concentrations but not of AUC, indicate non-linear pharmacokinetics over this dose range. The non-linearity may be due to a dose-dependent absorption or bioavailability, but is most probably explained by saturation of roxithromycin serum protein binding. This is in agreement with the observed dose-dependent increase in renal clearance of roxithromycin during the first 8 hours (Tremblay et al. 1988a).

In contrast, Puri et al. (1986) demonstrated a dose-related increase in both $t_{1/2}$ and amount of drug excreted in the urine (table XII).

In comparative pharmacokinetic studies the elimination half-life of roxithromycin was found to be 6 to 9 times longer than that of erythromycin (Kees et al. 1988; Segre et al. 1988).

With multiple dosing regimens of 150mg twice daily or 300mg every day, the elimination half-life of roxithromycin was significantly increased from 8.3 to 12.4 hours for the 150mg dose group after 11 days of multiple dosing. However, on day 11 it was similar to that of the 300mg dose group. About 8% of the administered dose was excreted in urine after single or repeated administration.

Administration of roxithromycin after food resulted in a significant prolongation of the mean elimination half-life (8.1 *vs* 9.1 hours) [Segre et al. 1988].

9.2 Influence of Age on Pharmacokinetics

The main pharmacokinetic features of roxithromycin as a function of age are shown in table XIV.

9.2.1 Infants and Children

In a study of Albin et al. cited by Bégué et al. (1987) the plasma pharmacokinetics of roxithromycin were analysed in 18 children as a function of age, following administration of 2.5 mg/kg twice daily for 5 days. There were no significant differences in the peak plasma concentrations between a single dose on day 1 and multiple doses of roxithromycin as determined after the last dose on day 6. In the 3 different age groups (i.e. 1 to 18 months; 18 months to 5 years; 5 to 13 years), there was no accumulation of the compound as demonstrated by the absence of significant differences in the level of C_{min} at days 1 and 6. The mean elimination half-life was about 20 hours in all age groups and the mean AUC ranged from 58 to 63 mg/L • h.

Another study of Kafetzis et al. (1988a) also analysed the effects of different ages and doses on the pharmacokinetics of roxithromycin in 24 infants and children suffering from a respiratory tract infection requiring macrolide therapy. In the first and second groups ages ranged from 1 to 12 months, and in the third group from 1 to 8 years. In groups 1 and 3 the dose of roxithromycin was 2.5 mg/kg every 12 hours and in group 2 it was 5 mg/kg every 12 hours. In each patient the duration of therapy was dependent on the course of the infectious disease, but the kinetic study was performed after the first dose, and before and after the last dose. Results showed that steady-state was reached by the time of the kinetic study, and that there was no accumulation of the compound; no difference between the troughs before the second and the last dose was in fact observed. The plasma concentrations observed for infants and children treated with 2.5 mg/kg were lower (4.77 and 5.9 mg/L) than those previously reported for adults receiving the recommended dosage of 150mg twice daily. In contrast, those recorded for infants receiving 5 mg/kg were higher (14.9 mg/L). It is therefore suggested that the paediatric dosage of roxithromycin should be 2.5 to 5.0 mg/kg twice daily.

9.2.2 Elderly Patients

The pharmacokinetics of a single dose of roxithromycin 300mg in healthy young and elderly volunteers were studied by Puri and Lassman (1987). A significant increase in the AUC and half-life was observed in the elderly group compared with the young group. The slower elimination in elderly patients may be due to decreased renal and/or hepatic function. The single *vs* multiple dose kinetics of roxithromycin 150mg in the elderly were studied by Nilsen et al. (1988). There were no changes in the elimination half-life of roxithromycin during multiple dosing (150mg twice daily for 6 days), but a significant increase in the elimination half-life was observed compared with young volunteers.

Table XIV. Effects of age on oral roxithromycin pharmacokinetics (mean ± SD)

Subjects	No.	Mean age/ gestational age	Oral dosage[a]	C_{max} (mg/L)	t_{max} (h)	$t_{½}$ (h)	CL_R (L/h)	AUC (mg/L · h)	Ke (h^{-1})	A_{ur} (%)	Assay	Reference
Children	5	1-18m	2.5 per kg bid/10	10.1 ± 1	1.36 ± 0.1	19.8 ± 37		61.5 ± 8.5[b]			HPLC	Bégué et al. (1987)
	7	18m-5y	2.5 per kg bid/10	8.7 ± 2.2	1.6 ± 0.17	21.0 ± 4.2		58 ± 14[b]				
	6	5-13y	2.5 per kg bid/10	8.9 ± 2.8	1.64 ± 0.25	20.8 ± 2.8		63 ± 21[b]				
	8	1-12m	2.5 per kg bid[c]	4.77 ± 0.53	1.78 ± 0.43	14.6 ± 4.8		43.5 ± 7.7[b]			Micro	Kafetzis et al (1988a)
	9	1-12m	5.0 per kg bid[c]	14.9 ± 2.9	2.06 ± 0.57	10.4 ± 2.4		98.0 ± 16.0[b]				
	7	1-8y	2.5 per kg bid[c]	5.9 ± 1.5	2.00 ± 0.38	9.0 ± 1.5		49 ± 11[b]				
Young		19-37y	300/1	9.68 ± 1.81	1.64 ± 1.21	11.2 ± 4.44	0.36 ± 0.10	122.56 ± 26.19	0.07 ± 0.02	9.49 ± 3.08[d]		Puri & Lassman (1987)
Elderly		60-79y	300/1	10.79 ± 1.94	2.06 ± 1.79	15.46 ± 7.05	0.22 ± 0.07	197.32 ± 67.80	0.06 ± 0.03	9.18 ± 3.36[d]		
Elderly	12		150/1	9.1 ± 1.2	2.27 ± 0.64	26.7 ± 3.0	0.06 ± 0.01[e]	148 ± 27[e]		1.7 ± 0.01[e]	HPLC	Nilsen et al. (1988)
			150 qd/11	11.29 ± 0.97	1.05 ± 0.20	27.2 ± 3.5	0.26 ± 0.07[e]	83 ± 9.8[b]		10.4 ± 2.1[e]		

a Dose (mg)/no. of doses.
b 0-12 hours.
c Mean duration of treatment 4.1 days (8.2 doses).
d 0-48 hours.
e 0-8 hours.
f 0-60 hours.

Abbreviations: Ke = rate constant for unchanged drug appearing in urine; CL_R = renal clearance; A_{ur} = amount of drug excreted in urine (percentage of administered dose); y = years; m = months; HPLC = high performance liquid chromatography; micro = microbiological assay; also see table II.

Steady-state levels were reached by day 4, when the plasma concentrations ranged from 4.92 to 5.68 mg/L, that is, slightly higher than those observed in young people.

These results do not justify a dosage modification in elderly patients. A possible mechanism to account for the multiple dose kinetics of roxithromycin in elderly volunteers is the saturation of the binding of roxithromycin to α_1-acid glycoprotein when the serum drug concentrations rise during multiple dosing, producing an increased free drug fraction available for distribution and elimination. This is in agreement with the abovementioned non-linear kinetics of roxithromycin in healthy young volunteers (Puri & Lassman, 1987; Tremblay et al. 1988a) and in the elderly (Nilsen et al. 1988) after an increase in the single dose from 150 to 450mg.

9.3 Influence of Various Pathophysiological States on Pharmacokinetics

A summary of pharmacokinetic data of roxithromycin in various pathophysiological states is shown in table XV.

9.3.1 Renal Diseases

The pharmacokinetics of roxithromycin after a single 300mg oral dose have been studied in patients with severe renal insufficiency compared with healthy volunteers (Puri & Lassman 1987). No significant differences were noted for C_{max} and t_{max} between normal and renally impaired subjects. A significant increase in the AUC and $t_{1/2}$ was observed in renal insufficiency. As expected, the total amount of roxithromycin excreted in the urine and the renal clearance of the antibiotic were reduced. These differences, although significant, may not be clinically important when the drug is given in a dosing regimen of 150mg twice daily. These observations have also been confirmed for the 300mg single dose by Tremblay et al. (1988c) in patients with renal insufficiency, as defined by a creatinine clearance (CL_{CR}) ranging from 4.4 to 71.7 ml/min. No correlation was observed between the values of the AUC and $t_{1/2}$ and CL_{CR}, probably because renal clearance accounts for a low percentage of the total clearance. As a result, there is no indication for dose modification in renal insufficiency.

9.3.2 Liver Disease

The pharmacokinetics of roxithromycin have also been assessed in patients with alcoholic cirrhosis (Lebrec et al. 1988). After a single dose of 150mg, the elimination half-life was significantly prolonged (25.2 hours) in comparison with that of healthy volunteers. However, C_{max}, t_{max} and AUC were similar to those of healthy subjects. The value of renal clearance (0.42 L/h) and amount of drug excreted in the urine mostly unmetabolised (28mg) were increased, thus partially compensating for the reduction in hepatic clearance.

These differences are not considered clinically relevant and no dose modification is necessary in these patients since the trough plasma concentrations at 12 hours post administration do not vary, and duration of treatment with such a drug is likely to be short.

9.3.3 Other Pathophysiological Conditions

Pharmacokinetic parameters in pregnancy were modified compared with non-pregnant subjects: maternal mean peak serum concentration (C_{max} = 1.90 mg/L) was lower, while elimination half-life (13.3 hours) and AUC (94.74 mg/L • h) were similar to those in healthy volunteers (Bergogne-Bérézin et al. 1987).

In healthy postpartum women given a single dose of roxithromycin 300mg, the peak concentration in milk was 0.53 mg/L in a 2- to 10-hour interval after dosing; the milk AUC was less than 5% of concurrent plasma AUC, indicating that the amount of roxithromycin cleared from plasma to milk was very small. Less than 0.05% (0.14mg of the administered dose) was recovered in the milk (Puri & Lassman 1987).

This small amount of drug is unlikely to produce any clinically significant effect in a breast-feeding infant.

Table XV. Summary of the effects of various pathophysiological states on oral roxithromycin pharmacokinetics (mean ± SD or range)

Oral dosage[a]	Pathophysiological state	No.	C_{max} (mg/L)	t_{max} (h)	$t_{1/2}$ (h)	CL_{CR} (ml/min)	CL_R (L/h)	AUC (mg/L · h)	A_{ur} (%)	Assay	Reference
300/1	Healthy volunteers		8.7 ± 0.68	1.4 ± 0.86	7.4 ± 2.30	116.1 ± 16.3	0.57 ± 0.18	110.6 ± 21.4[b]	14.0 ± 3.6[b]	Micro	Puri & Lassmann (1987)
	Severe renal insufficiency		10.2 ± 2.26	2.2 ± 1.08	16.0 ± 5.06	10.22 ± 2.62	0.04 ± 0.03	191.8 ± 51.9[b]	0.2 ± 0.1[b]		
150/1	Healthy volunteers	12	7.9 ± 0.66	1.93 ± 0.51	10.5 ± 1.4		0.22 ± 0.03[c]	81 ± 10[c]	11.6 ± 0.3[c]	HPLC	Tremblay et al. (1988c)
	Renal insufficiency	12	15.7 ± 1.4	2.04 ± 0.43	17.9 ± 2.4	4.4-71.7	0.03 ± 0.001[c]	211 ± 29[c]	0.4 ± 0.01[c]		
150/1	Alcoholic cirrhosis	10	5.8 ± 4.42	2.13 ± 2.50	25.2 ± 6.0		0.42 ± 0.38[c]	118 ± 91.7[c]	18.7 ± 10.5[c]	HPLC	Lebrec et al. (1988)
150 bid[d]/12	Pregnant women	23	1.90	1	13.3			94.7		Micro	Bergogne-Bérézin et al. (1987b)

a Dose (mg)/no. of doses.
b 0-48 hours.
c 0-72 hours.
d Following a 300mg loading dose.

Abbreviations: CL_{CR} = creatinine clearance; A_{ur} = amount of drug excreted in urine (percentage of administered dose); HPLC = high performance liquid chromatography; micro = microbiological assay; also see table II.

10. Azithromycin

Azithromycin (CP-62,993) is a new semisynthetic macrolide antibiotic which differs structurally from erythromycin by a methyl-substituted nitrogen at position 9a in the macrolide ring. This modification has produced an improvement of the *in vitro* spectrum and potency compared with erythromycin (Aronoff et al. 1987; Czinn et al. 1986; Retsema et al. 1987; Ridgway 1986; Walsh et al. 1987). Increased stability to acidic environment compared with erythromycin has also been reported by Fiese and Steffen (1987).

The preliminary evaluation of azithromycin in man has shown that after a single 500mg dose the oral bioavailability is about 40% with peak concentrations of 0.38 mg/L at about 2 hours after oral administration (Shepard et al. 1987). Azithromycin penetrates extensively into tissues. At 18 to 36 hours after a total oral dose of 500mg (i.e. 2 doses of 250mg every 12 hours), azithromycin concentrations in prostate (1.2 to 2.2 mg/kg), tonsils (3.9 to 4.5 mg/kg), and assorted tissues largely exceeded corresponding serum concentrations. Following administration of a single oral 500mg dose approximately 18 hours before surgery, azithromycin concentrations in gynaecological tissues (2.7 to 3.5 mg/kg) were higher than those in serum and largely exceeded the MIC_{90} for most relevant pathogens.

The volume of distribution at steady-state and clearance were 23 L/kg and 44.1 L/h respectively. The serum elimination half-life was 41 hours between 24 and 72 hours after dosing. The urinary excretion (0 to 14 days) was 6.1% and 15% following oral and intravenous administration, respectively.

The long serum elimination half-life and high tissue concentrations of azithromycin suggest the efficacy of a once-daily treatment for skin/soft tissue, respiratory and sexually transmitted infections.

11. Pharmacokinetic Drug Interactions

It is well known that macrolide antibiotics may interact with several compounds and possibly modify their pharmacokinetics. However, not all the macrolides may be considered as a potential source for severe drug interactions. For example, troleandomycin has proven to be the most commonly implicated compound among this class of antibiotics, while josamycin was seldom involved and midecamycin, its derivative miocamycin, and spiramycin have not so far been considered as potentially hazardous in this respect (Descotes et al. 1985a; Paire & Lavarenne 1982). Available data strongly suggest that the possible mechanism of interaction may be recognised in an inhibition of hepatic drug-metabolising enzymes: troleandomycin has been shown in rats and in humans to induce microsomal enzymes, namely cytochrome P450 isoenzymes, which actively transform the antibiotic by demethylation and oxidation into a nitroso-alkane derivative which forms a stable inactive complex with the iron of cytochrome P450 (Pessayre et al. 1981, 1985). Therefore, troleandomycin may in some way affect the oxidative metabolism of other drugs.

Indeed, the administration of therapeutic doses of this antibiotic may lead to a consistent decrease of antipyrine (phenazone), theophylline and methylprednisolone clearance (Larrey et al. 1983a; Paire & Lavarenne 1982; Szefler et al. 1980; Weinberger et al. 1977). Many drug interactions have been reported in subjects treated with troleandomycin: severe ischaemic accidents were observed in patients receiving both the macrolide and ergotamine (Larcan 1979); women safely treated for long periods with oral contraceptives developed a cholestatic jaundice when the macrolide was added (Miguet et al. 1980).

The addition of troleandomycin may also induce theophylline intoxication, by increasing the elimination half-life by 70% (Brazier et al. 1980; Weinberger et al. 1977), or the onset of signs of carbamazepine overdosage in stabilised epileptic patients treated with the tricyclic compound (Dravet et al. 1977; Mesdjian et al. 1980). Nevertheless, the reduced activity of the P450 enzymes is not immediate, and the concomitant administration of a single dose of troleandomycin and antipyrine in humans (Pessayre et al. 1985) or theophylline in rabbits (Hemsworth & Renton 1981) did not prolong the elimination half-life of these two drugs.

Similarly, oleandomycin, erythromycin and several erythromycin derivatives induced microsomal enzymes and were found to form stable cytochrome P450-metabolite complexes in rats, both *in vitro* and *in vivo*, albeit to a lesser extent (Delaforge et al. 1983; Descotes et al. 1985a; Larrey et al. 1983a). When administered in humans, erythromycin failed to decrease antipyrine clearance significantly (Larrey et al. 1983b). However, erythromycin (at least the base and ethylsuccinate) seems able to affect the clearance of theophylline, with an increase in plasma concentrations and half-life (Descotes et al. 1985a; Iliopolou et al. 1982; May et al. 1982; Paulsen et al. 1987; Pessayre et al. 1985; Prince et al. 1981). Moreover, a case has been described with elevated serum theophylline concentration occurring shortly after erythromycin therapy was discontinued, rather than when the two drugs were given together, suggesting the possible importance of monitoring theophylline clearance after discontinuing erythromycin treatment (Wiggins et al. 1986). Nevertheless, some authors have observed no major influence of this macrolide on theophylline kinetics (Kimelblatt & Slaughter 1980; Maddux et al. 1982; Pfeifer et al. 1979). It is possible that these discrepancies depend on the macrolide derivative used (Descotes et al. 1985a), or on initial theophylline concentration (Paulsen et al. 1987). An individual variability may also be expected in situations where drug-metabolising enzymes are both induced and inactivated (May et al. 1982; Pessayre et al. 1985; Pfeifer et al. 1979). Therefore, erythromycin derivatives may provoke severe interactions in some subjects, such as arterial spasms when combined with ergotamine (Lagier et al. 1979), theophylline intolerance (Cummings et al. 1977), or haemorrhage through slowing warfarin clearance (Bachmann et al. 1984; Bartle 1980). Moreover, erythromycin seems to modify the pharmacokinetics of carbamazepine (Wong et al. 1983) and cyclosporin (Freeman et al. 1987; Kessler et al. 1986), and may reduce methylprednisolone elimination (Laforce et al. 1983). However, decreased erythromycin serum and tissue concentrations and a reduced plasma AUC were observed after concomitant administration of theophylline, probably due to increased renal clearance (Hildebrandt et al. 1987; Iliopoulou et al. 1982) or to a delay in both absorption and elimination, suggesting the risk of inducing subtherapeutic concentrations of the antibiotic (Paulsen et al. 1987). Phenobarbitone may also increase the biliary excretion rate of unmetabolised antibiotic (Manzo et al. 1980), while thiopronine, a mucolytic compound, may increase concentrations of erythromycin in the lung. The mechanism of this last interaction is not fully understood but is probably related to increased vasobronchial permeability (Coppi & Alberti 1984).

Spiramycin, josamycin, midecamycin and roxithromycin have failed to form stable complexes with cytochrome P450 (Delaforge et al. 1988; Larrey et al. 1983a; Pessayre et al. 1985). Interestingly, Delaforge et al. (1983) suggested that the presence in macrolide antibiotics of some structural factors, such as a non-hindered, readily accessible *N*-dimethylamino group or hydrophobicity of the molecule, may play an important role in the explanation of these different behaviours with hepatic enzymes (Delaforge et al. 1983; Selles et al. 1983).

Drug interactions have not been reported with spiramycin and midecamycin (Lavarenne et al. 1981; Paire & Lavarenne 1982; Pessayre et al. 1985). No significant interaction with theophylline was observed with josamycin and roxithromycin, and although slightly increased serum theophylline concentrations were reported with these 2 macrolides, this interaction does not seem to justify a modification in the dosage of the antiasthmatic compound (Descotes et al. 1985b; Jiménez Baos et al., 1983; Ruff et al. 1984; Saint-Salvi et al. 1987; Selles et al. 1983). Roxithromycin seems to have no effect on carbamazepine (Saint-Salvi et al. 1987), unlike josamycin, which impairs the apparent clearance and increases the half-life of this antiepileptic drug (Albin et al. 1982; Vincon et al. 1987). Moreover josamycin, as well as erythromycin (Kessler et al. 1986), may inhibit the clearance of cyclosporin (Kreft-Jais et al. 1987).

In conclusion, drug interactions with macrolides deserve careful attention, although not all the compounds are potentially hazardous in this respect. However, with few exceptions (e.g. midecamycin, miocamycin and roxithromycin), macrolide antibiotics should not be administered to patients receiving long term treatment with xanthine derivatives or carbamazepine. Although there are few available data, care must also be taken in concomitant administration of these antibiotics with ergot alkaloids, oral contraceptives and (probably) cyclosporin. Finally, the possibility that additional drugs should be added to this list cannot yet be ruled out.

12. Conclusion

In the use of antibiotics, the concentrations achieved in the infected tissues and fluids are of fundamental importance: the high lipid solubility of macrolides, and their low degree of ionisation at pH values in blood and tissue fluids, allow these drugs to cross membrane barriers readily and to concentrate in tissues. However, a variety of limiting factors, including those relating to biological and chemical drug equivalency and specificity and the sensitivity of the analytical methodology, have particular relevance to the interpretation of pharmacokinetic data concerning implications for clinical use. Indeed, much of the available pharmacokinetic data concerning erythromycin and its formulations or analogues is derived by microbiological assays that do not distinguish between the parent drug and its metabolites, or between the free drug and the protein-bound fraction or unhydrolysed forms. Recently, non-microbiological assay techniques have been used for measuring levels of macrolides, and the results obtained did not differ from those obtained with bioassays. This is also true in the case of erythromycin esters and the rapidity with which they are hydrolysed *in vivo* and *in vitro*.

A comparison of bioavailability data of the different formulations or the semisynthetic derivatives, and the clinical significance of antibiotic level measured, are particularly difficult to evaluate.

Macrolides are usually administered orally and their oral absorption varies considerably among subjects; moreover, the chemical structure and coating may influence their pharmacokinetics and, as a result, the tissue distribution of the drugs. Among pharmacokinetic parameters, one of the most relevant factors is the extreme variability of the half-life of macrolides, which ranges from 1.5 hours for josamycin to 14 hours for roxithromycin and 41 hours for azithromycin. The longer half-life is one of the major improvements achieved with the new compounds.

It has been pointed out that drugs with long half-lives may have an advantage in tissue distribution, since there is more time for diffusion of molecules out of the vascular space due to prolonged serum concentrations. Macrolide serum or tissue concentrations associated with therapeutic effectiveness *in vivo* have not clearly correlated with MIC values observed *in vitro* for sensitive pathogens: the determination of macrolide serum and tissue concentrations remains a valid approach for pharmacokinetic studies, but it appears to have limited usefulness in clinical drug monitoring.

Future improvements in macrolides will come only from modification of the chemical structure to increase stability while retaining microbiological activity, obviating side effects and improving tissue penetration.

An important example of such a development in recent years is roxithromycin, which has microbiological activity equivalent to erythromycin, has a prolonged half-life, is relatively acid stable and is highly bound to serum proteins. All these parameters may explain the high serum and tissue concentrations and the relative therapeutic efficacy of this new macrolide.

References

Acar JF, Saint-Salvi B, Blanc F. Concentrations of roxithromycin in tear fluid and saliva after repeated dosing. British Journal of Clinical Practice 42 (Suppl. 55): 82, 1988

Albin H, Vincon G, Pehourcq F, Dangoumau J. Influence de la josamycine sur la pharmacocinétique de la carbamazèpine. Thérapie 37: 151-157, 1982

Andrews JM, Ashby JP, Wise R. Factors affecting the *in vitro* activity of roxithromycin. Journal of Antimicrobial Chemotherapy 20 (Suppl. B): 31-38, 1987

Armstrong JR, Cook FE, Robinson JR. Concentration of anti-

biotic and chemotherapeutic agents in the ejaculum. Journal of Urology 100: 72-76, 1968
Aronoff SC, Laurent C, Jacobs MR. *In vitro* activity of erythromycin, roxithromycin and CP-62993 against common pediatric pathogens. Journal of Antimicrobial Chemotherapy 19: 275-276, 1987
Auckenthaler RW, Zwahlen A, Waldvogel FA. Macrolides. In Peterson & Varholf (Eds) The antimicrobial agents annual/2, pp. 116-130, Elsevier, Amsterdam, 1987
Austin KL, Mather LE, Philpot CR, McDonald PJ. Intersubject and dose-related variability after intravenous administration of erythromycin. British Journal of Clinical Pharmacology 10: 273-279, 1980
Bachmann K, Schwartz JI, Forney Jr R, Frogameni A, Jauregui LE. The effect of erythromycin on the disposition kinetics of warfarin. Pharmacology 28: 171-176, 1984
Barlam T, Neu HC. *In vitro* comparison of the activity of RU 28965, a new macrolide, with that of erythromycin against aerobic and anaerobic bacteria. Antimicrobial Agents and Chemotherapy 25: 529-531, 1984
Bartle WR. Possible warfarin-erythromycin interaction. Archives of Internal Medicine 140: 985-987, 1980
Bass JW, Steele RW, Wiebe RA, Dierdorft EP. Erythromycin concentration in middle ear exudate. Pediatrics 48: 417-422, 1971
Baumueller A, Hoyme U, Madsen PO. Rosaramicin – a new drug for the treatment of bacterial prostatitis. Antimicrobial Agents and Chemotherapy 12: 240-242, 1977
Bégué P, Kafetsis DA, Albin H, Safran Ch. Pharmacokinetics of roxithromycin in paediatrics. Journal of Antimicrobial Chemotherapy 20 (Suppl. B): 101-106, 1987
Bégué P, Lacombe H, Cotin G, Chaviere F, Chrétien P, et al. Diffusion of roxithromycin into tonsillar tissue in children. British Journal of Clinical Practice 42 (Suppl. 55): 78-79, 1988
Bergan T. Pharmacokinetics of tissue penetration of antibiotics. Reviews of Infectious Diseases 3: 45-66, 1981
Bergan T, Engeset A, Olszewski W. Does serum protein binding inhibit tissue penetration of antibiotics? Reviews of Infectious Diseases 9: 713-718, 1987
Bergan T, Engeset A, Olszewski W, Josefsson K, Larsen N. Penetration of erythromycin into human peripheral lymph. Journal of Antimicrobial Chemotherapy 10: 319-322, 1982
Bergan T, Tolas P, Oydvin B. Influence of food and hepatobiliary disease on the excretion of josamycin. Pharmacology 8: 336-343, 1972
Bergogne-Bérézin E. The tissue penetration of macrolides with particular reference to the respiratory tract. In Butzler & Kobayashi (Eds) Macrolides: a review with an outlook on future developments, pp. 43-53, Excerpta Medica, Amsterdam, 1986
Bergogne-Bérézin E. Tissue distribution of roxithromycin. Journal of Antimicrobial Chemotherapy 20 (Suppl. B): 113-120, 1987
Bergogne-Bérézin E, Berthelot G, Uzzan J, Ravina JH. Evaluation of placental transfer of roxithromycin in late pregnancy. 27th Interscience Conference on Antimicrobial Agents and Chemotherapy, New York, 4-7 October 1987. Abstract No. 10977, p. 285, 1987
Bergogne-Bérézin E, Morel C, Even P, Bernard Y, Kafe H, et al. Pharmacocinétique des antibiotiques dans les voies respiratoires. Nouvelle Presse Médicale 7: 2831-2836, 1978
Bosco U. Utilità di una preparazione di eritromicina in supposte nella pratica pediatrica. Minerva Pediatrica 17: 401-402, 1973
Botto H, Camay M, Chrétien P, Safran C. Study of the diffusion of roxithromycin into prostatic tissue after repeat oral dosing. British Journal of Clinical Practice 42 (Suppl. 55): 83, 1988
Brazier JL, Kofman J, Faucon G, Perrin-Fayolle M, Lepape A, et al. Retard d'élimination de la théophylline dû à la troléandomycine. Absence d'effet de la josamycine. Thérapie 35: 545-549, 1980
Brittain DC. Update on antibiotics I. Erythromycin. Medical Clinics of North America 71: 1147-1154, 1987
Brun Y, Forey F, Gamondes JP, Tebib A, Brune J, et al. Levels of erythromycin in pulmonary tissue and bronchial mucus compared to those of amoxycillin. Journal of Antimicrobial Chemotherapy 8: 459-446, 1981
Bryskier A, Chantot JF, Lasc JC. Classification and structure-activity relationships of macrolides with emphasis on new developments. In Butzler & Kobayashi (Eds) Macrolides: a review with an outlook on future developments, pp. 7-21, Excerpta Medica, Amsterdam, 1986
Carlier MB, Zenebergh A, Tulkens PM. Cellular uptake and subcellular distribution of roxithromycin and erythromycin in phagocytic cells. Journal of Antimicrobial Chemotherapy 20 (Suppl. B): 47-56, 1987
Carlone NA, Ciuffini AM, Del Mastro S, Bonino S. Determinazione microbiologica dei livelli tonsillari ed oculari di josamicina in soggetti ospedalizzati. Giornale Italiano di Chemioterapia 29 (Suppl. 1): 77-83, 1982
Carlone NA, Ciuffini AM, Tullio V, Sassella D. Uptake of roxithromycin by mouse peritoneal macrophages. In Berkarda & Kuemmerle (Eds) Progress in chemotherapy. Proceedings of the 15th International Congress of Chemotherapy, Istanbul, 19-24 July 1987. Antimicrobial Section Vol. 1: pp. 506-508, Ecomed, Landsberg, 1987
Chabbert Y. Etude *in vitro* sur la spiramycine. Annales de l'Institut Pasteur 89: 434-446, 1955
Chastre J, Brun P, Fourtillan JB, Soler P, Basset G, et al. Pulmonary disposition of roxithromycin (RU 28965), a new macrolide antibiotic. Antimicrobial Agents and Chemotherapy 31: 1312-1316, 1987
Chelvan P, Hamilton-Miller JMT, Brumfitt W. Biliary excretion of erythromycin after parenteral administration. British Journal of Clinical Pharmacology 8: 233-235, 1979
Chen ML, Chiou WL. Analysis of erythromycin in biological fluids by high-performance liquid chromatography with electrochemical detection. Journal of Chromatography 278: 91-100, 1983
Chow AW. Erythromycin. In Ristuccia & Cunha (Eds) Antimicrobial therapy, pp. 209-218, Raven Press, New York, 1984
Clauzel AM, Simeon de Buochberg M, Jars N, Michel FB. Etude du passage de la midécamycine dans les expectorations. Nouvelle Presse Médicale 10: 1658, 1981
Concia E, Cruciani M, Barzaghi N, Bartucci F, Sassella D. Diffusion of roxithromycin into suction skin blister fluid. British Journal of Clinical Practice 42 (Suppl. 55): 86-87, 1988
Coppi G, Alberti D. Thiopronine and lung levels of erythromycin. Journal of Antimicrobial Chemotherapy 14: 307-308, 1984
Coyne TC, Shum S, Chun AHC, Jeansonne L, Shirkey HC. Bioavailability of erythromycin ethylsuccinate in pediatric patients. Journal of Clinical Pharmacology 18: 194-202, 1978
Cummings LH, Kozak PP, Gillman A. Erythromycin's effect on theophylline blood levels. Pediatrics 59: 144-145, 1977
Czinn S, Carr H, Aronoff S. Susceptibility of *Campylobacter pyloridis* to three macrolide antibiotics (erythromycin, roxithromycin [RU 28965], and CP-62,993) and rifampicin. Antimicrobial Agents and Chemotherapy 30: 328-329, 1986
De Grandi P, Comte R, Van Moos G, Grutter F, Pêchère JC. Concentrations of roxithromycin in plasma and gynaecological tissues following repeated oral administrations. British Journal of Clinical Practice 42 (Suppl. 55): 84-85, 1988
Delaforge M, Jaouen M, Manguy D. Dual effects of macrolide antibiotics on rat liver cytochrome P-450. Induction and formation of metabolite-complexes: a structure-activity relationship. Biochemical Pharmacology 32: 2309-2318, 1983
Delaforge M, Sartori E, Mansuy D. Effects of roxithromycin on rat hepatic P-450 cytochromes: comparison with troleandomycin and erythromycin. British Journal of Clinical Practice 42 (Suppl. 55): 67-69, 1988
De Louvois J. Factors influencing the assay of antimicrobial drugs

in clinical samples by the agar plate diffusion method. Journal of Antimicrobial Chemotherapy 9: 253, 1982

Descotes J, André P, Evreux JC. Pharmacokinetic drug interactions with macrolide antibiotics. Journal of Antimicrobial Chemotherapy 15: 659-664, 1985a

Descotes J, Ghanassia JP, Simonet R, Evreux JCL. Influence of josamycin on caffeine disposition in human healthy volunteers. In Ishigami (Ed.) Recent advances in chemotherapy. Proceedings of the 14th International Congress of Chemotherapy, Kyoto, 23-28 June 1985. Antimicrobial Section 2, pp. 1481-1482, University of Tokyo Press, Tokyo, 1985b

Dette GA, Knothe H. Kinetics of erythromycin uptake and release by human lymphocytes and polymorphonuclear leucocytes. Journal of Antimicrobial Chemotherapy 18: 73-82, 1986

Dette GA, Knothe H, Herrmann G. Kinetics of erythromycin binding to human serum. In Periti & Gialdroni Grassi (Eds) Current chemotherapy and immunotherapy. Proceedings of the 12th International Congress of Chemotherapy, Florence, 19-24 July 1981. Vol. II, pp. 911-912, American Society for Microbiology, Washington D.C., 1981

Dette GA, Knothe H, Herrmann G. Erythromycin binding to human serum. Biochemical Pharmacology 31: 1081-1087, 1982

Dewever M. Determination of roxithromycin concentrations in the mucosa of the maxillary sinus. British Journal of Clinical Practice 42 (Suppl. 55): 81, 1988

Disanto AR, Chodos DJ. Influence of study design in assessing food effects on absorption of erythromycin base and erythromycin stearate. Antimicrobial Agents and Chemotherapy 20: 190-196, 1981

Disanto AR, Tsering KY, Chodos DJ, DeSante DA, Albert KS, et al. Comparative bioavailability evaluation of erythromycin base and its salts and esters. I. Erythromycin estolate capsules versus enteric-coated erythromycin base tablets. Journal of Clinical Pharmacology 20: 437-443, 1980

Disse B, Gundert-Remy U, Weber E, Andrassy K, Stetzen W, et al. Pharmacokinetics of erythromycin in patients with different degrees of renal impairment. International Journal of Clinical Pharmacology, Therapy and Toxicology 24: 460-464, 1986

Dow J, Lemar M, Frydman A, Gaillot J. Automated high-performance liquid chromatographic determination of spiramycin by direct injection of plasma, using column-switching for sample clean-up. Journal of Chromatography 344: 275-283, 1985

Dravet C, Mesdjian E, Cenraud B, Roger J. Interaction carbamazépine-troléandomycine: une nouvelle interaction médicamenteuse? Nouvelle Press Médicale 6: 567-569, 1977

Ducci M, Scalori V, del Tacca M, Soldani G, Bernardini C, et al. The pharmacokinetics of two erythromycin esters in plasma and in saliva following oral administration in humans. International Journal of Clinical Pharmacology, Therapy and Toxicology 19: 494-497, 1981

Duthu GS. Interspecies correlation and the pharmacokinetics of erythromycin, oleandomycin, and tylosin. Journal of Pharmaceutical Sciences 74: 943-946, 1985

Fagioli A, Cruciani E, Riario Sforza G, Ferrone G, Di Silverio F. Livelli tissutali prostatici di josamicina. Giornale Italiano di Chemioterapia 29 (Suppl. 1): 85-87, 1982

Falchi M, Teodori F, Carraro A, Cioce C, Scaglione F, et al. Penetration of erythromycin into tonsillar tissue. Current Medical Research and Opinion 9: 611-615, 1985

Fiese EF, Steffen SH. Comparison of the acid stability of azithromycin (CP-62,993) and erythromycin A. 27th Interscience Conference on Antimicrobial Agents and Chemotherapy, New York, 4-7 October 1987. Abstract No. 229, p. 136, 1987

Fioretti M, Bandera M, Rimoldi R. Attività terapeutica e comportamento farmacocinetico della miocamicina a livello dell'apparato respiratorio. Giornale Italiano di Chemioterapia 31: 145-148, 1984

Fourtillan JB, Lefèbvre MA, Ghanassia JP. Pharmacokinetic handling of josamycin and its metabolites during oral repeated dosing in man. In Spitzy & Karrer (Eds) Proceedings of the 13th International Congress of Chemotherapy, Vienna, 1983. Vol. 5, pp. SS 4.4/1-2, 36/11-14, Egermann Druckereigesellschaft, 1983

Fourtillan JB, Lefèbvre MA, Gobin P. Josamycin chemical determination in biological fluids. Giornale Italiano di Chemioterapia 29 (Suppl. 1): 103-108, 1982

Fraschini F, Braga PC, Gagliardi V, Falchi M, Scaglione F, et al. Farmacocinetica della josamicina nell'uomo e distribuzione in vari compartimenti. Giornale Italiano di Chemioterapia 29 (Suppl. 1): 69-76, 1982

Fraschini F, Scaglione F, Cantarella Marchi E, Scarpazza P, Falchi M, et al. Plasma and tissue concentrations of miocamycin in humans. In Ishigami (Ed.) Recent advances in chemotherapy. Proceedings of the 14th International Congress of Chemotherapy, 23-28 June 1985. Antimicrobial Section 2, pp. 1447-1449, University of Tokyo Press, Tokyo, 1985

Fraser DG. Selection of oral erythromycin product. American Journal of Hospital Pharmacy 37: 1199-1205, 1980

Freeman DJ, Martell R, Carruthers SG, Keown PA, Stiller CR. Cyclosporin-erythromycin interaction in normal subjects. British Journal of Clinical Pharmacology 23: 776-778, 1987

Fukaya K, Shomura S, Kitai S, Murata S, Umemura K. Absorption, metabolism and excretion of 9,3″-diacetyl-midecamycin (MOM) in humans. Acta Toxicologica et Therapeutica 2: 45-64, 1981

Fukaya K, Watanabe S, Fujita M. Absorption and excretion of miocamycin tablets and dry syrup. In Ishigami (Ed.) Recent advances in chemotherapy. Proceedings of the 14th International Congress of Chemotherapy, Kyoto, 23-28 June 1985. Antimicrobial Section 2, pp. 1450-1451, University of Tokyo Press, Tokyo, 1985

Gaillot J, Lemar M. Eléments de pharmacocinétique de la spiramycine chez l'homme. Réunion interdisciplinaire Chimiotherapie antiinfective 3-12-1981, Vol. 43, p. 4, Paris, 1981

Galioto GB, Ortisi G, Nevio E, Bartucci F, Privitera G. Concentrations of roxithromycin (RU 28965) in serum and tonsil after single and multiple doses. In Berkarda & Kuemmerle (Eds) Progress in chemotherapy. Proceedings of the 15th International Congress of Chemotherapy, Istanbul, 19-24 July 1987. Antimicrobial Section Vol. 1, pp 191-193, Ecomed, Landsberg 1987

Garrod LP, Lambert HP, O'Grady F. Macrolides and lincosamides. In Fifth (Ed.) Antibiotic and chemotherapy, pp. 183-201, Churchill Livingstone, London, 1981

Ghanassia JP, Modai J, Fourtillan JB. Pharmacokinetics of josamycin in young adults and geriatric patients. In Periti & Gialdroni Grassi (Eds) Current chemotherapy and immunotherapy. Proceedings of the 12th International Congress of Chemotherapy, Florence, 19-24 July 1981. Vol. II, pp. 89-90, American Society for Microbiology, Washington, 1985

Gordon RC, Regamey C, Kirby WMM. Serum protein binding of erythromycin, lincomycin and clindamycin. Journal of Pharmaceutical Sciences 62: 1074-1077, 1973

Gribble MJ, Chow AW. Erythromycin. Medical Clinics of North America 66: 79-89, 1982

Griffith RS, Black HR. Erythromycin. Medical Clinics of North America 54: 1199-1215, 1970

Grove D, Randall WA. Assay methods of antibiotics. Medical Encyclopedia, Inc., New York, 1955

Hall KW, Nightingale CH, Gibaldi M, Nelson E, Bates TR, et al. Pharmacokinetics of erythromycin in normal and alcoholic liver disease subjects. Journal of Clinical Pharmacology 22: 321-325, 1982

Hammond JB, Griffith RS. Factors affecting the absorption and biliary excretion of erythromycin and two of its derivatives in humans. Clinical Pharmacology and Therapeutics 2: 308-312, 1961

Hand LW, Boozer RM, King-Thompson NL. Antibiotic uptake

by alveolar macrophages of smokers. Antimicrobial Agents and Chemotherapy 27: 42-45, 1985

Hand WL, King-Thompson N, Holman JW. Entry of roxithromycin (RU 965), imipenem, cefotaxime, trimethoprim, and metronidazole into human polymorphonuclear leukocytes. Antimicrobial Agents and Chemotherapy 31: 1553-1557, 1987

Heimdahl A, Nord CE. Impact of erythromycin on the normal human flora and colonization of the oral cavity, throat, and colon. In Periti & Gialdroni Grassi (Eds) Current chemotherapy and immunotherapy. Proceedings of the 12th International Congress of Chemotherapy, Florence, 19-24 July 1981. Vol. II, pp. 914-916, American Society for Microbiology, Washington D.C., 1981

Hemsworth TC, Renton KW. Depression of theophylline metabolism and elimination by troleandomycin and erythromycin. Biochemical Pharmacology 30: 1299-1304, 1981

Hildebrandt R, Moller H, Gundert-Remy U. Influence of theophylline on the renal clearance of erythromycin. International Journal of Clinical Pharmacology, Therapy and Toxicology 25: 601-604, 1987

Hovi T, Heikinheimo M. Effect of concomitant food intake on absorption kinetics of erythromycin in healthy volunteers. European Journal of Clinical Pharmcology 28: 231-233, 1985

Hoyme U, Baumueller A, Madsen PO. Antibiotics excreting in canine vaginal and urethral secretions. Investigative Urology 16: 35-38, 1978

Hudson D, Yoshihara G, Kirby W. Spiramycin. Archives of Internal Medicine 97: 57-61, 1956

Ikeda C, Kikuchi Y, Matsui H, Tachibana A. Effects of food on bioavailability of josamycin and josamycin propionate. In Ishigami (Ed.) Recent advances in chemotherapy. Proceedings of the 14th International Congress of Chemotherapy, Kyoto, 23-28 June 1985. Antimicrobial Section 2, pp. 1483-1484, University of Tokyo Press, Tokyo, 1985

Iliopolou A, Aldhous ME, Johnston A, Turner P. Pharmacokinetic interaction between theophylline and erythromycin. British Journal of Clinical Pharmacology 14: 495-499, 1982

Inouye S, Niida T. Discovery and development of midecamycin. In Periti & Gialdroni Grassi (Eds) Current chemotherapy and immunotherapy. Proceedings of the 12th International Congress of Chemotherapy, pp. 887-889, American Society for Microbiology, Washington D.C., 1981

Iwasawa T. Basic and clinical assessments of midecamycin. Chemotherapy 21: 870-881, 1973

Jiménez Baos R, Cadòrniga Carro R, Moreno Ubeda M, Casado de Frias E. Effects of josamycin on serum levels of theophylline. In Spitzy & Karrer (Eds) Proceedings of the 13th International Congress of Chemotherapy, Vienna, 28 August-2 September, 1983. Vol. 5, pp. 36/61-36/65, Egermann Druckereigesellschaft, 1983

Jones RN, Barry AL, Thornsberry C. *In vitro* evaluation of three new macrolide antimicrobial agents, RU 28965, RU 29065 and RU 29702, and comparison with other orally administered drugs. Antimicrobial Agents and Chemotherapy 24: 209-215, 1983

Josefsson K, Digranes A, Schreiner A. Influence of food on absorption of enteric-coated pellets of erythromycin base and of tablets of erythromycin stearate. In Spitzy & Karrer (Eds) Proceedings of the 13th International Congress of Chemotherapy, Vienna, 28 August-2 September 1983. Vol. 5, PS4.4/1-3, pp. 107/11-14, Egermann Druckereigesellschaft, 1983a

Josefsson K, Graffner C, Magni L. Reproducibility of erythromycin serum levels when given in enteric-coated pellets. In Spitzy & Karrer (Eds) Proceedings of the 13th International Congress of Chemotherapy, Vienna, 28 August-2 September 1983. Vol. 5, PS4.4/1-4, pp. 107/15-107/18, Egermann Druckereigesellschaft, 1983b

Josefsson K, Steinbakk M, Bergan T, Midtvedt T, Magni L. Pharmacokinetics of a new, microencapsulated erythromycin base after repeated oral doses. Chemotherapy 28: 176-184, 1982

Josselyn LE, Sylvester JC. Absorption of erythromycin. Antibiotics and Chemotherapy 3: 63-69, 1953

Kafetzis DA, Krotsi-Laskari M, Tremblay D, Saint-Salvi B. Multiple dose pharmacokinetics in infants and children treated with roxithromycin. British Journal of Clinical Practice 42 (Suppl. 55): 58, 1988a

Kafetzis DA, Ligatsikas C, Saint-Salvi B, Lenfant B, Blanc F. Concentrations of roxithromycin in tonsil and adenoid tissues after single and repeated administrations to children. British Journal of Clinical Practice 42 (Suppl. 55): 80, 1988b

Kamme C, Kahlmeter G, Melander A. Evaluation of spiramycin as a therapeutic agent for elimination of nasopharyngeal pathogens. Scandinavian Journal of Infectious Diseases 10: 135-142, 1978

Katsumi K, Sekizawa Y, Inoue M. In vitro antibacterial activity of a 9,3″-di-O-acetyl-midecamycin (MOM), a new macrolide antibiotic. Journal of Antibiotics 34: 436-442, 1981

Kees F, Grobecker H, Fourtillan JB, Tremblay D, Saint-Salvi B. Comparative pharmacokinetics of single dose roxithromycin (150mg) versus erythromycin stearate (500mg) in healthy volunteers. British Journal of Clinical Practice 42 (Suppl. 55): 51, 1988

Kernbaum S. La spiramycine. Utilisation en thérapeutique humaine. Seminares Hopitalières Paris 58: 289-297, 1982

Kessler M, Louis J, Renoult E, Vigneron B, Netter P. Interaction between cyclosporin and erythromycin in a kidney transplant patient. European Journal of Clinical Pharmacology 30: 633-634, 1986

Kimelblatt BJ, Slaughter RL. Lack of effect of intravenous erythromycin lactobionate on theophylline clearance. Journal of Allergy and Clinical Immunology 65: 314-315, 1980

Kosmidis J, Marosis K. Concentration of erythromycin in sputum of patients with chronic bronchitis. Chemioterapia 4 (Suppl. 2): 346, 1985

Kreft-Jais C, Billaud EM, Gaudry C, Bedrossian J. Effect of josamycin on plasma cyclosporine levels. European Journal of Clinical Pharmacology 32: 327-328, 1987

Kroboth PD, Brown A, Lyon JA, Kroboth FJ, Juhl RP. Pharmacokinetics of single-dose erythromycin in normal and alcoholic liver disease subjects. Antimicrobial Agents and Chemotherapy 21: 135-140, 1982

Kucers A, Bennet NMcK. Erythromycin. In The use of antibiotics. A comprehensive review with clinical emphasis, 4th ed., pp. 851-882, William Heinemann Medical Books, London, 1987

Kunin CM. A guide to use of antibiotics in patients with renal disease. Annals of Internal Medicine 67: 151-158, 1967

Laforce CF, Szeffler SJ, Miller MF, Elbing W, Brenner M. Inhibition of methylprednisolone elimination in the presence of erythromycin therapy. Journal of Allergy and Clinical Immunology 72: 34-39, 1983

Lagier G, Castot A, Riboulet G, Boesch C. Un cas d'ergotisme mineur semblant en rapport avec une potentialisation de l'ergotamine par l'ethylsuccinate d'érythromycine. Thérapie 34: 515-521, 1979

Lamy P, Anthoine D, Zuck P, Weber M, Baudesson D. Etude pharmacocinétique de la spiramycine en pathologie infectieuse respiratoire. Annales Médicale de Nancy 16: 109-112, 1977

Larcan A. L'ergotisme thérapeutique. Journal of Pharmacology 10: 413-430, 1979

Larrey D, Funck-Brentano C, Breil P, Vitaux J, Théodore C, et al. Effects of erythromycin on hepatic drug-metabolizing enzymes in humans. Biochemical Pharmacology 32: 1063-1068, 1983a

Larrey D, Tinel M, Pessayre D. Formation of inactive cytochrome P-450 Fe(II)-metabolite complexes with several erythromycin derivatives but not with josamycin and midecamycin in rats. Biochemical Pharmacology 32: 1487-1493, 1983b

Lassman HB, Puri SK, Ho I, Sabo R, Barry A. Influence of food on the absorption of RU 28965 (a new macrolide antibiotic) from film-coated tablets in healthy men. In Butzler & Kobayashi (Eds) Macrolides: a review with an outlook on future developments, pp. 138-142, Excerpta Medica, Amsterdam, 1986
Lavarenne J, Paire M, Talon O. Influence d'un nouveau macrolide, la midécamycine, sur les taux sanguins de théophylline. Thérapie 36: 451-456, 1981
Lebrec D, Benhamou JP, Fourtillan JB, Tremblay D, Saint-Salvi B, et al. Roxithromycin: pharmacokinetics in patients suffering from alcoholic cirrhosis. British Journal of Clinical Practice 42 (Suppl. 55): 63, 1988
Lee CC, Anderson RC, Chen KK. The excretory products of *N*-methyl-^{14}C-erythromycin in rats. Journal of Pharmacology and Experimental Therapeutics 117: 274-280, 1956
Le Roux Y, Desnottes JF, Frydman AM, Kaplan PH, Gaillot J, et al. Pharmacokinetics of spiramycin after single and multiple administration of a one-hour 500mg i.v. infusion in healthy volunteers. In Ishigami (Ed.) Recent advances in chemotherapy. Proceedings of the 14th International Congress of Chemotherapy, Kyoto, 23-28 June 1985. Antimicrobial Section 1, pp. 734-735, University of Tokyo Press, Tokyo, 1985
Lin C, Chung M, Gural R, Schuessler D, Kim M, et al. Pharmacokinetics and metabolism of rosaramicin in humans. Antimicrobial Agents and Chemotherapy 26: 522-526, 1984a
Lin C, Kim H, Marco A, Radwanski E, Symchowicz S. Pharmacokinetics and metabolism of ^{14}C rosaramicin in dogs. Antimicrobial Agents and Chemotherapy 29: 753-756, 1986
Lin C, Kim H, Schuessler D, Oden E, Symchowicz S. High-pressure liquid chromatographic method for determination of rosaramicin in humans. Antimicrobial Agents and Chemotherapy 18: 780-783, 1980
Lin C, Puar S, Schuessler D, Prananik BN, Symchowicz S. Isolation and identification of a metabolite of rosaramicin in human urine. Drug Metabolism and Disposition 12: 51-56, 1984b
Macfarlane JA, Mitchell AAB, Walsh JM, Roverbson JJ. Spiramycin in the prevention of postoperative staphylococcal infections. Lancet 1: 1-4, 1968
Maddux MS, Leeds NH, Organek HW, Hasegawa GR, Bauman JL. The effect of erythromycin on theophylline pharmacokinetics at steady state. Chest 81: 563-565, 1982
Magliulo E, Bonizzoni D, Concia E. La diffusibilità degli antibiotici nel fluido interstiziale umano. Influenza del legame proteico nella metodica della 'skin-window'. Chemioterapia Antimicrobica 2: 368-377, 1979
Magliulo E, Gandini T, Fumarola D, Maggiolo F, Maggiolo M, et al. Studio sul potere di diffusione di due antibiotici macrolidi in fluidi extravascolari umani. Giornale Italiano di Chemioterapia 29 (Suppl. 1): 89-101, 1982
Malmborg AS. Effect of food on absorption of erythromycin. A study of two derivatives, the stearate and the base. Journal of Antimicrobial Chemotherapy 5: 591-599, 1979
Manzo L, Gregotti C, Richelmi P, Di Nucci A, Bertè F. Effects of phenobarbitone on the distribution, metabolism and biliary excretion of erythromycin in rats. Chemotherapy 26: 164-170, 1980
Martin JR, Johnson P, Miller MF. Uptake, accumulation, and egress of erythromycin by tissue culture cells of human origin. Antimicrobial Agents and Chemotherapy 27: 314-319, 1985
May DC, Jarboe CH, Ellenburg DT, Roe EJ, Karibo J. The effects of erythromycin on theophylline elimination in normal males. Journal of Clinical Pharmacology 22: 125-130, 1982
McDonald PJ. Macrolide antibiotics – pharmacology and the importance of formulation. In Butzler & Kobayashi (Eds) Macrolides: a review with an outlook on future developments, pp. 22-29, Excerpta Medica, Amsterdam, 1986
McDonald PJ, Mather LE, Story MJ. Studies on absorption of a newly developed enteric-coated erythromycin base. Journal of Clinical Pharmacology 17: 601-606, 1977
McLean A, Sutton JA, Salmo J, Chatelet D. Roxithromycin – pharmacokinetic and metabolism study in humans. British Journal of Clinical Practice 42 (Suppl. 55): 52-53, 1988
Meirovich CI, Montrull H, Strusberg AM, Brizuela N, Forti IN. Roxithromycin levels in synovial fluid. British Journal of Clinical Practice 42 (Suppl. 55): 88, 1988
Mesdjian E, Dravet C, Cenraud B, Roger J. Carbamazepine intoxication due to triacetyloleandomycin administration in epileptic patients. Epilepsia 21: 489-490, 1980
Miguet JP, Vuitton D, Pessayre D, Allemand H, Metreau JM, et al. Jaundice from troleandomycin and oral contraceptives. Archives of Internal Medicine 92: 434, 1980
Miller MF, Martin JR, Johnson P, Ulrich JT, Rdzok EJ, et al. Erythromycin uptake and accumulation by human polymorphonuclear leukocytes and efficacy of erythromycin in killing ingested Legionella pneumophila. Journal of Infectious Diseases 149: 714-718, 1984
Mini E, Mazzei T, Reali EF, Periti P. Penetration of the new macrolide roxithromycin (RU 28965) into lung tissue and suction blister fluid. In Berkarda & Kuemmerle (Eds) Progress in chemotherapy. Proceedings of the 15th International Congress of Chemotherapy, Istanbul, 19-24 July, 1987. Antimicrobial Section Vol. 1, pp. 1350-1352, Ecomed, Landsberg, 1987
Mitsuhashi S (Ed.). Drug action and drug resistance in bacteria, University Park Press, Tokyo, 1971
Nicholas P. Erythromycin: clinical review. I. Clinical pharmacology. New York State Journal of Medicine 77: 2088-2096, 1977
Nicoletti P, Novelli A, Mazzei T, Lamanna S, Periti P. Clinical, pharmacokinetic and antimicrobial evaluation of josamycin in comparison with other macrolide antibiotics. In Spitzy & Karrer (Eds) Proceedings of the 13th International Congress of Chemotherapy, Vienna, 28 August-2 September, 1983. Vol. 5, pp. SS 4.4/1-6, 36/29-32, Egermann Druckereigesellschaft, 1983a
Nicoletti P, Rizzo M, Mazzei T, Novelli A, Ciuffi M, et al. Aspetti farmacocinetici della miocamicina. Chemioterapia 2 (Suppl. 3): 140-141, 1983b
Nilsen OG. Comparative pharmacokinetics of macrolides. Journal of Antimicrobial Chemotherapy 20 (Suppl. B): 81-88, 1987
Nilsen O, Saint-Salvi B, Lenfant B, Tremblay D, Manuel C. Pharmacokinetics of roxithromycin in the elderly – linearity and repeat dose studies. British Journal of Clinical Practice 42 (Suppl. 55): 59-60, 1988
Nishimura T. Clinical studies of miocamycin (9,3″-diacetylmidecamycin) in children and adults. Chemioterapia 2 (Suppl. 5): 289-290, 1983
Okolicsanyi L, Venuti M, Strazzabosco M, Biral A, Orlando R, et al. Pharmacokinetics of josamycin in patients with liver cirrhosis and Gilbert's syndrome after repeated doses. International Journal of Clinical Pharmacology, Therapy and Toxicology 23: 434-438, 1985
Osono T, Umezawa H. Pharmacokinetics of macrolides, lincosamides and streptogramins. Journal of Antimicrobial Chemotherapy 16 (Suppl. A): 151-166, 1985
Paavolainen M, Kohonen A, Palva T, Renkonen OV. Penetration of erythromycin stearate into maxillary sinus mucosa and secretion in chronic maxillary sinusitis. Acta Oto-Laryngologica 84: 292-295, 1977
Paire M, Lavarenne J. Interactions médicamenteuses avec les macrolides: action comparée de deux macrolides sur l'activité des macrosomes hépatiques. Pathologie Biologie 30: 535-538, 1982
Patamasucon P, Kaojarern S, Kusmiesz H, Nelson JD. Pharmacokinetics of erythromycin ethylsuccinate and estolate in infants under 4 months of age. Antimicrobial Agents and Chemotherapy 19: 736-739, 1981
Paulsen O, Hoglund P, Nilsson L-G, Bengtsson H-I. The interaction of erythromycin with theophylline. European Journal of Clinical Pharmacology 32: 493-498, 1987
Periti P, Fini-Storchi O, Novelli A, Ninu MD, Bordonaro P, et

al. Penetrazione nella mucosa nasale della eritromicina somministrata per via orale sotto forma del sale mercaptosuccinato del propilestere (RV11 Pierrel). Farmaci e Terapia 3: 194-197, 1986a
Periti P, Marino C, Novelli A, Bordonaro P, Reali EF, et al. Valutazione farmacocinetica clinica della eritromicina propionato d,l-mercaptosuccinato (RV11 Pierrel). Farmaci e Terapia 3: 189-193, 1986b
Periti P, Mazzei T. Pharmacokinetics of roxithromycin in renal and hepatic failure and drug interactions. Journal of Antimicrobial Chemotherapy 20 (Suppl. B): 107-112, 1987
Pessayre D, Descatoire V, Konstantinova-Mitcheva M, Wandsheer JC, Cobert B, et al. Self induction by triacetyloleandomycin of its own transformation into a metabolite forming a stable 456nm-absorbing complex with cytochrome P-450. Biochemical Pharmacology 30: 553-558, 1981
Pessayre D, Larrey D, Funck-Brentano C, Benhamou JP. Drug interactions and hepatitis produced by some macrolide antibiotics. Journal of Antimicrobial Chemotherapy 16 (Suppl. H): 181-194, 1985
Pfeifer HJ, Greenblatt DJ, Friedman P. Effects of three antibiotics on theophylline kinetics. Clinical Pharmacology and Therapy 26: 36-40, 1979
Philipson A, Sabath LD, Charles D. Transplacental passage of erythromycin and clindamycin. New England Journal of Medicine 288: 1219-1221, 1973
Pignanelli M, Calderari G, Fraschini F, Moro GF, Tassarotti B. Concentrazioni di antibiotici macrolidici in alcuni tessuti ascellari. Dental Cadmos 3: 91-94, 1984
Pocidalo JJ, Albert F, Desnottes JF, Kernbaum S. Intraphagocytic penetration of macrolides: in-vivo comparison of erythromycin and spiramycin. Journal of Antimicrobial Chemotherapy 16 (Suppl. A): 167-173, 1985
Posti J, Salonen M. Effect of formulation factors and food intake on the bioavailability of erythromycin stearate. International Journal of Pharmacy 17: 225-253, 1983
Pozzi E, Ferrara A, Sardi A, Berti MA, Coppi G. Bioavailability studies on erythromycin administered by rectal and oral routes. Current Therapeutic Research 31: 530-535, 1982
Prince RA, Wing DS, Weinberger MM, Hendeles LS, Riegelman S. Effect of erythromycin on theophylline kinetics. Journal of Allergy and Clinical Immunology 68: 427-431, 1981
Prokesch RC, Hand LW. Antibiotic entry into human polymorphonuclear leukocytes. Antimicrobial Agents and Chemotherapy 21: 373-380, 1982
Puri SK, Lassman HB. Roxithromycin: a pharmacokinetic review of a macrolide. Journal of Antimicrobial Chemotherapy 20 (Suppl. B): 89-100, 1987
Puri SK, Lassman HB, Ho I, Sabo R, Barry A. Safety, tolerance, and pharmacokinetics of single and multiple oral doses of RU28695 (a new macrolide antibiotic) in healthy men. In Butzler & Kobayashi (Eds) Macrolides: a review with an outlook on future developments, pp. 128-137, Excerpta Medica, Amsterdam, 1986
Raeder K, Wildfeuer A, Schwedass A, Laufen H. Determination of josamycin in plasma, erythrocytes and leukocytes via high-performance liquid chromatography by direct injection of plasma or homogenized blood cells, using alternating sample clean-up columns. Journal of Chromatography 344: 416-421, 1985
Retsema J, Girard A, Schelkly W, Manousos M, Anderson M, et al. Spectrum and mode of action of azithromycin (CP-62, 993), a new 15-membered-ring macrolide with improved potency against Gram-negative organisms. Antimicrobial Agents and Chemotherapy 31: 1939-1947, 1987
Ridgway GL. Antimicrobial chemotherapy of chlamydial infection: where next? European Journal of Clinical Microbiology 5: 550-553, 1986
Rimoldi R, Mangiarotti P, De Rose V, Nonis A, Bertoletti R, et al. Penetration of roxithromycin into bronchial secretions. British Journal of Clinical Practice 41 (Suppl. 55): 74-77, 1988
Rolston KVI, LeBlanc B, Ho DH. In vitro activity of RU 28965, a new macrolide, compared to that of erythromycin. Journal of Antimicrobial Chemotherapy 17: 161-163, 1986
Ruff F, Prosper M, Pujet JC. Théophylline et antibiotiques. Absence d'interaction avec la josamycine. Thérapie 39: 1-6, 1984
Rutland J, Berend N, Marlin GE. The influence of food on the bioavailability of new formulations of erythromycin stearate and base. British Journal of Clinical Pharmacology 8: 343-347, 1979
Sabath LD, Anhalt JP. Assay of antimicrobics. In Lenette et al. (Eds) Manual of clinical microbiology, pp. 485-490, American Society for Microbiology, Washington D.C., 1980
Sabath LD, Gerstain DA, Bronwen Loder P, Finland M. Excretion of erythromycin and its enhanced activity in urine against Gram-negative bacilli with alkalinization. Journal of Laboratory and Clinical Medicine 72: 916-923, 1968
Saint-Salvi B, Tremblay D, Surjus A, Lefebvre MA. A study of interaction of roxithromycin with theophylline and carbamazepine. Journal of Antimicrobial Chemotherapy 20 (Suppl. B): 121-129, 1987
Saito A, Nasu M, Hara K, Sawatari K, Hayashi A, et al. Fundamental studies on mydecamycin (SF-837), a new macrolide antibiotic, and its application in respiratory tract infections. Chemotherapy 21(4): 762-771, 1973
Sanders SW, Jaeger H, Cunci R, Fujita M, Maurette JM. Single and multiple dose pharmacokinetics and tolerance of miocamycin in healthy European volunteers. In Ishigami (Ed.) Recent advances in chemotherapy. Proceedings of the 14th International Congress of Chemotherapy, Kyoto, 23-28 June 1985. Antimicrobial Section 2, pp. 1452-1453, University of Tokyo Press, Tokyo, 1985
Sawae Y, Kumagai Y, Ishimaru T. Antimicrobial activity and pharmacokinetics of miocamycin, and its clinical usefulness. In Berkarda (Ed.) Progress in chemotherapy. Proceedings of the 15th International Congress of Chemotherapy, Istanbul, 19-24 July, 1987. Antimicrobial Section Vol. 1, pp. 165-167, Ecomed, Landsberg, 1987
Selles JPh, Panis G, Jaber H, Bres J, Armando P. Influence of josamycine on theophylline kinetics. In Spitzy & Karrer (Eds) Proceedings of the 13th International Congress of Chemotherapy, Vienna, 28 August-2 September 1983, SS 4.4/1-3, pp. 36/15-20, Egermann Druckereigesellschaft, 1983
Segre G, Bianchi E, Zanolo G, Bartucci F, Sassella D. Influence of food on the bioavailability of roxithromycin versus erythromycin stearate. British Journal of Clinical Practice 42 (Suppl. 55): 55-57, 1988
Segui A, Milon D, Cormier M, Lepesant G. Erythromycin lactobionate: pharmacokinetics and uterine tissue levels. European Journal of Drug Metabolism and Pharmacokinetics 12: 153-160, 1987
Shadomy S, Tipple M, Paxton T. Josamycin and rosaramycin: in vitro comparisons with erythromycin and clindamycin. Antimicrobial Agents and Chemotherapy 10: 773-775, 1976
Shanson DC, McNabb WR, Ruby K. High dose erythromycin for preventing endocarditis. Lancet 1: 299-300, 1983
Shanson DC, Tidbury P, McNabb WR, Tadayon' M. The pharmacokinetics and tolerance of oral erythromycin stearate compared with erythromycin ethylsuccinate: implications for preventing endocarditis. Journal of Antimicrobial Chemotherapy 14: 157-163, 1984
Shepard RM. High pressure liquid chromatographic (HPCL) assay for azithromycin (CP-62993/XZ-450) in serum and tissues. Interscience Conference on Antimicrobial Agents and Chemotherapy, New York, 4-7 October, 1987. Abstract 238, p. 138, 1987
Shepard RM, Weidler DJ, Garg DC, Madsen PO, Cox CE, et al. Human pharmacokinetics of azithromycin (CP-62, 993/XZ-

450), a new macrolide with an extended half-life and high tissue penetration. Interscience Conference on Antimicrobial Agents and Chemotherapy, New York, 4-7 October, 1987. Abstract 239, p. 138, 1987

Shiiki K, Sakamoto H. Penetration of antimicrobial agents into saliva (clinical application as a therapeutic drug monitoring method). Progress in Chemotherapy. 15th International Congress of Chemotherapy, Istanbul, 19-24 July, 1987. Antimicrobial Section Vol. 1, pp. 211-213, Ecomed, Landsberg, 1987

Shomura T, Umemura K. Studies on absorption, distribution, metabolism and excretion of a new macrolide antibiotic SF-837. I. Absorption, metabolism and excretion of SF-837. Chemical and Pharmaceutical Bulletin 21: 1824-1831, 1973

Spitzy KH, Hitzenberger G. The distribution volume of some antibiotics. Antibiotics Annual 1957, 996-1003, 1958

Steigbigel NH. Erythromycin, lincomycin and clindamycin. In Mandel et al. (Eds) Anti-infective therapy, pp. 197-218, John Wiley and Sons, New York, 1985

Stoehr GP, Juhl RP, Veals J, Symchowicz S, Gural R, et al. The excretion of rosaramicin in breast milk. Journal of Clinical Pharmacology 25: 89-94, 1985

Strausbaugh LJ, Bolton WK, Dilworth JA, Guerrant RL, Sande MA. Comparative pharmacology of josamycin and erythromycin stearate. Antimicrobial Agents and Chemotherapy 10: 450-456, 1976

Stubbs C, Haigh JM, Kanfer I. Determination of erythromycin in serum and urine by high-performance liquid chromatography with ultraviolet detection. Journal of Pharmaceutical Sciences 74: 1126-1128, 1985

Sundberg L, Edén T, Ernston S. Penetration of erythromycin in Waldeyer's ring–adenoid tissue. Acta Oto-Laryngologica (Suppl. 384): 3-9, 1981

Sundberg L, Eden T, Ernstson S, Pahlitzsch R. Penetration of erythromycin through respiratory mucosa. A study using secretary otitis media as a mode. Acta Oto-Laryngologica 365 (Suppl.): 1-17, 1979

Szefler SJ, Rose JQ, Ellis EF, Spector SL, Green AW, et al. The effect of troleandomycin on methylprednisolone elimination. Journal of Allergy and Clinical Immunology 66: 447-451, 1980

Thompson PJ, Burgess KR, Marlin GE. Influence of food on absorption of erythromycin ethyl succinate. Antimicrobial Agents and Chemotherapy 18: 829-831, 1980

Taranger C, Pons M, Tamalet J, Videau D. Action de la spiramycine sur le pouvoir pathogène et la croissance de bactéries Gram-positif. Pathologie & Biologie 20: 961-964, 1972

Tremblay D, Bryskier A, Vuckovic M, Stockis A, Manuel C. RU 28965, nouveau macrolide semi-synthétique: biodisponibilité et profil pharmacocinétique après administration par voie orale. Pathologie Biologie 33: 502-506, 1985

Tremblay D, Jaeger H, Fourtillan JB, Manuel C. Pharmacokinetics of three single doses (150, 300, 450mg) of roxithromycin in young volunteers. British Journal of Clinical Practice 42 (Suppl. 55): 49-50, 1988a

Tremblay D, Meyer B, Saint-Salvi B, Robinet D. Influence of food on bioavailability of roxithromycin (RU 28965). 3rd World Conference of Clinical Pharmacology and Therapeutics, Stockholm. Abstract No. 1206, 1986

Tremblay D, Mignot A, Couraud L, Saux MC, Manuel C. Concentrations of roxithromycin in lung tissue after repeat dosing. British Journal of Clinical Practice 42 (Suppl. 55): 73, 1988b

Tremblay D, Verger C, Saint-Salvi B, Robinet D, Manuel C. Pharmacokinetics of roxithromycin in chronic renal insufficiency. British Journal of Clinical Practice 42 (Suppl. 55): 61-62, 1988c

Tserng KY, Wagner JG. Fluorometric determination of erythromycin and erythromycin propionate in whole blood or plasma and correlation of results with microbiological assay. Analytical Chemistry 48: 348-353, 1976

Tsuji K. Fluorimetric determination of erythromycin ethylsuccinate in serum by high performance liquid chromatographic post-column, on-stream derivatization and extraction method. Journal of Chromatography 158: 337-348, 1978

Twiss RJ, Berger WV, Gillette L, Arnonson AR, Siegel L. The biliary excretion of erythromycin (ilotycin). Surgery, Gynecology and Obstetrics 102: 355-357, 1956

Vaillant L, Lorette G, Loulergue J, Audurier A. Erythromycin ethylsuccinate: diffusion through interstitial dermal fluid. European Journal of Clinical Pharmacology 33: 529-530, 1987

Venho VMK, Palva ES, Konno K, Stenfors E. The value of comparative bioavailability studies of marketed drugs in drug control. An example with erythromycin stearate. Methods and Findings in Experimental and Clinical Pharmacology 9: 445-447, 1987

Videau D. La spiramycine: bactériologie, pharmacologie, pharmacocinétique et distribution tissulaire. Cahiers de Médicine Vétérinaire 47: 155-164, 1978

Villa P, Sassella D, Corada M, Bartosek I. Toxicity, uptake and subcellular distribution of roxithromycin and erythromycin base in rat hepatocytes. British Journal of Clinical Practice 42 (Suppl. 55): 64-66, 1988

Vincon G, Albin H, Demotes-Mainard F, Guyot M, Bistue C, et al. Effects of josamycin on carbamazepine kinetics. European Journal of Clinical Pharmacology 32: 321-323, 1987

Vosbeck K, James PR, Zimmermann W. Antibiotic action of phagocytosed bacteria measured by a new method for determining viable bacteria. Antimicrobial Agents and Chemotherapy 25: 735-742, 1984

Walsh M, Kappus EW, Quinn TC. In vitro evaluation of CP-62,993, erythromycin, clindamycin, and tetracycline against Chlamydia trachomatis. Antimicrobial Agents and Chemotherapy 31: 811-812, 1987

Walstad RA, Hellum KB. Penetration of erythromycin in respiratory tract infections. Acta Oto-Laryngologica (Suppl. 407): 50-54, 1984

Washington JA II, Wilson WR. Erythromycin: a microbial and clinical perspective after 30 years of clinical use (second of two parts). Mayo Clinic Proceedings 60: 271, 1985

Weinberger M, Hudgel D, Spector S, Chidseu C. Inhibition of theophylline clearance by troleandomycin. Journal of Allergy and Clinical Immunology 59: 228-231, 1977

Welling PG. Effect of food on bioavailability of drugs. Pharmacy International 1: 14-18, 1980

Welling PG, Tse FLS. The influence of food on the absorption of antimicrocial agents. Journal of Antimicrobial Chemotherapy 9: 7-27, 1982

Wiggins J, Arbab O, Ayres JG, Skinner C. Elevated serum theophylline concentration following cessation of erythromycin treatment. European Journal of Respiratory Diseases 68: 298-300, 1986

Wildfeuer A, Laufen H, Rader K. Activity of josamycin in human tissue and neutrophils. In Ishigami (Ed.) Recent advances in chemotherapy. Proceedings of the 14th International Congress of Chemotherapy, Kyoto, 23-28 June, 1985. Antimicrobial Section 2, pp. 1478-1480, University of Tokyo Press, Tokyo, 1985

Wiley PE. Macrolide antibiotics. In Kuemmerle et al. (Eds) Clinical chemotherapy, Vol. II, pp. 163-176, Thierne-Stratton Inc., New York, 1983

Wilson JT, Van Boxtel CJ. Pharmacokinetics of erythromycin in man. In Schonfeld (Ed.) Antibiotics and chemotherapy 25: 181-203, 1978

Wise R, Kirkpatrick B, Asby J, Andrews JM Pharmacokinetics and tissue penetration of roxithromycin after multiple dosing. Antimicrobial Agents and Chemotherapy 31: 1051-1053, 1987

Wollmer P, Rhodes CG, Pike VW, Silvester DJ, Pride NB, et al. Measurement of pulmonary erythromycin concentration in patients with lobar pneumonia by means of positron tomography. Lancet 2: 1361-1364, 1982

Wong YY, Ludden TM, Bell RD. Effect of erythromycin on carbamazepine kinetics. Clinical Pharmacology and Therapeutics 33: 460-464, 1983

Yakatan GJ, Poynor WJ, Harris RG, Martin A, Leonard RG, et al. Single-dose fasting bioequivalence assessment of erythromycin stearate tablets in man. Journal of Pharmacokinetics and Biopharmaceutics 7: 355-368, 1979

Yakatan GJ, Poynor WJ, Breeding SA, Lankford CE, Dighe SV, et al. Single- and multiple-dose bioequivalence of erythromycin pharmaceutical alternatives. Journal of Clinical Pharmacology 20: 625-638, 1980

Yakatan GJ, Rasmussen CE, Feis PJ, Wallen S. Bioinequivalence of erythromycin ethylsuccinate and enteric-coated erythromycin pellets following multiple oral doses. Journal of Clinical Pharmacology 25: 36-42, 1985

Young RA, Gonzalez JP, Sorkin EM. Roxithromycin: a review of its antibacterial activity, pharmacokinetic properties and clinical efficacy. Drugs 37: 8-41, 1989

Zini R, Fournet MP, Barre J, Tremblay D, Tillement JP. In vitro study of roxithromycin binding to serum proteins and erythrocytes in humans. British Journal of Clinical Practice 42 (Suppl. 55): 54, 1988

Authors' address: Professor *P. Periti*, Department of Preclinical and Clinical Pharmacology, University of Florence, Viale Morgagni, 65, 50134 Florence (Italy).

Clinical Pharmacokinetics 16: 283-311 (1989)
0312-5963/89/0005-0283/$14.50/0

Clinical Pharmacokinetics of Epidural and Spinal Anaesthesia

A.G.L. Burm
Department of Anaesthesiology, Leiden University Hospital, Leiden, The Netherlands

Contents

Summary 283
1. Local Anaesthetic Agents and their Physicochemical Properties 284
2. Mechanism, Sites of Action and Local Distribution 285
2.1 Sites of Action 285
2.2 Local Drug Distribution 286
3. Systemic Absorption 289
3.1 Local Blood Flow 289
3.2 Tissue Uptake and Binding 290
3.3 Extent of Absorption 290
3.4 Absorption Rates 290
4. Systemic Disposition 292
4.1 Distribution and Plasma Binding 292
4.2 Elimination 294
4.3 Effects of Epidural and Spinal Blockade 296
5. Concentration-Time Profiles: Factors Altering the Pharmacokinetics 296
5.1 Concentrations Following Single Injections 296
5.2 Concentrations During Continuous Epidural Anaesthesia 297
5.3 Factors with Possible Effect 297
6. Central Nervous System and Cardiovascular Toxicity 303
6.1 Threshold Concentrations and Margin of Safety 303
6.2 Effect of Plasma Binding 303
6.3 Influence of Acid-Base Balance 304
6.4 Dose Limitations 304
7. Conclusions and Perspectives 304

Summary

Epidural and spinal anaesthesia results from the interaction of local anaesthetics with nerve structures, primarily those located within the subarachnoid space. Local anaesthetics can reach the sites of action along various distribution pathways. Uptake into extraneural tissues (in particular epidural fat) and systemic absorption compete with neural tissue distribution and thereby affect the clinical potency and duration of action. Consequently, epidural doses must be much higher than spinal doses.

The systemic absorption of lignocaine (lidocaine), bupivacaine and etidocaine following lumbar epidural administration has been shown to be biphasic, with a rapid initial absorption phase followed by a much slower absorption phase. Initial absorption rates of lignocaine and bupivacaine following subarachnoid injection are much slower, but the late absorption rates are similar to those after epidural administration.

The tissue distribution characteristics of various amide-type agents are similar, because more extensive plasma binding offsets the greater tissue affinity of the more lipophilic compounds bupivacaine and etidocaine. The amide-type agents are predominantly eliminated by hepatic metabolism, except prilocaine, which is also metabolised elsewhere in the body. Ester-type agents are rapidly hydrolysed in blood and liver and are eliminated much faster than amide-type agents.

The blood concentrations attained depend primarily upon the dose administered. The addition of adrenaline (epinephrine) reduces the peak plasma drug concentrations; similarly, the age of the patient, disease states and drug interactions may alter the pharmacokinetics to various extents.

Because of the low dose requirements, systemic toxicity is not a problem during spinal anaesthesia. During epidural anaesthesia, however, the safety margin is relatively small, and systemic toxicity is very likely to occur after inadvertent intravascular injection of an epidural dose.

Epidural and spinal anaesthesia are commonly used anaesthetic techniques, finding application in the areas of surgery, obstetrics, and diagnosis and management of acute and chronic pain. Both techniques involve injection of a local anaesthetic solution close to the target nerve structures, primarily located within the subarachnoid space. Therefore, unlike general and intravenous anaesthetics, local anaesthetics are not dependent upon the general circulation for transport to their sites of action. However, they do enter the general circulation and systemic uptake is largely responsible for terminating their action. In addition, because local anaesthetics can produce systemic toxicity, uptake into the general circulation is of concern to those practising regional anaesthesia. Toxic effects are likely to occur after inadvertent intravascular injection of epidural doses, so that knowledge of the pharmacokinetics of local anaesthetic agents following local and intravascular injection is essential for the safe application of major regional blockades.

This article summarises the pharmacokinetic characteristics of the local anaesthetics currently used for epidural and spinal anaesthesia, and the implications for the time course of the neural blockade and systemic toxicity. For more detailed considerations, data and additional references on the pharmacokinetics following epidural and subarachnoid administration, as well as other routes, the reader is referred to a recent text by Tucker and Mather (1988). The pharmacokinetics in obstetric patients and neonates have been reviewed in a recent article in the Journal (Kanto 1986), and are therefore not considered in detail.

1. *Local Anaesthetic Agents and their Physicochemical Properties*

The local anaesthetics used in clinical practice are either amino-esters or amino-amides (table I; fig. 1). Of the amino-esters, procaine is more of historical interest, although it is still used for diagnostic differential spinal blocks. Chloroprocaine achieved great popularity in epidural anaesthesia for short procedures in outpatients and in obstetrics in some countries, but the safety of this agent has been questioned after reports of several cases of persistent neurological damage and prolonged sensory or motor deficits following epidural or accidental subarachnoid injection of large volumes (doses between 360 and 840mg) of chloroprocaine solutions (Moore et al. 1982; Ravindran et al. 1980; Reisner et al. 1980). Recent investigations suggest that these effects may have been due to the low pH and high sodium bisulphite concentrations in the solutions rather than to a neurotoxic action of chloroprocaine (Ford & Raj 1987; Gissen et al. 1984). Amethocaine (tetracaine) is still widely used for spinal anaesthesia.

Of the amino-amides lignocaine (lidocaine), mepivacaine and bupivacaine are used for both

Table I. Physicochemical properties and equi-effective anaesthetic concentrations of the major local anaesthetic agents used in epidural and/or spinal anaesthesia (from Arthur et al. 1987; Tucker & Mather 1988)

Agent	pKa (25°C)	Partition coefficient[a]	Protein binding (%)[b]	Equi-effective anaesthetic concentration (%)[c]
Esters				
Procaine	9.05	0.02	5.8	2
Chloroprocaine	8.97	0.14	?	2
Amethocaine	8.46	4.1	75.6	0.25
Amides				
Lignocaine (lidocaine)	7.91	2.9	64.3	1
Mepivacaine	7.76	0.8	77.5	1
Prilocaine	7.9	0.9	≈55	1
Bupivacaine	8.16	27.5	95.6	0.25
Etidocaine	7.7	141	94	0.25
Cinchocaine	7.9	?	?	?

a *N*-Heptane/pH 7.4 buffer.
b Data for procaine and amethocaine represent nerve homogenate binding; data for lignocaine, mepivacaine, bupivacaine and etidocaine represent plasma protein binding at a concentration of 2 mg/L.
c Data derived from rat sciatic nerve block procedures.

epidural and spinal anaesthesia. In addition, etidocaine is often used for epidural anaesthesia in some countries. Prilocaine is useful for epidural anaesthesia, but anxiety about possible development of methaemoglobinaemia has limited its use. This drug is also potentially useful for spinal anaesthesia, but specific formulations for subarachnoid administration are not available. Cinchocaine (dibucaine) is still used by some anaesthesiologists for spinal anaesthesia, but is too toxic for epidural administration. Carticaine, a thiophene derivative, has undergone limited clinical evaluation (Brinkløv 1977; Kaukinen et al. 1986), and ropivacaine, the stereochemically pure *S*-(-)-*n*-propyl homologue of mepivacaine and bupivacaine, is currently under investigation.

The physicochemical properties of the most commonly used local anaesthetic agents are shown in table I.

2. *Mechanism, Sites of Action and Local Distribution*

Nerve blockade is the clinical manifestation of an interaction of local anaesthetic molecules with the sodium channels in excitable nerve membranes, resulting in inhibition of sodium influx and consequent inhibition of the initiation and propagation of action potentials (Strichartz & Ritchie 1987). Experimental evidence suggests that the charged cationic form of the local anaesthetics is primarily responsible for this effect, and that these molecules can reach the sites of action on the sodium channels only from the axoplasmic side of the membrane. However, the uncharged neutral form may also contribute to the effects by gaining access to the sites of action via hydrophobic routes and/or by another mechanism, involving membrane perturbation.

2.1 Sites of Action

The nerve structures generally considered to be the principal sites of action of epidural and spinal anaesthesia are the intradural spinal nerve roots and the periphery of the spinal cord (Bromage 1975, 1978; Cousins & Bromage 1988; Covino & Scott 1985; Greene 1981).

Urban (1973) reported that during induction of epidural and spinal anaesthesia the anterolateral

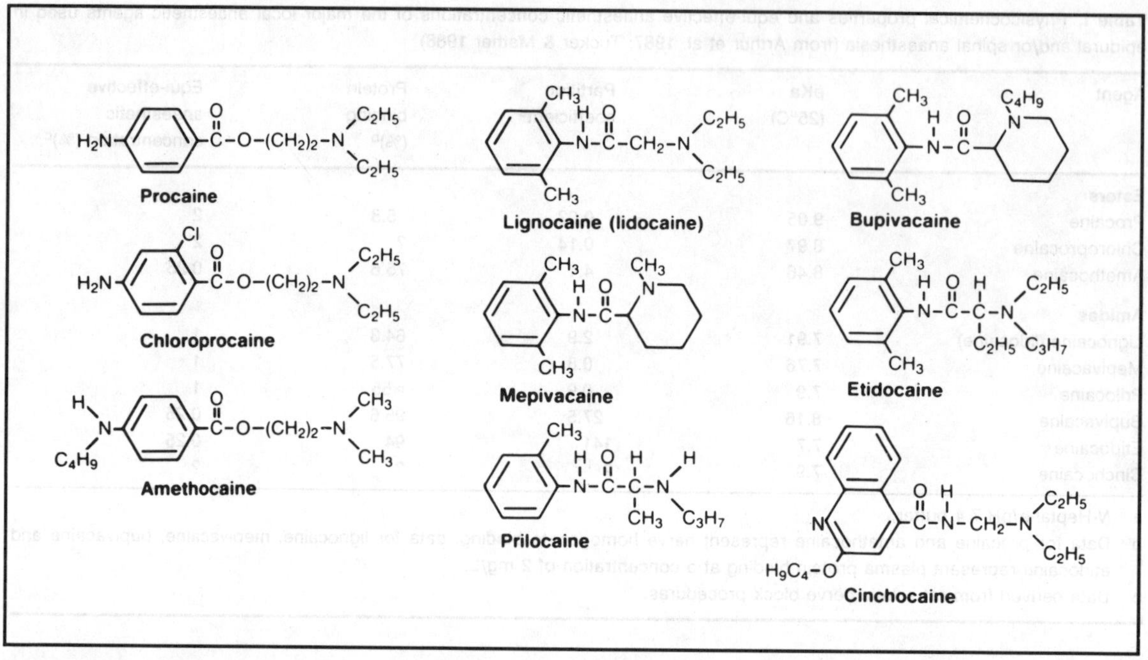

Fig. 1. Chemical structures of the major local anaesthetic agents used in epidural and/or spinal anaesthesia.

margins of analgesia substantiated a dorsal-to-ventral and cranial-to-caudal slanting course. This segmental pattern of onset of analgesia indicates that the initial action involves structures outside the cord (Urban 1973). Spinal cord involvement is indicated by studies of lower limb reflex changes during mid-thoracic epidural anaesthesia (Bromage 1974, 1975), and by observations that fine sensations such as light touch in caudal areas are not conducted past an area of segmental thoracic spinal anaesthesia (Greene 1981). Additional evidence is provided by the observations by Urban (1973) of non-segmental regression of analgesia, although this was not found by others (Forbes & Roizen 1978; Murphy et al. 1976). Electrophysiological studies in monkeys also demonstrated an action on the spinal cord, and furthermore indicated that the primary site of action may vary with the local anaesthetic and the dose (Cusick et al. 1980, 1982).

Electrophysiological studies in man indicated that neural pathways are not completely blocked (Lund et al. 1987a,b,c), but at present the results are difficult to interpret.

2.2 Local Drug Distribution

The segmental spread of epidural and spinal blocks may be expected to depend to a large extent upon the longitudinal distribution of the local anaesthetics within the epidural and subarachnoid spaces. This in turn is largely determined by physical spread, i.e. by bulk flow of solution during and after the injection. Extensive cephalic spread of local anaesthetics via upward CSF flow is unlikely, since their lipophilic properties should promote local uptake (Cousins & Mather 1984).

Once the drug is injected, further distribution to and from the target nerve structures may occur along various pathways.

2.2.1 Longitudinal Spread

Epidurograms, and external counting following injection of local anaesthetic solutions containing radiopaque materials or radioactive markers, indicate that solutions injected into the lumbar epidural space tend to spread more in a cephalic than in a caudal direction (Burn et al. 1973; Nishimura et al. 1959). Nishimura et al. (1959) and other authors (see Bromage 1975) reported a greater tendency towards cephalic spread in older patients, but this was not confirmed by Burn et al. (1973). In the latter study, caudal injection resulted in less extensive cephalic spread. Injection of larger volumes resulted in disproportionately smaller increases in longitudinal spread. The patients' height also affected the physical spread in that, in taller patients, a given volume of solution spread over a smaller number of spinal segments. The position of the patient during the injection and the rate of injection appeared to have little or no effect on the longitudinal spread. Varying degrees of lateral leakage were also observed, depending on the volume injected and, with smaller volumes, the age of the patient.

Following subarachnoid injection, physical spread appeared to vary strongly with the baricity (i.e. the density of the solution divided by the density of CSF) and, with hyperbaric solutions, the position of the patient during and after the injection (Kitahara et al. 1956).

Clinical studies of factors affecting the spread of analgesia are for the most part consistent with observations of the physical spread (Cousins & Bromage 1988; Greene 1985; Tucker & Mather 1988), but physical and analgesic spread are not synonymous and the relationship is not always clear. For detailed consideration of the various factors the reader is referred to other recent texts (Cousins & Bromage 1988; Greene 1985); they are also briefly considered in section 5.

2.2.2 Local Tissue Distribution

Local anaesthetics can enter the spinal roots and cord from the CSF by passive diffusion; deeper penetration of the cord most probably occurs via the spaces of Virchow-Robin (Greene 1983). In addition, spinal cord entry may involve distribution via spinal radicular arteries following uptake from the epidural space or CSF. Distribution via this route is suggested by the similarity in onset time for analgesia after subarachnoid and epidural injection of opioids (Cousins & Mather 1984).

Following epidural administration, local anaesthetics can enter the CSF by passive diffusion through the dura, in particular at the dural root sleeves, and possibly also by retrograde movement via the cyclic vacuolisation in the epithelial cells of arachnoid granulations (Bromage 1978; Cousins & Mather 1984). Another suggested pathway is centripetal spread via the subperineural and subpial spaces following seepage of solution into the paravertebral spaces. However, this is probably of secondary importance (Bromage 1978).

Uptake into extraneural tissues, such as epidural fat, limits the rate and extent of drug distribution to the nerves, and thereby reduces clinical potency. Although epidural fat concentrations are very poorly documented (Cohen 1968; Lebeaux & Tucker, cited in Tucker & Mather 1988), uptake into epidural fat is likely to be much more extensive after epidural than subarachnoid injection. This may largely explain the 5- to 10-fold higher dose requirements for lumbar epidural anaesthesia than for spinal anaesthesia. Uptake into epidural fat may also prolong the duration of blockade by forming a reservoir from which drug is slowly released, so maintaining concentrations in the nerves (Tucker & Mather 1988). Thus, with epidural anaesthesia, extensive uptake followed by slow release may lower the concentration gradient for egress of drug from the nerve. In contrast, during spinal anaesthesia, removal of drug from the subarachnoid space by diffusion through the dura and subsequent uptake into epidural fat helps to lower initial CSF concentrations.

Drug uptake into blood vessels within the spinal cord, as well as in other blood vessels such as the pia mater and epidural veins, interferes with drug distribution and ultimately effectively lowers intraneural drug concentrations. More rapid initial absorption of local anaesthetics following epidural compared with subarachnoid administration (see section 3) also contributes to the higher epidural dose requirements.

The rate and extent of drug distribution to and from the targets in the axonal membranes varies between local anaesthetics, depending upon their physicochemical properties. This has been considered in detail by Tucker and Mather (1988). Good correlations have been found *in vitro* between physicochemical properties (pKa, lipid solubility and protein binding) and the rate of onset of conduction blockade, potency and duration of action of various agents (Covino 1986; Covino & Vassallo 1976). *In vivo*, the relationships are altered by diffusion through non-nervous tissues, extraneural uptake and systemic absorption. The time of clinical onset of analgesia, determined by pin-prick, shows little variation between agents (Covino & Scott 1985). However, onset of motor blockade is slower than that of either sympathetic or sensory blockade, and differences also exist between agents in the rate of onset and the ultimate levels and intensities of motor block, in particular during epidural anaesthesia. For example, for comparable degrees of analgesia, motor block in the legs is considerably more profound with etidocaine after epidural administration than with bupivacaine. Variations in the onset of sensory and motor blockade may be related to differences in their location and slower diffusion into motor fibres, caused by heavy myelinisation and other Schwann cell coverings (Gissen et al. 1980; Wildsmith et al. 1985). The difference in sensory-motor dissociation between bupivacaine and etidocaine may be caused by the slower diffusion of bupivacaine into motor fibres, related to its higher pKa and lower lipid solubility (Gissen et al. 1982). However, the actual mechanism of this so-called differential blockade may be considerably more complex (Raymond & Gissen 1987).

2.2.3 CSF Concentrations

Concentration data providing information about the fate of local anaesthetics within the epidural and subarachnoid space are sparse. Concentration-time profiles have been determined in CSF in humans. However, since CSF was generally collected from a single site in the lumbar region, and because the distribution within CSF is inhomogeneous (Helrich et al. 1950), detailed pharmacokinetic evaluation is impossible.

Peak CSF concentrations about 2 orders of magnitude higher than corresponding blood concentrations, and higher than those needed to produce neural blockade, were reached in 10 to 30 minutes after epidural administration (Lund & Covino 1967; Meyer & Nolte 1978; Wilkinson & Lund 1970). Reported peak CSF concentrations vary between studies. For example, Lund and Covino (1967) reported an average peak CSF concentration of approximately 270 mg/L for lignocaine following epidural injection of a 600mg dose. In the same study, epidural injection of mepivacaine 600mg resulted in significantly higher peak CSF concentrations, which were approximately 400 mg/L on average. However, when lignocaine 300mg and mepivacaine 300mg were administered simultaneously the peak CSF concentrations of these agents were very similar, averaging approximately 150 mg/L after injection of a solution without adrenaline (epinephrine) and 120 mg/L after injection of a solution with adrenaline (Lund & Covino 1967). Simultaneous epidural administration of lignocaine 300mg and prilocaine 300mg also resulted in similar peak CSF concentrations of these agents, which were approximately 175 and 250 mg/L after injection of solutions with and without adrenaline (Lund & Covino 1967). Adrenaline therefore appeared to have inconsistent effects, although differences in the results after injection of solutions with or without that drug were not statistically significant. Large discrepancies exist between the measured CSF concentrations of bupivacaine. Thus, whereas Meyer and Nolte (1978) reported a mean peak CSF concentration of bupivacaine of approximately 240 mg/L following epidural administration of 3.75 mg/kg bupivacaine with adrenaline, Wilkinson and Lund (1970) reported peak concentrations of 30.6 mg/L on average after administration of bupivacaine 150mg with adrenaline. The discrepancy between these studies is difficult to interpret, but may in part be due to differences in the relative positions of the injection and sampling sites. The measured CSF concentrations indicate that local anaesthetics can rapidly penetrate the dura, although the amount that enters the subarachnoid space is probably small because of competing uptake into epidural fat and rapid systemic absorption.

Initial CSF concentrations after subarachnoid administration were much higher than the peak concentrations measured after epidural administration. For example, Lund and Cwik (1965) reported initial CSF concentrations of lignocaine and prilocaine varying from 1600 to 2000 mg/L on average, following subarachnoid injection of doses of 140 to 160mg. Bupivacaine concentrations in CSF, collected 5 minutes after subarachnoid injection of 15mg doses, varied from approximately 150 to 420 mg/L, depending in part upon the baricity of the injected solution (Biscoping 1986; Dennhardt & Konder 1983; Meyer & Nolte 1978). However, CSF concentrations also decreased rapidly due to spread away from the site of injection, tissue uptake and removal from the subarachnoid space (Greene 1981). Although comparison is difficult because sampling is not representative, the higher initial CSF concentrations after subarachnoid administration are consistent with the more rapid onset and the greater intensity of spinal anaesthesia compared with epidural anaesthesia.

2.2.4 *Tissue Concentrations*

The uptake of local anaesthetics into local tissues has been studied in dogs to a limited extent, following epidural injection of lignocaine and mepivacaine (Bromage et al. 1963, 1967) and subarachnoid administration of lignocaine and procaine (Cohen 1968). These studies showed extensive uptake into intradural spinal nerve roots and peripheral zones of the spinal cord, in particular the lateral and posterior columns. However, since concentrations were determined only at a single point in time the data provided no information on the rate of uptake. Although concentrations in various tissues appeared to be similar after both epidural and subarachnoid administration (Bromage 1978), tissue concentration-time profiles are likely to be different, as are the CSF concentration-time profiles and the time courses of blockade. With epidural administration, high concentrations of lignocaine and mepivacaine were also found in extradural spinal nerves, which suggests that these may be involved in epidural block. However, this is currently considered a non-essential feature (Bromage 1975, 1978). Furthermore, concentrations in the cervical region after epidural administration appeared to be lower than those in lower regions. This is in keeping with the time course of the spread of analgesia, as observed clinically, and with studies of the longitudinal physical spread of local anaesthetic solutions within the epidural space. CSF and tissue concentrations in the brain, measured after epidural injection, were small (Bromage et al. 1963).

3. *Systemic Absorption*

Vascular uptake occurs into the epidural veins and blood vessels within the subarachnoid space, in particular in the pia mater and the spinal cord (Bromage 1978; Greene 1983; Tucker & Mather 1988). A significant portion of a subarachnoid dose may be taken up into epidural veins following diffusion across the dura (Greene 1983). Transport to the general circulation occurs predominantly via the azygos collection system which empties into the superior vena cava (Bromage 1978; Tucker & Mather 1988).

The primary factors governing the absorption rate are local blood flow (perfusion) and competing uptake into and binding to local tissues. Diffusion is probably not rate-limiting in view of the lipophilic character of the local anaesthetics.

3.1 Local Blood Flow

The local perfusion during epidural and spinal anaesthesia is subject to modification by the effects of sympathetic blockade, including hypotension, vasodilatation of local blood vessels and, with higher levels of blockade, changes in cardiac output. Local anaesthetics can also alter local perfusion by a direct action on vascular smooth muscle, resulting in either vasoconstriction or vasodilatation, depending upon the local anaesthetic agent, its concentration and stereochemical configuration, the site of injection, the type of blood vessel (capacitance or resistance) and pre-existing vascular tone (Aps & Reynolds 1976, 1978; Blair 1975; Fairley & Reynolds 1981; Johns et al. 1985, 1986; Jorfeldt et al. 1970). Other factors that can influence local perfusion are hypovolaemia, local and systemic effects of added vasoconstrictors, systemic effects of local anaesthetics, effects of systemically administered drugs and cardiovascular changes due to pregnancy or disease, etc. (Cousins & Bromage 1988; Greene 1981).

The net effect on local perfusion is difficult to predict: recent studies of the effects of subarachnoid administration of various local anaesthetics on the spinal cord and spinal dural blood flows in animals have provided confusing results. In several studies administration of lignocaine, mepivacaine and amethocaine (tetracaine) did not produce significant effects on either total or regional spinal cord blood flow in dogs and cats (De Rosayro et al 1983; Dohi et al. 1984, 1987; Porter et al. 1985). However, in other studies in dogs, lignocaine and amethocaine increased both spinal cord and dural blood flows despite marked decreases in the mean arterial blood pressure (Kozody et al. 1985b,c). Changes occurred in particular in the lumbosacral segments, but not in the cervical segments. Decreases of spinal cord and dural blood flows have been observed following subarachnoid injection of bupivacaine in dogs and rats (Crosby 1985; Kozody et al. 1985c); addition of adrenaline to the local anaesthetic solution counteracted the increases in spinal cord and dural blood flow caused by lignocaine and amethocaine (Kozody et al. 1985b,c), but adrenaline had little effect when added to bupivacaine or when injected alone (Dohi et al. 1987; Kozody et al. 1984, 1985a).

In the study of Porter et al. (1985) neither lignocaine nor mepivacaine (with or without adrenaline) altered the total or segmental spinal cord blood flow in cats, but plasma concentrations of both drugs were markedly lower after administration of adrenaline-containing solutions. Confounding factors between the above studies include differences in species, volumes and doses administered, methods used to determine blood flows, times of the observations and administration of general anaesthetics. The consensus may be that whereas spinal cord blood flow tends to be resistant to alteration by local anaesthetics in the dose ranges in common clinical use, blood flow through other local tissue structures may be more readily affected, depending upon the local anaesthetic administered and the dose.

3.2 Tissue Uptake and Binding

In the initial period after injection, uptake of local anaesthetic into local tissues and fluids competes with vascular absorption. Later on, when gross local distribution has been completed, systemic absorption is likely to become directly dependent upon tissue/blood partitioning. Differences in absorption rates of various local anaesthetics can best be explained in terms of differences in the extent of local tissue uptake and binding, related to their physicochemical properties (Tucker & Mather 1988).

3.3 Extent of Absorption

Studies after epidural and subarachnoid administration of lignocaine and bupivacaine in man (Burm 1985; Burm et al. 1987b, 1988b) and subarachnoid administration of lignocaine in monkeys (Denson et al. 1981) showed that at least 95% of the dose ultimately entered the general circulation. This indicates that little or no metabolism occurs within the epidural and subarachnoid spaces. This will probably also be true for the other amide-type and ester-type agents. Even the presence of fresh blood in the CSF, due to a bloody tap, did not appear to result in significant metabolism of procaine (Schmidt 1964).

3.4 Absorption Rates

Absorption rates can be derived from the plasma concentration-time profiles after epidural or subarachnoid administration. However, the greatest caution should be exercised when interpreting or analysing the profiles and flip-flop kinetics should be anticipated (fig. 2). Accurate estimates of the absorption rates require additional data on the systemic disposition.

3.4.1 *Epidural Block*

Determination of the plasma concentration profiles of lignocaine, bupivacaine and etidocaine after both epidural and intravenous administration enabled Tucker and Mather (1975, 1979) to derive the absorption kinetics of these agents in human volunteers. They demonstrated that the absorption following epidural administration is biphasic. With all 3 agents a rapid initial absorption was followed by a much slower second phase. This biphasic absorption pattern was confirmed later by studies using stable isotope methods in surgical patients (Burm 1985; Burm et al. 1987b) [table II]. In these studies a small amount of a deuterium-labelled analogue was administered by rapid intravenous infusion after epidural administration of the unlabelled drug. Data on the systemic disposition were then derived from the plasma concentration-time profiles of the deuterium-labelled analogues, which had been shown previously to have disposition characteristics similar to the unlabelled drugs (Burm et al. 1988a). Subsequently, the data obtained were used to derive the absorption kinetics from the plasma concentration-time profiles of the unlabelled drugs.

The initial absorption rates appeared to be similar for all agents studied, whereas the later absorption rate was much slower for bupivacaine and etidocaine than for lignocaine (table II; fig. 3). The slower absorption of bupivacaine and etidocaine most probably reflects their greater tissue affinity; it is consistent with their longer duration of action and also with the observations of Lebeaux and Tucker (cited in Tucker & Mather 1988) that significant concentrations of etidocaine were still present in epidural fat 12 hours after epidural

Fig. 2. Plasma concentrations of bupivacaine and a deuterium-labelled analogue (bupivacaine-D_3) following epidural injection and intravenous infusion, respectively. In this trial the intravenous infusion (△; bupivacaine-D_3 14mg) was started 15 minutes after the epidural injection (□; bupivacaine 102mg). Note the slower decay of unlabelled drug, indicating that slow absorption rate-limits the elimination following epidural injection (flip-flop kinetics). [Burm et al. 1987b].

Table II. Mean absorption data of lignocaine (lidocaine) and bupivacaine following epidural and subarachnoid injection in premedicated surgical patients (after Burm et al. 1987b, 1988b)

	Epidural		Subarachnoid	
	lignocaine	bupivacaine	lignocaine	bupivacaine
f_1	0.38	0.28		0.35
$t_{½a1}$ (h)	0.16	0.12		0.83[a]
f_2	0.58	0.66	1.03	0.61
$t_{½a2}$ (h)	1.4	6.0[b]	1.2	6.8[c]
$f = f_1 + f_2$	0.96	0.94	1.03	0.96

a Significantly longer than $t_{½a1}$ for epidural bupivacaine ($p < 0.005$).
b Significantly longer than $t_{½a2}$ for epidural lignocaine ($p < 0.001$).
c Significantly longer than $t_{½a2}$ for subarachnoid lignocaine ($p < 0.02$).
Abbreviations: f_1, f_2 = fraction of the dose absorbed in the fast and slow absorption phases, respectively; $t_{½a1}$, $t_{½a2}$ = half-life of the fast and slow absorption phases; f = estimated total fraction of the dose ultimately absorbed into the general circulation.

injection, whereas corresponding lignocaine concentrations were much lower.

Addition of adrenaline to lignocaine and etidocaine solutions resulted in a 40% decrease in the fraction of the dose that was absorbed in the initial rapid phase, but did not significantly alter the absorption rates (Mather et al. 1976a; Tucker & Mather 1975, 1979).

3.4.2 *Subarachnoid Block*

Studies in surgical patients have demonstrated that the initial absorption rate of both lignocaine and bupivacaine was much slower after subarachnoid than after epidural administration (Burm 1985; Burm et al. 1988b) [table II]. In fact, no rapid absorption phase was detected after subarachnoid injection of lignocaine in most patients. The slower initial absorption following subarachnoid compared with epidural administration can be attributed to differences in the vascularities of the respective spaces. The epidural space is rich in epidural veins, draining the neural tissue of the cord, the CSF and the bony spinal canal, which offers the possibility of extensive uptake of local anaesthetic and rapid transport into the general circulation. In comparison, the perfusion of the subarachnoid space, in particular by blood vessels in the pia mater and the spinal cord, is less extensive, and local uptake of drug is therefore likely to be slower. The similarity of the late absorption rates following both methods of administration suggests that late uptake occurs from the same site, probably epidural fat (Tucker 1986).

Studies in monkeys have indicated that neither adrenaline nor phenylephrine altered the absorption kinetics of lignocaine (Denson et al. 1982; 1984c), but comparable data in humans are lacking.

4. *Systemic Disposition*

The distribution and elimination characteristics of intravenously administered lignocaine have been studied extensively, but relatively few studies have been performed with other local anaesthetic agents. These have been reviewed by Tucker and Mather (1979). Representative pharmacokinetic data for the commonly used amide-type local anaesthetics, determined in healthy male volunteers, are presented in table III.

4.1 Distribution and Plasma Binding

Although there is a wide variability in the lipid solubility of both ester-type and amide-type local anaesthetics, it is high enough to make it likely that tissue distribution will be perfusion-limited. The extent of distribution, based on free (unbound) drug concentration (V_{uss}) varies considerably between agents (table III). Distribution volumes based on total concentrations vary less, because the greater tissue affinity of the longer-acting agents is largely offset by a greater degree of plasma binding (see also table I).

At lower concentrations, amide-type agents are bound predominantly to high affinity, low capacity sites on α_1-acid glycoprotein and to a lesser extent to low affinity, high capacity binding sites, possibly on albumin (Denson et al. 1984a; Mather & Thomas 1978; McNamara et al. 1981; Routledge et al. 1980). For drug concentrations in the toxic range (see table IV), protein binding approaches saturation and unbound drug fractions are markedly increased (Denson et al. 1984a; Tucker et al. 1970). α_1-Acid glycoprotein concentrations are increased in the postoperative period, after trauma, in malignancy and in various disease states, and decreased in neonates, in pregnant patients and in women using oral contraceptives (Wood 1986). These changes are likely to be reflected in the degree of protein binding and consequently the apparent volume of distribution at steady-state (V_{ss}). The degree of protein binding also varies with plasma pH (Tucker et al. 1970). However, changes in protein binding should have little effect on V_{uss} or on the free plasma concentrations because only a small fraction of the total amount of drug in the body is bound to plasma proteins and because changes in the free fraction of the local anaesthetic in blood are effectively buffered by the large volume of distribution (Tucker 1986).

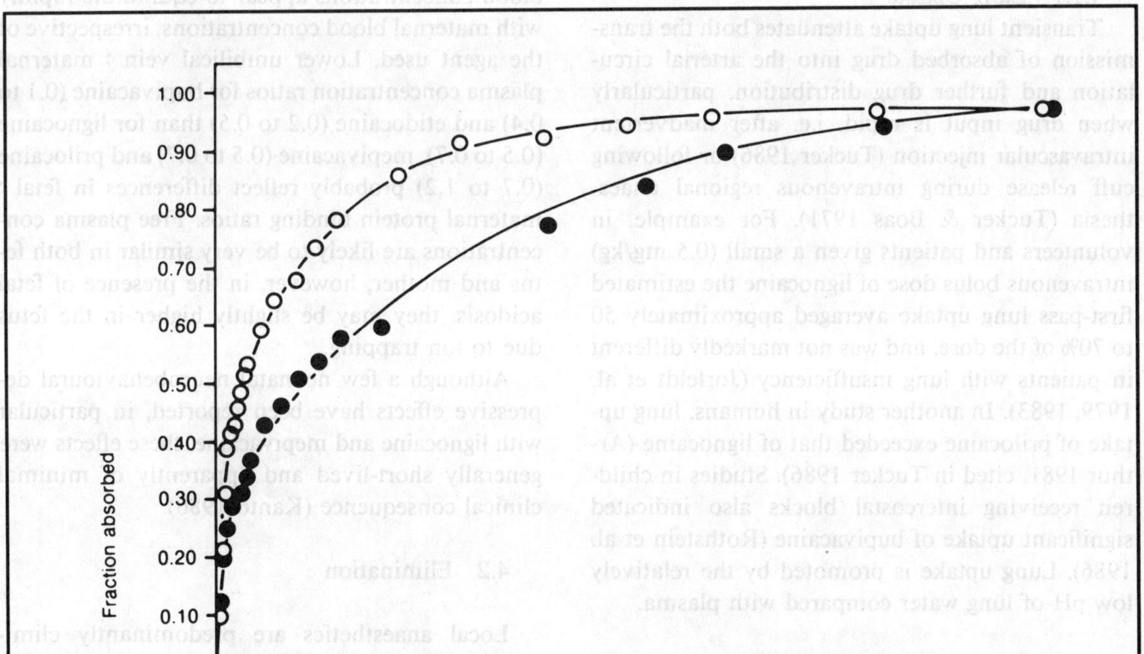

Fig. 3. Fraction of local anaesthetic absorbed into the general circulation as a function of the time after epidural administration in 2 patients. Individual data points represent values, determined by deconvolution; ○ = lignocaine; ● = bupivacaine. The curves through the data points were obtained by non-linear regression (after Burm et al. 1987b).

Table III. Pharmacokinetic variables describing the disposition kinetics of amide-type local anaesthetics in adult males (Tucker & Mather 1988)

Parameter	Prilocaine	Lignocaine	Mepivacaine	Bupivacaine	Etidocaine
λ	1.1	0.8	0.9	0.6	0.6
V_{ss} (L)[a]	191	91	84	73	134
V_{uss} (L)	?	253	382	1028	1478
CL (L/min)[a]	2.37	0.95	0.78	0.58	1.11
E_H	?	0.65	0.52	0.38	0.74
$t_{1/2}$ (h)	1.6	1.6	1.9	2.7	2.7
MBRT (h)	1.3	1.6	1.8	2.1	2.0

a Specified with respect to arterial total blood drug concentrations, with the exception of prilocaine data which are specified with respect to peripheral venous blood drug concentration.

Abbreviations: λ = blood/plasma concentration ratio; V_{ss} = volume of distribution at steady-state; V_{uss} = volume of distribution at steady-state based on unbound drug concentrations in plasma water; CL = mean total body clearance; E_H = estimated hepatic extraction ratio; $t_{1/2}$ = terminal elimination half-life; MBRT = mean body residence time.

4.1.1 Lung Uptake

Transient lung uptake attenuates both the transmission of absorbed drug into the arterial circulation and further drug distribution, particularly when drug input is rapid, i.e. after inadvertent intravascular injection (Tucker 1986) or following cuff release during intravenous regional anaesthesia (Tucker & Boas 1971). For example, in volunteers and patients given a small (0.5 mg/kg) intravenous bolus dose of lignocaine the estimated first-pass lung uptake averaged approximately 50 to 70% of the dose, and was not markedly different in patients with lung insufficiency (Jorfeldt et al. 1979, 1983). In another study in humans, lung uptake of prilocaine exceeded that of lignocaine (Arthur 1981, cited in Tucker 1986). Studies in children receiving intercostal blocks also indicated significant uptake of bupivaçaine (Rothstein et al. 1986). Lung uptake is promoted by the relatively low pH of lung water compared with plasma.

4.1.2 Placental Transfer

Of particular importance to the use of epidural anaesthesia in obstetrics is the transfer of these drugs through the placenta. This aspect has been considered in detail in a recent publication in the Journal (Kanto 1986) and by Tucker (1986). In summary, placental transfer of local anaesthetic agents is likely to be perfusion-limited and fetal blood concentrations appear to equilibrate rapidly with maternal blood concentrations, irrespective of the agent used. Lower umbilical vein : maternal plasma concentration ratios for bupivacaine (0.1 to 0.4) and etidocaine (0.2 to 0.5) than for lignocaine (0.5 to 0.7), mepivacaine (0.5 to 0.7) and prilocaine (0.7 to 1.2) probably reflect differences in fetal : maternal protein binding ratios. Free plasma concentrations are likely to be very similar in both fetus and mother; however, in the presence of fetal acidosis, they may be slightly higher in the fetus due to ion trapping.

Although a few neonatal neurobehavioural depressive effects have been reported, in particular with lignocaine and mepivacaine, these effects were generally short-lived and apparently of minimal clinical consequence (Kanto 1986).

4.2 Elimination

Local anaesthetics are predominantly eliminated by metabolism. The fraction of the dose that is excreted unchanged via the kidneys is generally less than 1 to 6% in adults (Tucker & Mather 1988), but in neonates this fraction is increased 10-fold with both lignocaine and mepivacaine (Kanto 1986; Mihaly et al. 1978; Moore et al. 1978).

Amide-type agents are predominantly cleared in the liver (Tucker et al. 1977b), but prilocaine also undergoes extensive metabolism elsewhere in the body (Arthur et al. 1979). Total blood clearances determined in healthy volunteers varied from 34.8 L/h for bupivacaine up to 142.2 L/h for prilocaine (table III), indicating that the total blood clearance of bupivacaine should be less sensitive to changes in liver blood flow, but more sensitive to changes in enzyme activity and plasma protein binding, than that of the other agents. On the other hand, the free drug clearance, and therefore free drug concentrations, should be less affected by changes in protein binding for bupivacaine than for high-clearance drugs such as etidocaine (Tucker 1988). Elimination half-lives in volunteers ranged from 1.6 to 2.7 hours, and are somewhat longer for bupivacaine and etidocaine than for the other amide-type agents.

Lignocaine clearance is relatively independent of age, weight, gender and race but it is altered by various disease states (Tucker 1986), and elimination half-lives are prolonged 2- to 3-fold in neonates (Kanto 1986). This prolongation is entirely accounted for by a relative increase in the volume of distribution of the drug, but in the case of mepivacaine, whose clearance is reduced to a greater extent than that of lignocaine by a reduction in enzyme activity, the decreased clearance also contributes to the prolonged half-life. Bupivacaine clearance following epidural or subarachnoid administration is reduced by 30 to 40% in elderly patients (Concilus et al. 1988; Veering et al. 1987a,b, 1988).

The impact of various disease states on the pharmacokinetics of lignocaine has been reviewed by Tucker and Mather (1988). Heart failure, hypotension and hypovolaemia are accompanied by marked reduction in clearance. Such reduced clearances are not accompanied by prolonged half-lives, because they are compensated for by concomitant decreases in the volume of distribution.

The clearance of lignocaine is reduced by about 40% in patients with severe liver cirrhosis (Thomson et al. 1973). Chronic hepatitis, in contrast to acute viral hepatitis, is associated with an increased clearance of lignocaine (Huet & Lelorier 1980; Williams et al. 1976). Since the volumes of distribution are also increased in liver disease, the half-life of lignocaine in patients with cirrhosis is markedly prolonged. On the other hand, renal disease appears to have little effect on the disposition of lignocaine (Thomson et al. 1973), and the influence of lung disease is not clear. The influence of disease on the disposition of other amide-type local anaesthetics has not been studied.

Various drugs, including halothane, propranolol, ephedrine and cimetidine, have been shown to alter the clearance of intravenously administered lignocaine (Tucker 1986; Tucker & Mather 1988). The clinical significance of this observation following epidural or subarachnoid administration is, however, not clear (see also section 5.3.6).

Ester-type agents are hydrolysed by cholinesterases in plasma and red cells, and by liver esterases. The clearance of these agents is extremely rapid in healthy subjects. Hydrolysis rates *in vitro* decrease in the order chloroprocaine > procaine > tetracaine (Foldes et al. 1965); half-lives in human plasma, determined *in vitro*, were less than 1 minute for chloroprocaine and procaine and somewhat longer in sera from neonates and patients with liver and kidney disease (Reidenberg et al. 1972). Hydrolysis rates are also reduced in patients with atypical cholinesterases. Ester hydrolysis is inhibited by neostigmine, bupivacaine and etidocaine in clinically relevant concentrations (Lalka et al. 1978; Raj et al. 1980).

The pharmacokinetics of procaine have been studied *in vivo* during and after a 1-hour continuous intravenous infusion (Seifen et al. 1979). In this study both clearance and volume of distribution decreased with increasing dose. Mean clearances were approximately 4.8 L/h/kg with the lower dose rate (1 mg/kg/min) and 2.4 L/h/kg with the higher (1.5 mg/kg/min). Elimination half-lives were 8.3 and 7.1 min, respectively.

4.2.1 Metabolites

The routes of metabolic breakdown of local anaesthetics have been described in detail in a recent publication by Tucker and Mather (1988) and will not be considered here. It is important, however, to realise that some of the metabolic products may retain much of the pharmacological activity of the parent drug and therefore measurement of such metabolites may be valuable, in particular during prolonged administration (Inoue et al. 1985). An example is monoethylglycinexylidide, one of the major metabolites of lignocaine, which has comparable antiarrhythmic and anti-convulsant activity to, and a slightly longer elimination half-life than lignocaine in humans (Tucker & Mather 1988). Metabolites can also be directly responsible for toxicity. For example, hydroxylation of *O*-toluidine, a metabolite of prilocaine, is responsible for the methaemoglobinaemia observed after administration of high doses (> 600mg) of prilocaine. The formation of derivatives of aminobenzoic acid from ester-type agents is responsible for the rare allergic reactions to this group of drugs.

4.3 Effects of Epidural and Spinal Blockade

Cardiovascular changes (including changes in cardiac output and regional blood flow), depending on the level of sympathetic blockade and the systemic effects of absorbed local anaesthetics and vasoconstrictors, may alter the distribution of local anaesthetics during epidural and spinal anaesthesia. Hepatic blood flow may also be decreased, an effect which has been demonstrated following epidural administration of lignocaine in volunteers (Kennedy et al. 1971). Maintenance of fluid balance may attenuate or prevent the effects of sympathetic blockade. For example, in sheep preloaded with adequate volumes of saline, spinal anaesthesia with amethocaine (analgesia level T1 to T6) did not result in significant haemodynamic changes, except for a 10% decrease in hepatic blood flow (Runciman et al. 1984).

Epidural blockade (sensory level T6 to T7) induced with amethocaine in healthy volunteers did not alter the disposition of etidocaine (Tucker & Mather 1975). Similarly, plasma concentration-time profiles of intravenously administered deuterated local anaesthetics in premedicated surgical patients receiving epidural anaesthesia with lignocaine or bupivacaine, or spinal anaesthesia with bupivacine (mean sensory level T8) did not differ significantly from those in volunteers without blockade (Burm et al. 1987b, 1988b). However, comparison of the plasma concentration-time profiles of deuterium-labelled lignocaine in patients receiving spinal blockade (level T5) with those in volunteers demonstrated markedly lower plasma concentrations during and immediately after the infusion (Burm et al. 1988b). This suggests a change in the distribution, possibly related to a more extensive sympathetic blockade in these patients, although transient changes in elimination cannot be ruled out.

5. *Concentration-Time Profiles: Factors Altering the Pharmacokinetics*

Since absorption rates are derived from the plasma or blood concentration-time profiles, examination of the profiles may provide worthwhile information regarding the impact of various factors on the absorption rate. However, since the concentration profiles after epidural or subarachnoid injection are also dependent upon systemic disposition, any change, or even a lack of change, should also be considered in relation to systemic disposition.

5.1 Concentrations Following Single Injections

Peak plasma or blood concentrations of the major local anaesthetic agents, and the times at which these are reached following various routes of administration, have been tabulated and reviewed by Tucker and Mather (1979, 1988). Reported maximum concentrations following epidural administration were generally reached in 10 to 30 minutes, with only marginal differences between agents. These peak concentrations, standardised for dose, varied widely, due in part to differences in sampling site (arterial versus venous) and the fluid analysed (blood or plasma). Typical peak plasma concentrations, measured in the average adult patient following administration of amide-type local anaesthetic, are presented in table IV. Concentrations of ester-type agents have only occasionally been determined. Chloroprocaine concentrations,

Table IV. Peak concentrations of amide-type local anaesthetics following epidural administration, and toxic threshold concentrations (after Mather & Cousins 1979)

Agent	Dose (mg)	C_{max} (mg/L)	C_{tox} (mg/L)	C_{tox}/C_{max}
Lignocaine (lidocaine)	400 (20 ml 2% plain)	3.5	5-6	1.6
	400 (20 ml 2% + Adr.)	2.4		2.3
Prilocaine	400 (20 ml 2% plain)	2.5	7-9	3.2
	400 (20 ml 2% + Adr.)	1.8		4.4
Mepivacaine	400 (20 ml 2% plain)	3.5	5-6	1.6
	400 (20 ml 2% + Adr.)	2.8		2.0
Etidocaine	200 (20 ml 1% plain)	0.8	≈2	2.5
	200 (20 ml 0.5% + Adr.)	0.6		3.3
Bupivacaine	100 (20 ml 1% plain)	0.8	≈1.6	2.0
	100 (20 ml 0.5% + Adr.)	0.6		2.7

Abbreviations: C_{max} = peak plasma drug concentration; C_{tox} = toxic threshold concentration; Adr. = adrenaline.

measured after epidural injection in obstetric patients for vaginal delivery (dose 468 ± 284mg) or caesarean section (dose 948 ± 347mg) were very low (< 0.1 mg/L) and decreased rapidly to undetectable levels (Kuhnert et al. 1980). Maximum concentrations after subarachnoid block are usually attained in 60 to 120 minutes, reflecting the slower initial absorption rate. With doses within the clinical range, peak plasma concentrations of lignocaine and bupivacaine are generally less than 1 and 0.1 mg/L, respectively (Axelsson & Widman 1981; Axelsson et al. 1986; Burm et al. 1983, 1987a; Giasi et al. 1979; Kuhnert et al. 1987b; Veering et al. 1988).

5.2 Concentrations During Continuous Epidural Anaesthesia

Concentration-time profiles during and after short-term intermittent epidural injections of lignocaine and etidocaine have been predicted from pharmacokinetic data obtained after single injections (Tucker & Mather 1975). These predictions indicated that systemic accumulation tends to be faster with the shorter-acting agents than with the longer-acting drugs. Concentration profiles measured in patients were fairly consistent with these predictions (Tucker & Mather 1979; Tucker et al. 1977a). Other studies indicate that systemic concentrations of the shorter-acting agents may rapidly approach the toxic threshold during prolonged surgical epidural anaesthesia (Moore et al. 1968; Takasaki et al. 1987). Systemic accumulation may be reduced by giving smaller 'top-up' doses at appropriate intervals, which should, however, not be too long in order to avoid marked regression (more than 1 or 2 dermatomes) between injections, which may result in tachyphylaxis (Cousins & Bromage 1988).

Long term epidural infusions of bupivacaine for prevention or relief of postoperative pain have been shown to result in prolonged and more extensive accumulation (Renck et al. 1976; Ross et al. 1980). The progressively increasing plasma concentrations probably reflect changes in plasma protein binding, related to increased levels of α_1-acid glycoprotein after surgery, so that elevated total plasma concentrations are probably not accompanied by similar elevations of the more important free drug concentrations (Tucker 1986). This may explain why serious toxic reactions did not occur in the study of Ross et al. (1980), even though total bupivacaine concentrations exceeded 3 mg/L in most patients after infusion for 44 hours.

Whereas the longer-acting agents bupivacaine and etidocaine demonstrate a lesser tendency to accumulate into the systemic circulation, predictions indicate that local accumulation of these agents may be more extensive despite longer dosing intervals (Tucker & Mather 1975). The clinical significance of this, however, is not clear.

5.3 Factors with Possible Effect

This section considers the impact of factors such as the site of injection, dose, patient characteristics, etc., on the time course of epidural and spinal blockade, and on the pharmacokinetics of the agents used.

5.3.1 Site of Injection

Plasma concentrations were comparable when measured after cervical, thoracic and lumbar epidural injections of a standard dose of lignocaine 200mg (Mayumi et al. 1983), indicating that absorption rates from these regions are similar. However, in clinical practice the doses required for cervical and thoracic epidural anaesthesia are generally smaller than those needed for lumbar epidural anaesthesia (Bromage 1978), and consequently higher concentrations should be anticipated after lumbar injection. Concentrations after caudal injection generally exceed those after lumbar administration, both because of the higher dose requirements and because the absorption from the caudal epidural space is faster, as has been demonstrated with mepivacaine and etidocaine (Lund et al. 1975; Tucker et al. 1972), but not with lignocaine (Mazze & Dunbar 1966). Injection in the thoracic or cervical region is rarely, if ever, used for spinal anaesthesia.

5.3.2 Dose and Concentration

Although the injection of larger volumes may result in a more extensive analgesic spread (Erdemir et al. 1965), the total dosage is probably a more important determinant of the spread of epidural and spinal anaesthesia than either the volume or concentration of local anaesthetic in the solution (Bromage 1962, 1978; Sheskey et al. 1983). Within the clinically useful dose range, increases in the dose generally result in disproportionately smaller increases in the number of blocked segments (Grundy et al. 1978; Park et al. 1982; Sheskey et al. 1983), and will, within limits, also speed the onset, enhance the intensity and prolong the duration of anaesthesia (Bridenbaugh et al. 1973; Buckley et al. 1978; Crawford 1964; Littlewood et al. 1979; Lund et al. 1973; Park et al. 1982; Scott et al. 1980; Sheskey et al. 1983).

Plasma concentrations are, within limits, independent of the concentration of the local anaesthetic in the solution and proportional to the dose (Lund et al. 1975; Scott et al. 1972; Van Kleef 1981). However, with fixed doses, caudal administration of more concentrated (2% *vs* 1%) mepivacaine solutions (Tucker et al. 1972) and lumbar epidural injection of more concentrated (1.5% *vs* 1%) etidocaine solutions (Lund et al. 1973, 1975) have been shown to result in higher plasma concentrations. Also, although peak etidocaine concentrations appeared to be proportional to the amount administered up to a dose of 300mg, further dose increments resulted in disproportionately larger increases in the plasma concentrations (Lund et al. 1975). The higher plasma concentrations with the more concentrated mepivacaine solutions and the disproportionate increases with higher etidocaine doses are thought to reflect a higher rate of absorption, due to saturation of local binding sites and/or greater vasodilatation (Lund et al. 1975; Tucker & Mather 1988).

The effects of dose and concentration on plasma concentrations after subarachnoid injection have not been studied extensively in humans, but in monkeys the absorption rate of lignocaine was independent of the concentration (Denson et al. 1983).

5.3.3 Rate of Injection

Increases in the rate of injection have minimal influence on the longitudinal physical or analgesic spread (Cousins & Bromage 1988; Greene 1985) or on plasma concentrations following epidural injection (Rosenberg et al. 1981; Scott et al. 1972).

5.3.4 Alkalisation and Carbonation

To speed the onset of epidural blockade some anaesthesiologists alkalise the acidic (pH 2.8 to 6.5; Moore 1981) local anaesthetic solutions, thereby increasing the fraction of un-ionised diffusible drug. However, although some authors reported a faster onset of action with lignocaine and bupivacaine (DiFazio et al. 1976; McMorland et al. 1986), others have noted disappointing results with chloroprocaine (Glosten et al. 1987; Ross et al. 1987).

Some investigators have reported that administration of carbonated solutions of lignocaine and prilocaine instead of the usual hydrochloride salt solutions produced earlier onset and improved the quality of the epidural block to a clinically useful degree, possibly by decreasing the intraneural pH and thereby increasing the fraction of active ionised drug (Bromage et al. 1967; Cousins & Bromage 1971). These observations, obtained from open studies, were confirmed later by a double-blind study (Nickel et al. 1986), although other double-blind studies only partially confirmed the improved quality, and did not corroborate the faster onset (Cole et al. 1985; Martin et al. 1981; Morison 1981). Carbonated bupivacaine solutions have no advantages over hydrochloride salt solutions (Brown et al. 1980a).

Alkalisation of lignocaine solutions did not alter the plasma concentrations achieved (DiFazio et al. 1986). Carbonation resulted in higher initial plasma concentrations, but did not significantly alter the peak concentrations of lignocaine or bupivacaine (Appleyard et al. 1974; Cousins & Bromage 1971). This suggests that carbonation results in a transient increase of the initial absorption rate, possibly by the vasodilatory effect of carbon dioxide and/or by increasing the fraction of un-ionised drug.

5.3.5 *Combining Local Anaesthetics*

Combinations of local anaesthetics, such as chloroprocaine plus bupivacaine or lignocaine plus bupivacaine, have been used with the objective of improvement in rapidity of onset combined with increased duration of blockade. However, the gains (if any) are small and the rationale for using combinations is questionable (Cousins & Bromage 1988; Seow et al. 1982).

When normalised for individual doses, blood concentrations of lignocaine and bupivacaine were similar after injection of a combination of the two agents and after injection of each drug alone (Seow et al. 1982). Since bupivacaine inhibits the hydrolysis of chloroprocaine, blood or plasma concentrations of the latter agent may be increased when a combination of these drugs is administered (Lalka et al. 1978; Raj et al. 1980).

5.3.6 *Additives*

Adrenaline and Phenylephrine

A vasoconstrictor, most commonly adrenaline, is often added to local anaesthetic solutions to slow the systemic absorption rate and thus prolong the duration of action. These agents may also modify the time course of blockade by interaction with adrenergic inhibitory systems in the spinal cord (Collins et al. 1981, 1983; Kraynack et al. 1983).

The addition of adrenaline may also enhance the intensity of epidural blocks, in particular motor blockade. This effect has been observed with lignocaine, bupivacaine and etidocaine (Bromage et al. 1964; Burm 1985; Murphy et al. 1976). Furthermore, it may speed the onset of action; this has been demonstrated with dilute solutions of bupivacaine (Eisenach et al. 1987) and with etidocaine (Murphy et al. 1976), although others have observed a slowing of the onset with lignocaine (Bromage et al. 1964).

Studies on the effect of adrenaline on the duration of epidural blockade have yielded variable results. In general, the addition of adrenaline (usually 5 μg/ml, but smaller amounts are used in obstetrics) prolonged the duration of epidural anaesthesia to a greater extent with lignocaine and mepivacaine than with prilocaine; comparatively little prolongation was noted with bupivacaine and etidocaine (Abboud et al. 1984, 1985, 1987; Abdel-Salam et al. 1975; Bridenbaugh et al. 1974; Bromage et al. 1964; Buckley et al. 1978; Burm 1985; Covino 1986; Littlewood et al. 1979; Murphy et al. 1976; Sinclair & Scott 1984). The effect of adrenaline may be greater when lower doses of local anaesthetics are administered (Covino 1986; Littlewood et al. 1979).

The effects of adrenaline on the duration of spinal anaesthesia also varied markedly between studies. Overall, it appears to prolong the duration of spinal blockade more consistently and to a greater extent when administered with amethocaine (Armstrong et al. 1983; Concepcion et al.

1984; Moore 1980; Park et al. 1975) than with lignocaine or bupivacaine (Burm 1985; Chambers et al. 1981, 1982; Leicht & Carlson 1986; Moore 1980; Moore et al. 1987; Racle et al. 1987a, 1988a; Spivey 1985).

Addition of phenylephrine increased the duration of spinal anaesthesia with amethocaine and lignocaine at least as much as addition of adrenaline (Armstrong et al. 1983; Concepcion et al. 1984; Leicht & Carlson 1986).

The addition of adrenaline has been shown to reduce peak plasma drug concentrations following epidural administration, but the effect varies with the type and dose of local anaesthetic (Braid & Scott 1965; Scott et al. 1972). Estimates vary widely, but indicate that with higher epidural doses, peak concentrations may be reduced on average by 30 to 40% with lignocaine and prilocaine, and 20 to 30% with mepivacaine, bupivacaine and etidocaine (Abdel-Salam et al. 1975; Appleyard et al. 1974; Braid & Scott 1965, 1966; Bridenbaugh et al. 1974; Burm et al. 1986; Laishley et al. 1988; Lund & Cwik 1966; Lund et al. 1975; Mather et al. 1976a; Matthes & Schabert 1966; Scott et al. 1972; Tucker et al. 1972; Wilkinson & Lund 1970). The increased effect with the shorter-acting agents is consistent with the greater prolongation of the duration of blockade, and is often attributed to a less extensive uptake into local tissues. Differences in vasoactive properties may also contribute to the diversity of the effects of adrenaline with various agents. Since the vasoactive properties vary with the dose, a smaller reduction by adrenaline of the absorption of the local anaesthetic may be seen with lower doses, as has been demonstrated with prilocaine (Braid & Scott 1966). Addition of adrenaline to a concentration of 5 μg/ml is often considered optimal in that it effectively reduces the peak plasma concentration while avoiding excessive systemic effects of adrenaline (Braid & Scott 1966; Scott et al. 1972). However, a recent study showed that the reduction of lignocaine concentrations is independent of the concentration of adrenaline in the range 1.7 to 5 μg/ml (Ohno et al. 1988). The above studies indicate that adrenaline has little or no effect on the time at which the peak concentrations are reached, although some authors reported a small prolongation. Phenylephrine 50 μg/ml was less effective than adrenaline 5 μg/ml in reducing the plasma concentrations of lignocaine (Stanton Hicks et al. 1973).

The effect of adrenaline on plasma concentrations after subarachnoid administration has been poorly investigated. Recent studies indicate that addition of adrenaline to hyperbaric lignocaine solutions reduces the peak concentrations by 30 to 50%, without altering the time to peak (Axelsson & Widman 1981; Burm et al. 1987a). Addition to hyperbaric bupivacaine solutions did not significantly alter the plasma concentration profiles (Burm et al. 1987a).

Clonidine

In a recent study by Racle et al. (1987a), the addition of clonidine prolonged the duration of spinal anaesthesia with bupivacaine to a greater extent than addition of adrenaline. This effect was considered to be related to an interaction of clonidine with the adrenergic inhibitory systems rather than to alteration of the local perfusion. The effects of clonidine on the plasma concentrations have not been investigated.

5.3.7 Baricity

Hyperbaric solutions containing glucose tend to spread further within the subarachnoid space than isobaric solutions, unless the patient is maintained in the sitting position for several minutes after injection (Brown et al. 1980b; Wildsmith et al. 1981). Other recent studies indicate that the quality of motor block may be poorer and the duration of action shorter with hyperbaric than with isobaric solutions (Axelsson et al. 1985; Möller et al. 1984).

Peak plasma concentrations of bupivacaine were attained later after injection of an isobaric solution than after a hyperbaric solution (Axelsson et al. 1986; Burm et al. 1983). Studies by Veering et al. (1987b, 1988) showed a similar tendency in younger but not in older patients. In contrast, the addition of glucose appeared to decrease the absorption rate of lignocaine in monkeys (Denson et al. 1983).

5.3.8 Patient Characteristics

Weight and Height

In general, the weight of the patient appears to have little or no effect on the spread of epidural or spinal anaesthesia (Cousins & Bromage 1988; Greene 1985) or on the plasma concentrations reached (Moore et al. 1976; Scott et al. 1972; Tucker et al. 1972). However, the epidural and spinal doses required to block a given number of spinal segments are likely to be somewhat higher in taller patients (Bromage 1978; Greene 1985). Nevertheless, correlations between plasma concentrations and the height of the patient after the administration of a fixed dose of mepivacaine were poor (Moore et al. 1976; Tucker et al. 1972).

Age

Various studies on the effects of ageing on the spread of epidural analgesia have demonstrated an enhanced spread and/or reduced dose requirements in patients older than 40 to 50 years compared with younger patients (Bromage 1969; Finucane et al. 1987; Grundy et al. 1978; Park et al. 1980, 1982; Sharrock 1978; Veering et al. 1987a). Analgesic spread has also been noted to be more extensive in older patients after subarachnoid injection (Bengtsson et al. 1983; Cameron et al. 1981; Freund et al. 1984; Pitkänen et al. 1984; Racle et al. 1988b; Veering et al. 1987b, 1988), although others reported no effect (Tuominen et al. 1987), and age did not show consistent effects on either the onset or the duration of analgesia.

The increased spread of analgesia is often attributed to a greater longitudinal spread of the solution. However, this has not been observed consistently in all studies on the physical spread (Burn et al. 1973; Cousins & Bromage 1988). Other pharmacokinetic and/or pharmacodynamic factors may also be responsible for, or contribute to, the observed effects of age.

Peak plasma concentrations after caudal or lumbar epidural administration of lignocaine and bupivacaine showed no correlation with age (Bowdle et al. 1986; Finucane et al. 1987; Freund et al. 1984; Veering et al. 1987a). Although Finucane et al. (1987) reported that peak concentrations were reached sooner in older patients, this effect was not observed by the other investigators. Terminal half-lives of lignocaine (Bowdle et al. 1986) and bupivacaine (Veering et al. 1987a) were 10 and 30% longer in elderly patients than in the young, respectively, and clearance of both lignocaine and bupivacaine was also reduced by 30 and 40%, respectively (fig. 4). The prolonged half-lives could indicate a slowing of the late absorption phase, but may also reflect changes in the systemic disposition, since the prolonged half-life of bupivacaine, observed by Veering et al. (1987a), was not accompanied by a longer duration of action. A decreased clearance of bupivacaine in elderly patients has also been observed during prolonged continuous epidural infusions (Concilus et al. 1988).

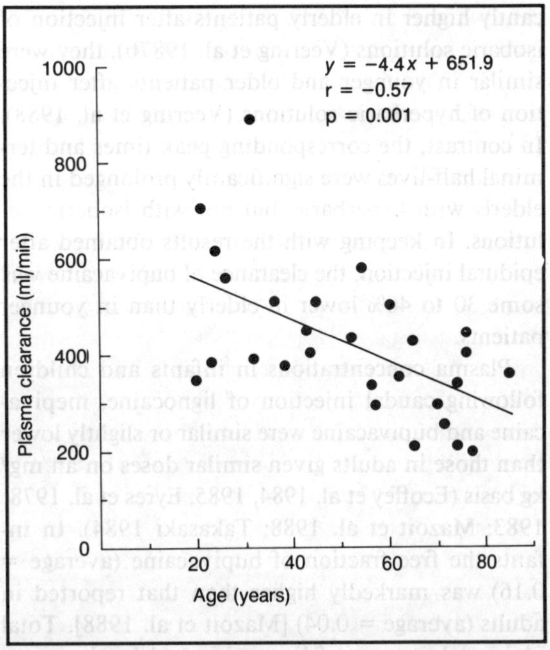

Fig. 4. Total plasma clearance of bupivacaine, determined after epidural injection, *versus* age (reprinted, with permission from the International Anesthesia Research Society, from Veering et al. 1987a).

Studies of the effects of age on the plasma concentration profiles after subarachnoid injection of bupivacaine yielded puzzling results in that, whereas peak plasma concentrations were significantly higher in elderly patients after injection of isobaric solutions (Veering et al. 1987b), they were similar in younger and older patients after injection of hyperbaric solutions (Veering et al. 1988). In contrast, the corresponding peak times and terminal half-lives were significantly prolonged in the elderly with hyperbaric, but not with isobaric, solutions. In keeping with the results obtained after epidural injection, the clearance of bupivacaine was some 30 to 40% lower in elderly than in younger patients.

Plasma concentrations in infants and children following caudal injection of lignocaine, mepivacaine and bupivacaine were similar or slightly lower than those in adults given similar doses on an mg/kg basis (Ecoffey et al. 1984, 1985; Eyres et al. 1978, 1983; Mazoit et al. 1988; Takasaki 1984). In infants the free fraction of bupivacaine (average = 0.16) was markedly higher than that reported in adults (average = 0.04) [Mazoit et al. 1988]. Total plasma clearances of lignocaine and bupivacaine, standardised for bodyweight, were slightly higher and terminal half-lives were similar to those in adults. The volumes of distribution, based on total plasma concentrations, were claimed to be markedly increased in both children and infants (Ecoffey et al. 1984, 1985; Mazoit et al. 1988). However, accurate determination of volume of distribution following caudal injection is not possible.

5.3.9 *Pregnancy*

Epidural (and probably spinal) dose requirements are reduced in pregnant women, possibly due to a greater sensitivity and/or enhanced diffusion, related to hormonal changes (Datta et al. 1983; Flanagan et al. 1987). Plasma concentrations of etidocaine in women in labour have been shown to be similar to those in non-pregnant women given a similar dose (Morgan et al. 1977).

5.3.10 *Disease*

The impact of disease states on the time course of epidural or spinal anaesthesia or on the plasma concentration-time profiles is not clear. Extrapolation of the findings after intravenous administration (see section 4.2) is difficult because of potentially compensating effects on the systemic absorption and the effects of sympathetic blockade. However, in patients with severely depressed hepatic function such as cirrhosis, prolonged and more extensive systemic accumulation is to be expected during intermittent epidural injection or continuous epidural infusion (Tucker & Mather 1988), and caution is required when using local anaesthetics in such patients.

5.3.11 *Drug Interactions*

Most of the current knowledge on the effects of systemically administered drugs on the pharmacokinetics of local anaesthetics has been derived from studies after intravenous administration. However, extrapolation to the situation during epidural or spinal anaesthesia is difficult, because the effect on the plasma concentration-time profiles may be offset by concomitant changes in the absorption and/or by predominant effects of sympathetic blockade. For example, pretreatment with cimetidine has been shown to reduce the plasma clearance and prolong the half-life of bupivacaine after intravenous administration (Noble et al. 1987), but did not alter the plasma concentration-time profile following epidural administration (Kuhnert et al. 1987a; O'Sullivan et al. 1988). Cimetidine increased the peak plasma concentration of lignocaine after epidural administration in 1 study (Dailey et al. 1985), but not in another (Webb & Ward 1983), although it prolonged the half-life of lignocaine in the latter study. Ranitidine did not significantly alter the plasma concentrations of epidurally administered lignocaine (Dailey et al. 1985) or bupivacaine (O'Sullivan et al. 1988). Intravenous injection of ephedrine has been shown to increase the clearance of lignocaine (Wiklund et al. 1977), but may also promote the absorption from the epidural space (Mather et al. 1976b).

Drugs that reduce the hepatic clearance of local anaesthetics mainly by enzyme inhibition, such as propranolol (Bax et al. 1985; Bowdle et al. 1987; Tucker et al. 1984), may be expected to result in more extensive systemic accumulation of local anaesthetics; however, controlled studies to confirm this expectation are lacking.

Many drugs have been shown to alter the degree of plasma protein binding *in vitro* (Denson 1987). The clinical significance of these findings, however, is questionable, because many studies were done with high, supratherapeutic concentrations, and because increased free drug fractions are not necessarily accompanied by increased free drug concentrations (Tucker 1986).

6. Central Nervous System and Cardiovascular Toxicity

Toxic effects associated with high blood concentrations can often be attributed to inadvertent intravascular injection, administration of excessive doses, or accumulation of local anaesthetic. With lignocaine, accumulation of metabolites, in particular monoethylglycinexylidide, may contribute to the toxicity during continuous epidural blockade. Intravascular injection of a full epidural dose will almost certainly result in toxicity. With the lower doses used in spinal anaesthesia, however, systemic toxicity is not a concern. Adverse effects of local anaesthetics, including systemic toxicity, have been reviewed by Reynolds (1987).

When toxicity develops slowly (as, for example, with gradually increasing plasma concentrations), mild effects such as circumoral and tongue numbness (not a CNS effect) or subjective and objective CNS effects such as lightheadedness, tinnitus, visual disturbances and slurred speech, usually precede severe CNS effects like unconsciousness, convulsions, coma and respiratory arrest (Scott 1975, 1986), which occur at higher concentrations. It should be emphasised, however, that in patients premedicated with anticonvulsant sedatives such as barbiturates or benzodiazepines, CNS toxicity may be masked (Reynolds 1987). In general, the cardiovascular system (CVS) appears to be more resistant to the toxic effects of local anaesthetics than the central nervous system. Blood levels associated with significant cardiovascular toxicity are higher than those associated with convulsions. However, the CVS : CNS toxicity ratio is likely to be smaller with bupivacaine than with lignocaine, as has been demonstrated in sheep (Kotelko et al. 1984). When plasma concentrations change abruptly, e.g. after rapid inadvertent intravascular injection of a full epidural dose, severe CNS and CVS effects may occur quickly without early warning signs.

6.1 Threshold Concentrations and Margin of Safety

Conservative estimates of the threshold blood drug concentrations associated with mild CNS effects in adults vary from 1.6 mg/L for bupivacaine up to 7 to 9 mg/L for prilocaine (table IV).

Estimates of the ratios of the toxic threshold concentration and average peak concentration (C_{tox} : C_{max}) measured after epidural injection of equivalent doses of plain local anaesthetic solutions range from 1.6 for lignocaine and mepivacaine up to 3.2 for prilocaine. When adrenaline is added to the solutions, estimated C_{tox} : C_{max} ratios are higher, varying from 2.0 for mepivacaine up to 4.4 for prilocaine (reflecting the slowing of the absorption by adrenaline and the lower C_{max} values) [Mather & Cousins 1984], but comparable data are not available for the ester-type agents. In 1 patient a total plasma concentration of 17 mg/L of chloroprocaine was measured following an apparent inadvertent intravenous injection which was not associated with systemic toxicity (Gross et al. 1981). In general, the much more rapid elimination of the ester-type agents compared with the amide types is an advantage, in particular during prolonged epidural anaesthesia. However, when plasma cholinesterase levels are low due to genetic variations, systemic toxicity cannot be excluded, even with correct administration of normal epidural doses of chloroprocaine (Smith et al. 1987).

6.2 Effect of Plasma Binding

Toxic effects are likely to be more closely related to free (unbound) plasma concentrations than to total blood or plasma concentrations (Denson et al. 1984b; Pieper et al. 1980). It should be emphasised, however, that the degree of protein binding is of only minor significance in controlling access of drug to the sites of toxicity, as explained by Tucker (1986). Thus, when drug input is gradual, changes in plasma protein binding probably have little influence on free drug concentrations, because they are effectively buffered by redistribution and, in some cases, clearance (Tucker 1988). Further, when drug input is rapid, such as after intravascular injection of a full epidural dose, plasma protein binding approaches saturation and a large proportion of the drug will be unbound (Tucker et al. 1970). Experiments with lignocaine and bupivacaine in rats have also indicated that binding to α_1-acid glycoprotein is rapidly reversible, so that uptake into the brain is not limited to the free drug (Pardridge et al. 1983; Terasaki et al. 1986). Consequently, massive first-pass extraction of toxic amounts of drug into the organs is to be expected after inadvertent intravascular injection.

6.3 Influence of Acid-Base Balance

The toxicity of local anaesthetics is closely related to acid-base status. In cats, toxicity was increased by acidosis and decreased by alkalosis (Englesson 1974; Englesson & Grevsten 1974), possibly through alteration of the fraction of ionised drug in brain cells. Changes in acid-base status due to metabolic and respiratory acidosis may also alter the uptake and egress of local anaesthetic into and from the brain and heart, but the effect depends on whether tissue acidosis is generated within these tissues or elsewhere. Simon et al. (1982, 1984) showed that brain uptake and brain blood partitioning of lignocaine was increased during drug-induced convulsions. In contrast, in sheep in which general systemic acidosis was induced, the uptake of lignocaine and bupivacaine in the heart (as expressed by the tissue/blood partition coefficient) decreased, as did the uptake of bupivacaine, but not lignocaine, in the brain (Nancarrow et al. 1987). In these studies tissue/blood partition coefficients were increased despite decreases in plasma protein binding.

6.4 Dose Limitations

Recommended maximum single doses of the local anaesthetics have been tabulated (Covino 1988). The recommended maximum doses for single epidural administration of the amide-type agents vary from 225mg for bupivacaine up to 600mg for prilocaine (solutions with adrenaline). The corresponding dose for chloroprocaine is 1000mg. These doses should, however, be interpreted in the light of the anaesthetist's experience, since their inadvertent injection is guaranteed to produce systemic toxicity. Therefore, slow injection or fractionated administration, in addition to other safety guidelines, is recommended, especially for inexperienced anaesthetists.

The recommended maximum doses for subarachnoid injection are 10mg for cinchocaine, 20mg for bupivacaine and amethocaine, and 100mg for lignocaine and mepivacaine (Covino 1988). Exceeding these doses may result in excessive spinal anaesthesia. Inadvertent intravascular injection should not normally result in overt toxicity.

7. *Conclusions and Perspectives*

Despite very extensive clinical experience, knowledge of the regional distribution of local anaesthetic drugs is fragmentary and to a large extent theoretical in nature.

Because of the small dose requirements systemic toxicity is not a concern with spinal anaesthesia. However, the safety margin is relatively small with epidural anaesthesia.

Of the amide-type agents, prilocaine has the most favourable pharmacokinetic characteristics and the widest safety margin. Yet it is infrequently used in epidural anaesthesia, probably because of its capacity to produce methaemoglobinaemia. However, with single doses (up to 600mg) this should not be a problem, although the drug is better avoided in obstetrics.

Ester-type agents have a distinct kinetic advantage over amide-type agents because they are rapidly eliminated. In the case of chloroprocaine, rapid elimination may assist tissue redistribution in lowering blood concentrations after an inadvertent intravascular injection, so that a possible toxic reaction is likely to be short-lived in healthy subjects. Furthermore, a high clearance limits the extent of systemic accumulation during intermittent administration.

An aspect which has not been considered is the stereoselectivity of the local anaesthetic agents. It has been known for many years that the enantiomers of mepivacaine, prilocaine, bupivacaine and etidocaine differ in their vasoactivity, absorption characteristics and *in vivo* anaesthetic potency and toxicity (Åberg 1972; Åkerman et al. 1966). Recent studies with mepivacaine in sheep have demonstrated considerable differences in the hepatic extraction and mean total body clearance of the enantiomers of mepivacaine (Runciman et al. 1984). In the absence of analytical methods capable of discriminating between the enantiomers, pharmacokinetic studies of these enantiomers following administration of racemic mixtures in humans have not been feasible. Recent developments in analytical chemistry, however, now make it possible to study the pharmacokinetics of individual enantiomers in humans.

Acknowledgements

The author would like to thank Professor J.G. Bovill, MD, PhD, FFARCSI; P.J. Hennis, MD, PhD; B.Th. Veering, MD; and Professor Joh. Spierdijk, MD, PhD, FFARCS (Hon.), for their encouragement and for reading and correcting parts of the text. The secretarial assistance of Mrs M.P.M. Toelen is gratefully acknowledged.

References

Abboud TK, David S, Nagappala S, Costandi J, Yanagi T, et al. Maternal, fetal and neonatal effects of lidocaine with and without epinephrine for epidural anesthesia in obstetrics. Anesthesia and Analgesia 63: 973-979, 1984

Abboud TK, DerSarkissian L, Terrasi J, Murakawa K, Zhu J, et al. Comparative maternal, fetal and neonatal effects of chloroprocaine with and without epinephrine for epidural anesthesia in obstetrics. Anesthesia and Analgesia 66: 71-75, 1987

Abboud TK, Sheikh-ol-Eslam A, Yanagi T, Murakawa M, Costandi J, et al. Safety and efficacy of epinephrine added to bupivacaine for lumbar epidural anesthesia in obstetrics. Anesthesia and Analgesia 63: 585-591, 1985

Abdel-Salam AR, Vonwiller JB, Scott DB. Evaluation of etidocaine in extradural block. British Journal of Anaesthesia 47: 1081-1086, 1975

Åberg G. Toxicological and local anaesthetic effects of optically active isomers of 2 local anaesthetic compounds. Acta Pharmacologica et Toxicologica 31: 273-286, 1972

Åkerman B, Astrom A, Ross S, Telc A. Studies on the absorption, distribution and metabolism of labelled prilocaine and lidocaine in some animal species. Acta Pharmacologica et Toxicologica 24: 389-403, 1966

Appleyard TN, Witt A, Atkinson RE, Nicholas ADG. Bupivacaine carbonate and bupivacaine hydrochloride: a comparison of blood concentrations during epidural blockade for vaginal surgery. British Journal of Anaesthesia 46: 530-533, 1974

Aps C, Reynolds F. The effect of concentration on vasoactivity of bupivacaine and lignocaine. British Journal of Anaesthesia 48: 1171-1174, 1976

Aps C, Reynolds F. An intradermal study of the local anaesthetic and vascular effects of the isomers of bupivacaine. British Journal of Clinical Pharmacology 6: 63-68, 1978

Armstrong IR, Littlewood DG, Chambers WA. Spinal anesthesia with tetracaine – effect of added vasoconstrictors. Anesthesia and Analgesia 62: 793-795, 1983

Arthur GR, Scott DHT, Boyes RN, Scott DB. Pharmacokinetic and clinical pharmacological studies with mepivacaine and prilocaine. British Journal of Anaesthesia 51: 481-485, 1979

Arthur GR, Wildsmith JAW, Tucker GT. Pharmacology of local anaesthetic drugs. In Wildsmith & Armitage (Eds) Principles and practice of regional anaesthesia, pp. 22-36, Churchill Livingstone, Edinburgh, London, Melbourne and New York, 1987

Axelsson KH, Sundberg AEA, Edström HH, Widman GB, Sjöstrand UH. Venous blood concentrations after subarachnoid administration of bupivacaine. Anesthesia and Analgesia 65: 753-759,1986

Axelsson K, Widman B. Blood concentration of lidocaine after spinal anaesthesia using lidocaine and lidocaine with adrenaline. Acta Anaesthesiologica Scandinavica 25: 240-245, 1981

Axelsson K, Widman GB, Sundberg AEA, Halgren S. A double-blind study of motor block in the lower limbs: studies with spinal anaesthesia with hyperbaric and glucose free 0.5% bupivacaine. British Journal of Anaesthesia 57: 960-970, 1985

Bax NDS, Tucker GT, Lennard MS, Woods HF. The impairment of lignocaine clearance by propranolol – major contribution from enzyme inhibition. British Journal of Clinical Pharmacology 19: 597-603, 1985

Bengtsson M, Edström HH, Löfström JB. Spinal analgesia with bupivacaine, mepivacaine and tetracaine. Acta Anaesthesiologica Scandinavica 27: 278-283, 1983

Biscoping J. Einfluss der Glucosekonzentration von Bupivacainlösungen auf die Lokalanaestheticaverteilung im Liquor bei Spinalanaesthesie. Regional Anaesthesie 9: 9-14, 1986

Blair MR. Cardiovascular pharmacology of local anaesthetics. British Journal of Anaesthesia 47 (Suppl.): 247-252, 1975

Bowdle TA, Freund PR, Slattery JT. Age-dependent lidocaine pharmacokinetics during lumbar peridural anesthesia with lidocaine hydrocarbonate and lidocaine hydrochloride. Regional Anesthesia 11: 123-127, 1986

Bowdle TA, Freund PR, Slattery JT. Propranolol reduces bupivacaine clearance. Anesthesiology 66: 36-38, 1987

Braid DP, Scott DB. The systemic absorption of local analgesic drugs. British Journal of Anaesthesia 37: 394-404, 1965

Braid DP, Scott DB. Effect of adrenaline on the systemic ab-

sorption of local anaesthetic drugs. Acta Anaesthesiologica Scandinavica 23 (Suppl.): 334-346, 1966
Bridenbaugh PO, Tucker GT, Moore DC, Bridenbaugh LD, Thompson GE. Etidocaine: clinical evaluation for intercostal nerve block and lumbar epidural block. Anesthesia and Analgesia 52: 407-412, 1973
Bridenbaugh PO, Tucker GT, Moore DC, Bridenbaugh LD, Thompson GE, et al. Role of epinephrine in regional block anesthesia with etidocaine: a double blind study. Anesthesia and Analgesia 53: 430-435, 1974
Brinkløv MM. Clinical effects of carticaine, a new local anesthetic. A survey and a double-blind investigation comparing carticaine with lidocaine in epidural analgesia. Acta Anaesthesiologica Scandinavica 21: 5-16, 1977
Bromage PR. Spread of analgesic solutions in the epidural space and their site of action: a statistical study. British Journal of Anaesthesia 34: 161-177, 1962
Bromage PR. Ageing and epidural dose requirements. Segmental spread and predictability of epidural analgesia in youth and extreme age. British Journal of Anaesthesia 41: 1016-1021, 1969
Bromage PR. Lower limb reflex changes in segmental epidural analgesia. British Journal of Anaesthesia 46: 504-508, 1974
Bromage PR. Mechanism of action of extradural analgesia. British Journal of Anaesthesia 47: 199-211, 1975
Bromage PR. Epidural analgesia, pp. 8-67, 85-91, 119-159, W.B. Saunders Company, Philadelphia, London, Toronto, 1978
Bromage PR, Burfoot MF, Crowell DF, Pettigrew RT. Quality of epidural blockade I. Influence of physical factors. British Journal of Anaesthesia 36: 342-352, 1964
Bromage PR, Burfoot MF, Crowell DE, Truant AP. Quality of epidural blockade III: carbonated local anaesthetic solutions. British Journal of Anaesthesia 39: 197-209, 1967
Bromage PR, Joyal AC, Binney JC. Local anaesthetic drugs: penetration from the spinal extradural space into the neuraxis. Science 140: 392-394, 1963
Brown DT, Morison DH, Covino BG, Scott DB. Comparison of carbonated bupivacaine and bupivacaine hydrochloride for extradural anaesthesia. British Journal of Anaesthesia 52: 419-422, 1980a
Brown DT, Wildsmith JAW, Covino BG, Scott DB. Effect of baricity on spinal anaesthesia with amethocaine. British Journal of Anaesthesia 52: 589-596, 1980b
Buckley FP, Littlewood DG, Covino BG, Scott DB. Effects of adrenaline and the concentration of solution on extradural block with etidocaine. British Journal of Anaesthesia 50: 171-175, 1978
Burm AGL. Pharmacokinetics and clinical effects of lidocaine and bupivacaine following epidural and subarachnoid administration in man, Ph.D. Thesis, pp. 99-177, University of Leiden, Leiden, 1985
Burm AGL, De Boer AG, Van Kleef JW, Vermeulen NPE, De Leede LGJ, et al. Pharmacokinetics of lidocaine and bupivacaine and stable isotope labelled analogues: a study in healthy volunteers. Biopharmaceutics and Drug Disposition 9: 85-95, 1988a
Burm AGL, Van Kleef JW, Gladines MPRR, Olthof G, Spierdijk J. Epidural anesthesia with lidocaine and bupivacaine: effects of epinephrine on the plasma concentration profiles. Anesthesia and Analgesia 65: 1281-1284, 1986
Burm AGL, Van Kleef JW, Gladines MPRR, Spierdijk J, Breimer DD. Plasma concentrations of lidocaine and bupivacaine after subarachnoid administration. Anesthesiology 59: 191-195, 1983
Burm AGL, Van Kleef JW, Gladines MPRR, Van Duinen M, Spierdijk J. Spinal anaesthesia with hyperbaric lidocaine and bupivacaine: effects of epinephrine on the plasma concentration profiles. Anesthesia and Analgesia 66: 1104-1108, 1987a
Burm AGL, Van Kleef JW, Vermeulen NPE, Olthof G, Breimer DD, et al. Pharmacokinetics of lidocaine and bupivacaine following subarachnoid administration in surgical patients: simultaneous investigation of absorption and disposition kinetics using stable isotopes. Anesthesiology 69: 584-592, 1988b
Burm AGL, Vermeulen NPE, Van Kleef JW, De Boer AG, Spierdijk J, et al. Pharmacokinetics of lidocaine and bupivacaine in surgical patients following epidural administration: simultaneous investigation of absorption and disposition kinetics using stable isotopes. Clinical Pharmacokinetics 13: 191-203, 1987b
Burn JM, Guyer PB, Langdon L. The spread of solution injected into the epidural space. A study using epidurograms in patients with the lumbosciatic syndrome. British Journal of Anaesthesia 45: 338-344, 1973
Cameron AE, Arnold RW, Ghoris MW, Jamieson V. Spinal analgesia using bupivacaine 0.5% plain. Anaesthesia 36: 318-320, 1981
Chambers WA, Littlewood DG, Logan MR, Scott DB. Effect of added epinephrine on spinal anesthesia with lidocaine. Anesthesia and Analgesia 60: 417-420, 1981
Chambers WA, Littlewood DG, Scott DB. Spinal anesthesia with hyperbaric bupvacaine: effect of added vasoconstrictors. Anesthesia and Analgesia 61: 49-52, 1982
Cohen EN. Distribution of local anesthetic agents in the neuraxis of the dog. Anesthesiology 29: 1002-1005, 1968
Cole CO, McMorland GH, Axelson JE, Jenkins LC. Epidural blockade for Caesarean section comparing lidocaine hydrocarbonate and lidocaine hydrochloride. Anesthesiology 62: 348-350, 1985
Collins JG, Kitahata LM, Homma E, Suzukawa M. Spinal cord effects of epinephrine. Anesthesia and Analgesia 60: 913-914, 1981
Collins JG, Matsumoto M, Kitahata LM. Suppression by spinally administered epinephrine of noxiously evoked dorsal horn neuron activity in cats: evidence for spinal epinephrine analgesia. Anesthesia and Analgesia 62: 253-254, 1983
Concepcion M, Maddi R, Francis D, Rocco A, Murray E, et al. Vasoconstrictors in spinal anesthesia with tetracaine – a comparison of epinephrine and phenylephrine. Anesthesia and Analgesia 63: 134-138, 1984
Concilus RR, Denson DD, Knarr D, Gregg RV, Raj PP. Bupivacaine clearance in continuous epidural infusions for postoperative pain relief. Regional Anesthesia 13: 69, 1988
Cousins MJ, Bromage PR. A comparison of the hydrochloride and carbonated salts of lignocaine for caudal analgesia in outpatients. British Journal of Anaesthesia 43: 1149-1155, 1971
Cousins MJ, Bromage PR. Epidural neural blockade. In Cousins & Bridenbaugh (Eds) Neural blockade in clinical anaesthesia and management of pain, 2nd ed., pp. 253-360, JB Lippincott, Philadelphia, London, New York, Sao Paolo, Mexico City, St. Louis, Sydney, 1988
Cousins MJ, Mather LE. Intrathecal and epidural administration of opioids. Anesthesiology 61: 276-310, 1984

Covino BG. Pharmacology of local anaesthetic agents. British Journal of Anaesthesia 58: 701-716, 1986
Covino BG. Clinical pharmacology of local anesthetic agents. In Cousins & Bridenbaugh (Eds) Neural blockade in clinical anaesthesia and management of pain, 2nd ed., pp. 111-144, J.B. Lippincott, Philadelphia, 1988
Covino BG, Scott DB. Handbook of epidural anaesthesia and analgesia, pp. 36-41, 66-76, Schulz Medical Information, Copenhagen, 1985
Covino BG, Vassallo HG. Local anesthetics. Mechanisms of action and clinical use, pp. 46-48, 75-89, Grune and Stratton, New York, San Francisco, London, 1976
Crawford OB. Comparative evaluation in peridural anesthesia of lidocaine, mepivacaine and L-67, a new local anaesthetic agent. Anesthesiology 25: 321-329, 1964
Crosby G. Local spinal cord blood flow and glucose utilization during spinal anesthesia with bupivacaine in conscious rats. Anesthesiology 63: 55-60, 1985
Cusick JF, Myklebust JB, Abram SE. Differential neural effects of epidural anesthetics. Anesthesiology 53: 299-306, 1980
Cusick JF, Myklebust JB, Abram SE, Davidson A. Altered neural conduction with epidural bupivacaine. Anesthesiology 57: 31-36, 1982
Dailey PA, Hughes SC, Rosen MA, Healy K, Cheek DBC, et al. Lidocaine levels during Cesarean section after pretreatment with ranitidine or cimetidine. Anesthesiology 63: A444, 1985
Datta S, Lambert DH, Gregus J, Gissen AJ, Covino BG. Differential sensitivities of mammalian nerve fibers during pregnancy. Anesthesia and Analgesia 62: 1070-1072, 1983
Dennhardt R, Konder H. Blut- und Liquorspiegel von Bupivacain bei Spinalanaesthesien. Regional Anesthesie 6: 72-75, 1983
Denson DD. Drug interactions with local anesthetics. In Langlöys (Ed.) Update regional anaesthesia, pp. 111-121, MAPAR Editions, Kremlin-Bicêtre, 1987
Denson DD, Bridenbaugh PO, Turner PA, Phero JC. Comparison of neural blockade and pharmacokinetics after subarachnoid lidocaine in the rhesus monkey. II: effects of volume, osmolality, and baricity. Anesthesia and Analgesia 62: 995-1001, 1983
Denson DD, Bridenbaugh PO, Turner PA, Phero JC, Raj PP. Neural blockade and pharmacokinetics following subarachnoid lidocaine in the rhesus monkey. I: effects of epinephrine. Anesthesia and Analgesia 61: 746-750, 1982
Denson DD, Coyle D, Thompson G, Myers J. Alpha$_1$-acid glycoprotein and albumin in human serum bupivacaine binding. Clinical Pharmacology and Therapeutics 35: 409-415, 1984a
Denson DD, Myers JA, Hartrick CT, Pitker CP, Coyle D, et al. The relationship between free bupivacaine concentration and central nervous system toxicity. Anesthesiology 61: A211, 1984b
Denson DD, Ritschel WA, Turner PA, Ohlweiler DF, Bridenbaugh PO. A comparison of intravenous and subarachnoid lidocaine pharmacokinetics in the rhesus monkey. Biopharmaceuticals and Drug Disposition 2: 367-380, 1981
Denson DD, Turner PA, Bridenbaugh PO, Thompson GA. Pharmacokinetics and neural blockade after subarachnoid lidocaine in the rhesus monkey. III: effects of phenylephrine. Anesthesia and Analgesia 63: 129-133, 1984c
De Rosayro AM, Tait AR, Labond V, Ketcham TR, Knight PR. The effect of subarachnoid lidocaine and epinephrine on spinal cord blood flow. Anesthesiology 59: A208, 1983
DiFaxio CA, Carron H, Grosslight KR, Moscicki JC, Bolding WR, et al. Comparison of pH-adjusted lidocaine solutions for epidural anesthesia. Anesthesia and Analgesia 65: 760-764, 1986
Dohi S, Matsumiya N, Takeshima R, Naito H. The effects of subarachnoid lidocaine and phenylephrine on spinal cord and cerebral blood flow in dogs. Anesthesiology 61: 238-244, 1984
Dohi S, Takeshima R, Naito H. Spinal cord blood flow during spinal anesthesia in dogs: the effects of tetracaine, epinephrine, acute blood loss and hypercapnia. Anesthesia and Analgesia 66: 599-606, 1987
Ecoffey C, Desparmet J, Berdeaux A, Maury M, Giudicelli JF, et al. Pharmacokinetics of lignocaine in children following caudal anaesthesia. British Journal of Anaesthesia 56: 1399-1402, 1984
Ecoffey C, Desparmet J, Maury M, Berdeaux A, Giudicelli JF, et al. Bupivacaine in children: pharmacokinetics following caudal anesthesia. Anesthesiology 63: 447-448, 1985
Eisenach JC, Grice SC, Dewan DM. Epinephrine enhances analgesia produced by epidural bupivacaine during labor. Anesthesia and Analgesia 66: 447-451, 1987
Englesson S. The influence of acid-base changes on central nervous system toxicity of local anesthetic agents I. An experimental study in cats. Acta Anaesthesiologica Scandinavica 18: 79-87, 1974
Englesson S, Grevsten S. The influence of acid-base changes on central nervous system toxicity of local anaesthetic agents. II. Acta Anaesthesiologica Scandinavica 18: 88-103, 1974
Erdemir HA, Soper LE, Sweet RB. Studies of factors affecting peridural anesthesia. Anesthesia and Analgesia 44: 400-404, 1965
Eyres RL, Bishop W, Oppenheim RC, Brown TCK. Plasma bupivacaine concentrations in children during caudal epidural analgesia. Anaesthesia and Intensive Care 11: 20-22, 1983
Eyres RL, Kidd J, Oppenheim R, Brown TCK. Local anaesthetic plasma levels in children. Anaesthesia and Intensive Care 6: 243-247, 1978
Fairley JW, Reynolds F. An intradermal study of the local anaesthetic and vascular effects of the isomers of mepivacaine. British Journal of Anaesthesia 53: 1211-1216, 1981
Finucane BT, Hammonds WD, Welch MB. Influence of age on vascular absorption of lidocaine from the epidural space. Anesthesia and Analgesia 66: 843-846, 1987
Flanagan HL, Datta S, Lambert DH, Gissen AJ, Covino BG. Effect of pregnancy on bupivacaine-induced conduction blockade in the isolated rabbit vagus nerve. Anesthesia and Analgesia 66: 123-126, 1987
Foldes FF, Davidson GM, Duncalf D, Kuwabara S. The intravenous toxicity of local anesthetic agents in man. Clinical Pharmacology and Therapeutics 6: 328-335, 1965
Forbes AR, Roizen MF. Does spinal anesthesia anesthetize the spinal cord? Anesthesiology 48: 440-455, 1978
Ford DJ, Raj PP. Peripheral neurotoxicity of 2-chloroprocaine and bisulfite in the cat. Anesthesia and Analgesia 66: 719-722, 1987
Freund PR, Bowdle TA, Slattery JT. Caudal anesthesia with lidocaine or bupivacaine: plasma local anesthetic concentration and extent of sensory spread in old and young patients. Anesthesia and Analgesia 63: 1017-1020, 1984
Giasi RM, D'Agostino E, Covino BG. Absorption of lidocaine following subarachnoid and epidural administration. Anesthesia and Analgesia 58: 360-363, 1979
Gissen AJ, Covino BG, Gregus J. Differential sensitivities of

mammalian nerve fibers to local anesthetic agents. Anesthesiology 53: 467-474, 1980
Gissen AJ, Covino BG, Gregus J. Differential sensitivity of fast and slow fibers in mammalian nerve. III: effect of etidocaine and bupivacaine on fast/slow fibers. Anesthesia and Analgesia 61: 570-575, 1982
Gissen AJ, Datta S, Lambert D. The chloroprocaine controversy: II. Is chloroprocaine neurotoxic? Regional Anesthesia 9: 135-145, 1984
Glosten B, Dailey P, Preston P, Shnider S, Ross B, et al. Epidural anesthesia with pH-adjusted 3% 2-chloroprocaine for postpartum tubal ligation. Anesthesiology 67: A630, 1987
Greene NM. Physiology of spinal anesthesia, 3rd ed., pp. 1-61, 265-273, Williams and Wilkins, Baltimore, London, 1981
Greene NM. Uptake and elimination of local anesthetics during spinal anesthesia. Anesthesia and Analgesia 62: 1013-1024, 1983
Greene NM. Distribution of local anesthetic solutions within the subarachnoid space. Anesthesia and Analgesia 64: 715-730, 1985
Gross TL, Kuhnert PM, Kuhnert BR, Pimental R. Plasma levels of 2-chloroprocaine and lack of sequelae following an apparent intravenous injection. Anesthesiology 54: 173-174, 1981
Grundy EM, Ramamurthy S, Patel KP, Mani M, Winnie AP. Extradural analgesia revisited: a statistical study. British Journal of Anaesthesia 50: 805-809, 1978
Helrich M, Papper EM, Brodie BB, Fink M, Rovenstine EA. The fate of intrathecal procaine and the spinal fluid level required for surgical anesthesia. Journal of Pharmacology and Experimental Therapeutics 100: 78-82, 1950
Huet P-M, Lelorier J. Effects of smoking and chronic hepatitis B on lignocaine and indocyanine green kinetics. Clinical Pharmacology and Therapeutics 28: 208-215, 1980
Inoue R, Suganuma T, Echizen H, Ishizaki T, Kushida K, et al. Plasma concentrations of lidocaine and its principal metabolites during intermittent epidural anesthesia. Anesthesiology 63: 304-310, 1985
Johns RA, DiFazio CA, Longnecker DE. Lidocaine constricts or dilates rat arterioles in a dose-dependent manner. Anesthesiology 62: 141-144, 1985
Johns RA, Seyde WC, DiFazio CA, Longnecker DE. Dose dependent effects of bupivacaine on rat muscle arterioles. Anesthesiology 65: 186-191, 1986
Jorfeldt L, Lewis DH, Löfström JB, Post C. Lung uptake of lidocaine in healthy volunteers. Acta Anaesthesiologica Scandinavica 23: 567-574, 1979
Jorfeldt L, Lewis DH, Löfström JB, Post C. Lung uptake of lidocaine in man as influenced by anaesthesia, mepivacaine infusion or lung insufficiency. Acta Anaesthesiologica Scandinavica 27: 5-9, 1983
Jorfeldt L, Löfström B, Pernow B, Wahren J. The effect of mepivacaine and lidocaine on forearm resistance and capacitance vessels in man. Acta Anaesthesiologica Scandinavica 14: 183-201, 1970
Kanto J. Obstetric analgesia: clinical pharmacokinetic considerations. Clinical Pharmacokinetics 11: 283-298, 1986
Kaukinen L, Kaukinen S, Kärkkäinen S. Epiduralanaesthesie mit Carticain bei Sectio caesarea. Ein Vergleich mit Bupivacain. Regional Anesthesie 9: 79-83, 1986
Kennedy WF, Everett GB, Cobb LA, Allen GD. Simultaneous systemic and hepatic hemodynamic measurements during high peridural anesthesia in normal man. Anesthesia and Analgesia 50: 1069-1078, 1971
Kitahara T, Kuri S, Yoshida J. The spread of drugs used for spinal anesthesia. Anesthesiology 17: 205-208, 1956
Kotelko DM, Shnider SM, Dailey DA, Brizgys RV, Levinson G, et al. Bupivacaine-induced cardiac arrhythmias in sheep. Anesthesiology 60: 10-18, 1984
Kozody R, Ong B, Palahniuk RJ, Wade JG, Cumming MO, et al. Subarachnoid bupivacaine decreases spinal cord blood flow in dogs. Canadian Anaesthetists' Society Journal 32: 216-222,1985a
Kozody R, Palahniuk RJ, Cumming MO. Spinal cord blood flow following subarachnoid tetracaine. Canadian Anaesthetists' Society Journal 32: 23-29, 1985b
Kozody R, Palahniuk RJ, Wade JG, Cumming MO, Pucci WR. The effect of subarachnoid epinephrine and phenylephrine on spinal cord blood flow. Canadian Anaesthetists' Society Journal 31: 503-508, 1984
Kozody R, Swartz J, Palahniuk RJ, Biehl DR, Wade JG. Spinal cord blood flow following subarachnoid lidocaine. Canadian Anaesthetists' Society Journal 32: 472-478, 1985c
Kraynack BJ, Gintautas J, Tjay H. Local anesthetic action of epinephrine and ephedrine. Regional Anesthesia 8: 32-33, 1983
Kuhnert BR, Kuhnert PM, Prochaska AL, Gross TL. Plasma levels of 2-chloroprocaine in obstetric patients and their neonates after epidural anesthesia. Anesthesiology 53: 21-25, 1980
Kuhnert BR, Zuspan KJ, Kuhnert PM, Syracuse CD, Brashear WT, et al. Lack of influence of cimetidine on bupivacaine levels during parturition. Anesthesia and Analgesia 66: 986-990, 1987a
Kuhnert BR, Zuspan KJ, Kuhnert PM, Syracuse CD, Brown DE. Bupivacaine disposition in mother, fetus, and neonate after spinal anesthesia for Caesarean section. Anesthesia and Analgesia 66: 407-412, 1987b
Laishley RS, Morgan BM, Reynolds F. Effect of adrenaline on extradural anaesthesia and plasma bupivacaine concentrations during Caesarian section. British Journal of Anaesthesia 60: 180-186, 1988
Lalka D, Vicuna N, Burrow SR, Jones DJ, Luddon DJ, et al. Bupivacaine and other amide local anesthetics inhibit the hydrolysis of chloroprocaine in human serum. Anesthesia and Analgesia 57: 534-538, 1978
Leicht CH, Carlson SA. Prolongation of lidocaine spinal anesthesia with epinephrine and phenylephrine. Anesthesia and Analgesia 65: 365-369, 1986
Littlewood DG, Buckley P, Covino BG, Scott DB, Wilson J. Comparative study of various local anaesthetic solutions in extradural block in labour. British Journal of Anaesthesia 51: 47S-52S, 1979
Lund C, Hansen OB, Mogenson T, Kehlet H. Effect of thoracic epidural bupivacaine on somatosensory evoked potentials after dermatomal stimulation. Anesthesia and Analgesia 66: 731-734, 1987a
Lund C, Selmar P, Hansen OB, Hjortsø NC, Kehlet H. Effect of epidural bupivacaine on somatosensory evoked potentials after dermatomal stimulation. Anesthesia and Analgesia 66: 34-38, 1987b
Lund C, Selmar P, Hansen OB, Kehlet H. Effect of intrathecal bupivacaine on somatosensory evoked potentials following dermatomal stimulation. Anesthesia and Analgesia 66: 809-813, 1987c
Lund PC, Bush DF, Covino BG. Determinants of etidocaine concentration in the blood. Anesthesiology 42: 497-503, 1975

Lund PC, Covino BG. Distribution of local anaesthetics in man following epidural anesthesia. Journal of Clinical Pharmacology 7: 324-329, 1967

Lund PC, Cwik JC. Citanest . . . a clinical and laboratory study. Anesthesia and Analgesia 44: 623-631, 1965

Lund PC, Cwik JC. A correlation of the differential penetration and the systemic toxicity of lidocaine, mepivacaine and prilocaine in man. Acta Anaesthesiologica Scandinavica 23 (Suppl.): 475-482, 1966

Lund PC, Cwik JC, Pagdanganan RT. Etidocaine – a new long-acting local anesthetic agent: a clinical evaluation. Anesthesia and Analgesia 52: 482-494, 1973

Martin R, Lamarche Y, Tétreault L. Comparison of the effectiveness of lidocaine hydrocarbonate and lidocaine hydrochloride with and without epinephrine in epidural anaesthesia. Canadian Anaesthetists' Society Journal 28: 217-223, 1981

Mather EL, Cousins MJ. Local anaesthetics and their current clinical use. Drugs 18: 185-205, 1979

Mather LE, Thomas J. Bupivacaine binding to plasma protein fractions. Journal of Pharmacy and Pharmacology 30: 653-654, 1978

Mather LE, Tucker GT, Murphy TM, Stanton-Hicks Md'A, Bonica JJ. The effects of adding adrenaline to etidocaine and lignocaine in extradural anaesthesia II: pharmacokinetics. British Journal of Anaesthesia 48: 989-994, 1976a

Mather LE, Tucker GT, Murphy TM, Stanton-Hicks Md'A, Bonica JJ. Hemodynamic drug interaction: peridural lidocaine and intravenous ephedrine. Acta Anaesthesiologica Scandinavica 20: 207-210, 1976b

Matthes H, Schabert P. Vergleichende Untersuchungen über Blutspiegel von Mepivacain nach Resorption aus verschiedenen Gewebe. Acta Anaesthesiologica Scandinavica 23 (Suppl.): 371-376, 1966

Mayumi T, Dohi S, Takahashi T. Plasma concentrations of lidocaine associated with cervical, thoracic and lumbar epidural anesthesia. Anesthesia and Analgesia 62: 578-580, 1983

Mazoit JX, Denson DD, Samii K. Pharmacokinetics of bupivacaine following caudal anesthesia in infants. Anesthesiology 68: 387-391, 1988

Mazze RI, Dunbar RW. Plasma lidocaine concentrations after caudal, lumbar epidural, axillary block and intravenous regional anesthesia. Anesthesiology 27: 574-579, 1966

McMorland GW, Douglas MJ, Jeffery WK, Ross PLE, Axelson JE, et al. Effect of pH adjustment of bupivacaine on onset and duration of epidural analgesia in parturients. Canadian Anaesthetists' Society Journal 33: 537-541, 1986

McNamara PJ, Slaughter RL, Pieper JA, Wyman MG, Lalka D. Factors influencing serum protein binding of lidocaine in humans. Anesthesia and Analgesia 60: 395-400, 1981

Meyer J, Nolte H. Liquorkonzentration von Bupivacain nach subduraler Applikation. Regional Anaesthesie 1: 38-40, 1978

Mihaly GW, Moore RG, Thomas T, Triggs EJ, Thomas D, et al. The pharmacokinetics and metabolism of the anilide local anaesthetics in neonates I. Lignocaine. European Journal of Clinical Pharmacology 13: 143-152, 1978

Möller IW, Fernandes A, Edström HH. Subarachnoid anaesthesia with 0.5% bupivacaine: effect of density. British Journal of Anaesthesia 56: 1191-1194, 1984

Moore DC. Spinal anesthesia: bupivacaine compared with tetracaine. Anesthesia and Analgesia 59: 743-750, 1980

Moore DC. The pH of local anesthetic solutions. Anesthesia and Analgesia 60: 833-834, 1981

Moore DC, Bridenbaugh LD, Bagdi PA, Bridenbaugh PO. Accumulation of mepivacaine hydrochloride during caudal block. Anesthesiology 29: 585-588, 1968

Moore DC, Chadwick HS, Ready LB. Epinephrine prolongs lidocaine spinal: pain in the operative site the most accurate method of determining local anesthetic duration. Anesthesiology 67: 416-418, 1987

Moore DC, Mather LE, Bridenbaugh PO, Bridenbaugh LD, Balfour RI, et al. Arterial and venous plasma levels of bupivacaine following epidural and intercostal nerve blocks. Anesthesiology 45: 39-45, 1976

Moore DC, Spierdijk J, Van Kleef JW, Coleman RL, Love GF. Chloroprocaine neurotoxicity: four additional cases. Anesthesia and Analgesia 61: 155-159, 1982

Moore RG, Thomas J, Triggs EJ, Thomas DB, Burnard ED, et al. The pharmacokinetics and metabolism of the anilide local anaesthetics in neonates III. Mepivacaine. European Journal of Clinical Pharmacology 14: 203-212, 1978

Morgan DJ, Cousins MJ, McQuillan D, Thomas J. Disposition and placental transfer of etidocaine in pregnancy. European Journal of Clinical Pharmacology 12: 359-365, 1977

Morison DH. A double-blind comparison of carbonated lidocaine and lidocaine hydrochloride in epidural anaesthesia. Canadian Anaesthetists' Society Journal 28: 387-389, 1981

Murphy TM, Mather LE, Stanton-Hicks Md'A, Bonica JJ, Tucker GT. The effects of adding adrenaline to etidocaine and lignocaine in extradural anaesthesia I: block characteristics and cardiovascular effects. British Journal of Anaesthesia 48: 893-898, 1976

Nancarrow C, Runciman WB, Mather LE, Upton RN, Plummer JL. The influence of acidosis on the distribution of lidocaine and bupivacaine into the myocardium and brain of the sheep. Anesthesia and Analgesia 66: 925-935, 1987

Nickel PM, Bromage PR, Sherrill DL. Comparison of hydrochloride and carbonated salts of lidocaine for epidural analgesia. Regional Anesthesia 11: 62-67, 1986

Nishimura N, Kitahara T, Kusakabe T. The spread of lidocaine and I-131 solution in the epidural space. Anesthesiology 20: 785-788, 1959

Noble DW, Smith KJ, Dundas CR. Effects of H_2-antagonists on the elimination of bupivacaine. British Journal of Anaesthesia 59: 735-737, 1987

Ohno H, Watanabe M, Saitoh J, Saegusa Y, Hasegawa Y, et al. Effect of epinephrine concentration on lidocaine disposition during epidural anesthesia. Anesthesiology 68: 625-628, 1988

O'Sullivan GM, Smith M, Morgan B, Brighouse D, Reynolds F. H_2-antagonists and bupivacaine clearance. Anesthesia 43: 93-95, 1988

Pardridge WM, Sakiyama R, Fierer G. Transport of propranolol and lidocaine through the rat blood-brain barrier. Journal of Clinical Investigation 71: 900-908, 1983

Park WY, Balingit PE, Macnamara TE. Effect of patient age, pH of cerebrospinal fluid, and vasopressor on onset and duratibn of spinal anesthesia. Anesthesia and Analgesia 54: 455-458, 1975

Park WY, Hagins FM, Rivat EL, Macnamara TE. Age and epidural dose response in adult man. Anesthesiology 56: 318-320, 1982

Park WY, Massengale M, Kim S-I, Poon KC, Macnamara TE.

Age and the spread of local anesthetic solutions in the epidural space. Anesthesia and Analgesia 59: 768-771, 1980
Pieper JA, Wyman MG, Goldreyer BN, Cannom DS, Slaughter RL, et al. Lidocaine toxicity: effect of total versus free lidocaine concentrations. Circulation 62 (III): 181, 1980
Pitkänen M, Haapaniemi L, Tuominen M, Rosenberg PH. Influence of age on spinal anaesthesia with isobaric 0.5% bupivacaine. British Journal of Anaesthesia 56: 279-284, 1984
Porter SS, Albin MS, Watson WA, Bunegin L, Pantoja G. Spinal cord and cerebral blood flow responses to subarachnoid injection of local anesthetics with and without epinephrine. Acta Anaesthesiologica Scandinavica 29: 330-338, 1985
Racle JP, Benkhadra A, Poy JY. Subarachnoid anaesthesia produced by hyperbaric lidocaine in elderly patients. British Journal of Anaesthesia 60: 831-835, 1988a
Racle JP, Benkhadra A, Poy JY, Gleizal B. Prolongation of isobaric bupivacaine spinal anesthesia with epinephrine and clonidine for hip surgery in the elderly. Anesthesia and Analgesia 66: 442-446, 1987a
Racle JP, Benkhadra A, Poy JY, Gleizal B. Effect of increasing amount of epinephrine during isobaric bupivacaine spinal anesthesia in elderly patients. Anesthesia and Analgesia 66: 882-886, 1987b
Racle JP, Benkhadra A, Poy JY, Gleizal B. Spinal analgesia with hyperbaric bupivacaine: influence of age. British Journal of Anaesthesia 60: 508-514, 1988b
Raj PP, Ohlweiler D, Hitt BA, Denson DD. Kinetics of local anesthetic esters and the effect of adjuvant drugs on 2-chloroprocaine hydrolysis. Anesthesiology 53: 307-314, 1980
Ravindran RS, Bond VK, Tasch MD, Gupta CD, Luerssen TG. Prolonged neural blockade following regional analgesia with 2-chloroprocaine. Anesthesia and Analgesia 59: 447-451, 1980
Raymond SA, Gissen AJ. Mechanisms of differential nerve block. In Strichartz GR (Ed.) Local anesthetics, pp. 95-164, Springer-Verlag, Berlin, Heidelberg, New York, London, Paris, Tokyo, 1987
Reidenberg MM, James M, Dring LG. The rate of procaine hydrolysis in serum of normal subjects and diseased patients. Clinical Pharmacology and Therapeutics 13: 279-284, 1972
Reisner LS, Hochman BN, Plumer MH. Persistent neurologic deficit and adhesive arachnoiditis following intrathecal 2-chloroprocaine injection. Anesthesia and Analgesia 59: 452-454, 1980
Renck H, Edström H, Kinnberger B, Brandt G. Thoracic epidural analgesia - II: prolongation in the early postoperative period by continuous injection of 1.0% bupivacaine. Acta Anaesthesiologica Scandinavica 20: 47-56, 1976
Reynolds F. Adverse effects of local anaesthetics. British Journal of Anaesthesia 59: 78-95, 1987
Rosenberg PH, Saramies L, Alila A. Lumbar epidural anaesthesia with bupivacaine in old patients: effects of speed and direction of injection. Acta Anaesthesiologica Scandinavica 25: 270-274, 1981
Ross BK, Hughes S, Glosten B, Shnider S, Preston P, et al. Evaluation of epidural pH-adjusted 2% 2-chloroprocaine for labor analgesia. Anesthesiology 67: A629, 1987
Ross RA, Clarke JE, Armitage EW. Postoperative pain prevention by continuous epidural infusion. A study of the clinical effects and the plasma concentrations obtained. Anaesthesia 35: 663-668, 1980
Rothstein P, Arthur GR, Feldman HS, Kopf GS, Covino BG. Bupivacaine for intercostal nerve blocks in children: blood concentrations and pharmacokinetics. Anesthesia and Analgesia 65: 625-632, 1986
Routledge PA, Barchowsky A, Bjornsson TD, Kitchell BB, Shand DG. Lidocaine plasma protein binding. Clinical Pharmacology and Therapeutics 27: 347-351, 1980
Runciman WB, Mather LE, Ilsley AH, Carapetis RJ, McLean CF. A sheep preparation for studying interactions between blood flow and drug disposition. II: experimental applications. British Journal of Anaesthesia 56: 1117-1129, 1984a
Runciman WB, Mather LE, Ilsley AH, Carapetis RJ, Upton RN. A sheep preparation for studying interactions between blood flow and drug disposition. III: effects of general and spinal anaesthesia on regional blood flow and oxygen tensions. British Journal of Anaesthesia 56: 1247-1258, 1984b
Schmidt KF. Metabolism of procaine in cerebrospinal fluid contaminated with blood. Anesthesiology 25: 563-564, 1964
Scott DB. Evaluation of the toxicity of local anaesthetic agents in man. British Journal of Anaesthesia 47: 56-61, 1975
Scott DB. Toxic effects of local anaesthetic agents on the central venous system. British Journal of Anaesthesia 58: 732-735, 1986
Scott DB, Jebson PJR, Braid DP, Örtengren B, Frisch P. Factors affecting plasma levels of lignocaine and prilocaine. British Journal of Anaesthesia 44: 1040-1049, 1972
Scott DB, McClure JH, Giasi RM, Seo J, Covino BG. Effects of concentration of local anaesthetic drugs in extradural block. British Journal of Anaesthesia 52: 1033-1037, 1980
Seifen AB, Ferrari AA, Seifen EE, Thompson DS, Chapman J. Pharmacokinetics of intravenous procaine infusion in humans. Anesthesia and Analgesia 58: 382-386, 1979
Seow LT, Lips FJ, Cousins MJ, Mather LE. Lidocaine and bupivacaine mixtures for epidural blockade. Anesthesiology 56: 177-183, 1982
Sharrock NE. Epidural anesthetic dose responses in patients 20 to 80 years old. Anesthesiology 49: 425-428, 1978
Sheskey MC, Rocco AG, Bizzarri-Schmid M, Francis DM, Edström H, et al. A dose-response study of bupivacaine for spinal anesthesia. Anesthesia and Analgesia 62: 931-935, 1983
Simon RP, Benowitz NL, Bronstein BS, Jacob P. Increased brain uptake of lidocaine during bicuculline-induced status epilepticus in rats. Neurology 32: 196-199, 1982
Simon RP, Benowitz NL, Culala S. Motor paralysis increases brain uptake of lidocaine during status epilepticus. Neurology 34: 384-387, 1984
Sinclair CJ, Scott DB. Comparison of bupivacaine and etidocaine in extradural blockade. British Journal of Anaesthesia 56: 147-153, 1984
Smith AR, Hur D, Resano F. Grand mal seizures after 2-chloroprocaine epidural anesthesia in a patient with plasma cholinesterase deficiency. Anesthesia and Analgesia 66: 677-678, 1987
Spivey DL. Epinephrine does not prolong lidocaine spinal anesthesia in term parturients. Anesthesia and Analgesia 64: 468-470, 1985
Stanton-Hicks M, Berger PU, Bonica JJ. Circulatory effects of peridural block: IV Comparison of effects of epinephrine and phenylephrine. Anesthesiology 39: 308-314, 1973
Strichartz GR, Ritchie JM. The action of local anesthetics on ion channels of excitable tissues. In Strichartz (Ed.) Local anesthetics, pp. 21-52, Springer-Verlag, Berlin, Heidelberg, New York, London, Paris, Tokyo, 1987

Takasaki M. Blood concentrations of lidocaine, mepivacaine and bupivacaine during caudal analgesia in children. Acta Anaesthesiologica Scandinavica 28: 211-214, 1984

Takasaki M, Oh-oka T, Doi K, Kosaka Y. Blood levels of mepivacaine during continuous epidural anesthesia. Anesthesia and Analgesia 66: 337-340, 1987

Terasaki T, Pardridge WM, Denson DD. Differential effect of plasma protein binding of bupivacaine on its in vivo transfer into the brain and salivary gland of rats. Journal of Pharmacology and Experimental Therapeutics 239: 724-729, 1986

Thomson PD, Melmar KL, Richardson JA, Cohn K, Steinbrunn W, et al. Lidocaine pharmacokinetics in advanced heart failure, liver disease and renal disease in humans. Annals of Internal Medicine 78: 499-508, 1973

Tucker GT. Pharmacokinetics of local anaesthetics. British Journal of Anaesthesia 58: 717-731, 1986

Tucker GT. Is plasma binding of local anaesthetics important? Acta Anaesthesiologica Belgica 39: 147-150, 1988

Tucker GT, Bax NDS, Lennard MD, Al-Asady S, Bharaj HS, et al. Effects of β-adrenoceptor antagonists on the pharmacokinetics of lignocaine. British Journal of Clinical Pharmacology 17: 21S-28S, 1984

Tucker GT, Boas RA. Pharmacokinetic aspects of intravenous regional anesthesia. Anesthesiology 34: 538-549, 1971

Tucker GT, Boyes RN, Bridenbaugh PO, Moore DC. Binding of anilide-type local anesthetics in human plasma: I. Relationships between binding, physicochemical properties, and anesthetic activity. Anesthesiology 33: 287-303, 1970

Tucker GT, Cooper S, Littlewood D, Buckley FP, Covino BG, et al. Observed and predicted accumulation of local anaesthetic agents during continuous extradural analgesia. British Journal of Anaesthesia 49: 237-242, 1977a

Tucker GT, Mather LE. Pharmacokinetics of local anaesthetic agents. British Journal of Anaesthesia 47: 213-224, 1975

Tucker GT, Mather LE. Clinical pharmacokinetics of local anaesthetics. Clinical Pharmacokinetics 4: 241-278, 1979

Tucker GT, Mather LE. Properties, absorption, and disposition of local anesthetic agents. In Cousins & Bridenbaugh (Eds) Neural blockade in clinical anesthesia and management of pain, 2nd ed., pp. 47-110, JB Lippincott, Philadelphia, London, New York, Sao Paolo, Mexico City, St Louis, Sydney, 1988

Tucker GT, Moore DC, Bridenbaugh PO, Bridenbaugh LD, Thompson GE. Systemic absorption of mepivacaine in commonly used regional block procedures. Anesthesiology 37: 277-287, 1972

Tucker GT, Wiklund L, Berlin-Wahlén A, Mather LE. Hepatic clearance of local anaesthetics in man. Journal of Pharmacokinetics and Biopharmaceutics 5: 111-122, 1977b

Tuominen M, Pitkänen M, Doepel M, Rosenberg PH. Influence of age and body mass on subarachnoid anaesthesia with tetracaine. Acta Anaesthesiologica Scandinavica 31: 474-478, 1987

Urban BJ. Clinical observations suggesting a changing site of action during induction and recession of spinal and epidural anesthesia. Anesthesiology 39: 496-503, 1973

Van Kleef JW. A clinical evaluation of bupivacaine (Marcaine®) 0.5% versus 0.75%, Ph.D Thesis, pp. 95-120, University of Leiden, Leiden, 1981

Veering BT, Burm AGL, Spierdijk J. Spinal anaesthesia with hyperbaric bupivacaine: effects of age on neural blockade and pharmacokinetics. British Journal of Anaesthesia 60: 187-194, 1988

Veering BT, Burm AGL, Van Kleef JW, Hennis PJ, Spierdijk J. Epidural anesthesia with bupivacaine: effect of age on neural blockade and pharmacokinetics. Anesthesia and Analgesia 66: 589-593, 1987a

Veering BT, Burm AGL, Van Kleef JW, Hennis PJ, Spierdijk J. Spinal anesthesia with glucose-free bupivacaine: effects of age on neural blockade and pharmacokinetics. Anesthesia and Analgesia 66: 965-970, 1987b

Webb TD, Ward DS. Elimination of lidocaine following regional block is inhibited by cimetidine. Anesthesiology 59: A213, 1983

Wiklund L, Tucker GT, Engberg G. Influence of intravenously administered ephedrine on splanchnic haemodynamics and clearance of lidocaine. Acta Anaesthesiologica Scandinavica 21: 275-281, 1977

Wildsmith JAW, Gissen AJ, Gregus J, Covino BG. Differential nerve blocking activity of amino-ester local anaesthetics. British Journal of Anaesthesia 57: 612-620, 1985

Wildsmith JAW, McClure JH, Brown DT, Scott DB. Effects of posture on the spread of isobaric and hyperbaric amethocaine. British Journal of Anaesthesia 53: 273-278, 1981

Wilkinson GR, Lund PC. Bupivacaine levels in plasma and cerebrospinal fluid following peridural administration. Anesthesiology 33: 482-486, 1970

Williams RL, Blaschke TF, Meffin PL, Melman KL, Rowland M. Influence of viral hepatitis on the disposition of two compounds with high hepatic clearance: lidocaine and indocyanine green. Clinical Pharmacology and Therapeutics 20: 290-299, 1976

Wood M. Plasma drug binding: implications for anesthesiologists. Anesthesia and Analgesia 65: 786-804, 1986

Author's address: Dr *A.G.L. Burm*, Department of Anaesthesiology, Leiden University Hospital, P.O. Box 9600, 2300 RC Leiden (The Netherlands).

Original Research Article

Clinical Pharmacokinetics 16: 312-316 (1989)
0312-5963/89/0005-0312/$02.50/0

Clearance of the Antihistamine Doxylamine Reduced in Elderly Men But Not in Elderly Women

H. Friedman, David J. Greenblatt, Joseph M. Scavone, Ethan S. Burstein, Hermann R. Ochs, Jerold S. Harmatz and *Richard I. Shader*

Division of Clinical Pharmacology, Departments of Psychiatry and Medicine, Tufts University School of Medicine and New England Medical Center, Boston, Massachusetts, USA, and the Medizinische Universitätsklinik, University of Bonn, Federal Republic of Germany

Summary *A single oral dose of doxylamine succinate 25mg was administered to 21 young (20 to 43 years) and 22 elderly (60 to 87 years) volunteers. Multiple plasma doxylamine concentrations were determined during a 30-hour period after each dose. Elderly and young women did not differ significantly in peak plasma doxylamine concentration (C_{max}) [116 vs 103 μg/L], time to C_{max} (t_{max}) [2.4 vs 2.4h], elimination half-life (12.2 vs 10.1h), volume of distribution (179 vs 176L) or clearance (191 vs 218 ml/min). C_{max} (107 vs 108 μg/L) and t_{max} (2.1 vs 1.6h) also did not differ between elderly and young men. However, elderly men had reduced doxylamine clearance (174 vs 240 ml/min, $p < 0.02$; 2.5 vs 3.2 ml/min/kg, $p < 0.07$) and prolonged half-life (15.5 vs 10.2h, $p < 0.05$). The reduced doxylamine clearance and prolonged half-life in elderly men, but not in elderly women, is similar to results for many other drugs which are transformed by oxidation.*

The H_1-antagonist doxylamine is available without prescription, and is extensively utilised as a night-time sedative or as a component of various cold preparations. As 'Bendectin', doxylamine was also prescribed for many years in a fixed combination with pyridoxine (vitamin B_6) for the treatment of nausea and vomiting associated with pregnancy (Friedman & Greenblatt 1985; Rickels et al. 1984).

The use of over-the-counter medications by the elderly is of considerable importance. Older persons frequently take non-prescription drugs for the treatment of allergic symptoms, minor viral respiratory infections, and sleeplessness (Greenblatt & Shader 1977; Lamy 1982). Previous studies demonstrate that healthy elderly individuals may have impaired clearance of a number of drugs, particularly those biotransformed by hepatic microsomal oxidation (Greenblatt et al. 1982b, 1986; Schmucker 1985; Vestal 1982). In some studies, the age-related decrement in metabolising capacity has been more evident in men than in women (Abernethy & Greenblatt 1983; Greenblatt et al. 1980, 1981, 1982a, 1983a,b, 1984a,b, 1987). These pharmacokinetic changes could lead to increased accumulation during long term treatment, as well as higher peak concentrations and delayed elimination following single doses, thereby increasing the likelihood of clinical toxicity. The present study evaluates the effect of age and gender on the pharmacokinetics of single doses of the antihistamine doxylamine.

Patients and Methods

A total of 43 healthy male and female volunteers participated after giving written informed consent (table I). Of these, 21 were 'young' (aged 20 to 43 years), and 22 were 'elderly' (aged 60 to 87 years). All young participants were healthy, active, ambulatory adults with no evidence of medical disease and receiving no other medications; young females were not taking oral contraceptives. Elderly volunteers were likewise active, ambulatory adults without active medical disease. One elderly man and 2 elderly women had cardiovascular disease which was being treated with oral medications and was fully compensated and stable. The other elderly subjects were taking no medication.

Procedure

Following an overnight fast, all subjects received a single oral dose of doxylamine hydrochloride 25mg (equivalent to 17.4mg of doxylamine base) with 100 to 200ml of tap water. Venous blood samples were drawn prior to administration and at various times up to 30 hours post-dose. The samples were centrifuged, and the serum or plasma separated and frozen until the time of assay.

Analysis of Samples

Concentrations of intact doxylamine in all samples were determined by gas chromatography with nitrogen phosphorus detection, using a previously described method (Friedman & Greenblatt 1985) with modifications, as follows. The internal standard brompheniramine (100ng) is added to a series of 15ml round-bottom glass culture tubes. Calibration standards for doxylamine are prepared by adding the following amounts of doxylamine base to consecutive tubes: 5, 10, 25, 50, 75, 100, 150 and 200ng. One millilitre of drug-free control serum or plasma is added to each of these calibration tubes. To all other tubes, containing only the internal standard, is added 1ml of 'unknown' serum or plasma. Samples are alkalinised with 1ml of 0.25 mol/L sodium hydroxide, extracted into 2ml of

Table I. Effect of age and gender on the pharmacokinetics of doxylamine

	Mean (± SE) value			
	young male	young female	elderly male	elderly female
Subject characteristics				
Number	9	12	12	10
Age (y)	34 ± 2[a]	30 ± 2[a]	66 ± 2[a]	73 ± 3[a]
Weight (kg)	76.5 ± 5.1	62.1 ± 3.6	71.3 ± 2.3	62.7 ± 2.4
Height (cm)	177 ± 2	165 ± 2	173 ± 2	164 ± 2
Percentage ideal weight	107 ± 6	110 ± 5	105 ± 4	113 ± 5
Cigarette smoking (no/yes)	6/3	10/2	8/4	9/1
Doxylamine pharmacokinetics				
C_{max} (μg/L)	108 ± 10	103 ± 8	107 ± 9	116 ± 13
t_{max} (h)	1.61 ± 0.26	2.4 ± 0.41	2.08 ± 0.29	2.40 ± 0.52
$t_{1/2}$ (h)	10.2 ± 0.7[b]	10.1 ± 1.1	15.5 ± 2.1[b]	12.2 ± 1.4
CL_{po} (ml/min)	240 ± 13[c]	218 ± 16	174 ± 19[c]	191 ± 24
(ml/min/kg)	3.22 ± 0.25[d]	3.69 ± 0.37	2.49 ± 0.28[d]	3.11 ± 0.42

Value of Student's independent t for young *vs* elderly of the same sex:
a $p < 0.001$.
b $p < 0.05$.
c $p < 0.025$.
d $p < 0.07$.
Abbreviations: C_{max} = peak plasma drug concentration; t_{max} = time to C_{max}; $t_{1/2}$ = elimination half-life; CL_{po} = oral clearance.

hexane-isoamyl alcohol (98 : 2) by agitation on a vortex mixer, and centrifuged. The organic layer is transferred to an automatic sampling vial, evaporated to dryness, and reconstituted in 0.2ml of toluene : isoamyl alcohol (85 : 15). The automatic sampler is programmed to inject 6μl of the solution on to the gas chromatograph (Hewlett Packard Model 5840A) under the described conditions.

The within-day replicability of identical samples (n = 6 at each concentration) is: 10.3% at 5 μg/L; 4.8% at 10 μg/L; 4.8% at 50 μg/L and 3.8% at 100 μg/L. A frozen quality control plasma sample, previously 'spiked' to contain 25 μg/L of doxylamine, was analysed along with each set of unknowns. The overall mean doxylamine concentration in the quality control sample measured across 21 analytical runs was 24.8 μg/L, with a coefficient of variation of 9.6%.

Kinetic and Statistical Analysis

The terminal log-linear phase of the serum or plasma doxylamine concentration curve was identified visually, and the slope (β) determined by linear regression analysis. This was used to calculate the apparent elimination half-life ($t_{1/2}$). Area under the curve (AUC) up to the final detectable concentration was determined by the linear trapezoidal method and extrapolated to infinity by addition of the final detectable concentration divided by β (Greenblatt & Koch-Weser 1975). Apparent oral clearance of doxylamine was calculated as the administered dose of doxylamine base (17.4mg) divided by total AUC. The peak plasma doxylamine concentration (C_{max}) and the time to C_{max} (t_{max}) were taken as indexes of the rate of doxylamine absorption.

Differences between young and elderly subjects of the same gender were evaluated by Student's independent t-test.

Results

Female subjects had lower values of height and bodyweight than did male subjects regardless of age; however, there were no significant differences attributable to age (table I). All 4 groups were comparable in percentage of ideal bodyweight, based on actuarial data (Abernethy & Greenblatt 1982). Between 1 and 4 subjects in each of the 4 groups were cigarette smokers.

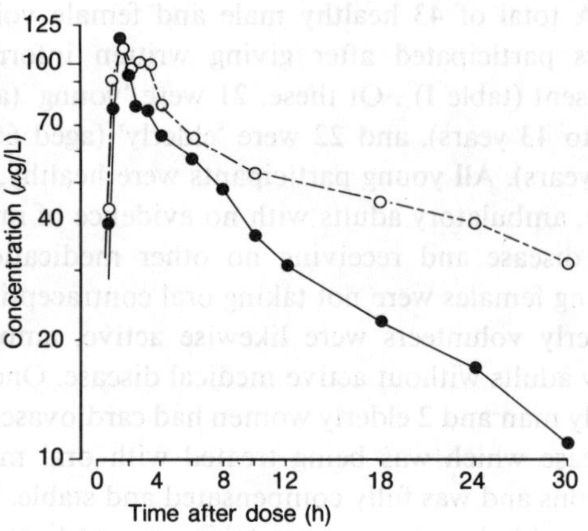

Fig. 1. Plasma doxylamine concentrations in representative young and elderly male volunteers; ● = age 30 years; ○ = age 66 years.

Figure 1 shows representative plasma doxylamine concentration curves. Among female subjects, C_{max} was higher in the elderly group (116 *vs* 103 μg/L), $t_{1/2}$ was longer (12.2 *vs* 10.1 hours), and clearance was lower (191 *vs* 218 ml/min) [table I]. However, none of these differences approached statistical significance. Although the statistical power of these comparisons was low ($p < 0.3$), the non-significance of the difference could not be attributed to an inadequate sample size. Further calculations indicated that, assuming the same difference in mean values between groups and the same relative standard deviations within groups, statistical significance at the $p < 0.05$ level would not be achieved with any finite sample size.

Among male volunteers, C_{max} and t_{max} were not significantly different between young and elderly groups. However, oral clearance of doxylamine was significantly reduced (174 *vs* 240 ml/min,

$p < 0.025$), and $t_{1/2}$ significantly prolonged (15.5 *vs* 10.2 hours, $p < 0.05$) in elderly *vs* young male volunteers, respectively (fig. 2). After correction for bodyweight, oral clearance of doxylamine was reduced in elderly *vs* young males (2.49 *vs* 3.22 ml/min/kg), although the level of statistical significance was not as great ($p < 0.07$).

Discussion

Although data in humans is limited, primate studies suggest that the antihistamine derivative doxylamine is biotransformed mainly by hepatic microsomal oxidation (Ganes et al. 1986; Holder et al. 1987; Slikker et al. 1986). The present study demonstrates that doxylamine clearance is significantly reduced, and elimination half-life is significantly prolonged, in healthy male subjects (mean age 66 years) in comparison with a group of healthy young male controls (mean age 34 years). However, among similar groups of young and elderly female volunteers, the trend towards longer half-life and lower clearance values in elderly as opposed to young subjects did not reach statistical significance. There were no significant differences attributable to age in peak plasma doxylamine concentration or the time to peak concentration, suggesting that age does not influence the rate of drug absorption from the gastrointestinal tract.

Although the effects of age on the pharmacokinetics of H_1-antagonists are not well established (Paton & Webster 1985), the findings with doxylamine are similar to results with a number of other drugs which undergo biotransformation by hepatic microsomal oxidation. Previous pharmacogeriatric studies of drugs metabolised by oxidative mechanisms indicate significant reductions of clearance, and prolongation of elimination half-life, in elderly *vs* young volunteers (Abernethy & Greenblatt 1983; Greenblatt et al. 1980, 1981, 1982a,b, 1983a, 1984a,b, 1987; Schmucker 1985; Vestal 1982). In many studies, the effect of age has been relatively

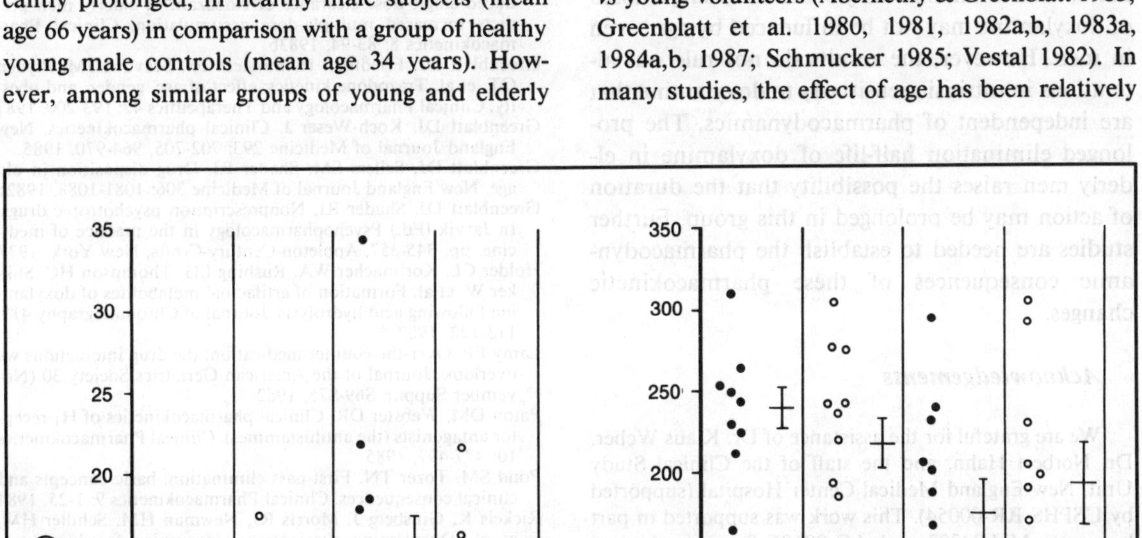

Fig. 2. Effect of age and gender on (**a**) elimination half-life and (**b**) clearance of doxylamine. Individual and mean (± SE) values are shown. See table I for statistical analysis.

gender-specific, with age effects far more pronounced in men than in women (Abernethy & Greenblatt 1983; Greenblatt et al. 1980, 1981, 1982a, 1983a,b, 1984a,b, 1987). For drugs metabolised by conjugation as opposed to oxidation, age effects are minimal.

Therapeutic Implications

Doxylamine clearance was reduced in elderly males, but peak plasma drug concentrations in men were not increased in the elderly. This is consistent with the observation that doxylamine clearance is considerably less than hepatic blood flow (Pond & Tozer 1984; Wilkinson 1987). If the intensity of drug action following single doses is related to C_{max}, then the pharmacokinetic findings as such suggest that the maximum intensity of action of single doses of doxylamine may not be influenced by age, even in men. However, the results do not rule out alterations in intrinsic sensitivity to doxylamine that are independent of pharmacodynamics. The prolonged elimination half-life of doxylamine in elderly men raises the possibility that the duration of action may be prolonged in this group. Further studies are needed to establish the pharmacodynamic consequences of these pharmacokinetic changes.

Acknowledgements

We are grateful for the assistance of Dr. Klaus Weber, Dr. Norbert Hahn, and the staff of the Clinical Study Unit, New England Medical Center Hospital (supported by USPHS RR-00054). This work was supported in part by grants MH-34223 and AG-00106 from the United States Public Health Service.

References

Abernethy DR, Greenblatt DJ. Pharmacokinetics of drugs in obesity. Clinical Pharmacokinetics 7: 108-124, 1982

Abernethy DR, Greenblatt DJ. Impairment of lidocaine clearance in elderly male subjects. Journal of Cardiovascular Pharmacology 5: 1093-1096, 1983

Friedman H, Greenblatt DJ. The pharmacokinetics of doxylamine: use of automated gas chromatography with nitrogen-phosphorus detection. Journal of Clinical Pharmacology 25: 448-451, 1985

Ganes DA, Hindmarsh KW, Midha KK. Doxylamine metabolism in rat and monkey. Xenobiotica 16: 781-794, 1986

Greenblatt DJ, Abernethy DR, Locniskar A, Harmatz JS, Limjuco RA, et al. Effect of age, gender, and obesity on midazolam kinetics. Anesthesiology 61: 27-35, 1984a

Greenblatt DJ, Abernethy DR, Matlis R, Harmatz JS, Shader RI. Absorption and disposition of ibuprofen in the elderly. Arthritis and Rheumatism 27: 1066-1069, 1984b

Greenblatt DJ, Abernethy DR, Shader RI. Pharmacokinetic aspects of drug therapy in the elderly. Therapeutic Drug Monitoring 8: 249-255, 1986

Greenblatt DJ, Allen MD, Harmatz JS, Shader RI. Diazepam disposition determinants. Clinical Pharmacology and Therapeutics 27: 301-312, 1980

Greenblatt DJ, Divoll M, Abernethy DR, Harmatz JS, Shader RI. Antipyrine kinetics in the elderly: prediction of age-related changes in benzodiazepine oxidizing capacity. Journal of Pharmacology and Experimental Therapeutics 220: 120-126, 1982a

Greenblatt DJ, Divoll M, Abernethy DR, Moschitto LJ, Smith RB, et al. Alprazolam kinetics in the elderly: relation to antipyrine disposition. Archives of General Psychiatry 40: 287-290, 1983a

Greenblatt DJ, Divoll M, Puri SK, Ho I, Zinny MA, et al. Clobazam kinetics in the elderly. British Journal of Pharmacology 12: 631-636, 1981

Greenblatt DJ, Divoll M, Puri SK, Ho I, Zinny MA, et al. Reduced single-dose clearance of clobazam in elderly men predicts increased multiple-dose accumulation. Clinical Pharmacokinetics 8: 83-94, 1983b

Greenblatt DJ, Friedman H, Burstein ES, Scavone JM, Blyden GT, et al. Trazodone kinetics: effect of age, gender, and obesity. Clinical Pharmacology and Therapeutics 42: 193-200, 1987

Greenblatt DJ, Koch-Weser J. Clinical pharmacokinetics. New England Journal of Medicine 293: 702-705, 964-970, 1985

Greenblatt DJ, Sellers EM, Shader RI. Drug disposition in old age. New England Journal of Medicine 306: 1081-1088, 1982b

Greenblatt DJ, Shader RI. Nonprescription psychotropic drugs. In Jarvik (Ed.) Psychopharmacology in the practice of medicine, pp. 345-357, Appleton-Century-Crofts, New York, 1977

Holder CL, Korfmacher WA, Rushing LG, Thompson HC, Slikker W, et al. Formation of artifactual metabolites of doxylamine following acid hydrolysis. Journal of Chromatography 419: 113-122, 1987

Lamy PP. Over-the-counter medication: the drug interactions we overlook. Journal of the American Geriatrics Society 30 (November Suppl.): S69-S75, 1982

Paton DM, Webster DR. Clinical pharmacokinetics of H_1-receptor antagonists (the antihistamines). Clinical Pharmacokinetics 10: 477-497, 1985

Pond SM, Tozer TN. First-pass elimination: basic concepts and clinical consequences. Clinical Pharmacokinetics 9: 1-25, 1984

Rickels K, Ginsberg J, Morris RJ, Newman HM, Schiller HM, et al. Doxylamine succinate in insomniac family-practice patients: a double-blind study. Current Therapeutic Research 35: 532-540, 1984

Schmucker DL. Aging and drug disposition: an update. Pharmacological Reviews 37: 133-148, 1985

Slikker W, Holder CL, Lipe GW, Korfmacher WA, Thompson HC, et al. Metabolism of ^{14}C-labeled doxylamine succinate (Bendectin) in the Rhesus monkey (Macaca mulatta). Journal of Analytical Toxicology 10: 87-92, 1986

Vestal RE. Pharmacology and aging. Journal of the American Geriatrics Society 30: 191-200, 1982

Wilkinson GR. Clearance approaches in pharmacology. Pharmacological Reviews 39: 1-47, 1987

Authors' address: Dr *David J. Greenblatt*, Division of Clinical Pharmacology, Tufts-New England Medical Center, Box 1007, 117 Harrison Avenue, Boston, MA 02111 (USA).

Original Research Article

Clinical Pharmacokinetics 16: 317-325 (1989)
0312-5963/89/0005-0317/$04.50/0

Co-Trimoxazole (Sulphamethoxazole plus Trimethoprim) Peritoneal Barrier Transfer Pharmacokinetics

Joseph E. Svirbely, Amadeo J. Pesce, Satwant Singh and *Ellen J. O'Flaherty*

Department of Pathology and Laboratory Medicine, University of Cincinnati Medical Center, Hemodialysis Unit, Veterans Administration Medical Center, and Department of Environmental Health, University of Cincinnati Medical Center, Cincinnati, Ohio, USA

Summary *The pharmacokinetics of co-trimoxazole (sulphamethoxazole plus trimethoprim) were studied in end-stage renal disease in patients undergoing treatment with continuous ambulatory peritoneal dialysis (CAPD) and free of peritonitis. Plasma and dialysate concentrations were monitored for 1 exchange after administration of a single oral or intraperitoneal dose of co-trimoxazole, and were fitted by a pharmacokinetic model that took into account the equilibrium nature of CAPD by including return from the peritoneum in oral studies and from the plasma in intraperitoneal studies. Clearances were calculated and compared by analysis of variance. There was a significant effect of direction of flow ($p < 0.01$), plasma-peritoneal clearances being larger than peritoneal-plasma clearances for both drugs. In addition, there was a significant difference ($p < 0.0001$) between sulphamethoxazole clearances and trimethoprim clearances, with the latter being greater in both directions.*

Continuous ambulatory peritoneal dialysis (CAPD) [Popovich et al. 1976] has become an accepted treatment for end-stage renal disease, despite the incidence of peritonitis which is a major complication and requires aggressive treatment with antibiotics. However, the latter, like many other drugs, display different characteristics in renal failure patients treated with CAPD from those in healthy subjects (Maher 1984).

The pharmacokinetics of several antibiotics have been studied in CAPD. These studies, using a variety of approaches, have arrived at different conclusions regarding peritoneal transfer. Somani et al. (1982), administering gentamicin either intraperitoneally or intravenously to CAPD subjects and measuring blood and dialysate concentrations over time, concluded that drug transfer from dialysate to blood was rapid and extensive, while reverse transfer was negligible. In contrast, Pancorbo and Comty (1981) calculated a plasma-to-dialysate clearance for gentamicin of 0.176 L/h after intraperitoneal administration. The pharmacokinetics of tobramycin (Bunke et al. 1983a), vancomycin (Blevins et al. 1984; Pancorbo & Comty 1982) and several cephalosporins (Bunke et al. 1983b; Gross et al. 1983; Local et al. 1981) have also been studied.

Peritoneal transfer processes (Maher 1980) and the resistances that limited their rates (Dedrick et al. 1982; Nolph et al. 1980) have been identified and characterised. Transfer across the peritoneal barrier occurs by both diffusion and ultrafiltration. Diffusion is the more rapid of the two, and is dependent on the area and permeability of the peritoneal barrier and on the free concentrations of solute in dialysate and in blood. Capillary permeability is inversely proportional to the square root of the molecular weight of the solute, and the distributed model of peritoneal transfer proposed by Flessner et al. (1984) leads to the expectation that this will also be true of the permeability of the peritoneal barrier. Permeability can also be expected to be influenced by the polarity of the solute. Lipophilic chemicals are transferred rapidly across lipoid barriers by diffusion, while polar or ionised solutes are hindered in their passage by interactions with charged elements within the barrier (Maher 1980) and the fact that ionised compounds are less lipophilic than their uncharged counterparts. If the peritoneal barrier were sufficiently impermeable to the ionised form of a solute, ionisation could in principle negate the availability of the solute for the diffusion process. Similarly, protein binding affects both diffusion and ultrafiltration, because bound drug is not available to either process due to the size of the drug-protein complex.

The purpose of this study is to define more clearly the importance of some of the parameters that influence drug transfer across the human peritoneal barrier. Transfers from plasma to peritoneum and from peritoneum to plasma were modelled within 1 exchange. The effect of partition coefficient and degree of ionisation on peritoneal transfer processes was investigated, in order to establish whether these factors influence transfer across the peritoneal barrier as they do that across other physiological barriers such as the blood-brain barrier and the transplacental barrier.

Co-trimoxazole (sulphamethoxazole plus trimethoprim) was chosen because the molecular weights and protein binding characteristics after 2 days are similar, while their pKa values, classification as acidic or basic drug, and partition coefficients are different. This allowed determination of the effect of these latter factors on transfer across the peritoneal barrier while molecular size and protein binding were controlled. The pharmacokinetics of co-trimoxazole in CAPD have been investigated before (Halstenson et al. 1984; Singlas et al. 1981), but the factors influencing peritoneal barrier transfer behaviour have not been previously described.

Patients and Methods

The pharmacokinetics of co-trimoxazole were studied following oral (PO) and intraperitoneal (IP) administration. Five adult male patients undergoing CAPD for end-stage renal disease were enrolled in the study, and 3 of these were the subject of the IP study. The patients were free of peritonitis both during and between studies. Experiments were monitored by the University of Cincinnati Committee on Human Research.

Before the PO study commenced, the overnight dialysate bag was drained, and vital signs were recorded. Fresh dialysate (2L, 1.5% dextrose) was instilled into the peritoneum and zero-time blood and dialysate samples were drawn immediately before 1 co-trimoxazole tablet containing sulphamethoxazole 800mg plus trimethoprim 160mg ('Bactrim-DS') was administered (study time zero). Dialysate and blood were sampled at 0.25, 0.5, 1, 1.5, 2, 4, 6, 12, 24 and 48 hours. Dialysate was exchanged after 6 hours and every 4 to 6 hours thereafter.

For the IP study, co-trimoxazole (sulphamethoxazole 800mg plus trimethoprim 160mg) ['Bactrim IV'] was added to fresh dialysate, and the contents of the bag were mixed. Zero-time blood and dialysate were drawn and dialysate containing co-trimoxazole was instilled into the peritoneum. Serial blood and dialysate samples were collected at 3 hours and the 48-hour samples were collected as in the PO study, except that additional samples were collected at 3 hours and the 48-hour samples were omitted. The first dialysate bag was exchanged for fresh dialysate free of co-trimoxazole after 6 hours, and no further drug was given. Patients received no other medications during the study.

Analysis

Concentrations of sulphamethoxazole, *N*-acetylsulphamethoxazole, and trimethoprim were tested in each sample. It should be noted that all patients studied were anuric during the course of the studies, making determination of the renal output of sulphamethoxazole and trimethoprim unnecessary. In order to calculate the percentage protein binding free sulphamethoxazole was measured in each plasma sample by splitting the sample and separating free from bound drug using the Amicon Micropartition System (Amicon Corporation, Danvers, Massachusetts).

Concentrations of free and total sulphamethoxazole and *N*-acetylsulphamethoxazole in plasma and dialysate were measured by a spectrophotometric method (Bratton & Marshall 1939). The sensitivity of the Bratton-Marshall procedure in this laboratory is 1 mg/L, linearity is to 500 mg/L, and the patients were kept free of substances which could interfere, such as other sulpha drugs. Furthermore, each run included a zero-time sample as a patient blank. With regard to reproducibility, a 50 mg/L spiked control run together with patient runs between January and May 1988, by 2 different technicians, yielded 29 control values with a mean of 46.6 ± 3.5 mg/L, with a coefficient of variation of 7.5%. A control was run with each batch of total sulphamethoxazole, free sulphamethoxazole, or *N*-acetylsulphamethoxazole during the study. Although hydroxysulphamethoxazole metabolites are theoretically capable of interfering with the Bratton-Marshall assay, concentrations are negligible during the first 6 hours after administration of an initial dose of sulphamethoxazole (Martea et al. 1987).

Trimethoprim concentrations in plasma and dialysate were measured by a high performance liquid chromatography (HPLC) method for trimethoprim developed in this laboratory (see Svirbely & Pesce 1987). The assay as reported demonstrated replication of $p = 0.96$, sensitivity 0.05 mg/L, linearity from 2 to 100 mg/L ($r = 0.99$), and freedom from interferences. In a separate experiment, the partition coefficients of sulphamethoxazole and trimethoprim between *n*-octanol and phosphate buffer (pH 7.52) were measured. *n*-Octanol was chosen as the organic phase because it approximates the partition characteristics of human tissue. The pH of 7.52 approximated the pH of dialysate during 80% of an exchange.

Pharmacokinetic Modelling

Blood and dialysate concentrations from the first exchange were generally fitted to a 1-compartment body model using the NONLIN84 pharmacokinetic modelling program (Metzler & Weiner 1985), with first-order exchange between blood and dialysate (table I). The 12-, 24- and 48-hour samples in the PO study were not used in this model, but the blood samples from that study including those taken at 12, 24 and 48 hours were used to calculate plasma elimination half-lives for sulphamethoxazole and trimethoprim and the apparent volumes of distribution of both drugs. Trimethoprim blood data alone from 3 patients in the PO study were better fitted by a 2-compartmental model if the 12-, 24- and 48-hour samples were included. However, when both the blood and dialysate trimethoprim data were modelled for the first exchange only, to determine plasma to peritoneal fluid and peritoneal fluid to plasma transfer rate constants and clearances, the data were better fitted by the 1-compartment equations in table I. For sulphamethoxazole, first-order appearance and disappearance of the acetylated metabolite and its elimination were incorporated into the equations. Input was either into the blood by first-order absorption from the gut (oral study) or directly into the peritoneal space at time zero (intraperitoneal study). First-order return from dialysate (oral study) and from plasma (intraperitoneal study) were included, allowing separation and calculation of plasma-peritoneal and peritoneal-plasma clearances for both sulphamethoxazole and trimethoprim. By using only the unbound fraction of each drug in modelling, the study eliminated any effect of protein binding on measured clearances. A constant percentage free fraction was used for unbound trimethoprim (Patel & Welling 1980) but the unbound fraction of sulphamethoxazole was measured because, according to Reidenberg et al. (1984), binding of basic drugs such as trimethoprim is unaltered by the acidosis found in renal disease, while

Table I. Sets of differential equations, parameters and constants used in modelling

Sulphamethoxazole data from oral study

$$DZ(1) = \left[k_{01} \cdot Z(2) \cdot f_u \cdot \frac{Vd}{Vp} \right] - k_{10} \cdot Z(1)$$

$$DZ(2) = \left[\frac{k_a \cdot D \cdot e^{-k_a t}}{Vd} \right] - k_{01} \cdot f_u \cdot Z(2) - k_m \cdot Z(2)$$

$$DZ(3) = k_m \cdot Z(2)$$

Trimethoprim data from oral study

$$DZ(1) = \left[k_{01} \cdot Z(2) \cdot f_u \cdot \frac{Vd}{Vp} \right] - k_{10} \cdot Z(1)$$

$$DZ(2) = \left[\frac{k_a \cdot D \cdot e^{-k_a t}}{Vd} \right] - k_{01} \cdot f_u \cdot Z(2)$$

Co-trimoxazole data from intraperitoneal study

$$DZ(1) = \left[k_{01} \cdot Z(2) f_u \cdot \frac{Vd}{Vp} \right] - k_{10} \cdot Z(1)$$

$$DZ(2) = k_{10} \cdot Z(1) \cdot \frac{Vd}{Vp}$$

Abbreviations: Z(1) = dialysate concentration; Z(2) = plasma concentration; Z(3) = metabolite concentration; DZ(1) = the derivative of the change in the dialysate level with time; DZ(2) = the derivative of the plasma level/dt; DZ(3) = the derivative of the metabolite level with respect to time; f_u = fraction unbound in plasma; Vd = volume of distribution; Vp = volume of peritoneal dialysate; k_m = apparent metabolism rate constant; k_{01} = plasma to peritoneal compartment transfer rate constant; k_{10} = peritoneal to plasma compartment transfer rate constant; t = time/dose interval; D = dose; k_a = absorption rate constant; $k_a \cdot D \cdot e^{-k_a t}/Vd$ = absorbance from gut.

the binding of acidic drugs such as sulphamethoxazole is decreased compared with that in healthy individuals.

The following kinetic parameters were estimated: apparent volume of distribution (Vd), apparent metabolic rate constant of sulphamethoxazole (k_m), plasma-peritoneal transfer rate constant (k_{01}) and peritoneal-plasma transfer rate constant (k_{10}). From these parameters, clearances were calculated as Vd × k_{01} for plasma-peritoneal clearance, and k_{10} × 2L for peritoneal-plasma clearance, 2L being the approximate volume of the dialysate. Criteria used to select or eliminate sets of differential equations and arrive at the models described by the equations in table I included comparison of correlation matrices of the estimates, eigenvalues of (A transpose A) matrices and calculations of the corrected sum of squares and sum of squared residuals, all generated by the NONLIN84 program as measures of the reliability of the modelling. Analysis of variance was performed on the clearance values, using the SAS statistical program (SAS 1985), to test for effect of direction (plasma-peritoneal *versus* peritoneal-plasma) and of drug (sulphamethoxazole *versus* trimethoprim).

Results

The partition coefficient of trimethoprim was 5.1 in the *n*-octanol buffer system. Sulphamethoxazole did not partition measurably into *n*-octanol. The mean protein binding of sulphamethoxazole was 54%, lower than the published figure of 66% (Patel & Welling 1980); percentage binding did not vary with concentration. Sample decay curves for 1 patient are shown in figure 1; these are typical of the pharmacokinetic behaviour and concentrations found with the other 4 patients. It should be noted that the sulphamethoxazole metabolite, *N*-acetyl-sulphamethoxazole, did not transfer across the peritoneal barrier from the plasma to the dialysate to a significant extent during the first exchange.

Pharmacokinetic data pooled from the oral and intraperitoneal studies are given in table II. Rate constants and clearances were first calculated sep-

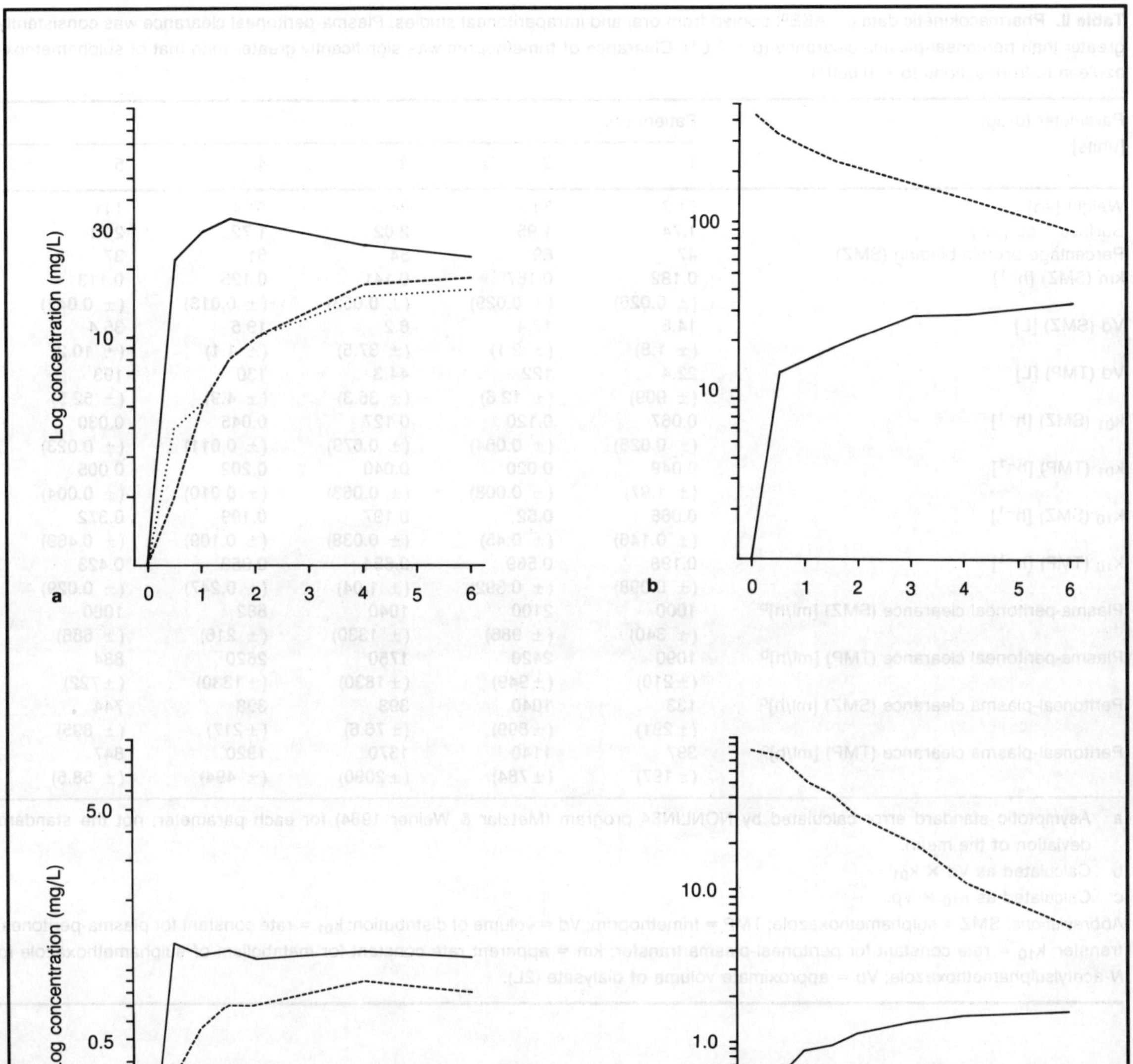

Fig. 1. Drug concentration data over the first exchange for 1 patient in both oral [(**a**) sulphamethoxazole; (**c**) trimethoprim] and intraperitoneal [(**b**) sulphamethoxazole; (**d**) trimethoprim] studies; (—) = plasma drug concentration; (---) = dialysate drug concentration; (...) = plasma *N*-acetylsulphamethoxazole concentration.

Table II. Pharmacokinetic data (± ASE[a]) pooled from oral and intraperitoneal studies. Plasma-peritoneal clearance was consistently greater than peritoneal-plasma clearance ($p < 0.01$). Clearance of trimethoprim was significantly greater than that of sulphamethoxazole in both directions ($p < 0.0001$)

Parameter (drug) [units]	Patient no.				
	1	2	3	4	5
Weight [kg]	61.3	84.2	86.2	61.4	141
Surface area [m^2]	1.74	1.95	2.02	1.72	2.71
Percentage protein binding (SMZ)	47	69	54	61	37
km (SMZ) [h^{-1}]	0.182 (± 0.026)	0.167 (± 0.029)	0.141 (± 0.053)	0.125 (± 0.013)	0.113 (± 0.042)
Vd (SMZ) [L]	14.6 (± 1.8)	17.4 (± 2.1)	8.2 (± 37.5)	19.5 (± 1.1)	35.4 (± 10.2)
Vd (TMP) [L]	22.4 (± 909)	122 (± 12.6)	44.3 (± 36.3)	130 (± 4.9)	193 (± 52.5)
k_{01} (SMZ) [h^{-1}]	0.067 (± 0.028)	0.120 (± 0.064)	0.127 (± 0.679)	0.045 (± 0.011)	0.030 (± 0.023)
k_{01} (TMP) [h^{-1}]	0.049 (± 1.97)	0.020 (± 0.008)	0.040 (± 0.063)	0.202 (± 0.010)	0.005 (± 0.004)
k_{10} (SMZ) [h^{-1}]	0.066 (± 0.146)	0.52 (± 0.45)	0.197 (± 0.038)	0.199 (± 0.109)	0.372 (± 0.469)
k_{10} (TMP) [h^{-1}]	0.198 (± 0.098)	0.569 (± 0.392)	0.684 (± 1.04)	0.959 (± 0.247)	0.423 (± 0.029)
Plasma-peritoneal clearance (SMZ) [ml/h][b]	1000 (± 340)	2100 (± 986)	1040 (± 1330)	882 (± 216)	1060 (± 686)
Plasma-peritoneal clearance (TMP) [ml/h][b]	1090 (±210)	2420 (±949)	1750 (±1830)	2620 (±1330)	884 (±722)
Peritoneal-plasma clearance (SMZ) [ml/h][c]	133 (±291)	1040 (±899)	393 (±76.6)	398 (±217)	744 (± 895)
Peritoneal-plasma clearance (TMP) [ml/h][c]	397 (±197)	1140 (±784)	1370 (±2090)	1920 (± 494)	847 (± 58.5)

a Asymptotic standard error calculated by NONLIN84 program (Metzler & Weiner 1984) for each parameter; not the standard deviation of the mean.

b Calculated as Vd × k_{01}.

c Calculated as k_{10} × Vp.

Abbreviations: SMZ = sulphamethoxazole; TMP = trimethoprim; Vd = volume of distribution; k_{01} = rate constant for plasma-peritoneal transfer; k_{10} = rate constant for peritoneal-plasma transfer; km = apparent rate constant for metabolism of sulphamethoxazole to *N*-acetylsulphamethoxazole; Vp = approximate volume of dialysate (2L).

arately for each study, and were combined for each of the 3 patients who participated in both studies, after analysis of variance had established that route of administration did not affect either rate constants or clearances. The reliability of the k_{01} and k_{10} transfer rate constants in table II as measured by a number of indicators was independent of the route of administration and acceptable for non-linear modelling. The results in table II show that plasma-peritoneal clearance was consistently greater than peritoneal-plasma clearance ($p < 0.01$), regardless of route of administration. Clearance of trimethoprim was found to be significantly higher than that of sulphamethoxazole in both directions across the peritoneal barrier ($p < 0.0001$).

Discussion

The rate of transfer across the peritoneal barrier should be inversely proportional to the square root of the molecular weight of the solute mass (Dedrick et al. 1982; Sorkin & Nolph 1981). The ratio of the square roots of the molecular weights of trimethoprim and sulphamethoxazole is 17 : 16, so close to unity that difference in molecular weight cannot explain the differences in clearance between the 2 drugs.

Protein binding restricts the amount of drug available for transfer, since only unbound drug passes freely across the peritoneal barrier. Trimethoprim is about 45% bound to plasma proteins (Patel & Welling 1980). Mean binding (± SD) of sulphamethoxazole to plasma proteins in the 5 patients in the current study was 54 ± 12% (table I). Any effect of plasma protein binding was eliminated in the study by modelling the movement of free rather than total drug. There is a lack of information on tissue binding and intrinsic distribution characteristic for co-trimoxazole (Patel & Welling 1980), but tissue binding in the central compartment, although it may affect the apparent volume of distribution, would not affect transperitoneal transfer of the drugs.

Polar molecules, with low lipid solubility, are hindered in their passage across lipoid barriers unless they are very small. Sulphamethoxazole is sufficiently polar that it did not partition measurably into the organic phase of the *n*-octanol/phosphate buffer system. Trimethoprim, however, has a partition coefficient of 5.1 in this system, representing fairly high lipid solubility for an orally administered drug. Thus, the greater clearance of trimethoprim, in both directions across the peritoneal barrier, is consistent with the relative polarities of the 2 drugs.

Degree of ionisation affects transfer in a way similar to polarity: the un-ionised form of the molecule is favoured over the ionised form as they move through the peritoneal barrier, because the latter interacts with charged groups within the barrier. Furthermore, because equilibrium across a lipoid barrier is established for un-ionised drug, the degree of ionisation of the drug in solution on either side of the barrier should control the transbarrier ratio of total drug concentrations at equilibrium.

The pKa of sulphamethoxazole, an acidic drug, is 5.7; that of trimethoprim, a basic drug, is 6.6. The Henderson-Hasselbach equation can be used to calculate the effect of pH on the degree of ionisation of co-trimoxazole in dialysate and in blood. The pH of dialysate in CAPD is 7.5 for 5 of the 6 hours of a typical exchange (Robson et al. 1981); at that level sulphamethoxazole would be 98.4% ionised and trimethoprim 11.2%. In blood also, sulphamethoxazole should be much more highly ionised than trimethoprim. At the typical blood pH of a CAPD patient (Teehan et al. 1981) of 7.35, sulphamethoxazole would be 97.8% ionised and trimethoprim must also contribute to its greater clearance in both directions across the peritoneal barrier.

Similar observations concerning the importance of polarity and degree of ionisation as determinants of peritoneal transfer rate in the rat were made by Torres et al. (1978). These investigators studied uptake from the peritoneum into the systemic circulation of compounds with varying partition coefficients, molecular weights and degrees of ionisation. In order to maximise the surface area of the peritoneum, they measured absorption from large volumes of fluid (50 ml) in female Sprague-Dawley rats weighing 200 ± 50g, utilising a dwell time of 1 hour. Uptake was strikingly dependent on both partition coefficient and molecular weight. Absorption of a series of barbiturates ranged from 96% for thiopentone, with a partition coefficient of 3.3, to 57% for barbitone with a partition coefficient of 0.001. The degree of ionisation also affected uptake. Absorption of a series of acidic compounds ranged from 76% for salicylate, almost completely ionised at physiological pH, to 95% for phenol, largely un-ionised. In the case of basic compounds, caffeine, mostly un-ionised, was 68% absorbed while atropine, mostly ionised at physiological pH, was 27% absorbed.

In the current study, the basic compound trimethoprim (89% un-ionised at pH 7.5) was 57% absorbed from the human peritoneum during the first hour of dialysate dwell time, while the acid sulphamethoxazole (only 1.6% un-ionised at dialysate pH) was only 27% absorbed during the first hour. These values are somewhat lower than those recorded by Torres et al. (1978). Apart from the species difference, the direction of net fluid flux in the 2 studies was different. Because an osmotically active compound was not included in the peritoneal instillate in the Torres et al. study, fluid flux favoured absorption; these authors measured an uptake of 10.5% of the 50ml instillate during the first hour. In the present study, net fluid flux was in the direction of transfer from plasma to peritoneum because the dialysate was osmotically active due to the addition of 1.5% dextrose. Pyle et al. (1981) estimated the net movement of fluid to be about 300ml in the course of a 4 to 6 hour exchange. This fluid flux constitutes a pressure which may overcome some of the resistance to transfer from plasma to peritoneum, but which itself constitutes a resistance to be overcome during peritoneal-plasma transfer. The result is that transfer in the direction of net fluid flux is favoured over transfer in the opposite direction. Thus, the net fluid flux from plasma to peritoneum in the current study is a reasonable explanation for the observation that plasma clearances were larger than peritoneal clearances. However, the net fluid flux, although demonstrating a mean of 300ml over 6 hours with a 1.5% dextrose dialysate, also demonstrates considerable variability (Pyle et al. 1981) which may account for some of the intrapatient variation in the clearances found in this study.

It should be emphasised that these clearances, calculated for transfer from plasma to peritoneum and from peritoneum to plasma, are not comparable to the net clearances calculated in studies in which the approach-to-equilibrium nature of CAPD was not taken into account. Net clearances, calculated using the formula:

Clearance = D/AUC

where D is the amount of drug absorbed or recovered from dialysate and AUC (area under the concentration/time curve) is determined directly from the plasma or serum concentration/time graph, are sensitive to dwell time; that is, to the extent to which return from peritoneum to plasma has influenced the AUC. At the beginning of an exchange the concentration gradient across the barrier favours plasma-peritoneal transfer in oral administration studies but at the end of an exchange the gradient equalises, aided by the flux of water into the dialysate.

While the approach used in the present study, and in others, is a grouped-parameter one in which a series of differential equations define transfer, Flessner et al. (1982) and Dedrick et al. (1984) have used physiological measurements such as pore radius and pore density to estimate capillary level solute permeability, and measurements and estimates for void fraction, retardation factor, tissue tortuosity, and tissue diffusivity to determine transport in the peritoneal barrier tissue space. This distributed model allows a thorough grasp of transfer phenomena, especially within the peritoneal barrier tissue, and is valuable for predicting methods of manipulating various parameters to respond to the demands of experimental or clinical conditions. However, the grouped-parameter approach used in the present study is capable of predicting plasma and peritoneal fluid concentrations more easily than the distributed model.

Based on the plasma data alone from the oral study, the apparent half-life of sulphamethoxazole ranged from 4.5 to 28.9 hours, which is similar to the range of elimination half-lives found in healthy individuals (Patel & Welling 1980). The mean metabolic rate constant for sulphamethoxazole (table II) was $0.15 \pm 0.03\ h^{-1}$, which corresponds to a half-life of metabolism of 4.5 hours. Thus, a large fraction of sulphamethoxazole elimination from the plasma is due to metabolism. Less than 10% of trimethoprim is metabolised (Patel & Welling 1980), and its half-life was 30.2 to 74.7 hours in patients in this study, substantially greater than in renally sufficent persons in whom the mean elimination half-life is approximately 12 hours (Patel & Welling 1980). The extent to which sulphamethoxazole is metabolised is the determining factor in its shorter half-life compared with trimethoprim.

The results demonstrate that transfer across the peritoneal barrier is similar in behaviour to transfer across many other barriers. This observation is consistent with the relative lipid solubilities and degrees of ionisation of sulphamethoxazole and trimethoprim.

Therapeutic Implications

The clinical implication of these findings is that co-trimethoxazole can be used effectively to treat sensitive intraperitoneal and systemic infections in CAPD patients. This finding agrees with those of other published studies (Halstenson et al. 1984; Singlas et al. 1981).

Our clinical experience in treating peritoneal infections with co-trimethoxazole is that the best strategy is to use both oral and intraperitoneal administration in order to obtain effective sulphamethoxazole concentrations in the peritoneum.

Acknowledgements

We would like to thank Dr S.A. Myre, Dr P.B. Hammond, Dr E. Foulkes, and F.M. Hassan for helpful discussion. We would also like to thank Bettye Morgan, R.N., and Audrey Dale, R.N., for helping with the clinical portions of the study.

Research was supported by grants from the Endowment Fund of the American Association for Clinical Chemistry and from the Kidney Foundation of Greater Cincinnati.

References

Blevins RD, Halstenson CE, Salemn NG, Matzke GR. Pharmacokinetics of vancomycin in patients undergoing continuous ambulatory peritoneal dialysis. Antimicrobial Agents and Chemotherapy 25: 603-606, 1984

Bratton AC, Marshall Jr EK. A new coupling component for sulfanilamide determination. Journal of Biological Chemistry 128: 537-550, 1939

Bunke CM, Aronoff GR, Brier ME, Sloan RS, Luft FC. Tobramycin kinetics during continous ambulatory peritoneal dialysis. Clinical Pharmacology and Therapeutics 34: 110-116, 1983a

Bunke CM, Aronoff GR, Brier ME, Sloan RS, Luft FC. Cefazolin and cephalexin kinetics in continous ambulatory peritoneal dialysis. Clinical Pharmacology and Therapeutics 33: 66-72, 1983b

Dedrick RL, Flessner MF, Collins JM, Schultz JS. Is the peritoneum a membrane? American Society of Artificial Interior Organs Journal 5: 1-8, 1982

Flessner MF, Dedrick RL, Schultz JS. A distributed model of peritoneal transport: theoretical considerations. American Journal of Physiology 246 (Regulatory Integrative Comparative Physiology 15): R597-R607, 1984

Gross ML, Somani P, Ribner BS, Raeader R, Freimer EH, et al. Ceftizoxime elimination kinetics in continous ambulatory peritoneal dialysis. Clinical Pharmacology and Therapeutics 34: 673-680, 1983

Halstenson CE, Blevins RB, Salem NG, Matzke GR. Trimethoprim-sulfamethoxazole pharmacokinetics during continuous ambulatory peritoneal dialysis. Clinical Nephrology 22: 239-243, 1984

Local FK, Munro AJ, Kerr DNS, Sussman M. Pharmacokinetics of intravenous and intraperitoneal cefuroxime in patients undergoing peritoneal dialysis. Clinical Nephrology 16: 40-43, 1981

Maher JF. Peritoneal transport rates: mechanisms, limitations, and methods for augmentation. Kidney International 18 (Suppl.): S117-S120, 1980

Maher JF. Pharmacokinetics in patients with renal failure. Clinical Nephrology 21: 39-46, 1984

Martea M, Hekster YA, Vree TB, Voets AJ, Berden JHM. Pharmacokinetics of cefradine, sulfamethoxazole, and trimethoprim and their metabolites in a patient with peritonitis and undergoing continuous ambulatory peritoneal dialysis. Pharmaceutisch Weekblad – Scientific Edition 9: 110-116, 1987

Metzler CM, Weiner DL. NONLIN84, a nonlinear estimation program, Statistical Consultants, Crestview Hills, Kentucky, 1984, 1985

Nolph KD, Miller F, Rubin J, Popovich R. New directions in peritoneal dialysis concepts and approaches. Kidney International 18 (Suppl.): S111-S116, 1980

Pancorbo S, Comty C. Pharmacokinetics of gentamicin in patients undergoing continuous ambulatory peritoneal dialysis. Antimicrobial Agents and Chemotherapy 19: 605-607, 1981

Pancorbo S, Comty C. Peritoneal transport of vancomycin in four patients undergoing continous ambulatory peritoneal dialysis. Nephron 31: 37-39, 1982

Patel RB, Welling PG. Clinical pharmacokinetics of co-trimoxazole. Clinical Pharmacokinetics 5: 405-423, 1980

Popovich RP, Moncrief JW, Decherd JF, Bomar JB, Pyle WK. The definition of a novel portable-wearable equilibrium technique. Abstract. American Society of Artificial Organs 64: 1976

Pyle WK, Moncrief JW, Popovich RP. Peritoneal transport evaluation in CAPD. In Moncrief & Popovich (Eds) CAPD update, pp. 35-52, Masson, New York, 1981

Reidenberg MM, Drayer DE. Alteration of drug-protein binding in renal disease. Clinical Pharmacokinetics 9 (Suppl. 1): 18-26, 1984

Robson M, Pinto T, Kao E, Oren A. The metabolism of lactate and bicarbonate in CAPD. In Atkins et al. (Eds) Peritoneal dialysis, pp. 212-216, Churchill Livingstone, Edinburgh, 1981

SAS Institute, Inc. SAS users guide: Statistics, Version 5 Edition, SAS Institute, Inc., Cary, North Carolina, 1985

Singlas E, Rottembourg J, de Martin A, Collins JN, Legrain M. Pharmacokinetics of co-trimoxazole using the peritoneal route: consequence for treatment of peritonitis in patients maintained on peritoneal dialysis. In Moncrief & Popovich (Eds) CAPD update, pp. 63-66, Masson, New York, 1981

Somani P, Shapiro RS, Stockard H, Higgins JT. Unidirectional absorption of gentamicin from the peritoneum during continuous ambulatory peritoneal dialysis. Clinical Pharmacology and Therapeutics 32: 113-121, 1982

Sorkin MI, Nolph KD. Dynamics of peritoneal transfer. In Atkins et al. (Eds) Peritoneal dialysis, pp. 12-21, Churchill Livingstone, New York, 1981

Svirbely JE, Pesce AJ. An HPLC method for trimethoprim utilizing solid phase column extraction. Therapeutic Drug Monitoring 9: 216-220, 1987

Teehan BP, Reichard GA, Sigler MH, Schleifer CR, Cupit MC, et al. Acid-base studies in continuous ambulatory peritoneal dialysis. In Moncrief & Popovich (Eds) CAPD update, p. 95, Masson, New York, 1981

Torres IJ, Litterst CL, Guarino AM. Transport of model compounds across the peritoneal membrane in the rat. Pharmacology 17: 330-340, 1978

Authors' address: *Joseph E. Svirbely*, Ohio River Division Laboratory, US Army Corps of Engineers, 5851 Mariemont Avenue, Cincinnati, OH 45227-0618 (USA).

Information for Authors

Manuscript Preparation: Articles are published in English. Submit 2 copies of the complete manuscript, including title page, text pages, references, tables, legends, footnotes and figures. Only typed copy, double-spaced on 1 side of preferably A4 (206mm × 294mm) typewriter paper with liberal margins is acceptable. Articles in the current issue of the Journal should be consulted for the general layout of the paper.

Subdivision of Articles: Manuscripts should be prepared and paginated in the following manner:

a) Title page
b) Summary
c) Text pages
   i) Original articles
      Introduction
      Methods
      Results
      Discussion
      Therapeutic Implications
   ii) Review articles
      Outline will be provided
d) Acknowledgements
e) List of references
f) Address for correspondence
g) Tables
h) Figures and legends
i) Footnotes

Title Page: There should be a separate title page with title, authors and institutions where the work was done, indicating the city, and a condensed running title of not more than 50 letters including spaces.

The name and address of author to whom correspondence should be addressed should appear separately at the end of the references.

Summary: For *original articles,* the summary should not exceed 150 words. It should be factual, not descriptive, and should present the reason for the study, the main findings (giving specific data if possible), and the principal conclusions. For *review articles,* the summary should be about 5% of the length of the article and should highlight the salient points discussed.

Results/Discussion/Implications (for Original Articles): Description of the experimental results should be succinct, but of sufficient detail to allow the experiment to be repeated by others. Conclusions and theoretical considerations must not appear in the results section, nor is a recapitulation of the results acceptable for the discussion section. Where relevant, a concise statement of the implications of the experimental results, particularly in the clinical use of drug(s), should appear as a separate section.

References: In the text, reference to published work is cited by author (alphabetically) and year — viz. (Hart 1986, 1987; Lind et al. 1980; Mariner & Jamieson 1976) . . . (Tipping 1982b; Wilson & Payne 1984b,c,d).

The list of references must be arranged alphabetically by first author's name (and initials if more than one author of the same name) or by second or third, etc. authors if more than one author of the same name and initials. If the sequence of the authors' names and initials is identical, the references should be arranged chronologically by year of publication. Only the first 5 authors are required.

Sample references are listed below. *Note:* titles of journals are *not* to be abbreviated. Supply inclusive pagination for all articles.

Journal article: Ashby J, Piddock LJV, Wise R. An investigation of the hydrophobicity of the quinolones. Journal of Antimicrobial Chemotherapy 16: 805-810, 1985

Silke B, Verma SP, Frais MA, Reynolds G, Jackson N, et al. Haemodynamic analysis of the effects of nicardipine and metoprolol alone and in combination in coronary artery disease. European Heart Journal 6: 930-938, 1985a

Silke B, Verma SP, Hussain M, Jackson NC, Hafizullah M, et al. Comparative haemodynamic effects of nicardipine and verapamil in coronary artery disease. Herz 10: 112-119, 1985b

Journal abstract: Sando H, Katagiri H, Okada M, Shoda R, Arai Y, et al. The effect of nifedipine and nicardipine on glucose tolerance, insulin and C-peptide. Abstract no. 262. Diabetes 32 (Suppl. 1): 6A, 1983

Book: Hart AH. Pharmacokinetics and metabolism of the benzamides. In Platts et al. (Eds) The benzamides: pharmacology and clinical aspects, Vol. 35, pp. 143-162, Raven Press, New York, 1986

Clinical Pharmacokinetics 16: 327-336 (1989)
0312-5963/89/0006-0327/$05.00/0

Clinical Pharmacokinetics-Pharmacodynamics of Anticancer Drugs

William E. Evans and *Mary V. Relling*

Pharmacokinetics and Pharmacodynamics Section, Pharmaceutical Division, St Jude Children's Research Hospital, Memphis, Tennessee, and Center for Pediatric Pharmacokinetics and Therapeutics, Departments of Clinical Pharmacy and Pediatrics, Colleges of Pharmacy and Medicine, University of Tennessee, Memphis, Tennessee, USA

Anticancer drugs typically have a narrow therapeutic index, often producing acute toxicity at dosages similar to those required for therapeutic efficacy. These toxicities may be severe and life-threatening (eg, neutropenia, thrombopenia), while the consequences of underdosing may be equally life-threatening. For drug-sensitive cancers, where it is essential to avoid underdosing of chemotherapy, more precise methods are needed to determine the maximum tolerated dosage in individual patients.

Several clinical trials have demonstrated a dose-response relationship for anticancer drugs, thus providing an impetus to investigate the relation between their pharmacokinetic profile and the therapeutic response. Recognition of a steep dose-response relationship for many of these agents, coupled with numerous studies describing large interpatient variability in their pharmacokinetics, provides a compelling rationale for systematic investigations of the clinical pharmacodynamics of cancer chemotherapy. Over the past 5 to 10 years several reports on this subject have been published, and representative studies are reviewed here. The major purpose of this article is to heighten awareness of pharmacokinetic and pharmacodynamic strategies for investigating the clinical activity of antineoplastic agents, and for adjusting the dosage of certain anticancer drugs in individual patients.

1. Clinical Response: Influence of the Drug Dose or Dose-Intensity

A number of investigators have demonstrated that the *intensity* of cancer chemotherapy regimens can have a significant influence on the response rate of several drug-sensitive cancers. In these reports, patients who received a higher percentage of the planned chemotherapy, a higher dosage (e.g. 2 mg/m^2 *versus* 1 mg/m^2) or a higher dose-intensity over a given time period (e.g. mg/m^2/week), were more likely to have a favourable clinical response. Examples of diseases and therapies for which such data have been reported are given in table I.

The importance of drug dose in cancer chemotherapy was extensively reviewed by Frei and Canellos (1980), and an impressive amount of new data has accumulated in the past 8 years. These observations provide important evidence that the relative intensity of cancer chemotherapy can have a significant influence on the clinical outcome of particular diseases. In other words, reducing the dose and/or delaying the time over which a treatment is given, so as to spare the patient mild toxicity or inconvenience, may be a great disservice to the patient, as it may reduce the probability of

Table I. Some examples of studies reporting the influence of dose-intensity on clinical response

Disease	Therapy	Reference
Acute lymphocytic leukaemia	Cyclophosphamide, MTX and mercaptopurine	Pinkel et al. (1971)
Breast cancer	Adjuvant CMF	Bonnadonna & Valagussa (1981); Hryniuk & Levine (1986)
Colorectal cancer	5-Fluorouracil	Hryniuk et al. (1987)
Hodgkin's disease	MOPP	Carde et al. (1983)
Metastatic breast cancer	CMF	Tannock et al. (1988)
Myeloma	Prednisone	Palmer et al. (1988)
Osteosarcoma	MTX	French Bone Tumour Study Group (1988)
Ovarian and endometrial cancer	Doxorubicin (adriamycin) and cisplatin (*cis*-platinum II)	Levin & Hryniuk (1987)
Small cell carcinoma of the lung	Cyclophosphamide, CCNU and MTX	Cohen et al. (1977)
	Etoposide	Hryniuk (1987)
Testicular cancer	Cisplatin (with vinblastine and bleomycin)	Samson et al. (1984)

Abbreviations: CMF = Cyclophosphamide, methotrexate (amethopterin), 5-fluorouracil; MOPP = mustine (mechlorethamine), vincristine, prednisone, procarbazine; CCNU = cyclohexyl-chloroethyl-nitrosourea; MTX = methotrexate (amethopterin).

cure. The overall importance of this concept and the problems associated with ignoring it were recently the subject of an editorial by the Director of the US National Cancer Institute (DeVita Jr 1986). It should be noted, however, that dose-intensity is only of importance in drug-sensitive cancers, and that prospective, randomised clinical trials are needed to clearly define the importance of dose-intensity for most of the examples described in table I (Henderson et al. 1988).

2. *Systemic Exposure as an Alternative Measure of Treatment Intensity*

The concept of measuring treatment intensity at a level beyond dose-intensity is depicted schematically in figure 1, and indicates that the amount and duration of systemic exposure to a given drug are determined by well-recognised pharmacokinetic variables, which are known to differ greatly from patient to patient. Therefore, even when one is able to ensure that the protocol (assumed optimal) dose of a drug is actually administered, systemic drug exposure [e.g. area under the serum concentration-time curve (AUC)], and therefore response, may be vastly different from patient to patient (figure 2). With antineoplastic regimens for which dose-intensity has been shown to be important, it seems logical that pharmacokinetic variability can be equally or more important.

This hypothesis is especially relevant for those anticancer drugs with highly variable pharmacokinetics, and essentially every antineoplastic agent we have studied has exhibited highly variable pharmacokinetic parameters, even within populations of patients with *normal* renal and liver function. For example, the clearance rate of methotrexate (amethopterin), etoposide, teniposide, doxorubicin (adriamycin), cyclophosphamide and bleomycin have been shown to differ by a factor of 2 to 10 among children with cancer (Crom et al. 1987). Similar variability has also been observed in adult patients (Bender et al. 1978), and for other pharmacokinetic parameters such as drug absorption (Zimm et al. 1983) and distribution (Evans et al 1983). Thus, even if one standardises the dose-intensity of these drugs to some predefined optimal level, a 2- to 10-fold range in drug clearance will yield a similarly wide range in systemic exposure to the drug.

Although it is recognised that drug concentration in serum is not necessarily equal to drug concentration in the tumour (as indicated in figure 1), it is clear that drug exposure at the systemic level is more likely to be correlated with that at the tumour level, than is simply the amount of administered drug. One might also argue that clinicians

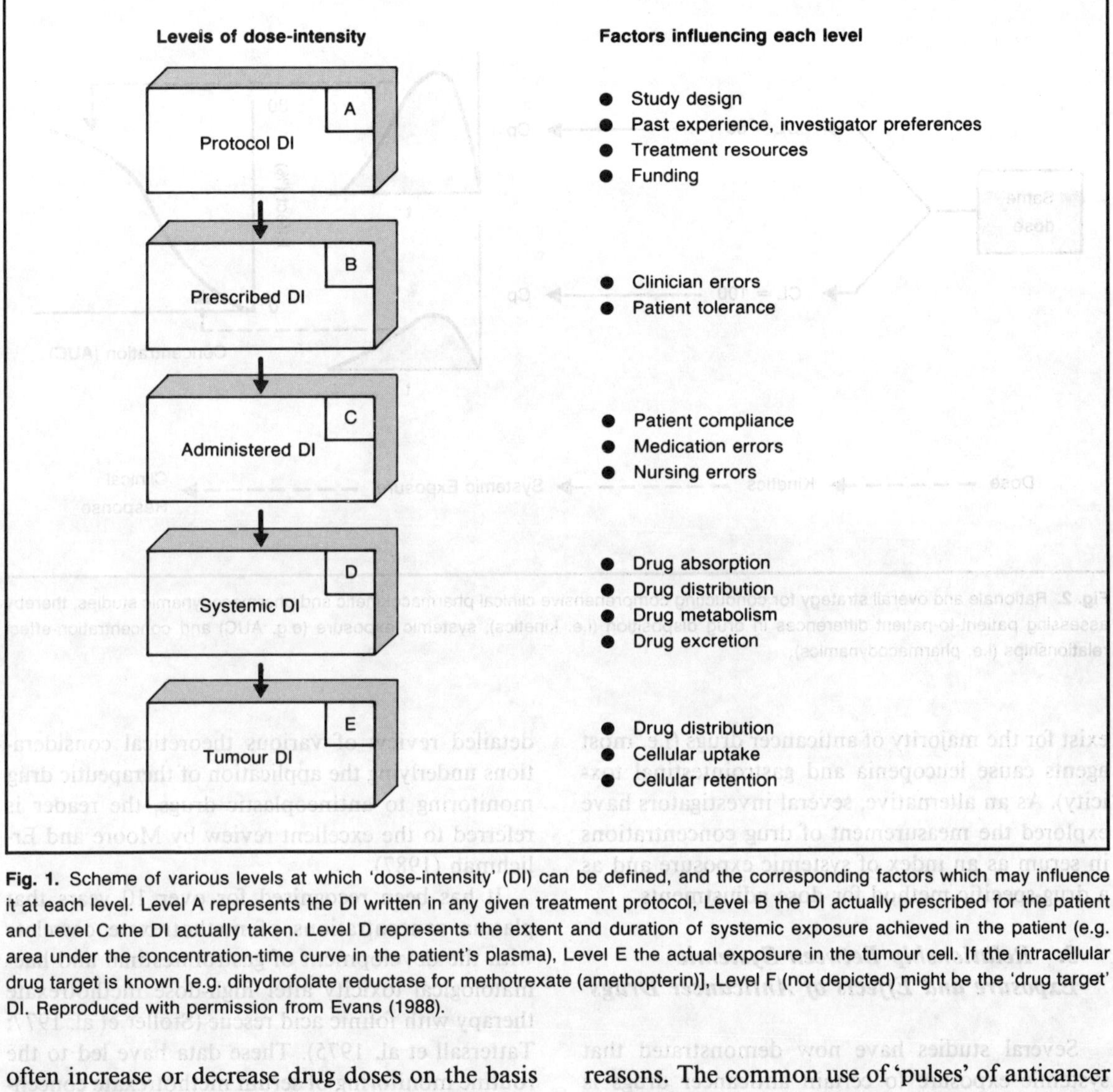

Fig. 1. Scheme of various levels at which 'dose-intensity' (DI) can be defined, and the corresponding factors which may influence it at each level. Level A represents the DI written in any given treatment protocol, Level B the DI actually prescribed for the patient and Level C the DI actually taken. Level D represents the extent and duration of systemic exposure achieved in the patient (e.g. area under the concentration-time curve in the patient's plasma), Level E the actual exposure in the tumour cell. If the intracellular drug target is known [e.g. dihydrofolate reductase for methotrexate (amethopterin)], Level F (not depicted) might be the 'drug target' DI. Reproduced with permission from Evans (1988).

often increase or decrease drug doses on the basis of some clinical measure of drug effects, thus adjusting for patient-to-patient differences in drug disposition. One such example is the alteration of the dose of acute lymphocytic leukaemia remission maintenance therapy to keep the circulating white blood cell count within a predefined range (i.e. 2000 to 4000 per μl). Although this strategy does offer a reasonable approach to determine which patients can tolerate higher doses of anticancer drugs, it falls short of being a solution to the problem for several reasons. The common use of 'pulses' of anticancer drugs, which result in nearly uniform leucopenia, in addition to the use of drug combinations rather than single agents, makes it difficult to adjust antineoplastic dosage based on clinical monitoring parameters alone. Ideally, one would have a specific measure of cytotoxic effect for each drug given in a combination regimen, thus providing a drug-specific end-point by which the dose of each drug could be individualised. Unfortunately, unique and sensitive measures of cytotoxicity do not currently

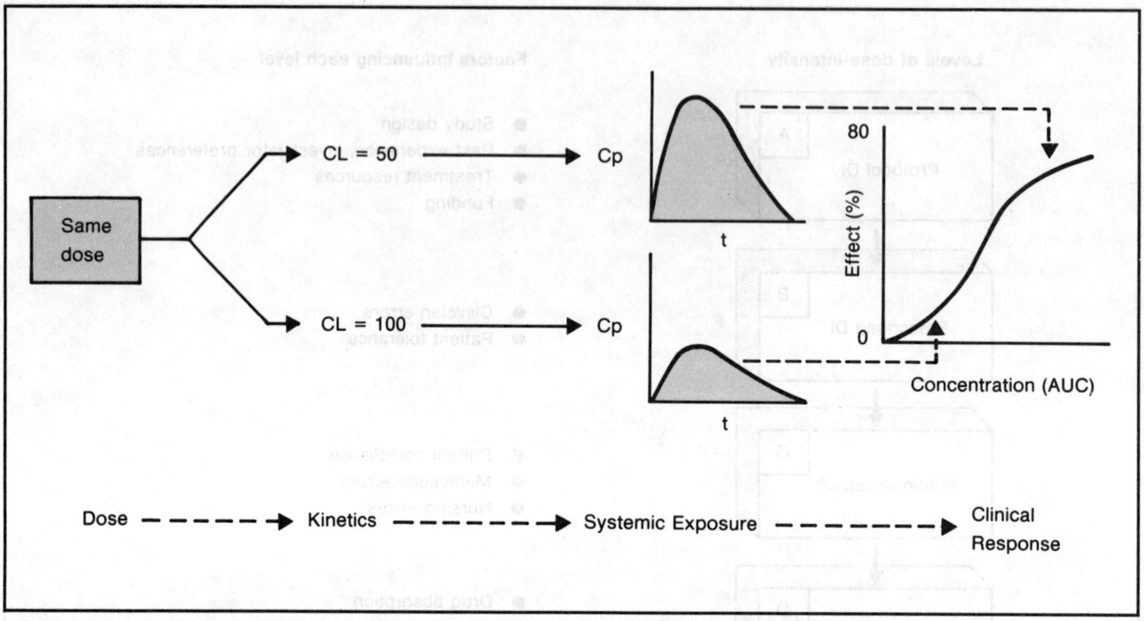

Fig. 2. Rationale and overall strategy for conducting comprehensive clinical pharmacokinetic and pharmacodynamic studies, thereby assessing patient-to-patient differences in drug disposition (i.e. kinetics), systemic exposure (e.g. AUC) and concentration-effect relationships (i.e. pharmacodynamics).

exist for the majority of anticancer drugs (i.e. most agents cause leucopenia and gastrointestinal toxicity). As an alternative, several investigators have explored the measurement of drug concentrations in serum as an index of systemic exposure and as a drug-specific method for dose adjustments.

3. *Relationship Between Systemic Exposure and Effects of Anticancer Drugs*

Several studies have now demonstrated that systemic exposure to certain anticancer drugs is correlated with either their toxicity, their efficacy, or both. These studies support the rationale behind the use of drug concentrations as a method to adjust drug dosages, and provide the impetus to conduct clinical pharmacokinetic studies with other drugs and for other types of cancer (Bertino 1987). Several representative pharmacokinetic studies are discussed below and a number of additional studies are summarised in table II, exemplifying how this body of knowledge has evolved. For a more detailed review of various theoretical considerations underlying the application of therapeutic drug monitoring to antineoplastic drugs, the reader is referred to the excellent review by Moore and Erlichman (1987).

It has been recognised for over 10 years that plasma concentrations of methotrexate correlate with the development of gastrointestinal and haematological toxicity after high-dose methotrexate therapy with folinic acid rescue (Stoller et al. 1977; Tattersall et al. 1975). These data have led to the routine monitoring of serum methotrexate concentrations as a prospective method for adjusting folinic acid rescue and preventing toxicity (Evans et al. 1986a).

More recently, clinical pharmacokinetic studies of high-dose methotrexate have been expanded to include an association between its pharmacokinetics and disease relapse in children with acute lymphocytic leukaemia (Borsi & Moe 1987; Evans et al. 1984, 1986b). Both higher systemic clearance of methotrexate and lower steady-state plasma drug concentrations (C^{ss}) were associated with a higher risk of early relapse. In a multivariate analysis of prognostic factors affecting outcome in acute lymphocytic leukaemia (including white blood cell count, age, sex, race and DNA index), systemic exposure to the drug (e.g. C^{ss}) was an independent and strong prognostic variable (Evans et al. 1986b). A randomised clinical trial is now under way at our institution to prospectively test whether the administration of higher dosages of methotrexate (and other anticancer drugs) will improve clinical response in acute lymphocytic leukaemia patients with rapid drug clearance.

As in the case of methotrexate, studies indicating a relationship between the pharmacokinetics of 5-fluorouracil and toxicity preceded those studies showing an association with oncolytic effectiveness. In patients with colorectal cancer given a continuous infusion of 5-fluorouracil for 6 days, there was an increased risk of leucopenia in individuals with 120-hour plasma drug concentrations greater than 1.5 μmol/L (Au et al. 1982). Subsequent studies by other investigators (Goldberg et al. 1988; Milano et al. 1988) have confirmed a relationship between toxicity and plasma AUC of 5-fluorouracil for the entire 5 days of therapy. In addition, in patients receiving this drug for colorectal cancer liver metastases, decreased plasma AUC was associated with an increase in the size of hepatic metastatic lesions (Milano et al. 1987). Thus, with 5-fluorouracil and possibly many other anticancer drugs, clinicians may be faced with the dilemma that the same high systemic exposure that results in more effective anti-tumour therapy also results in more toxicity. The goal is to define a level of systemic exposure which maximises the likelihood of therapeutic response while producing minimal (acceptable) toxicity, then to use pharmacokinetic principles to select a dosage which will yield a level of systemic exposure within this narrow range.

4. *Utility of Pharmacodynamic Studies in the Drug Development Process*

Pharmacodynamic principles are increasingly being applied to studies of anticancer agents in Phase I and Phase II clinical trials, as these represent a time in their clinical evaluation when the drugs are given as single agents. They also represent a critical stage in the drug development process when decisions are made about the dosages of these drugs for future clinical trials. Recently, the European Organization for Research and Treatment of Cancer (EORTC 1987) and National Cancer Institute (USA) investigators (Collins et al. 1986) have advocated the use of AUC as a pharmacokinetic guide to dose escalations in Phase I clinical trials. Even more recently, our laboratory has advocated the determination of 'maximum tolerated systemic exposure (MTSE)' in Phase I clinical studies, as a more informative alternative to the traditional 'maximum tolerated dosage (MTD)' (Evans 1988). Such data should lead to the use of dosages which are more likely to produce oncolytic responses in Phase II clinical trials (i.e. to avoid subtherapeutic dosages in clinical trials conducted to identify drug-responsive tumours).

This concept is exemplified in a Phase I-II study of continuous infusion teniposide in 26 children with refractory leukaemia and solid tumours (Rodman et al. 1987). As shown in figure 3, both oncolytic response and severe gastrointestinal toxicity were related to systemic exposure to teniposide (measured by plasma AUC or C^{ss}). Moreover, as has been reported by others, there was a poor correlation between dose and either response or toxicity, despite the fact that in this dose-finding trial, doses ranged from 300 to 750 mg/m^2/72h. Therefore, it is clear that assessment of pharmacokinetics and pharmacodynamics in Phase I and Phase II trials may provide more useful information regarding drug tolerance and efficacy, and thus provide an attractive alternative to determining the MTD (in mg per weight or body surface area). This approach to studying new anticancer drugs has been used by other investigators to define a relationship between systemic exposure and toxicity for drugs such as menogoril (Egorin et al. 1986), carboplatin (Egorin et al. 1984, 1985), and hexamethylene-bisacetrimide (Egorin et al. 1987b).

It should be acknowledged that not all studies have found a significant pharmacokinetic relationship for anticancer drugs and their efficacy or tox-

Table II. Summary of selected clinical pharmacodynamic studies with anticancer drugs

Drug	Type of study[a]	Pharmacokinetic parameter	Drug effect(s) measured	Pharmacodynamic relationship	Reference
Amsacrine (AMSA)	6 (of 19) adults with disseminated cancer given 30 or 40 mg/m^2	CL_s of ^{14}C-AMSA	Lowest measured granulocyte or platelet count	Lower CL_s associated with lowest granulocyte count	Hall et al. (1983)
Carboplatin	Adults with refractory tumours and renal dysfunction (n = 22)	Plasma AUC	Change in platelet count	Higher AUC associated with greater % drop in platelet count	Egorin et al. (1984)
	Adults with refractory tumours (n = 23)	Plasma AUC	Change in platelet count	Prospective validation of above relation between AUC and change in platelet count	Egorin et al. (1985)
Cisplatin	40 adults with various cancers given 80 mg/m^2	Total plasma platinum concentration	> 30% increase in serum creatinine or > 30% decrease in CL_{CR}	Higher C at 12 and 24h associated with nephrotoxicity	Campbell et al. (1983)
Cytosine arabinoside (ARA-C)	Adults with acute non-lymphocytic leukemia (n = 28)	4h Retention of ARA-CTP in leukaemic blasts (after *in vitro* incubation)	Complete remission (CR)	Greater cellular retention of ARA-CTP associated with higher % achieving CR and a longer duration of CR	Rustum & Preisler (1979); Rustum et al. (1987)
Etoposide	Adults with refractory cancer (n = 18)	Steady-state plasma concentration (C^{ss})	Surviving fraction of white blood cells	Lower surviving fraction of WBCs with higher C^{ss}	Bennett et al. (1987)
5-Fluorouracil	Adults with liver metastases from colorectal cancer (n = 9)	Plasma AUC	Change in platelet and WBC count	Higher AUC associated with decreased platelet and WBC count	Goldberg et al. (1988)
	(n = 42)	Total cycle plasma AUC	Probability of toxicity (mucositis, diarrhoea, leucopenia, or anaemia)	AUC for cycle > 30 mg/L · h associated with toxicity	Milano et al. (1988)
	(n = 6)	Plasma AUC corrected for dose	Hepatic tumour mass	Decreased AUC associated with increase in hepatic metastases	Milano et al. (1987)
	Colorectal cancer (n = 24)	CL and C^{ss}	Change in WBC count	Leucopenia more frequent with 120h C > 1.5 μmol/L or with low clearance	Au et al. (1982)
Hexamethylene-bisacetamide	Adults with refractory solid tumours (n = 20)	Plasma AUC	Change in platelet count	Higher AUC associated with a greater % decrease in platelet count	Egorin et al. (1987b)

Table II. Contd.

Drug	Type of study[a]	Pharmacokinetic parameter	Drug effect(s) measured	Pharmacodynamic relationship	Reference
Menogaril	Patients with refractory malignancies (n = 24)	Plasma AUC	Change in WBC and neutrophil count	Higher AUC associated with greater % decrease in WBC or absolute neutrophil counts	Egorin et al. (1986)
	Adults with liver dysfunction (n = 23)	Plasma AUC	Change in WBC and neutrophil count	Higher AUC associated with greater % decrease in WBC and neutrophil count	Egorin et al. (1987a)
Mercaptopurine (MP)	Children with ALL (n = 22 and n = 19)	Red cell concentration of MP metabolite (6TG nucleotide)	Absolute neutrophil count 14 days post-dose	Higher 6TG nucleotide RBC concentration associated with neutropenia	Lennard et al. (1983, 1986)
MTX (High-dose)	Children with ALL in first remission (n = 108)	Systemic clearance (CL_s)	Disease relapse	Higher CL_s associated with increased risk of early relapse	Evans et al. (1984)
	Children with ALL in first remission (n = 108), longer follow-up of same patients as above	C^{ss}	Disease relapse	$C^{ss} < 16$ μmol/L with 24h infusion of 1 g/m^2 associated with increased risk of early relapse	Evans et al. (1986b)
	Children with ALL in first or second remission (n = 58)	CL_s	Disease relapse	Higher CL_s in those who relapsed	Borsi & Moe (1987)
	Metastatic tumours and osteosarcoma (n > 100)	Plasma concentration at 48 hours	Toxicity (mucositis) myelosuppression, renal dysfunction)	48h concentration > 0.9 μmol/L associated with risk of toxicity	Tattersall et al. (1975); Stoller ete al. (1977); Evans et al. (1986a)
N-methyl-formamide	Adults with refractory solid tumours (n = 15)	Plasma AUC	Hepatotoxicity	Higher AUC associated with hepatotoxicity after IV doses	Rowinsky et al. (1988)
Teniposide	Children with refractory ALL or solid tumours (n = 23)	CL_s (C^{ss})	Oncolytic response (> 75% decrease in leukaemic blasts or PR for solid tumours)	C^{ss} higher (CL_s lower) in responders *vs* non-responders	Rodman et al. (1987)
Vincristine	Adults (n = 24) and children (n = 3) with cancer or ITP	Plasma AUC	Neurological exam	Higher cumulative AUC associated with more severe neurotoxicity	Desai et al. (1982)

a Patients and disease.

Abbreviations: ALL = acute lymphocytic leukaemia; AUC = area under the concentration-time curve; C = plasma drug concentration; C^{ss} = plasma drug concentration at steady-state; CL_{CR} = creatinine clearance; CL_s = systemic clearance; ITP = idiopathic thrombocytopenic purpura; PR = partial response; RBC = red blood cell; WBC = white blood cell; ARA-CTP = cytosine arabinoside triphosphate; 6TG = 6 thioguanine.

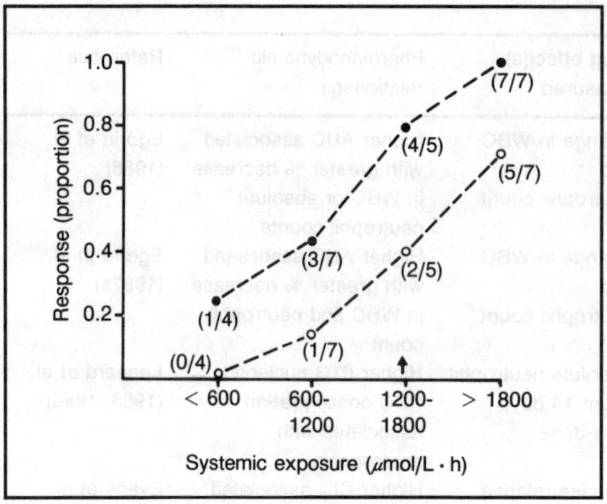

Fig. 3. Relation between teniposide systemic exposure (area under the concentration-time curve) and probability of oncolytic reponse (●) or grade 2 to 4 gastrointestinal toxicity (○). Arrow depicts a potential initial target level of systemic exposure, providing a high probability of response and acceptable toxicity. Developed from data published in Rodman et al. (1987). Figures in parentheses indicate the proportion of patients responding to treatment or experiencing toxic effects.

icity. For instance, in 40 patients with acute non-lymphocytic leukaemia treated with daunorubicin and cytosine arabinoside, there was no relationship between any measure of daunorubicin or daunorubicinol concentration in plasma, white blood cells or bone marrow cells, and either outcome or toxicity (Kokenberg et al. 1988). The same lack of a relationship has been described for cytosine arabinoside plasma AUC in patients with acute non-lymphocytic leukaemia (Rustum et al. 1987). There are several possible explanations for this lack. First, acute non-lymphocytic leukaemia, like many types of cancer, is probably a very heterogeneous disease, so that within a group of patients there may be many different tumour types which vary greatly in their drug-responsiveness. Secondly, as in the study of Kokenberg et al. (1988), if patients are treated with more than one drug, it is difficult to ascribe toxicity or response to the pharmacokinetics of any particular one of the agents they have received. Other reasons for failing to detect a pharmacokinetic relationship include the possibility that all patients in a trial were under- or over-dosed, that inappropriate pharmacokinetic or drug-effect parameters were measured, or that the researchers failed to assay for active drug or metabolites in the appropriate biological fluid. That these investigators (Rustum & Preisler 1979; Rustum et al. 1987) did document a relationship between cytosine arabinoside triphosphate retention in leukaemic blast cells and clinical response is an excellent example of the potential need to consider active metabolites and biological fluids other than serum when attempting to define the pharmacodynamics of anticancer drugs.

5. *Conclusions*

It is clear that the pharmacokinetics of most anticancer drugs are highly variable from patient to patient, and also within the same patient over a course of chemotherapy. Several studies cited in this article have demonstrated a significant relationship between the pharmacokinetics (e.g. AUC) of selected anticancer drugs and their clinical effects (e.g. toxicity or efficacy). These data suggest that use of clinical pharmacokinetic principles to individualise dosages of certain anticancer drugs could increase the probability of response or decrease the probability of toxicity, or both. However, in essentially all cases where significant concentration-effect relationships have been demonstrated, prospective randomised clinical trials are needed to rigorously assess the clinical importance of using pharmacokinetic and pharmacodynamic principles to individualise the dosages of anticancer drugs.

Acknowledgements

This work was supported in part by NIH MERIT award R37 CA 36401, Leukemia Program Project grant CA 20180, Solid Tumor Program Project grant CA 23066, Cancer Center CORE grant CA 21765, a Center of Excellence grant from the State of Tennessee, and ALSAC.

References

Au JLS, Rustum YM, Ledesma EJ, et al. Clinical pharmacological studies of concurrent infusion of 5-fluorouracil and thymidine in treatment of colorectal carcinomas. Cancer Research 42: 2930-2937, 1982

Bender RA, Zwelling LA, Doroshow JH, Locker GY, Hande KR, et al. Antineoplastic drugs: clinical pharmacology and therapeutic use. Drugs 16: 46-87, 1978

Bennett CL, Sinkule JA, Schilsky RL, et al. Phase I clinical and pharmacological study of 72-hour continuous infusion of etoposide in patients with advanced cancer. Cancer Research 47: 1952-1956, 1987

Bertino JR. Blood levels of cancer chemotherapeutic agents and clinical outcome. Journal of Clinical Oncology 5: 996, 1987

Bonnadonna G, Valagussa P. Dose-response effect of adjuvant chemotherapy in breast cancer. New England Journal of Medicine 304: 10-15, 1981

Borsi J, Revesz T, Schuler D. Prognostic importance of systemic clearance of methotrexate in childhood ALL. Cancer Chemotherapy and Pharmacology 19: 261-264, 1987

Borsi JD, Moe PJ. Systemic clearance of methotrexate in the prognosis of acute lymphocytic leaukemia in children. Cancer 60: 3020-3024, 1987

Campbell BA, Kalman SM, Jacobs C. Plasma platinum levels: relationship to cisplatin dose and nephrotoxicity. Cancer Treatment Reports 67: 169-172, 1983

Carde P, MacKintosh FR, Rosenberg SA. A dose and time response analysis of treatment of Hodgkin's disease with MOPP chemotherapy. Journal of Clinical Oncology 1: 146-153, 1983

Cohen MH, Creaven PJ, Fossieck BE, et al. Intensive chemotherapy of small cell bronchogenic carcinoma. Cancer Treatment Reports 61: 349-354, 1977

Collins JM, Zaharko DS, Dedrick RI, et al. Potential roles for preclinical pharmacology in Phase I clinical trials. Cancer Treatment Reports 70: 73-80, 1986

Crom WR, Glynn-Barnhart AM, Rodman JH, Christensen M, Relling MV, et al. Pharmacokinetics of anticancer drugs in children. Clinical Pharmacokinetics 12: 168-213, 1987

Desai ZR, Van den Berg HW, Bridges JM, et al. Can severe vincristine neurotoxicity be prevented? Cancer Chemotherapy and Pharmacology 8: 211-214, 1982

DeVita Jr. VT. Dose-response is alive and well. Journal of Clinical Oncology 4: 1157-1159, 1986

Egorin MJ, Conley BA, Forrest A, et al. Phase I study and pharmacokinetics of menogaril (NSC 269148) in patients. Cancer Research 47: 6104-6110, 1987a

Egorin MJ, Sigman LM, Van Echo DA, Forrest A, et al. Phase I clinical and pharmacokinetic study of hexamethylene bisacetamide administered as a five-day continuous infusion. Cancer Research 47: 617-623, 1987b

Egorin MJ, Van Echo DA, Olman EA, et al. Prospective validation of a pharmacologically based dosing scheme for carboplatin. Cancer Research 45: 6502-6506, 1985

Egorin MJ, Van Echo SJ, Tipping EA, et al. Pharmacokinetics and dosage reduction of carboplatin in patients with impaired renal function. Cancer Research 44: 5432-5438, 1984

Egorin MJ, Van Echo DA, Whitacre MY, et al. Human pharmacokinetics, excretion, and metabolism of the anthracycline antibiotic menogaril and their correlation with clinical toxicities. Cancer Research 46: 1513-1520, 1986

EORTC Pharmacokinetic and Metabolism Group. Pharmacokinetically guided dose escalation in Phase I clinical trials. Commentary and proposed guidelines. European Journal of Cancer and Clinical Oncology 23: 1083-1087, 1987

Evans WE. Clinical pharmacodynamics of anticancer drugs: a basis for extending the concept of dose-intensity. Blut 56: 241-248, 1988

Evans WE, Crom WR, Stewart CF, et al. Methotrexate systemic clearance influences probability of relapse in children with standard-risk acute lymphocytic leukemia. Lancet 1984: 359-62, 1984

Evans WE, Crom WR, Stewart CF, et al. Clinical pharmacodynamics of high-dose methotrexate in acute lymphocytic leukemia. New England Journal of Medicine 314: 471-477, 1986b

Evans WE, Crom WR, Yalowich J. Methotrexate. In Evans et al. (Eds) Applied pharmacokinetics: principles of therapeutic drug monitoring, 2nd ed., pp. 1009-1056, Applied Therapeutics, Inc., Spokane, Washington, 1986a

Evans WE, Hutson PR, Stewart CF, et al. Methotrexate cerebrospinal fluid and serum concentrations after intermediate-dose methotrexate infusion. Clinical Pharmacology and Therapeutics 33: 301-307, 1983

Frei III E, Canellos GP. Dose: a critical factor in cancer chemotherapy. American Journal of Medicine 69: 585-594, 1980

French Bone Tumour Study Group. Age and dose chemotherapy as major prognostic factors in a trial of adjuvant therapy of osteosarcoma combining two alternating drug combinations and early prophylactic lung irradiation. Cancer 61: 1304-311, 1988

Goldberg JA, Kerr DJ, Willmott N, et al. Pharmacokinetics and pharmacodynamics of locoregional 5-fluorouracil (5FU) in advanced colorectal liver metastases. British Journal of Cancer 57: 186-189, 1988

Hall SW, Friedman J, Legha SS, Benjamin RS, Gutterman JU, et al. Human pharmacokinetics of a new acridine derivative, 4′-(9-acridinylamino) methanesulfon-m-anisidide (NSC 249992). Cancer Research 43: 3422-3426, 1983

Henderson IC, Hayes DF, Gelman R. Dose-response in the treatment of breast cancer: a critical review. Journal of Clinical Oncology 6: 1501-1515, 1988

Hryniuk WM. Average relative dose intensity and the impact on design of clinical trials. Seminars in Oncology 14: 65-74, 1987

Hyrniuk WM, Figueredo A, Goodyear M. Applications of dose intensity to problems in chemotherapy at breast and colorectal cancer. Seminars in Oncology 14 (Suppl. 4): 3-11, 1987

Hryniuk WM, Levine M. Analysis of dose intensity for adjuvant chemotherapy trials in stage II breast carcinoma. Journal of Clinical Oncology 4: 1162-1170, 1986

Kokenberg E, Sonneveld P, Sizoo W, et al. Cellular pharmacokinetics of daunorubicin: relationships with the response to treatment in patients with acute myeloid leukemia. Journal of Clinical Oncology 6: 802-812, 1988

Lennard L, Keen D, Lilleyman JS. Oral 6-mercaptopurine in childhood leukemia: parent drug pharmacokinetics and active metabolite concentrations. Clinical Pharmacology and Therapeutics 40: 287-292, 1986

Lennard L, Rees CA, Lilleyman JS, Maddocks KL. Childhood leukemia: a relationship between intracellular 6-mercaptopurine metabolites and neutropenia. British Journal of Clinical Pharmacology 16: 359-363, 1983

Levin L, Hryniuk W. The application of dose intensity to problems in chemotherapy of ovarian and endometrial cancer. Seminars in Oncology 14 (Suppl. 14): 12-19, 1987

Milano G, Namer M, Boublil JL, et al. Relationship between systemic 5-FU passage and response in colorectal cancer patients treated with intrahepatic chemotherapy. Cancer Chemotherapy and Pharmacology 20: 71-74, 1987

Milano G, Roman P, Khater R, et al. Dose *versus* pharmacokinetics for predicting tolerance to 5-day continuous infusion of 5-FU. International Journal of Cancer 41: 537-541, 1988

Moore MJ, Erlichman C. Therapeutic drug monitoring in oncology: problems and potential in antineoplastic therapy. Clinical Pharmacokinetics 13: 205-227, 1987

Palmer M, Belch A, Hanson J, Brox L. Dose intensity analysis of melphalan and prednisone in multiple myeloma. Journal of the National Cancer Institute 80: 414-418, 1988

Pinkel D, Hernandez K, Borella L, et al. Drug dosage and remission duration in childhood lymphocytic leukemia. Cancer 37: 247-256, 1971

Rodman JH, Abromowitch M, Sinkule JA, Rivera GK, Evans WE. Clinical pharmacodynamics of continuous infusion teniposide: systemic exposure as a determinant of response in a Phase I trial. Journal of Clinical Oncology 5: 1007-1014, 1987

Rowinsky EK, Noe DA, Douglas WO, et al. Clinical pharmacology of oral and IV N-methylformamide: a pharmacologic basis for lack of clinical antineoplastic activity. Journal of the National Cancer Institute 80: 670-678, 1988

Rustum YM, Preisler HD. Correlation between leukemic cell retention of 1-β-D-arabinofuranosylcytosine 5′-triphosphate and response to therapy. Cancer Research 39: 39-49, 1979

Rustum YM, Riva C, Preisler HD. Pharmacokinetic parameters of ara-C and their relationship to intracellular metabolism of ara-C, toxicity, and response of patients with acute nonlymphocytic leukemia treated with conventional and high-dose ara-C. Seminars in Oncology 14 (Suppl. 1): 141-148, 1987

Samson MK, Rivkin SE, Jones SE, et al. Dose-response and dose survival advantage for high- versus low-dose cisplatin combined with vinblastine and bleomycin in disseminated testicular cancer. Cancer 53: 1029-1035, 1984

Stoller RG, Hande KR, et al. Use of plasma pharmacokinetics to predict and prevent methotrexate toxicity. New England Journal of Medicine 297: 630-634, 1977

Tannock IF, Boyd NF, DeBoer G, et al. A randomized trial of two dose levels of cyclophosphamide, methotrexate, and fluorouracil chemotherapy for patients with metastatic breast cancer. Journal of Clinical Oncology 6: 1377-1387, 1988

Tattersal MHN, Parker LM, Pitman SW, et al. Clinical pharmacology of high-dose methotrexate (NSC-740). Cancer Chemotherapy Reports (now Cancer Part 3 6: Treatment Reports) Part 3 6: 25-29, 1975

Zimm S, Collins JM, Riccardi R, et al. Variable bioavailability of oral mercaptopurine: is maintenance chemotherapy in acute lymphocytic leukemia being optimally administered? New England Journal of Medicine 308: 1005-1009,1983

Authors' address: Dr *William E. Evans*, St Jude Children's Research Hospital, 332 North Lauderdale Street, Memphis, TE 38105 (USA).

Clinical Pharmacokinetics 16: 337-364 (1989)
0312-5963/89/0006-0337/$14.00/0

Pharmacokinetics of the Newer Benzodiazepines

Pamela D. Garzone and *Patricia D. Kroboth*

Center for Pharmacodynamic Research and Department of Pharmacy Practice, University of Pittsburgh, Pittsburgh, Pennsylvania, USA

Contents

Summary 337
1. Assay Methods 339
2. Alprazolam 341
2.1 Structure-Activity Relationship 341
2.2 Pharmacokinetics 342
2.3 Drug Interactions 345
3. Triazolam 346
3.1 Structure-Activity Relationship 346
3.2 Pharmacokinetics 346
3.3 Drug Interactions 350
4. Midazolam 352
4.1 Structure-Activity Relationship 352
4.2 Pharmacokinetics 352
4.3 Influence of Surgery on the Pharmacokinetics of Midazolam 356
4.4 Drug Interactions 356
5. Loprazolam 358
5.1 Structure-Activity Relationship 358
5.2 Pharmacokinetics 358
5.3 Drug Interactions 361

Summary

The assay methods used to determine the concentrations of the newer benzodiazepines include electron-capture gas-liquid chromatography, high performace liquid chromatography with ultraviolet detection, gas chromatography-mass spectrometry, radioassay and radioreceptor assay. The method used frequently is the highly sensitive and specific electron-capture gas-liquid chromatography. Other methods are associated with limitations.

The triazolo- and imidazolebenzodiazepines differ structurally from the 'classical' benzodiazepines such as diazepam, and offer distinct differences in pharmacological activity and in time-course of effect. Alprazolam and triazolam, both 1,4-triazolobenzodiazepines, have high affinities for the benzodiazepine receptor as do midazolam and loprazolam, which are 1,4-imidazolebenzodiazepines.

Absorption is characteristically rapid, with peak alprazolam and triazolam concentrations occurring within 1 hour after oral administration. Sublingual administration results in peak alprazolam and triazolam concentrations that are higher and occur earlier than with the oral route.

The volume of distribution of alprazolam and triazolam is approximately 1L. Alprazolam is 70% bound to plasma proteins and the extent of binding is independent of concentration. Similarly, triazolam is approximately 85% bound to plasma proteins, variability in binding being explained by variations in α_1-acid glycoprotein concentration.

The 1,4-triazolo ring prevents the oxidative metabolism of the classical benzodiazepines which results in formation of active metabolites with long elimination half-lives. Alprazolam is extensively metabolised: 29 metabolites have been identified in the urine, and its major metabolite, α-hydroxyalprazolam, has pharmacological activity. α-Hydroxyalprazolam and 4-hydroxyalprazolam are detectable in plasma in amounts which account for less than 10% of the administered dose. Mean alprazolam elimination half-life in healthy adult subjects ranges from 9.5 to 12 hours; liver disease prolongs alprazolam elimination, but renal insufficiency does not. Triazolam also undergoes oxidation and subsequent glucuronidation. α-Hydroxytriazolam is the major metabolite, in addition to which 4-hydroxyalprazolam and α-4-hydroxytriazolam have been identified in plasma and urine. The elimination half-life of triazolam ranges between 1.8 and 5.9 hours, while that of the conjugated metabolites is short, approximately 3.8 hours. Accumulation of triazolam or its metabolites after multiple doses does not occur. Liver disease prolongs triazolam elimination from the body, but renal disease does not.

Factors such as age, gender, and obesity can influence the pharmacokinetics of alprazolam and triazolam. The reported drug-drug interactions with both agents are predominantly the result of inhibition of the microsomal enzyme system responsible for the hepatic metabolism and elimination of these benzodiazepines.

Midazolam and loprazolam are basic compounds; the imidazole ring allows for the preparation of aqueous injectable solutions that are stable and well tolerated. Both drugs are rapidly absorbed after oral administration. Peak midazolam concentrations occur in 20 to 60 minutes, while peak loprazolam concentrations are reached in 0.5 to 2 hours. Bioavailability of oral midazolam ranges from 34 to 68%. It is also rapidly absorbed after intramuscular administration, and the bioavailability then ranges from 40 to 100%. The absolute bioavailability of loprazolam in man has not been reported; however, approximately 70 to 75% of the oral dose is absorbed in animals.

The volume of distribution for both midazolam and loprazolam is large, 0.5 to 3 L/kg, with great intersubject variability. The plasma protein binding of midazolam is 95%, while loprazolam is 80% protein bound.

Midazolam undergoes hydroxylation and subsequent glucuronidation. The elimination half-life of midazolam is approximately 2 hours; however, there have been reports of prolonged elimination (> 8 hours) in subpopulations of subjects. The elimination half-life of α-hydroxymidazolam, the major midazolam metabolite, is approximately 1 hour.

Loprazolam is not as rapidly metabolised as midazolam. The major elimination pathway is N*-oxidation of the piperazine ring. Depending on the assay method, the elimination half-life for loprazolam has ranged between 4 and 15 hours. The longer half-life may reflect the activity of metabolites, with the actual value being between 4 and 7 hours. The most common type of drug-drug interaction reported for midazolam also involves the inhibition of the microsomal mixed function oxidase system responsible for the metabolism of that drug. Loprazolam interactions have not been extensively studied.*

Recently there has been a proliferation of new benzodiazepine compounds. These benzodiazepines differ structurally from chlordiazepoxide and diazepam, and also differ from these 'classical' benzodiazepines in pharmacological profile, including antidepressant properties and favourable sedative time-course. Table I lists some of the characteristics of the newer benzodiazepines. Figure 1 is a comparison of the plasma concentration *vs* time profiles of 4 of these agents.

Table I. Comparison of the newer benzodiazepines

Drug	K_i (nm)	Metabolic pathway	Overall elimination
1,4-Triazolobenzodiazepines			
Alprazolam	3.40	Oxidation	Intermediate
Triazolam	0.76	Oxidation	Ultrashort
1,4-Imidazolebenzodiazepines			
Midazolam	3.30	Oxidation	Short
Loprazolam		Oxidation	Intermediate

Abbreviation: K_i = affinity constant.

1. Assay Methods

Methods used to determine benzodiazepine plasma concentrations include electron-capture gas-liquid chromatography (GLC), high performance liquid chromatography (HPLC) with ultraviolet (UV) detection, gas chromatography-mass spectrometry (GC-MS), radioimmunoassay (RIA) and radioreceptor assay (RRA). The choice of assay method depends on the characteristics of the benzodiazepine, the expertise of the analyst, the equipment available, the desired sensitivity and specificity and the time involved in development and validation.

The GLC method of Greenblatt and colleagues has been frequently employed in the pharmacokinetic analysis of alprazolam (Greenblatt et al. 1981a). The limit of sensitivity ranges from 0.25 to 1 μg/L and the coefficient of variation is less than 6% (Ciraulo et al. 1986; Greenblatt et al. 1983a). Alprazolam metabolites cannot be detected and quantified using this assay method. Smith and Kroboth used an HPLC procedure that measures

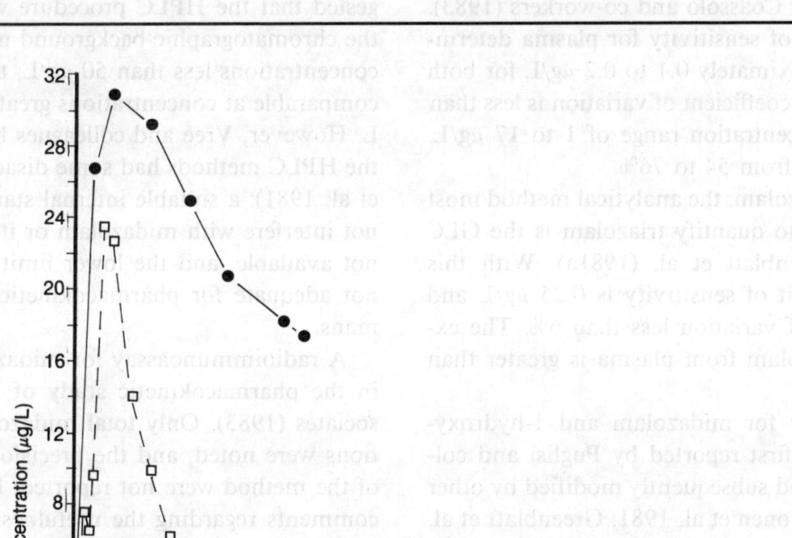

Fig 1. Time-course of plasma benzodiazepine concentrations after single oral doses of alprazolam 2mg (●) [adapted from Kroboth & Smith 1987], triazolam 0.5mg (○) [Kroboth et al., unpublished data], midazolam 7.5mg (□) [Garzone 1987] and loprazolam 1.0mg (■) [adapted from Swift et al. 1985].

alprazolam and its two primary metabolites, α- and 4-hydroxyalprazolam (Smith & Kroboth 1987). The extraction efficiency is 78% and the lower limit of quantitation is 1 μg/L. Relative standard deviations are 12% for alprazolam concentrations less than 5 μg/L, 5% for concentrations of 5 to 100 μg/L and less than 8% for α- and 4-hydroxyalprazolam concentrations of 1 to 50 μg/L.

Dehlin and colleagues also used an HPLC method to quantify triazolam and α-hydroxytriazolam (Dehlin et al. 1983). The lower limit of detection is 0.09 μg/L for triazolam and 0.05 μg/L for α-hydroxyalprazolam. The coefficients of variation at 2 and 0.5 μg/L are 3.1 and 6.3%, respectively. Some patients studied were taking other medications; these drugs did not interfere with the assay.

The simultaneous assay of triazolam and α-hydroxytriazolam by capillary gas chromatography has been reported by Coassolo and co-workers (1983). The lower limit of sensitivity for plasma determinations is approximately 0.1 to 0.2 μg/L for both compounds. The coefficient of variation is less than 4%. Over a concentration range of 1 to 17 μg/L, recovery ranged from 54 to 76%.

As with alprazolam, the analytical method most frequently used to quantify triazolam is the GLC method of Greenblatt et al. (1981a). With this method, the limit of sensitivity is 0.25 μg/L and the coefficient of variation less than 6%. The extraction of triazolam from plasma is greater than 95%.

A GLC assay for midazolam and 1-hydroxymidazolam was first reported by Puglisi and colleagues (1978) and subsequently modified by other investigators (Allonen et al. 1981; Greenblatt et al. 1981b). Recovery of midazolam averages 80 to 90%, while that of its metabolite averages 50 to 80%. The lower limit of sensitivity of this GLC method ranges from 2 to 5 μg/L and the coefficient of variation is less than 7% for concentrations between 5 and 100 μg/L. The GLC method of Arendt and colleagues permitted the quantification of midazolam, 1-hydroxymidazolam and 4-hydroxymidazolam (Arendt et al. 1984). With this method, sensitivity limits are approximately 1 to 3 μg/L for midazolam and 4-hydroxymidazolam and 5 to 10 μg/L for 1-hydroxymidazolam. Extraction procedure, internal standard, carrier gas and operating conditions vary among the reported GLC methods, accounting for the differences in sensitivity and specificity.

An HPLC method with UV detection for quantifying midazolam and 1-hydroxymidazolam was reported by Vasiliades and Sahawneh (1981). A C_{18} column is used in this reversed-phase assay which uses flurazepam as the internal standard. Within-run absolute recovery averages 78 ± 5%, and the coefficient of variation is 3 to 5% for midazolam and 4% for 1-hydroxymidazolam concentrations between 200 and 400 μg/L. The precision is 5% at midazolam concentrations of less than 50 μg/L, which compares with the coefficient of variation of 7% at midazolam concentrations of 3 and 5 μg/L reported for the GLC methods. The authors suggested that the HPLC procedure was better since the chromatographic background noise was less at concentrations less than 50 μg/L; the methods are comparable at concentrations greater than 100 μg/L. However, Vree and colleagues have stated that the HPLC methods had some disadvantages (Vree et al. 1981): a suitable internal standard that does not interfere with midazolam or its metabolites is not available, and the lower limit of detection is not adequate for pharmacokinetic studies in humans.

A radioimmunoassay for midazolam was used in the pharmacokinetic study of Avram and associates (1983). Only total midazolam concentrations were noted, and the precision and accuracy of the method were not reported. For this reason, comments regarding the usefulness of this procedure cannot be made.

A GC-MS method that is sensitive and specific for midazolam and 1-hydroxymidazolam was developed at Hoffmann LaRoche (Rubio et al. 1982). This method has a relative standard deviation of less than 6% at concentrations of 5 μg/L. Desmethylmidazolam, a minor metabolite, does not interfere with this procedure although, if present in sufficient quantities, it will interfere with electron-capture GLC or RIA assays.

Several assay procedures have been used in pharmacokinetic studies of loprazolam. The RRA is a method based on the displacement of specific ^{3}H-diazepam to a membrane fraction from rat brain by the benzodiazepine (Kreiger et al. 1983). Radioactivity measurements are made by liquid scintillation counting. In pharmacokinetic studies which used this method for the determination of loprazolam in plasma, concentrations were higher and the elimination half-life was prolonged compared with studies using GLC or HPLC (Jochemson et al. 1986). Similarly, the RIA method employed by McInnes et al. gave higher loprazolam concentrations than an HPLC-GC assay procedure (McInnes et al. 1985). Both the RRA and RIA assays are sensitive to loprazolam concentrations of 1 μg/L, but in both assays piperazine *N*-oxide loprazolam, desmethylloprazolam and 4-hydroxyloprazolam (3 metabolites of loprazolam) cross-react with loprazolam. This may account for the higher observed concentrations of loprazolam in these studies.

Stevens and colleagues used a specific HPLC method for extraction and separation of loprazolam and the internal standard; they then hydrolysed the benzodiazepine extracts to the corresponding benzophenones which were determined by gas chromatography with electron capture detection (Stevens et al. 1983). The lower limit of detection for loprazolam was 1 μg/L and the coefficient of variation averaged 8.5% for concentrations between 10 and 24 μg/L. At concentrations of 2.5 μg/L or less, the coefficient of variation was 20%. Levasseur et al. developed a GLC procedure in which the coefficient of variation for loprazolam concentrations between 1 and 15 μg/L was 9.8% (Levasseur et al. 1985). Like the method of Stevens and colleagues, it had a sensitivity limit of 1 μg/L.

In summary, the most frequently used assay procedure for quantifying the newer benzodiazepines is GLC with electron-capture detection. This method is very sensitive and specific. Other assay methods have been used, but are associated with limitations.

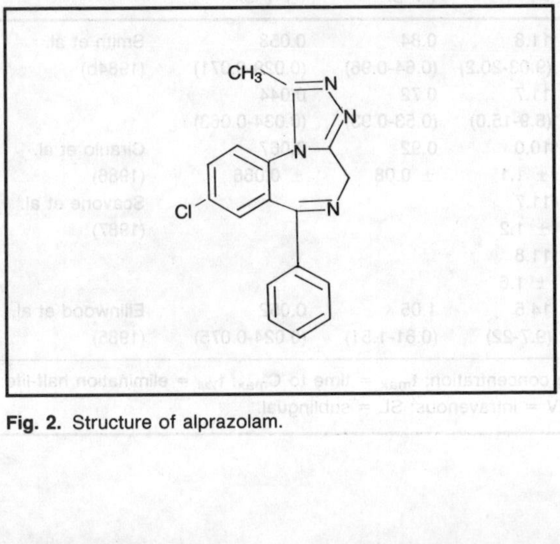

Fig. 2. Structure of alprazolam.

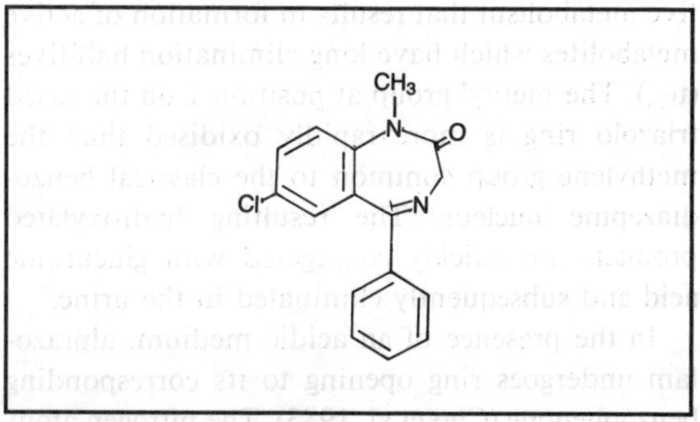

Fig 3. Structure of diazepam.

2. *Alprazolam*

2.1 Structure-Activity Relationship

Alprazolam (fig. 2) was the first of the class of compounds referred to as the 1,4-triazolobenzodiazepines. As such, the 1,4-triazolo ring (a 5-membered heterocycle fused on position 1,2 of the diazepine nucleus) is a departure from the classical benzodiazepines (fig. 3). The chlorine atom at position 8 on the phenyl ring along with the triazolo ring enhances alprazolam's potency. Pharmacologically, alprazolam is similar to diazepam; however, it has a higher binding affinity as determined by a ^{3}H-flunitrazepam binding assay for the benzodiazepine receptor (Sethy & Harris 1982). The K_i (affinity constant) of alprazolam is 3.4nm, compared with 5.3nm for diazepam.

The 1,4-triazolo ring prevents the usual oxidative metabolism that results in formation of active metabolites which have long elimination half-lives ($t_{1/2\beta}$). The methyl group at position 1 on the fused triazolo ring is more rapidly oxidised than the methylene group common to the classical benzodiazepine nucleus. The resulting hydroxylated products are quickly conjugated with glucuronic acid and subsequently eliminated in the urine.

In the presence of an acidic medium, alprazolam undergoes ring opening to its corresponding benzophenone (Cho et al. 1983). The nitrogen atom at position 2 of the triazolo ring is the most basic. Unlike midazolam, alprazolam is insoluble in water.

2.2 Pharmacokinetics

A summary of the pharmacokinetics of alprazolam is presented in table II.

2.2.1 Oral Absorption

In a single-dose study comparing the pharmacokinetics and pharmacodynamics of alprazolam with those of lorazepam and diazepam, mean peak plasma drug concentrations (C_{max}) of 40 μg/L were reached in 1.4 hours following a dose of alprazolam 0.028 mg/kg given as an oral suspension (Ellinwood et al. 1985). This time to peak concentration (t_{max}) is similar to the 1.7 hour t_{max} reported by Scavone and colleagues following administration of a 1mg oral tablet (Scavone et al. 1987). The same investigators reported a C_{max} of 14.4 μg/L after the 1mg tablet, which is consistent with the figure reported by Ciraulo and co-workers of 19 μg/L mean C_{max} after the administration of a single 1mg oral tablet (Ciraulo et al. 1986). Similarly, Smith and co-workers reported a C_{max} of 17.4 μg/L with this dose (Smith et al. 1984a). Average steady-state concentrations obtained in patients with panic disorders receiving multiple oral doses of 1mg (3, 6 and 9 mg/day) are 29.6, 61.5 and 102.9 μg/L, respectively (Ciraulo et al. 1986). Thus, alprazolam exhibits linear pharmacokinetics over the dosage ranges studied.

The influence of the dosing regimen on plasma alprazolam concentrations was evaluated by Smith and Kroboth (1987). Four treatment regimens were studied: (a) 2mg orally every 12 hours; (b) 1mg orally 4 times daily; (c) 0.25mg orally every hour up to 4mg total dose; and (d) placebo. C_{max} values for treatments (a), (b) and (c) on day 1 were 33.2, 25 and 32.3 μg/L, respectively ($p > 0.05$). The t_{max} for treatment (a) [1.7h] was significantly different from that for both treatment (b) [13.4h] and treat-

Table II. Pharmacokinetics of alprazolam in healthy subjects [mean (± SE) or range]

Dose (mg)	Route	$t_{1/2\alpha}$ (min)	C_{max} (μg/L)	t_{max} (h)	$t_{1/2\beta}$ (h)	Vd (L/kg)	CL (L/h/kg)	Reference
1.0	PO	18.9 (9.0-29.7)	17.4 (10.9-21.2)	1.17 (0.67-2.5)	11.8 (9.03-20.2)	0.84 (0.64-0.96)	0.053 (0.029-0.071)	Smith et al. (1984b)
1.0	IV		23.7 (17.6-27.5)	0.17 (0.17-0.2)	11.7 (8.9-15.0)	0.72 (0.53-0.93)	0.044 (0.034-0.063)	
1.0	PO		19.0 ± 2.0	1.30 ± 0.4	10.0 ± 1.1	0.92 ± 0.08	0.067 ± 0.066	Ciraulo et al. (1986)
1.0	SL		17.3 ±1.2	1.17 ± 0.25	11.7 ± 1.2			Scavone et al. (1987)
1.0	PO		14.4 ± 1.4	1.73 ±0.28	11.8 ± 1.6			
0.028/kg	PO (solution)		40.0 (25-62)	1.45 (0.33-3.5)	14.5 (9.7-22)	1.05 (0.61-1.51)	0.052 (0.024-0.075)	Ellinwood et al. (1985)

Abbreviations: $t_{1/2\alpha}$ = absorption half-life; C_{max} = peak plasma drug concentration; t_{max} = time to C_{max}; $t_{1/2\beta}$ = elimination half-life; Vd = apparent volume of distribution; CL = clearance; PO = oral; IV = intravenous; SL = sublingual.

ment (c) [15h]. Accumulation of alprazolam was seen with each regimen after 4 days of treatment; C_{max} increased to 56, 54.1 and 50.6 μg/L for treatments (a), (b) and (c), respectively.

The absorption half-life ($t_{½\alpha}$) is significantly longer in young than in elderly women (31.9 *vs* 13.1 minutes) [Greenblatt et al. 1983a]. In addition, peak plasma alprazolam concentrations are lower (15.7 *vs* 25.9 μg/L) and occur later (1.8 *vs* 0.6h) in young than in elderly women. In young men, the $t_{½\alpha}$ is slightly longer (23.2 minutes) than in elderly men (19.9 minutes) [$p > 0.05$]. However, C_{max} and t_{max} values are not significantly different between these 2 groups.

In a randomised crossover study, the effects of food on serum alprazolam concentrations were evaluated in male volunteers after the administration of a 1mg single oral tablet (Smith & Schoenfeld 1981a). The mean t_{max} was 1.6 hours when subjects were fasted 12 hours before and 4 hours after drug administration, and 2.5 hours when the subjects received alprazolam with a standard meal. Although absorption appeared to be slowed by the presence of food, the difference in t_{max} was not statistically significant.

2.2.2 Sublingual Absorption

When compared with tablets given orally (PO) the absorption of sublingual alprazolam (SL) is more rapid; peak concentrations are higher (17.3 μg/L SL *vs* 14.9 μg/L PO) and occur earlier (1.17h SL *vs* 1.73h PO) [Scavone et al. 1987]. These differences, however, are not statistically significant.

2.2.3 Systemic Bioavailability

In a crossover study, 6 men received oral and intravenous doses to assess the absolute bioavailability of alprazolam (Smith et al. 1984a). The fraction absorbed (f) was 0.92, indicating that alprazolam is fully bioavailable following oral administration. Systemic bioavailability data after other routes of administration, e.g. intramuscular, are not available.

2.2.4 Distribution

The volume of distribution (Vd) for alprazolam is approximately 0.8 L/kg after a 1mg oral tablet in healthy subjects (Smith et al. 1984a). The apparent Vd in patients who have panic disorders is 0.92 L/kg (Ciraulo et al. 1986) and is consistent with that in the healthy subjects.

In obese subjects, the Vd of alprazolam (114L) is significantly greater than in controls (73L) following a 0.5mg single oral tablet (Abernethy et al. 1983). Similarly, the Vd was significantly larger in young (1.17 L/kg) *vs* elderly men (0.97 L/kg) [Greenblatt et al. 1983a]. Age did not influence the Vd of alprazolam in women. When the data from this study were pooled into 2 groups, the mean Vd for women was 1.1 L/kg compared with 1.07 L/kg in men. Therefore, it appears that gender does not change the Vd of alprazolam. Its Vd is unchanged in alcoholic liver disease (Juhl et al. 1984).

The plasma protein binding of alprazolam to albumin was evaluated along with other benzodiazepines by Moschitto and Greenblatt (1983). The mean free fraction (% unbound) was 31.6%; little change was observed over the concentration range from 10 to 10,000 μg/L. The unbound fraction reported by Ciraulo (29%) is in agreement with Moschitto's findings (Ciraulo et al. 1986). The free fraction of alprazolam is not significantly influenced by age or gender (Greenblatt et al. 1983a). However, alprazolam free fraction is significantly higher (35.7%) in renal failure patients than in control subjects (31.9%) [Ochs et al. 1986]. The reduced plasma protein binding observed in this clinical setting may be due to the underlying disease or to medications used to treat the disease.

The octanol : buffer partition ratio for alprazolam is 18, indicating that it is highly lipophilic (Greenblatt et al. 1983c). Consistent with this, peak brain alprazolam concentrations were reached 1 minute after an intravenous (IV) dose and 15 minutes after an oral dose of 2.23 mg/kg in mice; brain concentrations equalled blood concentrations 15 minutes after alprazolam administration (Thomas & Judy 1976). ^{14}C-alprazolam was detected in low concentrations in the mouse fetus 15 minutes and 8 hours after an oral dose of 2.23 mg/kg (Thomas & Judy 1976). The transfer of alprazolam into human milk has not been determined.

2.2.5 Metabolism and Elimination

Alprazolam undergoes hydroxylation via the microsomal enzyme system. It is extensively metabolised: 29 metabolites have been identified in the urine, with only about 20% of the administered dose excreted as unchanged alprazolam (Reineke et al. 1978). The major metabolite is α-hydroxyalprazolam, which accounts for 17% of the total ^{14}C activity recovered in the urine (Eberts et al. 1980). The other metabolites recovered in the urine are 4-hydroxyalprazolam (0.3%), α-4-dihydroxyalprazolam (0.2%), 3-methyltriazolyl (0.9%) and analogues of the chlorobenzophenone (17%). Approximately 94% of the total dose is recovered within 72 hours.

α-Hydroxyalprazolam has pharmacological activity (K_i value of 4.2nm) as determined by the *in vitro* ^3H-flunitrazepam binding assay (Sethy & Harris 1982). In contrast, both 4-hydroxyalprazolam and α-4-dihydroxyalprazolam have low affinity for the receptor, as indicated by their K_i values of 24 and 34nm, respectively. The α-hydroxyalprazolam and 4-hydroxyalprazolam metabolites are present in the plasma in quantities less than 10% of unchanged alprazolam concentrations (Smith & Kroboth 1987). Therefore, it is unlikely that α-hydroxyalprazolam contributes to alprazolam's *in vivo* activity.

Mean elimination half-lives of alprazolam in healthy adult subjects range from 9.5 to 12 hours (Eberts et al. 1980; Scavone et al. 1987; Smith & Kroboth 1987; Smith et al. 1984a). A similar mean $t_{½\beta}$ of 10 hours was observed in patients with panic disorders (Ciraulo et al. 1986). α-Hydroxyalprazolam has been reported to have a $t_{½\beta}$ of 1 to 2 hours after administration to volunteers (Hengen et al. 1982). This contrasts with the mean observed α-hydroxyalprazolam $t_{½\beta}$ of 15.1 hours reported by Smith and Kroboth (1987) after administration of alprazolam. The latter $t_{½\beta}$ estimate most probably reflects formation rate, which is slower than elimination rate.

The accumulation ratio, calculated as the ratio of area under the concentration-time curve (AUC) of oral alprazolam (2mg every 12 hours) on day 4 to that on day 1, was determined for alprazolam, 4-hydroxyalprazolam and α-hydroxyalprazolam (Smith & Kroboth 1987): the figures were 2.05, 2.23 and 2.65, respectively. Based on these results, the extent of accumulation of alprazolam and its metabolites appears to be similar, and minimal metabolite accumulation would be expected with long term therapy.

In 1 study of alprazolam in subjects of varying ages, elderly men (> 62 years of age) had a significantly longer $t_{½\beta}$ than young men (19.0 *vs* 11.1h); clearance was also lower in elderly men (0.04 *vs* 0.08 L/h/kg). However, the $t_{½\beta}$ and total clearance did not differ between young and elderly women (10.8 *vs* 13.5h and 0.08 *vs* 0.06 L/h/kg) [Greenblatt et al. 1983a]. A second study, which evaluated the pharmacokinetics and pharmacodynamics of alprazolam during multiple-dose administration, demonstrated no differences in pharmacokinetic parameter estimates between men and women. Mean elimination half-lives during the washout period following 4 days of dosing were 22.1 hours in elderly women and 26.1 hours in elderly men; mean apparent oral clearance values were 0.039 and 0.037 L/h/kg for elderly women and men, respectively (McAuley et al. 1987).

Similarly, the $t_{½\beta}$ of alprazolam is significantly prolonged in obese subjects compared with controls (22 *vs* 11h) [Abernethy et al. 1983]. Clearance (CL) is also reduced (3.98 *vs* 5.28 L/h), but the difference is not significant. Smoking has been reported to accelerate the elimination of alprazolam following a 0.5mg dose given every 8 hours for 8 days (Smith et al. 1983b). The $t_{½\beta}$ was 9.5 hours in smokers compared with 14.2 hours in nonsmokers; again, this difference was not significant.

In patients with renal insufficiency, there was no difference in the $t_{½\beta}$ of alprazolam between patients (11.5h) and control subjects (11.3h) [Ochs et al. 1986]. Similarly, there was no difference in CL (0.07 L/h/kg). However, in alcoholic liver disease patients, the $t_{½\beta}$ of alprazolam was significantly prolonged (19.7h) and CL reduced (0.04 L/h/kg) when compared with age- and sex-matched controls (11.4h and 0.07 L/h/kg, respectively) [Juhl et al. 1984]. These data suggest that alprazolam accumulation would not occur in patients with renal disease, but that dosage adjustments would be necessary in patients with liver disease, based on alterations in pharmacokinetics.

Studies in animals have shown that alprazolam does not induce or inhibit the liver enzyme system (Philopoulos et al. 1980).

2.3 Drug Interactions

Most of the interactions that have been documented with alprazolam are with drugs that inhibit or induce the mixed function oxidase system. One study investigated whether propranolol, which reduces hepatic blood flow and inhibits liver enzymes, affects the pharmacokinetics of alprazolam, diazepam and lorazepam (Ochs et al. 1984a). Six healthy subjects were given a single oral dose of alprazolam 1mg either alone or after receiving 80mg of propranolol 3 times daily for 48 hours. Peak plasma alprazolam concentrations were lower (12.5 *vs* 15.9 μg/L) and t_{max} occurred later (2.4 *vs* 1.6h) with the concurrent administration of propranolol than with alprazolam alone. Alprazolam $t_{1/2\beta}$ and CL were not significantly different in the 2 treatments (15.9 *vs* 18.5h and 0.06 *vs* 0.05 L/h/kg, respectively). Propranolol had little effect on the pharmacokinetics of alprazolam, although the interaction needs further investigation because alprazolam was administered as a single oral dose.

Conversely, dextropropoxyphene, which is also known to inhibit the mixed function oxidase system, significantly impairs the clearance of alprazolam (Abernethy et al. 1985). Eight healthy subjects received a single dose of oral alprazolam 1mg on 2 occasions; once with dextropropoxyphene 65mg every 6 hours beginning 12 hours prior to alprazolam administration, and once alone as the control treatment. Dextropropoxyphene did not alter alprazolam peak concentration (18.7 μg/L with dextropropoxyphene and 20 μg/L alone) or Vd (1.2 L/kg). Although t_{max} was delayed in the dextropropoxyphene-treated group (2.2h) compared with the controls (0.64h), the difference was not significant. However, oral alprazolam CL was reduced from 0.08 to 0.05 L/h/kg and $t_{1/2\beta}$ prolonged from 11.6 to 18.3 hours with the concurrent administration of dextropropoxyphene ($p < 0.005$). The clinical implications of this pharmacokinetic interaction were not established in the study. The expected outcome of concomitant dextropropoxyphene and alprazolam administration would be a longer time to reach steady-state concentrations of alprazolam, and elevated alprazolam concentrations at steady-state.

In a single-dose study evaluating the effect of cimetidine administration on alprazolam and triazolam, Abernethy and colleagues reported that cimetidine (300mg every 6 hours beginning 12 hours before alprazolam ingestion) had no effect on C_{max} (16 μg/L) or t_{max} (1.1h) [Abernethy et al. 1983]. Cimetidine reduced the Vd of alprazolam from 1.52 to 1.34 L/kg, a difference of borderline significance ($p < 0.1$). The free fraction of alprazolam (30%) was not altered, but CL was significantly reduced from 0.1 to 0.06 L/h/kg. Associated with the reduced clearance, alprazolam $t_{1/2\beta}$ was significantly prolonged from 12.4 to 16.6 hours. These results suggest that cimetidine has little influence on alprazolam absorption but alters its elimination. Therefore, concurrent administration of cimetidine with multiple doses of alprazolam would result in elevated steady-state plasma alprazolam concentrations.

When cimetidine was administered for 2 weeks (1g daily) before alprazolam ingestion (0.5mg 3 times daily for 1 week), more extensive alprazolam accumulation occurred than had been predicted in Abernethy's single-dose study (Pourbaix et al. 1985). C_{max} was significantly higher in the alprazolam-cimetidine group (33.1 μg/L) compared with the alprazolam group (18.2 μg/L) but t_{max} was the same (2h). Alprazolam $t_{1/2\beta}$ was increased from 12.2 to 14.2 hours and the Vd reduced from 93.9 to 62.2L after cimetidine pretreatment. These differences were not significant. However, alprazolam CL was significantly reduced from 0.3 to 0.19 L/h/kg and $AUC_{0\rightarrow\infty}$ increased from 294 to 508 μg/L · h after cimetidine. Based on these results, a reduced daily dosage of alprazolam or increased dosing interval is suggested when the 2 drugs are given together.

The potential interaction between alprazolam and metronidazole, an imidazole antibiotic which may impair microsomal drug oxidising capacity, has also been evaluated (Blyden et al. 1988). In this single-dose study, metronidazole did not alter any pharmacokinetic variable of alprazolam.

The influence of low oestrogen oral contraceptives on the pharmacokinetics of 4 benzodiazepines, including alprazolam, has been evaluated (Stoehr et al. 1984). Subjects included women who had been taking oral contraceptives for a minimum of 3 months, and age- and weight-matched control women. Alprazolam 1mg was given as a single oral tablet. There was no significant difference between groups in peak plasma alprazolam concentrations (18.0 *vs* 21.3 μg/L), t_{max} (2.1 *vs* 1.5h), or Vd (1.03 *vs* 1.1 L/kg). The mean rate constant for elimination was lower in the oral contraceptive user group than in the controls (0.056 *vs* 0.072h^{-1}). Correspondingly, this difference was also reflected in the $t_{1/2\beta}$ of alprazolam (12.4 *vs* 9.6h) and CL (0.06 *vs* 0.07 L/h/kg). Alprazolam AUC was significantly greater in the users of oral contraceptives at 326 *vs* 241 μg/L • h, a finding consistent with the reduced CL and prolonged $t_{1/2\beta}$. Consequently, the time required to reach steady-state alprazolam concentrations would be longer in oral contraceptive users.

3. Triazolam

3.1 Structure-Activity Relationship

Like alprazolam, triazolam belongs to the group of benzodiazepines referred to as the 1,4-triazolobenzodiazepines. Consequently the same 5-membered heterocycle at the 1,2 position of the diazepine ring is present (fig. 4). In addition, the electronegative chlorine atom at position 8, present in both alprazolam and triazolam, is necessary for benzodiazepine activity.

The chlorine atom on the phenyl ring at position 2′ in the triazolam structure is the only substituent not present in the alprazolam structure. This halogen is responsible for the increased biological potency of triazolam; the K_i value for triazolam is 0.76 versus 3.4 for alprazolam.

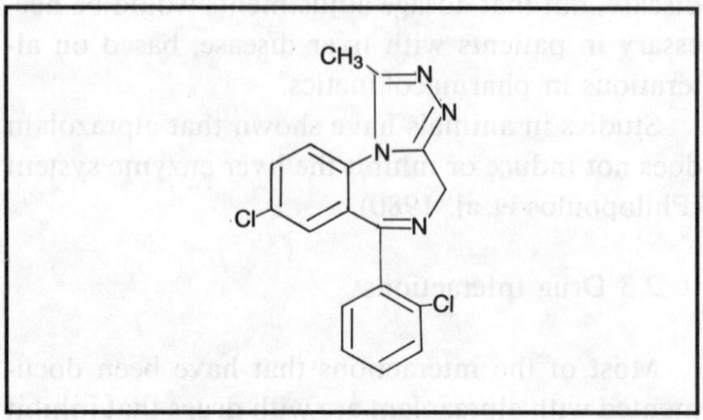

Fig. 4. Structure of triazolam.

Unlike the imidazole ring present in midazolam, the triazolo ring is not basic. For this reason, the preparation of water-soluble salts is not possible; this limits the usefulness of triazolam as an injectable preparation.

The triazolo ring and the attached methyl group are responsible for the rapid oxidation by liver enzymes, resulting in a short elimination half-life and conversion to metabolites that are rapidly excreted.

Similar to other 1,4-benzodiazepines, triazolam exists as a pH-dependent equilibrium mixture of ring opened and closed forms (Konishi et al. 1982).

3.2 Pharmacokinetics

A summary of pharmacokinetic parameter estimates for triazolam is given in table III.

3.2.1 Absorption

Oral Absorption

Triazolam is rapidly absorbed following the administration of oral tablets, reaching peak plasma concentrations (range of 2 to 10 μg/L) within 2 hours (Eberts et al. 1981; Friedman et al. 1986; Scavone et al. 1986). Approximately 85% of the oral dose is absorbed (Eberts et al. 1981).

Peak triazolam concentrations have been reported to be higher (8.2 *vs* 4.1 μg/L) and occur earlier (0.8 *vs* 2.1h) in elderly than in young women

(Greenblatt et al. 1983b). This difference has not been observed between young and elderly men. Different results were seen in a study conducted by Smith and co-workers (Smith et al. 1983a). The mean peak concentration in elderly women was 5.66 μg/L compared with 6.1 μg/L observed in young women. Associated with the higher peak triazolam concentrations in young women was a reduction in the oral CL (0.28 L/h/kg) compared with that of the elderly women (0.33 L/h/kg). The t_{max} was 0.65 and 1.85 hours in young and elderly women, respectively. Again, no significant differences were observed between the young and elderly men who were studied.

The absorption of triazolam is subject to diurnal variation (Smith et al. 1986). The mean t_{max} observed following an oral dose of triazolam 0.5mg in the evening was 2.32 hours compared with 1.75 hours after daytime administration. The $t_{1/2\alpha}$ determined from NONLIN curve fitting was significantly longer after evening administration (21.9 *vs* 13.3 minutes, respectively). Also, the lag time was significantly greater after the evening dose when compared to the daytime dose (33.6 and 17.8 minutes, respectively). C_{max} values (3.99 and 3.34 μg/L) did not differ. The authors suggested that the faster daytime absorption of triazolam was related to the longer predose fasting period before the morning dose (12h) compared with the evening (4h). The slower absorption rate observed in the evening is probably of little clinical significance.

A crossover study was conducted in 16 healthy adult men to evaluate the effects of a 12-hour fast or a meal on the bioavailability of an orally administered triazolam 0.5mg tablet (Smith & Schoenfeld 1981b). Average peak triazolam concentrations were higher (5.76 *vs* 4.39 μg/L; $p = 0.05$) and occurred earlier (1.13 *vs* 2.14h; $p < 0.01$) in the fasted than in the fed treatment. The AUC of triazolam was significantly greater at 0 to 2 hours (7.75 *vs* 5.10 μg/L • h; $p = 0.01$) when subjects were fasted. No significant difference in $AUC_{0\rightarrow\infty}$ or triazolam elimination was observed. Therefore, administering triazolam after a meal reduces the apparent rate, but not the extent, of absorption.

Factors such as obesity, smoking status, or gender (between the ages of 20 and 58 years) have little influence on the absorption characteristics of triazolam (Abernethy et al. 1984; Ochs et al. 1987; Smith et al. 1983a).

Sublingual Absorption

In a crossover study comparing the triazolam 0.5mg tablet administered by the sublingual and oral routes, C_{max} (3.9 μg/L SL *vs* 4.7 μg/L PO) but not t_{max} (1.2h) was significantly different. Based

Table III. Pharmacokinetics of triazolam in healthy subjects [mean (±SE) or range]

Dose (mg)	Route	$t_{1/2\alpha}$ (min)	C_{max} (μg/L)	t_{max} (h)	$t_{1/2\beta}$ (h)	Vd (L/kg)	CL (L/h/kg)	Reference
0.5	SL		4.70 ±0.45	1.22 ±0.30	4.06 ±0.72			Scavone et al. (1986)
0.5	PO		3.90 ±0.43	1.25 ±0.23	3.65 ±0.55			
0.5	PO		4.41 (1.67-9.39)	1.30 (0.5-4.0)	2.56 (1.13-4.44)			Friedman et al. (1986)
0.5	PO	13.28 ±6.90	3.99 ±1.47	1.75 ±1.05	2.94 ±1.05	1.31 ±0.39	0.33 ±0.113	Smith et al. (1986)
0.5	PO	10.00 (1-19)	5.00 (0.75-12.0)	1.20 (0.25-2.0)	2.60 (1.8-3.9)			Jochemsen et al. (1983)

Abbreviations: see table II.

on the increased AUC for sublingual triazolam compared with oral administration, bioavailability was 28% greater. A study of a sublingual tablet formulation also demonstrated that the AUC for the sublingual route is approximately 20% greater than for the oral tablet formulation (Kroboth et al. 1986). The absorption profile following sublingual administration suggests that a fraction of the triazolam dose is absorbed sublingually, while some is first swallowed and then absorbed.

3.2.2 Systemic Bioavailability

The bioavailability of triazolam after oral and sublingual administration was determined in a 3-way crossover which included an intravenous treatment. In all 3 treatments, a single dose of 0.25mg was administered. Following the oral tablet, the mean absolute bioavailability was 44%; the sublingual tablet resulted in a 53% absolute bioavailability (Kroboth et al. 1986). These values were lower than anticipated from previous studies. Since more than 85% of a radiolabelled dose is recovered in the urine (Eberts et al. 1981), the results of this study suggest that orally administered triazolam undergoes non-hepatic presystemic metabolism.

3.2.3 Distribution

The apparent Vd of triazolam is approximately 1 L/kg (range of 0.7 to 1.7 L/kg) [Eberts et al. 1981]. No differences are observed between obese and normal weight subjects, men and women or young and elderly subjects (Abernethy et al. 1984; Smith et al. 1983a). The apparent Vd (97L) was not significantly changed after 7 days of multiple triazolam doses (Dehlin et al. 1983).

Plasma protein binding of triazolam was evaluated over a concentration range of 10 to 10,000 μg/L (Moschitto & Greenblatt 1983). In this study, triazolam was 78% protein bound and the extent of binding was independent of concentration. Eberts and co-workers demonstrated that triazolam was 89% bound over a concentration range from 20 to 1000 μg/L and that binding was independent of concentration (Eberts et al. 1981). Furthermore, binding to serum albumin was only 49%, indicating that triazolam binds to other serum proteins. The percentage of unbound triazolam reported by Jochemsen and colleagues similarly ranged from 7.8 to 11.8% (mean 9.9%) in 8 healthy volunteers (Jochemsen et al. 1983). Smoking has no effect on the percentage of unbound triazolam (Ochs et al. 1987).

Kroboth and colleagues studied the characteristics of triazolam binding to albumin and α_1-acid glycoprotein in patients on haemodialysis and continuous ambulatory peritoneal dialysis (Kroboth et al. 1984). Mean α_1-acid glycoprotein concentrations were lower in the first samples (1090 mg/L) than in the second samples (1378 mg/L) collected 1 week later. Correspondingly, the percentage of unbound triazolam was lower in the second sample (9.1% *vs* 11.0%). Linear regression analysis of the binding ratio and α_1-acid glycoprotein concentrations demonstrated that α_1-acid glycoprotein concentrations explain 64% of the variability in the triazolam binding ratio. Thus, conditions that influence α_1-acid glycoprotein concentrations, such as uraemia, will also influence the percentage of unbound triazolam.

Triazolam would be expected to cross readily into the central nervous system because of its high lipid solubility (Greenblatt et al. 1983c). ^{14}C-triazolam studies performed in monkeys have shown high radioactivity in the brain 1 hour after an oral dose of 0.5 mg/kg (Kitagawa et al. 1979).

There are no data regarding the placental transfer of triazolam or its passage into breast milk in humans. However, data obtained from pregnant rats suggest that triazolam crosses the placenta, resulting in fetal concentrations within 0.5 hour after administration (Kitagawa et al. 1979). Similarly, triazolam concentrations have been measured in the milk of lactating rats. These *in vitro* studies suggest similar results would be seen in humans.

3.2.4 Metabolism and Elimination

Triazolam, like alprazolam, undergoes hydroxylation and subsequent conjugation with glucuronic acid (Eberts et al. 1981). The major metabolite is α-hydroxytriazolam. The ratio of unconjugated to conjugated triazolam peak concentrations is approximately 20%, indicating that this major metabolite undergoes rapid conversion to its glucuronide conjugate. The C_{max} values for α-hydroxytriazolam glucuronic acid range from 2.68 to 10.22 μg/L (mean 6.13 μg/L) following a 0.88mg oral dose. The t_{max} ranges from 0.75 to 2.5 hours (mean 1.25 hour). Although α-hydroxytriazolam has been reported to have potent pharmacological activity in animals (Sethy & Harris 1982), its rapid inactivation by glucuronidation most probably prevents it from contributing to triazolam's activity. In addition to α-hydroxytriazolam, 4-hydroxytriazolam has been identified in the plasma, along with α-hydroxytriazolam and the conjugated form of both. The formation of 4-hydroxytriazolam glucuronic acid is also rapid; the mean C_{max} and t_{max} are 6.13 μg/L and 2.5 hours, respectively.

Six urinary metabolites of triazolam have been identified (Eberts et al. 1981). The major one is α-hydroxytriazolam, which accounts for 69% of the urinary ^{14}C activity. 4-Hydroxytriazolam accounts for 11% of the activity, and 3-dichlorotriazolyl benzophenone analogues account for the remainder.

The $t_{½β}$ of triazolam ranges between 1.8 and 3.9 hours (mean 2.6 hours) in healthy adult subjects following the administration of a 0.5mg oral dose (Jochemsen et al. 1983). This is in agreement with Friedman and co-workers who reported an overall mean $t_{½β}$ of 2.6 hours (range 1.13 to 4.4 hours) in a population analysis of triazolam pharmacokinetics (Friedman et al. 1986). Although the route of administration (oral *vs* sublingual) does not influence the $t_{½β}$ of triazolam, time (day or evening) of administration does (Smith et al. 1986). With evening administration, $t_{½β}$ is significantly prolonged (3.77 *vs* 2.94h; $p < 0.05$) compared with daytime administration. Following the administration of multiple doses of triazolam in elderly subjects, the $t_{½β}$ was 1.4 hours on day 1 and 1.37 hours on day 7, providing evidence for the lack of accumulation (Dehlin et al. 1983).

Smoking does not influence the elimination of the drug (Ochs et al. 1987). Mean triazolam $t_{½β}$ is not significantly different between young (3h) and elderly (4.6h) men or young (2.7h) and elderly (3.2h) women (Greenblatt et al. 1983b). There is a significant difference between elderly men (3.38h) and elderly women (2.41h) [Smith et al. 1983a]. Although age may not influence the $t_{½β}$ of triazolam, clearance is correlated with age (Greenblatt et al. 1983b). The decrease in clearance with increasing age is accompanied by higher peak triazolam concentrations and an increase in the total AUC. These age-related changes have been explained by the reduced hepatic oxidising capacity in the elderly, together with an age-related reduction in hepatic blood flow. However, there is a poor correlation of $t_{½β}$ and clearance of antipyrine (phenazone) with those of triazolam (r = 0.34 and 0.44, respectively). The authors suggested that the antipyrine test had limited value in identifying individuals with high or low triazolam clearance values.

In morbidly obese subjects, triazolam $t_{½β}$ is significantly longer (4.1h) than in the matched normal-weight subjects (2.6h), and is associated with a reduced clearance (Abernethy et al. 1984).

The effects of end-stage renal disease on triazolam elimination were investigated by Kroboth et al. (1985). There was no difference in $t_{½β}$ between controls (2.6h) and dialysis subjects (2.29h). Based on this information, it appears that dosage adjustment in this group of patients would not be necessary.

The pharmacokinetics of triazolam were evaluated in 8 biopsy-proven cirrhotic patients and in age-, weight- and gender-matched healthy subjects after night-time administration of a 0.25mg oral tablet (Kroboth et al. 1987). No significant differences were observed for C_{max} or t_{max} between healthy subjects and patients with cirrhosis (1.43 *vs* 1.62 μg/L and 2 *vs* 1.9h, respectively).

Although the apparent oral clearance of triazolam varied widely in the subjects studied, it was reduced from 0.4 L/h/kg in healthy subjects to 0.3 L/h/kg in patients with cirrhosis. This was accompanied by an increase in $AUC_{0\to\infty}$ from 9.51 to 15.5 μg/L • h in the cirrhotic patients. Apparent oral clearance of triazolam for the cirrhotic patients was directly correlated with albumin concentration (r^2 = 0.59; p = 0.027) and indocyanine green elimination rate (r^2 = 0.65; p = 0.015), and inversely related to partial thromboplastin time (r^2 = 0.81; p = 0.002).

Bakti and co-workers also evaluated the pharmacokinetics of triazolam in 8 patients with biopsy-proven cirrhosis and 8 age-matched controls (Bakti et al. 1987). Mean peak triazolam concentrations of 3.6 μg/L occurred at 1.3 hours after the administration of a 0.25mg oral dose in healthy subjects. In the patients with cirrhosis, C_{max} was 3.1 μg/L and not significantly different from the control subjects; t_{max} was the same as in the control group, 1.3 hours. The median $t_{1/2\beta}$ of triazolam was 3.9 hours in controls *vs* 9.7 hours in cirrhotic patients ($p < 0.01$). The free fraction of the drug was significantly larger in the cirrhotic patients (17%) than in the control subjects (14%; $p < 0.001$). The clearance of free triazolam in cirrhotic patients and control subjects was 0.9 L/h/kg and 1.43 L/h/kg, respectively; this reduction in clearance was significant. In addition, free triazolam clearance was correlated with the aminopyrine breath test ($r^2 = 0.77$; $p < 0.001$) but marginally correlated with the fractional clearance of indocyanine green ($r^2 = 0.48$; $p < 0.05$). Thus, the presence of cirrhosis decreases the clearance of triazolam. This reduction is correlated with severity of disease, and consequently dosage adjustments may be necessary.

The elimination half-lives of the conjugated α-hydroxy and 4-hydroxytriazolam metabolites are short, approximately 3.8 hours (Eberts et al. 1981). Accumulation of these metabolites would not be expected to occur even after multiple doses.

In the rat, triazolam therapy (0.5 mg/kg for 14 days) did not induce the hepatic oxidising enzymes (Kitagawa et al. 1979).

3.3 Drug Interactions

In a study designed to evaluate the influence of renal disease on the pharmacokinetics of triazolam, the influence of aluminium hydroxide gel was also investigated (Kroboth et al. 1985). Dialysis patients served as their own controls and were given triazolam and triazolam plus aluminium hydroxide gel on 2 separate occasions. Triazolam C_{max} was higher when it was coadministered with aluminium hydroxide gel (6.4 μg/L) than when administered alone (4.04 μg/L). In addition, $AUC_{0\rightarrow\infty}$ was significantly greater after antacid administration (29.6 compared with 23.2 μg/L • h). No differences in t_{max} were observed. The authors suggested that the aluminium hydroxide gel enhanced the absorption of triazolam; the higher gastric pH prevented the hydrolysis of triazolam to its open ring benzophenone, allowing for greater absorption of the ring-closed triazolam. Subsequent analysis of these same data revealed that higher α_1-acid glycoprotein concentrations during the aluminium hydroxide plus triazolam treatment explained a significant portion of the variability in the apparent oral clearance of triazolam (Kroboth & Smith, submitted for publication).

In a single-dose study of triazolam plus the concurrent administration of cimetidine 300mg every 6 hours beginning 12 hours prior to triazolam ingestion, total triazolam CL was reduced from 0.35 to 0.23 L/h/kg and the $AUC_{0\rightarrow\infty}$ was increased from 25 to 38 μg/L • h (Abernethy et al. 1983). The $t_{1/2\beta}$ of 3.2 hours was not prolonged by cimetidine. The observed results were believed to be due to a reduction in the first-pass metabolism of triazolam and subsequent increased systemic bioavailability.

Pourbaix and colleagues evaluated the effects of long term administration of cimetidine 1g daily for 2 weeks on the pharmacokinetics of oral triazolam 0.5g taken every night for 1 week (Pourbaix et al. 1985). Cimetidine resulted in statistically significant increases in triazolam C_{max} (7.8 *vs* 11.8 μg/L), $t_{1/2\beta}$ (2.23 *vs* 3.74h) and AUC (31.3 *vs* 68.9 μg/L • h). The oral clearance was significantly reduced from 0.29 to 0.13 L/h/kg. The authors suggested that the observed results were due to inhibition of metabolism and reduction in hepatic blood flow by cimetidine.

To further discern whether pH or effects on the liver are responsible for the observed changes in the pharmacokinetics of triazolam when cimetidine is administered concurrently, Cox and colleagues administered triazolam 0.5mg solution by intraduodenal infusion to 4 healthy subjects in a 4-way crossover study; the treatments were triazolam, triazolam pH 6.0 with cimetidine pretreatment, triazolam solution at pH 2.3 (containing the triazolobenzophenone) and triazolam solution at pH 6.0 (containing negligible triazolobenzophenone) [Cox et al. 1986]. The rate and extent of systemic absorption of triazolam was not significantly different for solutions at pH 2.3 and pH 6.0. These findings suggest that changes in gastric pH due to cimetidine or antacid administration have little effect on the absorption of triazolam. When the cimetidine treatment was compared to control, there were significant changes in triazolam's pharmacokinetics. C_{max} and $AUC_{0\to\infty}$ were increased after the administration of cimetidine, while little effect was observed on the $t_{1/2\beta}$. The lack of effect on the $t_{1/2\beta}$ was due to a reduction in both clearance and Vd/F. Thus, cimetidine may reduce the intestinal metabolism of triazolam or its distribution, but not its absorption characteristics.

Several studies have investigated the potential interaction between ethanol and triazolam, since ethanol inhibits cytochrome P450-mediated oxidative biotransformation in addition to causing psychomotor impairment, with conflicting results. The first report by Ochs and co-workers found no significant differences between control subjects and those given ethanol concurrently, with regard to triazolam C_{max} (5.4 μg/L), t_{max} (1.5h), $t_{1/2\beta}$ (2.6h) and apparent oral CL (0.4 *vs* 0.47 L/h/kg) [Ochs et al. 1984b]. In a subsequent study $AUC_{0\to\infty}$ was significantly different in the control (6.7 μg/L • h) and triazolam-ethanol (8.2 μg/L • h) treatments (Dorian et al. 1985). The difference in AUC was accompanied by a reduction in CL (37.8 *vs* 31.9 L/h, respectively). C_{max} (1.8 *vs* 2.2 μg/L) and $t_{1/2\beta}$ (2.6 *vs* 2.8h) were not statistically different. The observed increase in plasma triazolam concentrations is predictable, given the enzyme inhibitory effects of ethanol.

Other drugs known to be inhibitors of the mixed function oxidase system would be expected to alter the pharmacokinetics of triazolam. For example, macrolide antibiotics form complexes with cytochrome P450 and inactivate it (Pessayre 1983). Consequently, the potential interaction between triazolam and erythromycin, a macrolide antibiotic, was investigated (Phillips et al. 1986). Plasma triazolam concentrations after coadministration with erythromycin 333mg 3 times daily for 3 days were higher at all sampling times than concentrations when triazolam was taken alone, expressed as a 51% higher AUC ($p < 0.05$). In addition, triazolam CL was reduced by 52%, its $t_{1/2\beta}$ was prolonged from 3.6 to 5.9 hours and Vd was decreased from 155 to 111L. C_{max} was greater after erythromycin pretreatment, but not significantly so. Both metabolic inhibition and reduction in first-pass metabolism may have contributed to the observed outcome.

Isoniazid, the antitubercular agent, can also impair the hepatic enzyme oxidising capacity (Muakkassah et al. 1981). The effect of isoniazid on the kinetics of triazolam was evaluated in healthy adult subjects who received, on 2 occasions, a single dose of oral triazolam 0.5mg alone or coadministered with isoniazid base 90mg taken twice daily beginning 3 days before the study day and continuing for 24 hours after triazolam administration (Ochs et al. 1983). Isoniazid increased the peak plasma triazolam concentrations from 5.9 μg/L in the control subjects to 7.1 μg/L, but this difference was not significant. The triazolam t_{max}, 1.04 hours, was not altered with the concurrent administration of isoniazid. Triazolam $t_{1/2\beta}$ was significantly prolonged from 2.54 to 3.32 hours, and apparent oral CL was reduced from 0.41 to 0.24 L/h/kg in the isoniazid treatment group. Consequently, the total AUC increased from 26.5 μg/L • h in the control group to 38.6 μg/L • h in the isoniazid group ($p < 0.01$). The authors suggested that these observations were due to reduced first-pass hepatic extraction of triazolam, resulting in an increased systemic availability of the oral dose.

Triazolam was also evaluated in the low-dose oestrogen oral contraceptives-benzodiazepine interaction study conducted by Stoehr et al. (1984). Peak triazolam concentrations occurred later in the oral contraceptive users (1.5 hours) compared with the matched control group (1 hour) but this difference was not significant. Triazolam $AUC_{0\to\infty}$ was increased from 19.4 to 28.9 μg/L • h and clearance was reduced from 0.43 to 0.29 L/h/kg in the oral contraceptive user group. Again, these changes were not statistically significant. No changes were observed in any other pharmacokinetic parameters

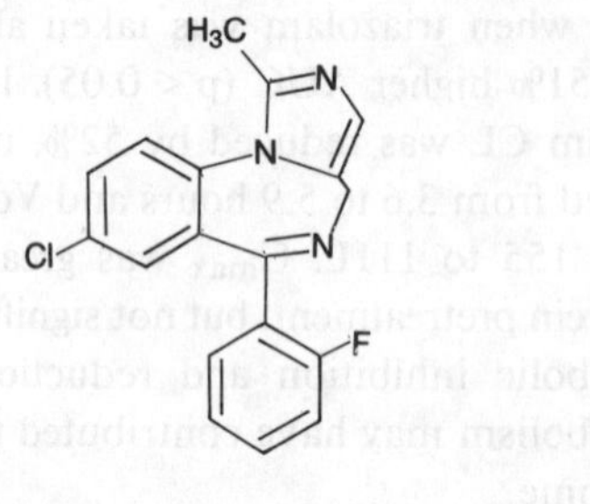

Fig. 5. Structure of midazolam.

that were determined. The clinical relevance of the interaction is unknown, since this was a single-dose study.

4. Midazolam

4.1 Structure-Activity Relationship

The structure of midazolam is shown in figure 5. Several features distinguish it from other benzodiazepines, including its water solubility and basic nature. Like triazolam, it has a short duration of action. The fused imidazole ring increases stability against hydrolysis, delaying degradation and subsequent loss of potency. These characteristics allow for the preparation of aqueous injectable solutions that are stable and well tolerated when administered parenterally.

Other substituents that are present for the 1,4-triazolobenzodiazepines are also present in the midazolam structure. For example, the methyl group at position 1 on the imidazole ring is responsible for the short $t_{½\beta}$ of midazolam. It is more rapidly oxidised by hepatic enzymes than the methylene group at position 4 of the classical benzodiazepine nucleus. Both the fused imidazole ring at position 1,2 on the diazepine nucleus and the chlorine atom at position 8 on the phenyl ring also increase the biological activity of midazolam. The drug has a low K_i value of 3.3nm; this implies a high affinity for benzodiazepine receptors (Gerecke 1983). Like alprazolam and triazolam, midazolam exists in equilibrium with an open ring benzophenone in acidic medium (Tuzel et al. 1984).

Thus, midazolam has characteristics that differ from other currently available benzodiazepines: (1) basic properties that enable the manufacturer to prepare stable, water-soluble salts; (2) short elimination half-life; and (3) enhanced potency (compared with the classical benzodiazepines), related to its high affinity for benzodiazepine receptors.

4.2 Pharmacokinetics

A summary of the pharmacokinetic parameters of midazolam, obtained from published studies, appears in table IV.

4.2.1 Absorption

Oral Absorption

At physiological pH, midazolam becomes very lipophilic (Greenblatt et al. 1983c), which contributes to rapid gastrointestinal absorption. Peak concentrations following the administration of single oral doses of midazolam maleate occur in 20 to 60 minutes (Allonen et al. 1981; Heizmann et al. 1983; Sjövall et al. 1983). In studies that have assessed the pharmacokinetic characteristics of midazolam using a compartmental analysis approach, the reported absorption half-lives have been less than 14 minutes (Allonen et al. 1981; Heizmann et al. 1983; Smith et al. 1981). Peak plasma concentrations range from 50 to 250 μg/L following oral doses of 7.5, 10 and 15mg. A non-linear relationship between oral dose and plasma concentration was first reported by Heizmann et al. and subsequently verified by Bornemann and colleagues (Bornemann et al. 1985; Heizmann et al. 1981). The C_{max} increased proportionally at doses of 7.5mg (34 μg/L) to 15mg (67 μg/L) but increased disproportionately to the 30mg dose (212 μg/L). Ingestion of midazolam 1 hour before or with a meal did not significantly alter its t_{max} (1h), C_{max} (63 μg/L) or $AUC_{0\rightarrow\infty}$ (200 μg/L · h) compared with administration to subjects in the fasting state (Bornemann et al. 1986). However, a reduction in the rate and extent of absorption was observed when midazolam was ingested 1 hour after a meal. This may be clinically important if onset of effect is delayed.

Table IV. Pharmacokinetics of midazolam in healthy subjects [mean (±SD)]

Dose	Route	$t_{½α}$ (min)	C_{max} (μg/L)	t_{max} (h)	$t_{½β}$ (h)	Vd (L/kg)	CL (L/h)	Reference
5mg	IV		112.6 ±16.1		2.09 ±0.84	1.14 ±0.57	27.78 ±6.81	Smith et al. (1981)
0.15 mg/kg	IV		329.0 ±53.22		2.29 ±0.42		19.38 ±5.16	Heizmann et al. (1983)
10mg	PO	53.09 ±30.62	77.5 ±27.28	0.67 ±0.45	1.36 ±1.08	0.38 ±0.12		Smith et al. (1981)
15mg	PO	13.80 ±22.2	154.0 ±51.0		2.10 ±0.5		38.7 ±9.24	Allonen et al. (1981)
20mg	PO		263.8 ±106.0	0.33 ±0.112	1.9 ±0.39			Heizmann et al. (1983)

Abbreviations: see table II.

Intramuscular Absorption

Midazolam, as the hydrochloride and lactate salt, is rapidly absorbed after intramuscular administration. Appearance in the systemic circulation occurs within 5 minutes and the drug reaches peak concentrations at 20 to 30 minutes (Crevoisier et al. 1981; Smith et al. 1984a). Peak concentrations of 25 to 200 μg/L have been reported following doses of 5, 10 and 12.5mg.

Rectal Absorption

Mean peak plasma midazolam concentrations of 99 μg/L were reached within 20 minutes (mean 16 minutes) in children given a 0.3 mg/kg solution administered rectally (Saint Maurice et al. 1986).

4.2.2 Systemic Bioavailability

Systemic bioavailability (f) of oral midazolam ranges from 34 to 68%; the differences in reported values are subject to the influence of dose-dependency (Allonen et al. 1981) and age of subjects in the study (Greenblatt et al. 1984). Bioavailability for a 15mg oral dose ranged between 35 and 67%, compared with 28 and 36% for a 7.5mg oral dose (Allonen et al. 1981). Greenblatt and colleagues reported a significantly higher absolute systemic bioavailability in elderly men (0.5) than in young subjects (0.41) [Greenblatt et al. 1984]. In this study, bioavailability was inversely related to total clearance. No significant differences between young and elderly women were observed. Comparison of the f values determined for a 10mg oral midazolam solution (0.35) and tablet (0.38) did not reach statistical significance (Smith et al. 1981). The results of this study indicate the extent of first-pass extraction of midazolam from the liver. Following IM administration, the systemic bioavailability is reported to be 0.4 to 1.0 (Smith et al. 1984). Crevoisier and colleagues reported 0.82 to 0.91 absolute bioavailability for both the hydrochloride and lactate salts (Crevoisier et al. 1981).

4.2.3 Distribution

In healthy subjects, midazolam has a short distribution phase half-life of between 5 and 30 minutes (Sjövall et al. 1983; Smith et al. 1984a). The Vd is characteristically large, 0.4 to 2.0 L/kg, with considerable intersubject variation. Smoking does not influence the Vd of midazolam, but evidence of the effect of age on the Vd of the drug is conflicting. Greenblatt and colleagues did not observe age-related effects after correcting for bodyweight in young and elderly men (Greenblatt et al. 1984). However, Servin and co-workers reported a significant increase ($p < 0.05$) in Vd in elderly subjects (> 80 years of age, 3 L/kg) compared with young subjects (30 years of age, 1.4 L/kg) [Servin et al. 1987], and bodyweight, gender, pregnancy and renal insufficiency have been reported to increase the Vd of the drug (Greenblatt et al. 1984; Kanto et al. 1983; Vinik et al. 1983).

Midazolam has been reported to be 94 to 96% protein bound in tests using equilibrium dialysis (Allonen et al. 1981; Greenblatt et al. 1984; Vinik et al. 1983). The free fraction is significantly higher (6.5%; $p < 0.005$) in renal failure patients than in control subjects (3.9%) [Vinik et al. 1983]. Smoking, age, bodyweight and gender do not alter the protein binding of midazolam.

Smith and colleagues evaluated the uptake of midazolam into red blood cells in healthy volunteers of 21 and 22 years of age (Smith et al. 1981). At plasma concentrations of 2 μg/L there was negligible entry. However, as plasma midazolam concentrations increased, red blood cell content increased non-linearly, with erythrocyte midazolam concentrations of 2, 36 and 41 μg/L at plasma concentrations of 42, 81 and 88 μg/L, respectively. In an elderly (63 to 84 years) population the red cell uptake of midazolam was linear over a plasma concentration range of 8 to 1064 μg/L, averaging approximately 5% (Smith et al. 1984a).

Penetration of midazolam into cerebrospinal fluid (CSF) was evaluated by Sjövall and co-workers (1983). A single oral dose of 15mg IM injection of 0.075 mg/kg or IV dose of 0.075 mg/kg was administered to patients undergoing surgery with spinal anaesthesia. CSF samples were obtained via lumbar puncture at regular intervals beginning 6 minutes after drug administration and continuing for at least 4 hours, and in some cases up to 18 hours. Concentrations of midazolam in the CSF were measured using gas chromatography with electron capture. Midazolam was not detected in the CSF following oral or IM administration. A measurable amount of midazolam (2 to 4 μg/L) appeared in the CSF as early as 8 minutes after drug administration in 4 of 26 patients who received the IV dose. CSF midazolam concentrations of 6 μg/L were detectable 50 minutes after administration.

Maternal and fetal midazolam concentrations were evaluated in women undergoing elective caesarean section who had been given a single oral dose of midazolam 15mg as a sedative (Kanto et al. 1983). Concentrations of midazolam were measurable in only 1 of 13 patients 12 hours after receiving the dose; the venous plasma concentration was 12 μg/L and umbilical venous and arterial serum concentrations were 7 μg/L. In the women given a premedication dose of midazolam 0.05 mg/kg IM 18 to 45 minutes before surgery, mean maternal peak serum concentrations 30 minutes after drug administration were 28 μg/L (range 20 to 36 μg/L) with corresponding mean venous and arterial umbilical concentrations of 22 and 13 μg/L, respectively. Apgar scores of the newborn infants at 1 and 5 minutes were greater than 7 in both groups.

4.2.4 Metabolism and Elimination

Midazolam is biotransformed by microsomal oxidation. It undergoes hydroxylation and subsequent glucuronidation (Allonen et al. 1981). The major metabolite is α-hydroxymidazolam, which is pharmacologically active but less so than the parent compound (Ziegler et al. 1983). The $t_{1/2\beta}$ of this metabolite is approximately 1 hour. Also formed in parallel and in smaller amounts are 4-hydroxymidazolam and 1,4-dihydroxymidazolam, which are excreted as glucuronide conjugates. The hepatic clearance of midazolam has been reported to be approximately 50% of hepatic blood flow (Greenblatt et al. 1981).

The high plasma clearance of midazolam (24 to 51 L/h) suggests that its elimination is perfusion and enzyme-capacity limited (Heizmann et al. 1983). Total plasma clearance has been reported to be higher in the supine (36.96 L/h) than the ambulant (19.02 L/h) position, and greater in the evening (27.78 L/h) than in the morning (19.02 L/h) under ambulant conditions (Klotz & Ziegler 1982). These results suggest that the positional differences are the result of the increase in hepatic blood flow accompanying the supine position. Time of day differences were postulated to be due to diurnal variation influence on the metabolising capacity of the liver enzymes. Using a prolonged midazolam infusion administered to 5 healthy adult men, Klotz and Reimann (1984) further evaluated any time-dependent pharmacokinetic effects. Although the mean plasma clearance was higher for daytime (40.86 L/h) than evening (36.06 L/h), there were no significant differences. No temporal change in protein binding was observed. Total plasma midazolam clearance is reduced in elderly subjects (Greenblatt et al. 1984).

The $t_{1/2\beta}$ of midazolam has been reported to be in the range of 1 to 2.5 hours in healthy subjects (Heizmann & Ziegler 1981; Heizmann et al. 1983; Smith et al. 1981). Dundee and colleagues reported that 8% (9 of 115 surgical patients evaluated) of the patients who received a dose of midazolam 0.3 mg/kg IV had a $t_{1/2\beta}$ greater than 8 hours (Dundee et al. 1986a). In an additional group of 102 patients, 5 (5%) had elimination half-lives greater than 8 hours. Defective hepatic metabolism, reflecting polymorphic oxidation, was believed to be the cause of the prolonged $t_{1/2\beta}$ in these subjects. Klotz and colleagues tested this hypothesis in patients known to be extensive or poor metabolisers of sparteine, a compound with genetically determined polymorphic metabolism (Klotz et al 1986). All 23 subjects were phenotyped with an oral test dose of sparteine. A single dose of midazolam 0.075mg IV was administered, and plasma and urine samples were analysed for midazolam and α-hydroxymidazolam. The $t_{1/2\beta}$ of midazolam was 2.2 hours in the extensive metabolisers and 4.4 hours in the poor metabolisers. The lower $t_{1/2\beta}$ in the poor metabolisers was accompanied by an increase in apparent volume of distribution at steady-state (Vd_{ss}) [0.7 L/kg to 1.5 L/kg] although CL was higher in the poor metabolisers (23.5 L/h) than that in the extensive metabolisers (18.6 L/h). No significant changes were observed for α-hydroxymidazolam. The findings do not support the hypothesis that the metabolism of midazolam is controlled by the gene responsible for sparteine metabolism; however, other genetic factors may be involved. Likewise, changes in Vd or other physiological factors such as surgical stress may influence the $t_{1/2\beta}$ of midazolam.

The elimination of midazolam is prolonged significantly in elderly (age 60 to 74 years) compared with young (age 24 to 33 years) men (5.6 *vs* 2.1 hours) [Greenblatt et al. 1984]. In elderly women, midazolam clearance is reduced and $t_{1/2\beta}$ prolonged, but not significantly (Avram et al. 1983; Greenblatt et al 1984). Likewise, $t_{1/2\beta}$ is prolonged in obese subjects, although this is related to the attendant increase in Vd (from 1.7 to 2.7 L/kg) since clearance was unchanged (28.3 *vs* 31.8 L/h in non-obese subjects). Smoking has been shown not to alter the $t_{1/2\beta}$ or CL of midazolam (Ochs et al. 1985).

In patients with biopsy-proven alcoholic cirrhosis, the $t_{1/2\beta}$ of midazolam following a single 0.075 mg/kg IV dose was significantly longer than that in age- and weight-matched control subjects (3.9 *vs* 1.6 hours) [Macgilchrist et al. 1987]. Clearance was also reduced in the cirrhotic patients (0.34 *vs* 0.61 L/h/kg in controls).

Similarly, in another study evaluating the pharmacokinetics of an orally administered dose of midazolam 15mg in compensated alcoholic liver cirrhosis, the $t_{1/2\beta}$ was 3.8 hours (range 2.9 to 5.2 hours) for midazolam and 3.7 hours (range 2.4 to 6.8 hours) for α-hydroxymidazolam (Rinetti et al. 1985).

Total midazolam clearance in chronic renal failure patients (0.68 L/h/kg) was significantly higher than in matched control subjects (0.4 L/h/kg) [Vinik et al. 1983]. Clearance of unbound midazolam was similar in both groups (10.56 and 11.34 L/h/kg). The absence of pharmacokinetic changes in these patients suggests that dose modification may not be necessary in renal failure patients.

When given to rats in high doses (9 mg/kg/day), midazolam has been shown to induce liver enzymes (White et al. 1987). Allen and co-workers investigated whether or not midazolam, in therapeutic doses, produced similar effects in humans (Allen et al. 1987). Plasma concentrations of antipyrine were determined before midazolam administration and after 10 days of administering an oral dose of midazolam 15mg. There was no change in the C_{max} (16.5 mg/L), $t_{1/2\beta}$ (10h), $AUC_{0\rightarrow\infty}$ (250 mg/L • h) or CL (0.042 L/kg/h) of antipyrine. This study demonstrated that doses of 7.5 to 15mg, equivalent to < 0.2 mg/kg/day, were not likely to alter human drug metabolising enzyme activity.

4.3 Influence of Surgery on the Pharmacokinetics of Midazolam

Physiological changes related to surgery, e.g. decreased cardiac output, decreased organ perfusion, decreased glomerular filtration, impaired hepatic enzyme activity and haemodilution, can significantly alter a drug's disposition in the body. Midazolam has been used both as an induction agent prior to surgical procedures and as a sedative following surgery. Consequently, several investigators have evaluated the influence of surgery on the pharmacokinetic variables of midazolam. In 67 surgical patients divided into 2 groups according to age and given midazolam 0.3 mg/kg IV either for induction or for sedation, Harper et al. reported a prolonged distribution and $t_{1/2\beta}$ in patients undergoing major (intra-abdominal or thoracic) versus minor (gynaecological or endoscopic) procedures (Harper et al. 1985). The distribution $t_{1/2}$ increased from 18 to 30 minutes and the $t_{1/2\beta}$ increased from 3.2 to 3.8 hours. The prolonged $t_{1/2\beta}$ was more pronounced (4.1 *vs* 2.4h) in older patients (mean 65 years of age) undergoing minor procedures than in young (mean 33 years of age) patients undergoing either minor or major procedures. The changes in the $t_{1/2\beta}$ were accompanied by changes in midazolam clearance; the type of operation had no influence, but younger patients had a higher clearance (0.4 L/h/kg) than the older patients (0.32 L/h/kg). The Vd was significantly greater in young patients undergoing major compared to minor surgery (2.1 L/kg *vs* 1.2 L/kg). Vd was not different in the older patients undergoing either minor or major procedures (1.7 L/kg). According to the authors, the prolonged $t_{1/2\beta}$ seen with age was the result of a decrease in clearance rather than changes in volume of distribution. The changes in Vd in young patients undergoing major procedures were believed to be related to changes in midazolam plasma protein binding, biological fluid compartments, or alterations in regional blood flow. In 6 patients not included in the data reported, the $t_{1/2\beta}$ was abnormally long, ranging between 10.5 and 18.6 hours. The authors believed the findings to be consistent with a subgroup of the population being poor metabolisers of midazolam.

The influence of cardiopulmonary bypass surgery on the pharmacokinetics of midazolam was investigated by Kanto et al. (1985). Samples were drawn through a radial artery cannula before and after injection of midazolam 0.075 mg/kg or 0.15 mg/kg, in addition to samples obtained during extracorporeal circulation and the postperfusion period. Midazolam distribution $t_{1/2}$ was approximately 3.5 minutes. There was a rapid decrease in midazolam concentrations at the beginning of extracorporeal circulation followed by increased plasma concentrations during the postperfusion period. The apparent $t_{1/2\beta}$ of midazolam during the postperfusion period was 4.5 hours. When compared with results in healthy adults, the disappearance of midazolam from plasma in patients undergoing cardiac surgery was similar (3.5 *vs* 5 minutes) while midazolam elimination from the body in the postperfusion period was prolonged (4.5 *vs* 2h).

Persson et al. (1987) evaluated the pharmacokinetics of midazolam following a 0.3 mg/kg injection in 15 women, 36 to 53 years of age, undergoing hysterectomy. Plasma CL (28.98 L/h), Vd (1.9 L/kg) and $t_{1/2\beta}$ (3.1h) were consistent with those reported in healthy volunteers. The authors felt this to indicate that surgery has negligible influence on the pharmacokinetics of midazolam.

These studies suggest that surgery influences the pharmacokinetics of midazolam to some extent. The changes are more apparent in elderly patients than in young, and are related to the physiological changes that occur during surgery.

4.4 Drug Interactions

Drug interactions with midazolam have not been extensively studied. Pharmacodynamic interactions have been reported to occur with alcohol (increase in midazolam effect on immediate recall and iconic memory), physostigmine (reversal of midazolam's hypnotic effects), aspirin and probenecid (more rapid onset of thiopentone induction) and ketamine (decrease in psychotic sequelae and increase in heart rate and blood pressure) [Caldwell & Gross 1982; Cartwright & Pingel 1984; Dundee et al. 1986b; Suhhan & Hindmarch 1983].

The interaction between midazolam and the H_2-antagonists cimetidine and ranitidine, and between midazolam and antacid, has been extensively investigated. In the study conducted by Elwood et al. (1983), midazolam plasma concentrations were consistently higher for the first 6 hours following ranitidine administration. There was a difference in the $AUC_{0\rightarrow\infty}$ between control (187 μg/L • h) and ranitidine treatments (310 μg/L • h; $p < 0.01$). The reason postulated for this difference was that the increase in gastric pH associated with ranitidine administration increased the absorption of midazolam.

The effects of cimetidine, ranitidine and magnesium trisilicate mixture on the pharmacokinetics of midazolam and temazepam (a benzodiazepine with a low liver extraction ratio) were investigated by Elliot et al. (1984). Both ranitidine and cimetidine increased the relative bioavailability of midazolam by approximately 70%. Peak plasma midazolam concentration was significantly greater in the cimetidine and ranitidine treatments but t_{max} was unchanged. Plasma concentrations and relative bioavailability of temazepam were unchanged. The authors concluded that both ranitidine and cimetidine affect liver function, and midazolam is more susceptible to altered liver function than temazepam.

In the study conducted by Fee and co-workers, plasma midazolam concentrations following a 15mg oral dose were highest after cimetidine pretreatment, intermediate after ranitidine pretreatment and lowest with no pretreatment (Fee et al. 1987). The mean absolute bioavailability of midazolam was increased after cimetidine (0.56; $p < 0.01$) and ranitidine (0.54; $p < 0.05$) compared with the control value (0.43). No significant change in $t_{1/2\beta}$ was demonstrated. These alterations were explained by a reduction in hepatic clearance of midazolam when concentrations of the H_2-antagonists were high and midazolam was undergoing absorption; less of the midazolam dose would undergo first-pass metabolism, resulting in increased systemic bioavailability.

Garzone (1987) evaluated the effects of cimetidine, ranitidine and a magnesium-aluminium hydroxide antacid pretreatment on the pharmacokinetics of midazolam. The stable isotope $^{15}N_3$-midazolam was administered as a 5mg IV dose simultaneously with a single 7.5mg oral tablet. In the ranitidine treatment, the $t_{1/2\alpha}$ of midazolam was decreased (not significantly) by approximately 30%, from 18 to 12.5 minutes. C_{max} of oral midazolam increased after cimetidine, decreased after antacid, and was unaltered after ranitidine. Likewise, t_{max} (1.7h) was essentially unchanged in each treatment group, except after the administration of cimetidine when t_{max} increased to 2.1 hours. Again, the difference was not significant. The $t_{1/2\beta}$ of midazolam was prolonged after cimetidine from 2.34 to 2.89 hours. In addition, the prolonged $t_{1/2\beta}$ was accompanied by a decrease in oral midazolam clearance (from 0.47 to 0.41 L/h/kg); these changes were not significant. Ranitidine and antacid had no effect on either $t_{1/2\beta}$ or CL. Oral midazolam $AUC_{0\rightarrow\infty}$ increased from 81.84 μg/L • h in the control study period to 169.18, 117.32, and 99.51 μg/L • h after pretreatment with cimetidine, ranitidine and antacid, respectively ($p < 0.0001$). Absolute bioavailability was significantly greater in the cimetidine (0.56) and ranitidine (0.43) pretreatment groups compared to the control group (0.34; $p < 0.0002$). These observed differences were postulated to be the result of inhibition of midazolam metabolism due to the effect of cimetidine on oxidative metabolism. The influence of ranitidine on the absorption rate of midazolam may have been related to its effect on midazolam's first-pass metabolism; i.e. while midazolam was undergoing absorption, ranitidine would be preferentially transported to the liver, thereby decreasing the hepatic clearance of midazolam and resulting in increased systemic absorption and bioavailability. Enhanced absorption due to gastric pH changes caused by the H_2-antagonists was discounted, although gastric pH determinations were not made.

Salonen et al. (1986) studied the effect of a single dose of cimetidine 400mg given 2 hours prior to oral midazolam 15mg in healthy adult male volunteers. A significant difference was found between the C_{max} (76 *vs* 105 μg/L) and $AUC_{0\rightarrow\infty}$ (212 *vs* 289 μg/L • h), but not t_{max} (2.6 *vs* 2.1h) or $t_{1/2\beta}$ (3 *vs* 4h) in the cimetidine group compared to control.

The effects of cimetidine and ranitidine on steady-state midazolam concentrations were evaluated by Klotz et al. (1985). Steady-state concentrations were achieved by an intravenous bolus dose of midazolam 0.05 mg/kg followed by a constant infusion of 0.025 mg/kg/h for 10 hours. On 3 separate occasions, subjects received single doses of ranitidine 300mg, cimetidine 800mg or placebo in a random order. Cimetidine significantly increased the mean steady-state plasma concentrations of midazolam from 56.7 to 71.3 μg/L ($p = 0.004$). The steady-state plasma midazolam concentration after ranitidine was not different from that after placebo (61.8 μg/L).

Only one published study failed to detect a clinically or statistically significant interaction between midazolam and the H_2-antagonists (Greenblatt et al. 1986). The authors emphasised that the sample may have been too small to detect any differences, and that there is considerable variation in the metabolism of midazolam.

Based on the results of these studies, the conclusion may be drawn that the H_2-antagonists alter midazolam pharmacokinetic variables; however, the alterations are not always predictable because of the large intersubject variability in midazolam disposition. The results also reflect the influence of study design and sample size on the ability to detect differences.

Experiments in rats have provided indirect biochemical evidence (increased Ca^{++} uptake into synaptosomes was increased by benzodiazepines under depolarising conditions) of a theoretically possible interaction between benzodiazepines and calcium channel antagonists (Mendelson et al. 1984). A study was undertaken by Handel and colleagues to evaluate the potential interaction of nitrendipine on the pharmacokinetics and pharmacodynamics of midazolam under steady-state conditions (Handel et al. 1988). Subjects received a loading dose of midazolam 0.07 mg/kg IV, followed by a constant infusion of 0.035 mg/kg/h for 6 hours on 2 separate occasions, with a solution of placebo or nitrendipine 20mg ingested 2 hours after the start of the infusion. The concurrent administration of nitrendipine did not change the midazolam concentration-time profile.

5. *Loprazolam*

5.1 Structure-Activity Relationship

Loprazolam is a 1,4-imidazolebenzodiazepine and, like midazolam, has a basic heterocycle ring at the 1,2 position of the diazepine ring (fig. 6). It differs from midazolam in several aspects: (1) a nitro group at position 8 on the diazepine nucleus; (2) a carboxy group at position 1 of the fused imidazole ring; (3) a piperazine ring at position 2 of the imidazole ring system. Consequently, loprazolam is not metabolised as rapidly as midazolam, and its major route of metabolism is *N*-oxidation. However, as with midazolam, the presence of the imidazole ring allows for the preparation of water-soluble salts.

5.2 Pharmacokinetics

Table V summarises the pharmacokinetics of loprazolam.

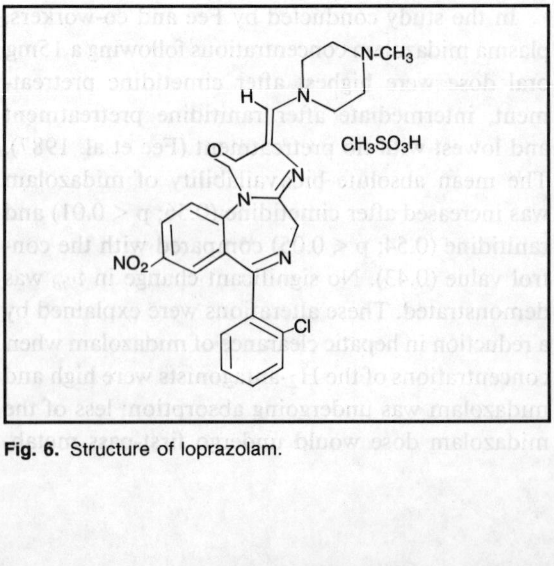

Fig. 6. Structure of loprazolam.

Table V. Pharmacokinetics of loprazolam in healthy subjects [mean (± SD) or range]

Dose	Route	C_{max} (μg/L)	t_{max} (h)	$t_{½β}$ (h)	CL (L/h/kg)	Reference
1.0mg	PO	6.0 ± 2.6	(0.5-2.0)			Stevens et al. (1985)
2.0mg	PO	11.30 ± 2.9	(0.5-2.0)	6.80 ± 2.9		
1.0mg[a]	PO	3.10 (1.3-4.4)	3.00 (2-12)	14.80 (10.6-22.1)	0.23	Jochemsen et al. (1986)
0.5mg[b]	PO	2.27 (1.58-3.28)	2.75 (1.5-6.0)	10.95 (5.48-17.28)		Ford et al. (1987)
1.0mg[b]	PO	5.28 (3.44-7.61)	1.56 (1-2)	11.81 (5.38-19.36)		
2.0mg	PO	9.70 ± 4.30	2.40 ± 0.90	6.30 ± 1.10		Stevens et al. (1983)
2.0mg	PO	9.60 ± 1.50	2.40 ± 0.30	7.50 ± 0.70		Krieger et al. (1983)

a Radioreceptor assay.
b Loprazolam only, no metabolites.
Abbreviations: see table II.

5.2.1 Absorption

Oral Absorption

In a crossover-designed study comparing doses of oral loprazolam 1 and 2mg, concentrations in the plasma were measurable at 0.5 hour (3 μg/L) and were still detectable 24 hours after dosing (< 2 μg/L) [Stevens et al. 1985]. The peak concentrations after the 2mg oral dose (11.3 μg/L) were significantly higher than the C_{max} achieved after the 1mg dose (6.0 μg/L). The t_{max} for both doses ranged from 0.5 to 2 hours. Similarly, Levasseur and colleagues reported a mean C_{max} of 6.1 μg/L and t_{max} of 1.8 hours (Levasseur et al. 1985). In these 2 studies, the doses had been administered in the morning and blood samples drawn accordingly. When given in the evening, oral doses of 0.5 and 1mg produced C_{max} values of 2.27 and 5.28 μg/L at 2.75 and 1.56 hours, respectively (Ford et al. 1987).

Stevens and associates reported a mean C_{max} of 9.7 μg/L and t_{max} of 2.4 hours following a single night-time oral dose of 2mg (Stevens et al. 1983). Similarly, Krieger and colleagues observed a mean C_{max} of 9.6 μg/L occurring at 2.4 hours (Krieger et al. 1983). There has been no direct comparison between daytime and night-time loprazolam administration, but these studies suggest that C_{max} is higher and delayed when it is given at night. Large intersubject variation was present in the studies and, in addition, different assay methodologies were used to quantify loprazolam concentrations. This may explain the observed differences.

With repeated dosing (2mg nightly for 8 days), C_{max} (11.5 μg/L) on day 8 was not statistically different from that on day 1 (9.7 μg/L) [Stevens et al. 1983]. The t_{max} was also similar on day 1 to that on day 8 (2.2 *vs* 2.4h). Multiple oral doses of 1mg for 7 days resulted in a mean C_{max} of 4.6 μg/L (McInnes et al. 1985). This was similar to the mean C_{max} of 4.1 μg/L observed after the first dose. The t_{max} was 5.0 and 5.5 hours, respectively. The lag time ranged from 1 to 1.5 hours. The slower rate of absorption observed in this study may have been due to the influence of food, since the dose was given 2 hours after the evening meal. No controlled study evaluating the effect of food on the rate and extent of loprazolam absorption has been published.

The data from the multiple dose studies were used to calculate the accumulation factor (R) for loprazolam. The R that was calculated was greater than 1.0 (range 1.07 to 1.14). Similarly, Ford and colleagues predicted R to be 1.16 based on the results of a single loprazolam dose in healthy subjects (Ford et al. 1987). Accumulation would thus be expected to occur with repeated dosing. The differences observed in C_{max} after repeated dosing ranged from 11 to 35%, depending on the assay used, although statistical significance was not reached. Furthermore, $AUC_{0\rightarrow\infty}$ was 11 to 30% greater after repeated administration, providing further evidence of accumulation.

In elderly versus young subjects, mean loprazolam C_{max} values were not significantly different (2.4 *vs* 2.3 μg/L for a 0.5mg dose and 5.2 *vs* 5.3 μg/L for a 1mg dose), nor was t_{max} (2.67 *vs* 2.75h and 2.19 *vs* 1.56h, respectively) [Ford et al. 1987]. This suggests that age has little influence on the absorption of loprazolam.

The influence of gender, bodyweight or smoking on absorption characteristics of loprazolam has not been reported.

5.2.2 Systemic Bioavailability

Absolute bioavailability data in humans are not available. In animals, approximately 70 to 75% of the oral dose is absorbed (Illing et al. 1983a). It is estimated that 70% of an oral dose is absorbed in humans.

5.2.3 Distribution

After oral administration, the Vd of loprazolam is 283L, assuming 100% absorption (Levasseur et al. 1985). Vd/F was found to be higher in young (313L) than in elderly (285L) subjects following a single oral dose of 0.5mg (Ford et al. 1987), and after a single oral dose of 1mg was 285 and 268L, respectively. Only the observed differences after the 0.5mg dose were statistically significant. Other factors, such as gender or disease processes known to influence the Vd of other benzodiazepines, have not been reported for loprazolam.

The plasma protein binding of loprazolam in humans is approximately 80%, as determined by equilibrium dialysis (Illing et al. 1983a). The influence of gender, age or disease processes on loprazolam binding to plasma proteins has not been determined.

In rats, whole body autoradiography and tissue distribution studies with ^{14}C-loprazolam have demonstrated loprazolam concentrations in the brain (Illing et al. 1983a). The liver, kidneys and intestine had the highest concentrations of loprazolam.

Traces of loprazolam were found in 4 of 14 lactating women following a single night-time dose of 1mg (Kesson et al. 1983). Blood and breast milk samples were collected at 2 and 12 hours after drug administration. Loprazolam concentrations were determined by radioimmunoassay (RIA). The mean loprazolam concentration in breast milk was 2.9 μg/L after 2 hours and 0.9 μg/L after 12 hours. Corresponding plasma concentrations were 6.0 and 3.9 μg/L, respectively. Placental transfer of loprazolam has not been studied.

5.2.4 Metabolism and Elimination

The metabolic pathway of loprazolam differs somewhat depending on the species used in the evaluation. In rats, the major metabolic pathway is hydroxylation of the diazepine ring, with the reduction and subsequent acetylation of the nitro group. In humans, *N*-oxidation of the piperazine ring is the major pathway. Following the administration of ^{14}C-loprazolam (approximately 30μCi) in humans, more than 90% of the radioactivity present 2 hours post dose was accounted for by equal amounts of loprazolam and its piperazine-*N*-oxide metabolite (Illing et al. 1983a). The radioactivity present after 24 hours was not extractable and consisted of polar material. Up to 22% of a single oral dose of loprazolam 2mg was found in human bile as loprazolam and the piperazine-*N*-oxide metabolite (Illing et al. 1983b). 92% of the total radioactivity of ^{14}C-loprazolam was recovered in urine

(39%) and faeces (53%) after 14 days (Illing et al. 1983a).

Secondary peaks in the plasma concentration/time profiles have been observed following loprazolam administration in some studies (McInnes et al. 1985; Stevens et al. 1985) but not in others (Ford et al. 1987; Swift et al. 1985). Enterohepatic recycling could account for this observation. In addition, the effects of food and assay methodology (HPLC/GC *vs* RIA) also need to be considered.

The $t_{1/2\beta}$ of loprazolam ranges from 4 to 7 hours, making it an intermediate-acting benzodiazepine. This $t_{1/2\beta}$ was reported in the studies which utilised HPLC and GC. A $t_{1/2\beta}$ of 15 hours has been reported in the studies using RIA methodology (Jochemsen et al. 1986). This value may be due to the detection of loprazolam metabolites. Similar results were observed by Krieger and colleagues, who reported higher loprazolam concentrations and a longer time to reach steady-state (4 days *vs* 2 days) when a radioreceptor assay was used compared with chromatographic methods (Krieger et al. 1983).

The $t_{1/2\beta}$ of loprazolam is not influenced by time of day of administration (day *vs* evening), although no well-designed study has been done. It was slightly prolonged (7.8 *vs* 6.3h) after multiple doses, but this difference was not significant (Stevens et al. 1985). This trend was also reported by Krieger et al. (1985).

In elderly hospitalised patients, there is also a trend towards a more prolonged $t_{1/2\beta}$ (12.7h) than in young patients (10.9h) [Ford et al. 1987]. However, Swift and colleagues found a significant difference between elderly (19.8h) and young subjects (11.2h) [Swift et al. 1985]. The intersubject variability in this study was high; the $t_{1/2\beta}$ ranged from 8.7 to 14.4 hours in the young and 9.5 to 30.7 hours in the elderly. This variability may reflect differences in rates of metabolic elimination, accumulation of drug, changes in volume of distribution or protein binding alterations of drug in elderly patients.

Ford and colleagues also analysed plasma samples for the piperazine-*N*-oxide metabolite in the 2 subject groups (Ford et al. 1987). There was a significant increase in $t_{1/2\beta}$ in the elderly *vs* young subjects (14.9 *vs* 11.6h, respectively). The accumulation of this metabolite after multiple doses has not been evaluated.

A proportional increase in $AUC_{0\rightarrow24}$ is observed following single oral doses of 0.5 to 2mg for both loprazolam and its *N*-oxide metabolite, suggesting that elimination is linear and independent of dose (Stevens et al. 1985).

There is evidence in animals that hepatic enzyme induction occurs at high doses (64 mg/kg for 6 months in the rat and 6.3 mg/kg for 12 months in the dog) [Ankier et al. 1983]. In humans, the enzyme induction potential was evaluated following the administration of oral loprazolam 1mg at night for 15 or 30 nights. Antipyrine $t_{1/2\beta}$ was unchanged before and after loprazolam in both study periods. Thus, it is unlikely that loprazolam induces microsomal enzyme activity in humans.

The influence of renal or hepatic disease on the pharmacokinetics of loprazolam has not been determined.

5.3 Drug Interactions

There is a paucity of information on loprazolam interactions. The effect of the concurrent administration of alcohol and loprazolam was evaluated using effect measurements (McManus 1983). There was no evidence of a hangover effect of loprazolam or potentiation of the effects of loprazolam by alcohol. It would be expected that drugs known to inhibit or induce the microsomal liver enzyme system could potentially interact with and alter the pharmacokinetic characteristics of loprazolam.

References

Abernethy DR, Greenblatt DJ, Divoll M, Moschitto LJ, Harmatz JS, et al. Interaction of cimetidine with the triazolobenzodiazepines alprazolam and triazolam. Psychopharmacology 80: 275-278, 1983

Abernethy DR, Greenblatt DJ, Divoll M, Smith RB, Shader RI. The influence of obesity on the pharmacokinetics of oral alprazolam and triazolam. Clinical Pharmacokinetics 9: 177-183, 1984

Abernethy DR, Greenblatt DJ, Morse DS, Shader RI. Interaction of propoxyphene with diazepam, alprazolam, and lorazepam. British Journal of Clinical Pharmacology 19: 51-57, 1985

Allen JG, Alderson K, Galloway DB, Hallett C. The effect of midazolam (Hypnovel) administration on antipyrine pharmacokinetics in humans. Xenobiotica 17: 875-879, 1987

Allonen H, Ziegler G, Klotz U. Midazolam kinetics. Clinical Pharmacology and Therapeutics 30: 653-661, 1981
Ankier SI, Barclay SP, Warrington SJ. Loprazolam (RV31158)–lack of effect on hepatic microsomal enzyme activity in man. Correspondence. British Journal of Clinical Pharmacology 16: 200-201, 1983
Arendt RM, Greenblatt DJ, Garland WA. Quantitation by gas chromatography of the 1- and 4-hydroxy metabolites of midazolam in human plasma. Pharmacology 29: 158-164, 1984
Avram MJ, Frazen RJ, Caldwell NJ. Midazolam kinetics in women of two age groups. Clinical Pharmacology and Therapeutics 34: 505-508, 1983
Bakti G, Fisch HU, Karlaganis G, Minder C, Bircher J. Mechanism of the excessive sedative response of cirrhotics to benzodiazepines: model experiments with triazolam. Hepatology 7: 629-638, 1987
Blyden GT, Scavone JM, Greenblatt DJ. Metronidazole impairs clearance of phenytoin but not of alprazolam or lorazepam. Journal of Clinical Pharmacology 28: 240-245, 1988
Bornemann LD, Crews T, Chen SS, Twardak S, Patel IH. Influence of food on midazolam absorption. Journal of Clinical Pharmacology 26: 55-59, 1986
Bornemann LD, Min BH, Crews T, Rees MMC, Blumenthal HP, et al. Dose dependent pharmacokinetics of midazolam. European Journal of Clinical Pharmacology 29: 91-95, 1985
Caldwell CB, Gross JB. Physostigmine reversal of midazolam induced sedation. Anesthesiology 57: 125, 1982
Cartwright PO, Pingel SM. Midazolam and diazepam in ketamine anesthesia. Anesthesia 39: 439-442, 1984
Cho MJ, Scahill TA, Aster JB. Kinetics and equilibrium of the reversible alprazolam ring-opening reaction. Journal of Pharmaceutical Sciences 72: 356-362, 1983
Ciraulo DA, Barnhill JG, Boxenbaum HG, Greenblatt DJ, Smith RB. Pharmacokinetics and clinical effects of alprazolam following single and multiple oral doses in patients with panic disorder. Journal of Clinical Pharmacology 26: 292-298, 1986
Coassolo Ph, Aubert C, Cano JP. Simultaneous assay of triazolam and its main hydroxy metabolite in plasma and urine by capillary gas chromatography. Journal of Chromatography 274: 161-170, 1983
Cox SR, Kroboth PD, Anderson DH, Smith RB. Mechanism for the interaction between triazolam and cimetidine. Biopharmaceutics and Drug Disposition 7: 567-575, 1986
Crevoisier C, Eckert M, Heizmann P, Thurneysen DJ, Ziegler WH. Relation entre l'effet clinique et la pharmacocinétique du midazolam aprés administration IV et IM. Arzneimittel-Forschung 31: 2211-2215, 1981
Dehlin O, Bjornson G, Borgesson L. Abrahamsson L, Smith RB. Pharmacokinetics of triazolam in geriatric patients. European Journal of Clinical Pharmacology 25: 91-94, 1983
Dorian P, Sellers CM, Kaplan HL, Hamilton C, Greenblatt DJ, et al. Triazolam and ethanol interaction: kinetic and dynamic consequences. Clinical Pharmacology and Therapeutics 37: 558-562, 1985
Dundee JW, Collier PS, Carlisle RJT, Harper KW. Prolonged midazolam elimination half-life. British Journal of Clinical Pharmacology 21: 425-429, 1986a
Dundee JW, Halliday WJ, McMurray TJ. Aspirin and probenecid pretreatment influences the potency of thiopentone and the onset of action of midazolam. European Journal of Anesthesiology 3: 247-251, 1986b
Eberts FS, Pilopoulos Y, Reineke LM, Vliek RW. Disposition of ^{14}C-alprazolam, a new anxiolytic-antidepressant in man. Abstract. Pharmacologist 22: 279, 1980
Eberts FS, Pilopoulos Y, Reineke LM, Vliek RW. Triazolam disposition. Clinical Pharmacology and Therapeutics 29: 81-93, 1981
Ellinwood EH, Heatherly DG, Nikardo AM, Bjornsson TD, Kilts C. Comparative pharmacokinetics and pharmacodynamics of lorazepam, alprazolam and diazepam. Psychopharmacology 86: 392-399, 1985
Elliott P, Dundee JW, Elwood RJ, Collier PS. The influence of H_2 receptor antagonists on the plasma concentrations of midazolam and temazepam. European Journal of Anesthesiology 1: 245-251, 1984
Elwood RJ, Hildebrande PJ, Dundee JW, Collier PS. Ranitidine influences the uptake of oral midazolam. British Journal of Clinical Pharmacology 15: 743-745, 1983
Fee JP, Collier PS, Howard PJ, Dundee JW. Cimetidine and ranitidine increase midazolam bioavailability. Clinical Pharmacology and Therapeutics 41: 80-84, 1987
Ford S, Ankier SI, Corless D, Bevan CD, Pidgen AW, et al. Pharmacokinetics of loprazolam and its principal metabolite in young subjects and elderly hospital patients. Xenobiotica 8: 1001-1009, 1987
Friedman H, Greenblatt DJ, Burstein ES, Harvatz JS, Shader RI. Population study of triazolam pharmacokinetics. British Journal of Clinical Pharmacology 22: 639-642, 1986
Garzone PD. Stable isotope technology in drug-drug interactions: the effects of cimetidine, ranitidine, and antacid on the pharmacokinetics of midazolam, Ph.D dissertation, University of Pittsburgh, 1987
Gerecke M. Chemical structure and properties of midazolam compared with other benzodiazepines. British Journal of Clinical Pharmacology 16: 11S-16S, 1983
Greenblatt DJ, Abernethy DR, Locniskar A, Harmatz JS, Limjuco RA, et al. Effect of age, gender and obesity on midazolam's kinetics. Anesthesiology 61: 27-35, 1984
Greenblatt DJ, Arendt RM, Abernethy DR, Giles HG, Sellers EM, et al. *In vitro* quantitation of benzodiazepine lipophilicity: relation to *in vivo* distribution. British Journal of Anaesthesiology 55: 985-989, 1983c
Greenblatt DJ, Divoll M, Abernethy DR, Moschitto LJ, Smith RB, et al. Alprazolam kinetics in the elderly: relation to antipyrine disposition. Archives of General Psychiatry 40: 287-290, 1983a
Greenblatt DJ, Divoll M, Abernethy DR, Moschitto LJ, Smith RB, et al. Reduced clearance of triazolam in old age: relation to antipyrine oxidizing capacity. British Journal of Clinical Pharmacology 15: 303-309, 1983b
Greenblatt DJ, Divoll M, Moschitto LJ, Shader RI. Electron-capture gas chromatographic analysis of the triazolobenzodiazepines alprazolam and triazolam. Journal of Chromatography 225: 202-207, 1981a
Greenblatt DJ, Locniskar A, Ochs HR, Lauven PM. Automated gas chromatography for studies of midazolam pharmacokinetics. Anesthesiology 55: 176-179, 1981b
Greenblatt DJ, Locniskar A, Scavone JM, Blyden GJ, Ochs HR, et al. Absence of interaction of cimetidine and ranitidine with intravenous and oral midazolam. Anesthesia and Analgesia 65: 176-180, 1986
Handel J, Ziegler G, Gemeinhardt A, Stuber H, Fischer C, et al. Lack of effect of nitrendipine on the pharmacokinetics and pharmacodynamics of midazolam during steady state. British Journal of Clinical Pharmacology 25: 243-250, 1988
Harper KW, Collier PS, Dundee JW, Elliot P, Halliday NJ, et al. Age and nature of operation influence the pharmacokinetics of midazolam. British Journal of Anaesthesiology 57: 866-871, 1985
Heizmann P, Eckert M, Ziegler WH. Pharmacokinetics and bioavailability of midazolam in man. British Journal of Clinical Pharmacology 16: 43S-49S, 1983
Heizmann P, Ziegler WH. Excretion and metabolism of ^{14}C-midazolam in humans following oral dosing. Arzneimittel-Forschung 31: 2220-2222, 1981
Hengen N, Hoffman E, Schick C. Liquid chromatographic assay of the new benzodiazepine derivative GP 55129 in plasma and

urine after application to humans. Naunyn-Schmiedeberg's Archives of Pharmacology 319 (Suppl.): R88, 1982

Illing HPA, Bevan CD, Robinson JD, Chamberlain J, Fromson JM. Metabolism of loprazolam in rat, dog and man *in vivo*. Xenobiotica 13: 539-553, 1983b

Illing HPA, Ings RMJ, Johnson KI, Fromson JM. Disposition of ^{14}C-loprazolam in animals and man. Xenobiotica 13: 439-449, 1983a

Jochemsen R, Van Rijn PA, Hazelzet TGM, Van Boxtel CJ, Breimer DD. Comparative pharmacokinetics of midazolam and loprazolam in healthy subjects after oral administration. Biopharmaceutics and Drug Disposition 7: 53-61, 1986

Jochemsen R, Wesselman JGJ, Van Boxtel CJ, Hermans J, Breimer DD. Comparative pharmacokinetics of brotizolam and triazolam in healthy subjects. British Journal of Clinical Pharmacology 16 (Suppl. 2): 291S-298S, 1983

Juhl RP, Van Thiel DH, Dittert LW, Smith RB. Alprazolam pharmacokinetics in alcoholic liver disease. Journal of Clinical Pharmacology 24: 113-119, 1984

Kanto J, Djovall S, Erkkola R, Hiberg J, Kangas L. Placental transfer and maternal midazolam kinetics. Clinical Pharmacology and Therapeutics 33: 786-791, 1983

Kanto J, Himberg JJ, Heikkila H, Arola M, Jalonen J, et al. Midazolam kinetics before, during and after cardiopulmonary bypass surgery. International Journal of Clinical Pharmacy Research 2: 123-126, 1985

Kesson CM, Gray JMD, Lawson DH. A pilot study into the secretion of loprazolam in human breast milk. In Loprazolam clinical workshop, p. 31, Medicine Publishing Foundation, Oxford, 1983

Kitagawa H, Esumi Y, Krurosawa S, Sekine S, Yokoshima T. Metabolism of 8-chloro-6-(o-chlorophenyl)-1-methyl-4H-s-triazolo [4,3a] [1,4] benzodiazepine, triazolam, a new central depressant, I: absorption, distribution and excretion in rats, dogs, and monkeys. Xenobiotica 9: 415-428, 1979

Klotz U, Arvela P, Rosenkranz B. Effect of single doses of cimetidine and ranitidine on the steady-state plasma levels of midazolam. Clinical Pharmacology and Therapeutics 38: 652-655, 1985

Klotz U, Mikus G, Zekorn C, Eichelbaum M. Pharmacokinetics of midazolam in relation to polymorphic sparteine oxidation. British Journal of Clinical Pharmacology 22: 618-620, 1986

Klotz U, Reimann IW. Chronopharmacokinetic study with prolonged infusion of midazolam. Clinical Pharmacokinetics 9: 469-474, 1984

Klotz U, Ziegler G. Physiologic and temporal variation in hepatic elimination of midazolam. Clinical Pharmacology and Therapeutics 32: 107-112, 1982

Konishi M, Hirai K, Mori Y. Kinetics and mechanisms of the equilibrium reaction of triazolam in aqueous solution. Journal of Pharmaceutical Sciences 71: 1328-1334, 1982

Krieger J, Perianu M, Bertagna C, Mangen P, Kurtz D. Hypnotic benzodiazepines: relationship between sleep parameters and pharmacokinetics of loprazolam. Drug Development and Research 3: 143-152, 1983

Kroboth PD, Smith RB, Rosanske T, Hamilton JM, McAuley JW, et al. Triazolam route of administration studies, I: pharmacokinetics. Abstract. Pharmaceutical Research 3(S): 111, 1986

Kroboth PD, Smith RB, Silver MR, Rault R, Sorkin MI, et al. Effects of end stage renal disease and aluminium hydroxide on triazolam pharmacokinetics. British Journal of Clinical Pharmacology 19: 839-842, 1985

Kroboth PD, Smith RB, Sorkin MI, Silver M, Rault R, et al. Triazolam protein binding correlation with alpha-1 acid glycoprotein concentration. Clinical Pharmacology and Therapeutics 36: 379-383, 1984

Kroboth PD, Smith RB, Van Thiel DH, Juhl RP. Nighttime dosing of triazolam in patients with liver disease and normal subjects: kinetics and daytime effects. Journal of Clinical Pharmacology 27: 555-560, 1987

Levasseur FA, Caille G, Elie R, Vezina M, Lariviere L. Electron-capture gas chromatographic determination of loprazolam in plasma and a pharmacokinetic application. Biopharmaceutics and Drug Disposition 6: 381-387, 1985

Macgilchrist AJ, Birnie GG, Cook A, Scohie G, Murray T, et al. Pharmacokinetics and pharmacodynamics of intravenous midazolam in patients with severe alcoholic cirrhosis. Gut 27: 190-195, 1987

McAuley JW, Hamilton JM, Kroboth PD, Smith RB. Alprazolam in elderly: kinetics and dynamics during multiple dosing. Abstract. Pharmaceutical Research 4(S): 99, 1987

McInnes GT, Banting EA, Ings RMJ, Robinson J, Ankier SI. Pharmacokinetics and pharmacodynamics following single and repeated nightly administration of loprazolam, a new benzodiazepine hypnotic. British Journal of Clinical Pharmacology 19: 649-656, 1985

McManus IC. The interaction of loprazolam and alcohol in a volunteer study. In Loprazolam clinical workshop, p. 30, Medicine Publishing Foundation, Oxford, 1983

Mendelson WB, Skolnick P, Martin JV, Luu MD, Wagner R, et al. Diazepam-stimulated increase in the synaptosomal uptake of $^{45}Ca^{++}$: reversal by dihydropyridine calcium channel antagonists. European Journal of Pharmacology 104: 181-183, 1984

Muakkassah SF, Bidlack WR, Lang WCT. Mechanism of the inhibitory action of isoniazid on microsomal drug metabolism. Biochemistry and Pharmacology 30: 1651-1658, 1981

Moschitto LJ, Greenblatt DJ. Concentration-independent plasma protein binding of benzodiazepines. Journal of Pharmacy and Pharmacology 35: 179-180, 1983

Ochs HR, Greenblatt DJ, Arendt RM, Hubbel W, Shader RI. Pharmacokinetic non-interaction of triazolam and ethanol. Journal of Clinical Psychopharmacology 4: 106-107, 1984b

Ochs HR, Greenblatt DJ, Burstein ES. Lack of influence of cigarette smoking on triazolam's pharmacokinetics. British Journal of Clinical Pharmacology 23: 759-763, 1987

Ochs HR, Greenblatt DJ, Knuchel M. Differential effect of isoniazid on triazolam oxidation and oxazepam conjugation. British Journal of Clinical Pharmacology 16: 743-746, 1983

Ochs HR, Greenblatt DJ, Knuchel M. Kinetics of diazepam, midazolam and lorazepam in cigarette smokers. Chest 87: 223-226, 1985

Ochs HR, Greenblatt DJ, Labedzki L, Smith RB. Alprazolam kinetics in patients with renal insufficiency. Journal of Clinical Psychopharmacology 6: 292-294, 1986

Ochs HR, Greenblatt DJ, Verburg-Ochs B. Propranolol interaction with diazepam, lorazepam and alprazolam. Clinical Pharmacology and Therapeutics 36: 451-455, 1984a

Persson P, Nilsson A, Hartvey P, Tamsen A. Pharmacokinetics of midazolam in total IV anaesthesia. British Journal of Anaesthesiology 59: 548-556, 1987

Pessayre D. Effects of macrolide antibiotics on drug metabolism in rats and humans. International Journal of Clinical Pharmacology Research 111: 449-458, 1983

Phillips JP, Antale EJ, Smith RB. A pharmacokinetic drug interaction between erythromycin and triazolam. Journal of Clinical Psychopharmacology 6: 297-299, 1986

Philopoulos Y, Eberts FS, Vliek RW, Russell RR, Collin RJ. Metabolism of alprazolam. Enzyme induction study with rat hepatic microsomal mixed function oxidase. Upjohn Technical Report, 1980

Pourbaix S, Desager JP, Hulhoven R, Smith RB, Harvengt C. Pharmacokinetic consequences of long term coadministration of cimetidine and triazolobenzodiazepines, alprazolam and triazolam in healthy subjects. International Journal of Clinical Pharmacology, Therapy and Toxicology 23: 447-451, 1985

Puglisi CV, Meyer JC, D'Arconte L, Brooks MA, deSilva JAF. Determination of water soluble imidazo-1,4-benzodiazepines in blood by electron-capture gas liquid chromatography and in urine by differential pulse polarography. Journal of Chromatography 14: 81-96, 1978

Reineke LM, Vliek RW, Eberts FS. Metabolism of alprazolam. Urine metabolite profile in human, dog and rat. Upjohn Technical Report, 1978

Rinetti M, Ascalone V, Colombi Zinelli L, Cisternino M. A pharmacokinetic study on midazolam in compensated liver cirrhosis. International Journal of Clinical Pharmacy Research 6: 405-411, 1985

Rubio F, Miwa BJ, Garland WA. Determination of midazolam and two metabolites of midazolam in human plasma by gas chromatography-negative chemical-ionization mass spectrometry. Journal of Chromatography 233: 157-165, 1982

Saint Maurice C, Meistelman C, Rey E, Esteve C, DeLauture D, et al. The pharmacokinetics of rectal midazolam for premedication in children. Anesthesiology 65: 536-538, 1986

Salonen M, Aantau E, Aaltonen L, Kanto J. Importance of the interaction of midazolam and cimetidine. Acta Pharmacologica et Toxicologica 58: 91-95, 1986

Scavone JM, Greenblatt DJ, Friedman H, Shader RI. Enhanced bioavailability of triazolam following sublingual *versus* oral administration. Clinical Pharmacology 26: 208-210, 1986

Scavone JM, Greenblatt DJ, Shader RI. Alprazolam kinetics following sublingual and oral administration. Journal of Clinical Psychopharmacology 7: 332-334, 1987

Servin F, Enriquez I, Fournet M, Failler JM, Favinotti R, et al. Pharmacokinetics of midazolam used as an intravenous induction agent for patients over 80 years of age. European Journal of Anesthesiology 4: 1-7, 1987

Sethy VH, Harris DW. Determination of biological activity of alprazolam, triazolam and their metabolites. Journal of Pharmacy and Pharmacology 34: 115-116, 1982

Sjövall S, Kanto J, Himberg JT, Hovi-Viander M, Salo M. CSF penetration and pharmacokinetics of midazolam. European Journal of Clinical Pharmacology 25: 247-251, 1983

Smith MT, Eadie MJ, O'Rourke Brophy T. The pharmacokinetics of midazolam in man. European Journal of Clinical Pharmacology 19: 271-278, 1981

Smith MT, Heazlewood V, Eadie MJ, O'Rourke Brophy T, Tyrer JH. Pharmacokinetics of midazolam in the aged. European Journal of Clinical Pharmacology 26: 381-388, 1984a

Smith RB, Divoll M, Gillespie WR, Greenblatt DJ. Effect of subject age and gender on the pharmacokinetics of oral triazolam and temazepam. Journal of Clinical Psychopharmacology 3: 172-176, 1983a

Smith RB, Gwilt PR, Wright CE. Single and multiple dose pharmacokinetics of oral alaprazolam in healthy smoking and nonsmoking men. Clinical Pharmacy 2: 139-143, 1983b

Smith RB, Kroboth PD. Influence of dosing regimen on alprazolam and metabolite serum concentration and tolerance to sedative and psychomotor effects. Psychopharmacology 93: 105-112, 1987

Smith RB, Kroboth PD, Phillips JP. Temporal variation in triazolam pharmacokinetics and pharmacodynamics after oral administration. Journal of Clinical Pharmacology 26: 120-124, 1986

Smith RB, Kroboth PD, Vanderlugt JT, Phillips JP, Juhl RP. Pharmacokinetics and pharmacodynamics of alprazolam after oral and IV administration. Psychopharmacology 84: 452-456, 1984b

Smith RB, Schoenfeld MJ. Effect of food on the bioavailability of Xanax (alprazolam) following a single oral 1.0mg dose. Upjohn Technical Report, 1981a

Smith RB, Schoenfeld MJ. The effect of food on the bioavailability of 0.5mg Halcion administered as a single dose. Upjohn Technical Report, 1981b

Stevens LA, Bevan CD, Salmon J, Krieger J, Perianu M, et al. Single and repeated dose kinetics of the hypnotic agent loprazolam in healthy volunteers. European Journal of Clinical Pharmacology 25: 651-655, 1983

Stevens LA, Pidgen AW, Bevan CD, Ings RMJ, Lawrence JR, et al. Correlation of the clinical pharmacodynamics of loprazolam with serum concentrations. Xenobiotica 15: 623-631, 1985

Stoehr GP, Kroboth PD, Juhl RP, Wender DB, Phillips JP, et al. Effect of oral contraceptives on triazolam, temazepam, alprazolam and lorazepam kinetics. Clinical Pharmacology and Therapeutics 36: 683-690, 1984

Suhhan Z, Hindmarch I. The effects of midazolam in conjunction with alcohol on iconic memory and free recall. Neuropsychobiology 9: 230-234, 1983

Swift CG, Swift MR, Ankier SI, Pidgen A, Robinson J. Single dose pharmacokinetics and pharmacodynamics of oral loprazolam in the elderly. British Journal of Clinical Pharmacology 20: 119-128, 1985

Thomas RC, Judy RW. Tissue levels of alprazolam–^{14}C(U-31889) in the mouse as determined by whole body section autoradiography. Upjohn Company, 1976

Tuzel IH, Skinner JM, Wyler-Plaut R. Injectable midazolam. Investigational drug brochure. Hoffmann-LaRoche Inc., 1984

Vasiliades J, Sahawneh TH. Determination of midazolam by high performance liquid chromatography. Journal of Chromatography 225: 266-271, 1981

Vinik HR, Reves JG, Greenblatt DJ, Abernethy DR, Smith LR. The pharmacokinetics of midazolam in chronic renal failure patients. Anesthesiology 59: 390-394, 1983

Vree TB, Baars AM, Booij LHD, Driessen JJ. Simultaneous determination and pharmacokinetics of midazolam and its hydroxymetabolites in plasma and urine of man and dog by means of high-performance liquid chromatography, Arzneimittel-Forschung 31: 2215-2219, 1981

White SM, Allen JG, Altman JFB. The effects of midazolam administration on the pharmacokinetics of antipyrine in the rat. Xenobiotica 17: 869-873, 1987

Ziegler WH, Schalch E, Leishman B, Eckert M. Comparison of the effects of intravenously administered midazolam, triazolam and their hydroxy metabolites. British Journal of Clinical Pharmacology 16: 63-69, 1983

Authors' address: *Pamela D. Garzone*, Center for Pharmacodynamic Research, 527 Salk Hall, University of Pittsburgh, Pittsburgh, PA 15261 (USA).

Clinical Pharmacokinetics 16: 365-386 (1989)
0312-5963/89/0006-0365/$11.00/0

Clinical Pharmacokinetic Considerations in the Treatment of Patients with Leprosy

K. Venkatesan

Central JALMA Institute for Leprosy, Agra, India

Contents

Summary 365
1. Fundamental Pharmacokinetic Properties of Antileprosy Drugs 367
1.1 Dapsone 367
1.2 Rifampicin 370
1.3 Clofazimine 371
1.4 Ethionamide and Prothionamide 375
1.5 Thiacetazone 375
1.6 Isoniazid 376
1.7 Pyrazinamide 377
2. Side Effects of Antileprosy Drugs 377
2.1 Dapsone 377
2.2 Rifampicin 378
2.3 Clofazimine 378
2.4 Ethionamide and Prothionamide 378
2.5 Thiacetzaone 378
3. Pharmacokinetics in Various Pathophysiological States 378
4. Implications for the Treatment of Leprosy 379

Summary *On the basis of the efficacy of the available agents, the World Health Organization has recommended only 4 drugs for combined chemotherapy of leprosy: rifampicin, dapsone, clofazimine and ethionamide/prothionamide. Thiacetazone and isoniazid are also used to a lesser extent by some physicians. Pyrazinamide may find a place in treating 'persister' bacilli.*

Dapsone is absorbed slowly after oral administration. Peak plasma drug concentration is reached at about 4 hours; absorption half-life is 1.1 hours; elimination half-life is about 30 hours. Oral availability is around 90%. Dapsone is approximately 70% protein-bound, while its monoacetylated metabolite is amost entirely bound. Dapsone crosses the placenta and is excreted into breast milk. It is metabolised via acetylation and N*-hydroxylation, but acetylation polymorphism has no effect on dapsone handling by leprosy patients. Dapsone penetrates into sciatic nerves of experimental animals but its presence has not been demonstrated in Schwann cells.*

Oral doses of rifampicin are rapidly and completely absorbed. The bioavailability is greater when the drug is given before meals; peak concentrations occur at 1 to 2 hours. 80 to 90% of rifampicin is bound to plasma proteins, and the drug is found in saliva, cerebrospinal fluid and breast milk. Its main metabolite, desacetyl rifampicin, also exhibits antimycobacterial activity in tuberculosis. Rifampicin induces its own metabolism, as well as that of dapsone and steroids. Absorption of dapsone and rifampicin is reported to be reduced in leprosy patients.

Clofazimine has been in use in leprosy treatment since 1960. In higher doses it exerts an anti-inflammatory action which is useful in treating leprosy patients in reaction. Oral absorption of the drug is slow and dose-dependent; faecal excretion also increases with dose. Single- and multiple-dose studies have shown a plasma half-life of around 10 days. Bioavailability of the drug is higher when given with food than when fasting; the peak plasma concentration occurs at 4 to 8 hours when the drug is administered with breakfast. After absorption, the drug is thought to circulate in protein-bound form, accounting for the fact that it is deposited in various tissues. Uneven distribution and prolonged retention in the tissues are special features of clofazimine metabolism. One unconjugated and 2 conjugated metabolites have been detected in urine, and the urinary excretion of both the parent compound and its metabolites is around 1% of the dose. Clofazimine crosses the placental barrier and is excreted into breast milk, but does not cross the blood-brain barrier. Small amounts of the drug are found in sebum and sweat.

The pharmacokinetic properties of ethionamide and prothionamide are similar in man. Both are absorbed rapidly and completely following oral administration. Peak plasma concentration of prothionamide occurs at around 18 minutes; plasma half-life is about 2 hours. The sulphoxide metabolite of the drug is active against Mycobacterium leprae.

The pharmacokinetics of thiacetazone, isoniazid and pyrazinamide are reviewed briefly. All 3 drugs are well absorbed after oral administration.

Haematological, dermatological and neurological effects and gastrointestinal symptoms are some of the side effects of the drugs reviewed. These may not pose serious problems at therapeutic dosages in leprosy, but the increased incidence of hepatotoxicity on combining rifampicin and ethionamide/prothionamide causes serious concern.

Rifampicin increases the excretion of dapsone, although this is not of therapeutic significance. Dapsone plus clofazimine reduces the absorption of rifampicin, while rifampicin plus dapsone does not affect absorption of clofazimine. Isoniazid treatment lowers the tissue concentration of clofazimine and increases its urinary excretion.

The modern era of leprosy chemotherapy began in the 1940s with the introduction of the sulphones (Faget et al. 1943), of which dapsone (4,4′-diaminodiphenyl sulphone) remains the mainstay of treatment even today, as one of the main components of various multidrug regimens advocated by physicians everywhere. However, the widespread emergence of dapsone-resistant strains of *Mycobacterium leprae* in lepromatous leprosy patients on dapsone monotherapy (WHO 1977) has forced leprologists to develop a rationally sound combination chemotherapy involving companion antileprosy drugs. The bacteriological and pharmacological activities of these drugs have been evaluated and compared by Colston et al. (1978a). Dapsone, clofazimine (a phenazine derivative), rifampicin and ethionamide/prothionamide are the only bactericidal drugs being considered as candidates for limited duration multidrug regimens (WHO 1982). Thiacetazone (thiosemicarbazone) and acedapsone (diacetyl dapsone), which exerts its antibacterial activity on conversion to dapsone, are reported to be useful in treating leprosy patients (Colston et al. 1978a; Zuidema et al. 1986). The usefulness of isoniazid is debatable (Freerksen 1975; Molesworth 1975; Pattyn et al. 1981; Shepard 1967), but pyrazinamide may prove helpful for the treatment of 'persister' bacilli in multi-bacillary leprosy cases (Katoch et al. 1988). The structures and the important bacteriological and pharmacological properties of the major drugs are given in figure 1 and table I. This review deals with the fundamental pharmacokinetic properties of the above-mentioned antileprosy drugs, and with their particular considerations in the treatment of leprosy patients.

1. Fundamental Pharmacokinetic Properties of Antileprosy Drugs

1.1 Dapsone

1.1.1 Absorption and Bioavailability

The rate of absorption of dapsone is rather slow, with a mean absorption half-life ($t_{½\alpha}$) of 1.1 hours [absorption rate constant (k_a) = $0.6h^{-1}$] after a single oral dose of 100mg (Ahmad & Rogers 1980a). An incomplete absorption of about 70 to 80% has been suggested on the basis of the findings of isotope studies in leprosy patients (Alexander et al. 1970). The absolute oral availability of dapsone has been reported to be 86 to 104% in healthy volunteers after a single oral dose of 100mg (Pieters & Zuidema 1987).

Concentration-time profiles in healthy volun-

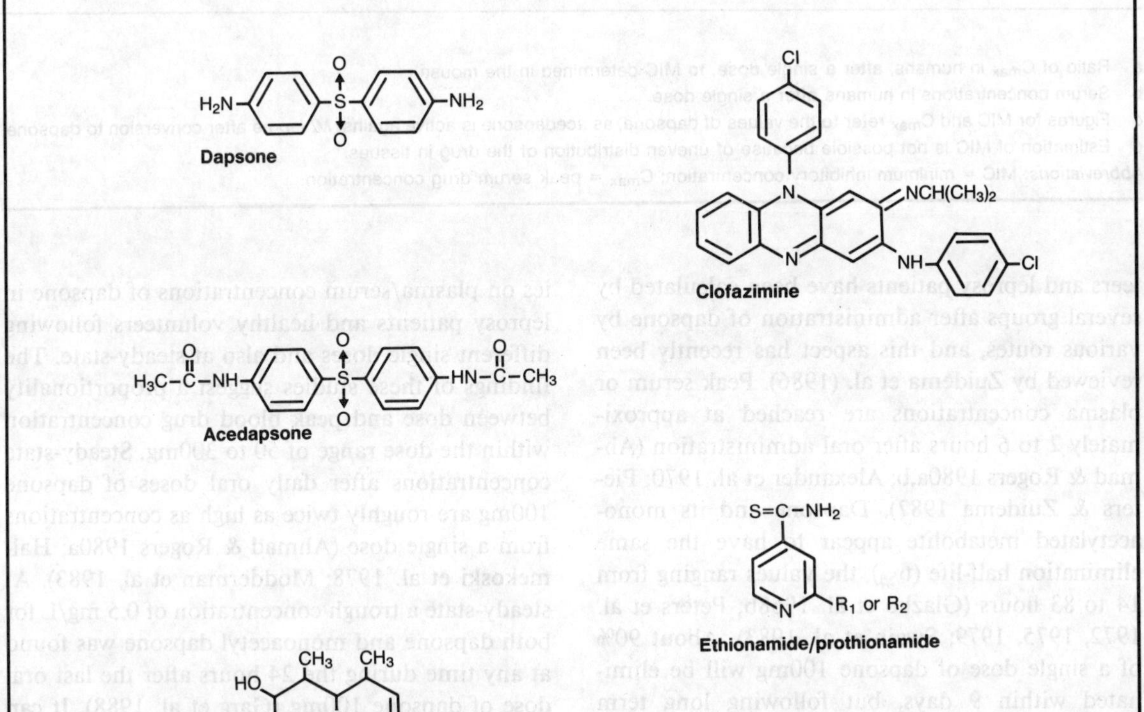

Fig. 1. Structure of common antileprosy drugs.

Table I. Bacteriological and pharmacological properties of common antileprosy drugs

Drug	MIC	Dose (mg)	Ratio of C_{max} to MIC[a]	No. of days during which C_{max} exceeds MIC[b]	Bactericidal activity
Dapsone	0.003	100	500	1	Low
Acedapsone	0.003	225	15	200	None
Rifampicin	0.3	600	30	1	High
Clofazimine[d]		50-100			Low
Ethionamide	0.05	375-500	60	1	Intermediate
Prothionamide	0.05	375-500	40	1	Intermediate
Thiacetazone	0.2	150	8	2	None

a Ratio of C_{max} in humans, after a single dose, to MIC determined in the mouse.
b Serum concentrations in humans after a single dose.
c Figures for MIC and C_{max} refer to the values of dapsone, as acedapsone is active against *M. leprae* after conversion to dapsone.
d Estimation of MIC is not possible because of uneven distribution of the drug in tissues.
Abbreviations: MIC = minimum inhibitory concentration; C_{max} = peak serum drug concentration.

teers and leprosy patients have been calculated by several groups after administration of dapsone by various routes, and this aspect has recently been reviewed by Zuidema et al. (1986). Peak serum or plasma concentrations are reached at approximately 2 to 6 hours after oral administration (Ahmad & Rogers 1980a,b; Alexander et al. 1970; Pieters & Zuidema 1987). Dapsone and its monoacetylated metabolite appear to have the same elimination half-life ($t_{1/2\beta}$), the values ranging from 14 to 83 hours (Glazko et al. 1968b; Peters et al. 1972, 1975, 1979; Swain et al. 1983). About 90% of a single dose of dapsone 100mg will be eliminated within 9 days, but following long term administration the drug has been detected in the body for up to 35 days after discontinuation of treatment (Lang 1979).

Dapsone concentration-time profiles in healthy volunteers after an intravenous infusion of the drug have recently been reported by Pieters and Zuidema (1987). The various pharmacokinetic parameters reported in studies of single-dose oral administration and intravenous infusion are shown in table II.

Zuidema et al. (1986), reviewing the pharmacokinetics of dapsone, mentioned a number of studies on plasma/serum concentrations of dapsone in leprosy patients and healthy volunteers following different single doses and also at steady-state. The findings of these studies suggest a proportionality between dose and peak blood drug concentration within the dose range of 50 to 300mg. Steady-state concentrations after daily oral doses of dapsone 100mg are roughly twice as high as concentrations from a single dose (Ahmad & Rogers 1980a; Halmekoski et al. 1978; Modderman et al. 1983). At steady-state a trough concentration of 0.5 mg/L for both dapsone and monoacetyl dapsone was found at any time during the 24 hours after the last oral dose of dapsone 100mg (Garg et al. 1988). It can be seen that at steady-states achieved by daily oral doses of dapsone 100mg, the serum or plasma concentration at any time will be about 150 times greater than the minimum inhibitory concentration (MIC) for *M. leprae* in blood (as determined in mice), and this fact is therapeutically significant.

Steady-state serum drug concentrations in leprosy patients following repeated intramuscular injections of dapsone 375mg in oily vehicle (UNICEF injection) have been reported by Modderman et al. (1983). During the week following the final injection, dapsone concentrations of 1 mg/L (300 times greater than MIC) were maintained. A monthly intra-adipose injection (in the gluteal subcutaneous fat layer) of rounded double-pyramidal crystals of defined size in an aqueous vehicle has been reported to result in an absorption rate which is sufficiently sustained for therapeutic purposes in terms of serum concentration well above MIC for *M. leprae* (Zuidema et al. 1986); this parenteral approach may be clinically useful, as it permits supervised monthly administration.

Monoacetyl dapsone and acedapsone are known prodrugs of dapsone. Intramuscular injection of acedapsone 225mg in benzyl benzoate/castor oil (4 : 6) results in blood concentrations of 0.02 to 0.08 mg/L during a 75-day period (George & Balakrishnan 1986; Glazko et al. 1968a), 6 to 25 times higher than the MIC for dapsone. In the context of the frequent emergence of dapsone resistance under such low therapeutic concentrations of the drug, its usefulness in leprosy chemotherapy is questioned by Zuidema et al. (1986). Repeated monthly injections of monoacetyl dapsone 700mg (equivalent to dapsone 600mg) produce blood concentrations between those of dapsone and monoacetyl dapsone (in the range of 0.5 to 1 mg/L) and are 180 to 300 times higher than the MIC (Zuidema et al. 1984).

1.1.2 Distribution and Protein Binding

While about 70 to 80% of dapsone is bound to plasma proteins, its main metabolite monoacetyl dapsone is almost entirely protein bound (Ahmad & Rogers 1980b; Biggs et al. 1979; Modderman et al. 1983; Peters et al. 1981). It has also been reported that monoacetyl dapsone is 20-25-fold more highly bound than dapsone (Glazko et al. 1969).

Dapsone seems to be widely distributed throughout the tissues, concentrations of the drug being nearly the same as those in blood (Chatterjee & Poddar 1957; Peters et al. 1977). Dapsone readily penetrates into the sciatic nerves of dogs and sheep, concentrations in nerve tissues equalling total plasma concentration (Allen et al. 1975). However, penetration of the drug into Schwann cells of nerves was not demonstrable in mice with advanced neuropathy (Boddingius & Stolz 1981).

The salivary glands are highly permeable for dapsone and particularly monoacetyl dapsone. Saliva concentrations of dapsone are about 18 to 27% of the blood concentration (Zuidema & Van Ginneken 1983a,b). Dapsone crosses the placenta (Hocking 1968), but no serious harmful effects on the child *in utero* have been reported (Jopling 1978). It is excreted in breast milk (Sanders et al. 1982); however, despite its presence in the urine of breast-

Table II. Pharmacokinetic parameters of dapsone (single dose) in healthy volunteers

No. of subjects	Dose (mg)[a]	Route	C_{max} (mg/L)[b]	$t_{1/2\beta}$ (h)[a]	k_e (h^{-1})[a]	k_a (h^{-1})	AUC (0-48h) (mg/L · h)[b]	Vd (L/kg)[a]	F (%)[a]	Reference
5	48.3 ± 2.0	IV	0.65-1.17	22.4 ± 5.6	0.033 ± 0.008		13.3-37.5	0.98 ± 0.12		Pieters & Zuidema (1987)
5	100	PO	1.12-2.28	21.7 ± 5.7	0.034 ± 0.009		24.0-75.4		93 ± 8	Pieters & Zuidema (1987)
1	100	PO	1.9	30	0.02	0.6		1.5		Ahmad & Rogers (1980a)

a Mean ± SD.
b Range.
Abbreviations: C_{max} = peak serum drug concentration; $t_{1/2\beta}$ = terminal half-life; k_e = elimination rate constant; k_a = absorption rate constant; AUC (0-48h) = area under the concentration-time curve from zero time to 48 hours post-dose; Vd = apparent volume of distribution; F = bioavailability; IV = intravenous; PO = oral.

fed infants, only 2 cases of neonatal haemolysis have been reported (Hocking 1968; Sanders et al. 1982). It has been suggested by Jopling (1978) that the presence of antileprosy drugs in the milk may protect the child from leprosy infection.

1.1.3 Metabolism and Excretion

Acetylation and *N*-hydroxylation are the 2 main pathways of dapsone metabolism (Glazko et al. 1969; Karim et al 1981; Zuidema et al. 1986). While the parent compound is easily acetylated to monoacetyl dapsone, further acetylation of the metabolite does not occur to any significant extent (Jones & Ovenell 1979; Lammintausta et al. 1979; Murray et al. 1971). A constant equilibrium between acetylation and deacetylation is reached within a few hours after the oral administration of either dapsone or monoacetyl dapsone (Gelber et al. 1971). However, deacetylation is a rather slow process compared with acetylation (Zuidema et al. 1986), probably owing to the extensive protein binding of monoacetyl dapsone. Acedapsone is also deacetylated *in vivo* to form monoacetyl dapsone and dapsone (Glazko et al. 1968b). Both the prodrugs exert their antibacterial effect only after conversion to dapsone. Individual variability in acetylation because of the genetically determined *N*-acetyl transferase activity has been shown to be of 3 acetylator phenotypes, viz. 'slow', 'fast' and 'intermediate' (Gelber et al. 1971; Peters et al. 1972, 1975, 1979). However, this acetylation polymorphism does not seem to affect the pharmacokinetic parameters of the drug (Zuidema et al. 1986).

Hydroxylation is the other main pathway of metabolism of dapsone. Probably about 2 to 7% of *N*-hydroxyl dapsone is excreted in the free form and 30 to 50% in the conjugated form. A high renal clearance of these metabolites has been suggested (Zuidema et al. 1986).

Five to 15% of the dapsone dose is excreted as unchanged drug (Ellard 1966; Gelber et al. 1971). The amount of monoacetyl dapsone excreted in urine is very small, and acedapsone does not appear to be excreted as such (Zuidema et al. 1986).

Monoacetyl dapsone and other *N*-substituted sulphones are much less effective than dapsone in terms of antibacterial action (Bawden & Tute 1981), and probably do not contribute to the therapeutic effect in leprosy as indicated by an absence of a relationship between acetylation status and the development of resistance in leprosy patients (Balakrishnan & Ramu 1977; Gelber & Rees 1975; Peters et al. 1976). The concentrations of NOH metabolites in blood are extremely low and their contribution to the effect in leprosy can be ignored (Zuidema et al. 1986).

1.2 Rifampicin

The semi-synthetic antibiotic rifampicin is the 3-(4-methyl-1-piperazinyl-iminomethyl) derivative of rifamycin SV. Of the available antileprosy drugs, rifampicin possesses the highest bactericidal activity against *M. leprae*, having an MIC of 0.3 mg/L in mice (table I).

1.2.1 Absorption and Bioavailability

The absorption of orally administered rifampicin is both rapid and nearly complete. The rate of absorption is not dose-related, since the time required for the drug to reach its peak serum concentration has been found to be the same at different dosage levels (Acocella 1978; Lecaillon et al. 1981). The mean values of the absorption half-life of rifampicin in leprosy patients after a single oral dose of 600mg are reported to be 0.56 to 0.67 hour (Mehta et al. 1985). The peak plasma concentration is attained after 1 to 4 hours and reaches values of approximately 6 and 9 mg/L after single oral doses of 450 and 600mg, respectively. The peak serum concentration and area under the concentration-time curve (AUC) are greater if rifampicin is taken before breakfast than after; but the serum concentrations remain above MIC (for *M. tuberculosis*) for the same length of time in both cases (Riess 1969; Siegler et al. 1974).

Using high performance liquid chromatography (HPLC), Acocella et al. (1985) have calculated the pharmacokinetics of rifampicin in 4 male patients attending a chest clinic. For an oral dose of 8.1 ± 0.7 mg/kg bodyweight, the reported parameters were: peak plasma drug concentration (C_{max}) = 6.3

± 0.5 mg/L, time to reach C_{max} (t_{max}) = 3.2 ± 0.2 hours, area under the concentration-time curve (AUC) [0-12h] = 36.0 ± 5.5 mg/L • h and elimination half-life ($t_{1/2\beta}$) = 4.7 ± 1.9 hours, while corresponding figures for its major metabolite desacetyl rifampicin were C_{max} = 0.8 ± 0.1 mg/L, t_{max} = 5.0 ± 1.0 hours and AUC = 4.9 ± 1.3 mg/L • h (± standard error). The pharmacokinetic parameters reported in a study in leprosy patients by Mehta et al. (1985) do not appear to vary much from those reported in patients with chest ailments by Acocella et al. (1985).

During continuous administration of rifampicin the serum concentration and half-life are usually higher after the first dose than subsequent doses (Furesz 1970; Maggi et al. 1969). Steady-state concentrations are not reached until after a relatively long time; the high liposolubility of the drug may account for this observation (Seydel 1970). The maximal induction of rifampicin metabolism, and presumably that of the hepatic microsomal enzyme system in general, is probably attained after about 7 daily doses (300, 450 and 600mg) of the drug (Acocella et al. 1971; Immanuel et al. 1985).

1.2.2 Distribution and Protein Binding

Rifampicin diffuses rapidly from plasma into the other body fluids, tissues and organs. In the liver, bile, gallbladder and urine, rifampicin reaches concentrations which are higher than those found in the blood, and salivary concentrations are approximately 20% of the serum concentration (Pawlowska & Pniewski 1979). Rifampicin has been shown to cross the blood-brain barrier (Pilheu & Sippel 1975) and the placental barrier (Rocker 1977). A study in Japanese women has shown that values for t_{max} for rifampicin are about the same in cord blood and maternal blood and that the fetal serum concentrations at birth range between 12 and 33% of those in the maternal serum (Kenny & Strates 1981). The ability of rifampicin to cross the placental barrier does not result in adverse effects to the fetus.

A mean plasma protein binding rate of 88.9 ± 0.9% has been reported in healthy subjects (Boman & Ringberger 1974). The percentage of protein binding has been found to be unrelated to the plasma concentration of the drug (Kenny & Strates 1981).

1.2.3 Metabolism and Excretion

In a review of the pharmacokinetics of rifampicin by Acocella (1978), the drug is metabolised into compounds such as 25-desacetyl rifampicin, rifampicin quinone, desacetyl rifampicin quinone, 3-formyl rifampicin SV, 3-formyl desacetyl rifampicin and a few others. The modern technique of HPLC has made it possible to study rifampicin and its metabolites separately yet simultaneously (Gidoh & Tsutsumi 1981; Lecaillon et al. 1978). These metabolites are eliminated from the system through the bile and also the urine. The major metabolite, 25-desacetyl rifampicin, has been shown to be active against *M. tuberculosis* as rifampicin itself (Acocella 1978). The quantity of rifampicin and 3 of its metabolites – 25-desacetyl rifampicin, 3-formyl rifampicin SV and 3-formyl desacetyl rifampicin – recovered in the urine has been found to rise from 3% of the dose after oral administration of 150mg to approximately 12% after a 600mg dose (Lecaillon et al. 1981).

1.3 Clofazimine

Clofazimine [3-(*p*-chloroanilino)-10-(*p*-chlorophenyl)-2,10-di-hydro-2-(isopropylimino) phenazine] is active against *M. leprae* in mice and in humans (Browne et al. 1981; Pettit & Rees 1966; Shepard 1976; Shepard & Chang 1964). In addition, this drug possesses anti-inflammatory properties when used in higher doses, which has been found useful in treating lepromatous leprosy in the reactive phase (Browne 1965).

1.3.1 Absorption and Bioavailability

The exact mechanism of clofazimine absorption from the gastrointestinal tract is not clear. Studies carried out on various laboratory animals have revealed a species variation: absorption is good in mice, rats and monkeys, decidedly poorer in rabbits and guinea-pigs and practically negligible in dogs (Barry et al. 1960; Vischer 1969).

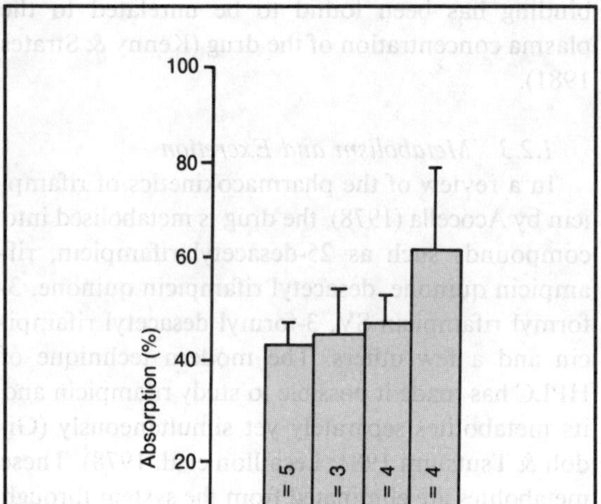

Fig. 2. Percentage absorption of clofazimine from the alimentary tract in relation to single oral doses of clofazimine; n = number of leprosy patients in age group; error bar denotes upper range of SD. Student's t-test: 100mg *vs* 600mg $p < 0.01$, 100mg *vs* 400mg $p > 0.01 < 0.05$, 100mg *vs* 300mg $p = 0.1$ (after Mathur et al. 1985).

In humans, only about 20% of the crystalline substance is absorbed after oral administration, but this figure rises to 50% when the micronised form of the drug is used, and may reach 85% with oral administration in the form of a suspension in oil. Very slow absorption from the site of intramuscular injection has limited drug administration to the oral route (Vischer 1969).

Faecal excretion of clofazimine by humans is variable; on average 11 to 59% of a single dose is excreted in 3 days (Levy 1974). Dose-dependent absorption in leprosy patients has also been reported by Mathur et al. (1985) in a study on faecal excretion in relation to various single doses of the drug. While 70% of a single dose of clofazimine 100mg ('Lamprene' capsule) was absorbed from the gut, only about 45% was absorbed after administration of a single dose of 600mg (fig. 2).

In 6 subjects in whom it was assessed, maximum plasma drug concentrations occurred between 4 and 8 hours after a single oral dose of clofazimine 200mg, taken 10 minutes after breakfast (Lanyi et al. 1987). The mean plasma concentration was 407.6 ± 136.81 ng/g as determined by a thin layer chromatographic method described by Lanyi and Dubois (1982). The mean AUC (0-264h) for plasma was 16.05 ± 0.398 μg/g · h, but AUC was lower when the drug was administered in the fasting state. Oral administration of clofazimine to healthy volunteers with food containing proteins and fat resulted in an increase in bioavailability by about 62% compared with administration in fasting conditions (fig. 3).

A few studies have been published on plasma concentrations of clofazimine in leprosy patients employing spectrophotometric methods based on that described by Barry et al. (1960). An average plasma concentration of 1.15 mg/L has been reported in leprosy patients receiving a daily dose of 300mg (Balakrishnan et al. 1976; Venkatesan et al. 1980). Leprosy patients receiving clofazimine 100mg thrice weekly or 100, 300 or 400mg daily

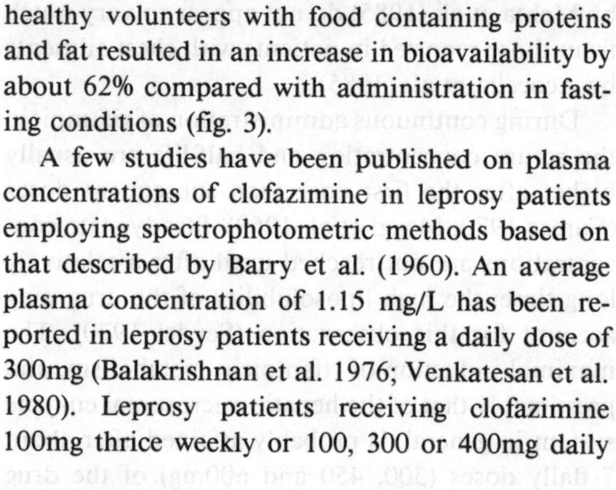

Fig. 3. Mean plasma concentration-time curves of clofazimine in healthy subjects (n = 3) after a single oral dose of 200mg with (●) and without (○) breakfast after overnight fast; ▨ = area showing an increase in bioavailability in terms of AUC (0-264h) [after Lanyi et al. 1987].

for varying periods have plasma drug concentrations of 0.5, 0.7, 1.0 and 1.4 mg/L, respectively (Mansfield 1974). A single oral dose of clofazimine 300mg given to leprosy patients has been shown to result in a plasma drug concentration of 0.2 mg/L (Banerjee et al. 1974); this low concentration has been suggested to be due either to incomplete absorption from the gut or to rapid hepatic removal of the absorbed drug via the portal vein (first-pass effect). The above findings indicate that, as after a single dose, the plasma concentration of the drug is also dose-related during continued administration, although there does not appear to be a linear relationship between dosage and plasma concentrations.

1.3.2 Distribution and Protein Binding

The distribution of clofazimine is relatively slower than the absorption (Vischer 1969). Clofazimine and related phenazines have been reported to show very selective tissue distribution in humans and experimental animals (Barry et al. 1959; Byrne et al. 1969). A significant proportion of these drugs is found in adipose tissue and in cells of the reticuloendothelial system, where they can be seen concentrated in phagosome-type inclusions and ultimately as crystals of pure drug (Conalty & Jackson 1962). Presumably, clofazimine after absorption circulates bound to plasma proteins and is engulfed in this form by the cells of the reticuloendothelial system, where it remains after digestion of the protein (Vischer 1969).

At autopsies performed on 3 leprosy patients, clofazimine was found predominantly in the mesenteric lymph node, adrenals, subcutaneous fat, liver, bile, gallbladder, spleen, small intestine, muscle, bone and skin, and to a small extent in nerve tissue. In these patients, who had received clofazimine in varying doses of up to 300mg daily for 35 to 243 days, the brain concentration was near zero (Mansfield 1974). In another autopsy study 'ghosts' of clofazimine crystals have been found in histological sections of intestinal mucosa (Desikan & Balakrishnan 1976). Yet another detailed autopsy study by Balakrishnan et al. (1976) showed high clofazimine content in spleen, small intestine and mesenteric lymph node, relatively low concentration in liver, omentum and lungs, and an absence of drug in brain tissue. There was a fairly sharp fall in the skin concentration of clofazimine in the first 2 months following cessation of treatment, but traces of clofazimine (about 4 μg/g) were found in the skin even after 1 to 2 years. Dose and duration of treatment did not appear to influence the amount of drug in the skin (Balakrishnan et al. 1976).

Little is known about the penetration of the drug into nerves. McDougall & Jones (1981) noticed foamy perineural macrophages containing amorphous material, histologically identified as lipofuscin, in a nerve biopsy of a leprosy patient in the reactive phase, and interpreted this as evidence of previous clofazimine treatment.

Based on an observation that infants born to mothers who had received the drug during pregnancy were deeply pigmented at birth, Waters (1969) reported that clofazimine crosses the placenta. There is no report of any teratogenic effect associated with the drug (Schulz 1971). Clofazimine is excreted in breast milk to such an extent as to colour the milk (personal observation). Experimental studies in female mice, rats, guinea-pigs and rabbits have shown similar observations (Vischer 1969).

1.3.3 Metabolism and Excretion

The exact manner in which clofazimine is metabolised in humans is still not fully known. At least 3 metabolites have been detected in urine of leprosy patients receiving clofazimine 300mg daily. Two of the metabolites are conjugated; they are 3-(B-D-glucopyranosiduronic acid)-10-(*p*-chlorophenyl)-2,10-dihydro-2-isopropyl iminophenazine and 3-(*p*-chloroanilino)-10-(*p*-chlorophenyl)-4,10-dihydro-4-(B-D-glucopyranosiduronic acid)-2-isopropyl iminophenazine. The third metabolite, an unconjugated one, is 3-(*p*-hydroxy anilino)-10-(*p*-chlorophenyl)-2,10-dihydro-2-isopropyl iminophenazine (fig. 4).

These metabolites are excreted in very small amounts constituting only 0.6% of the daily dose (assuming 70% drug absorption), while about 1%

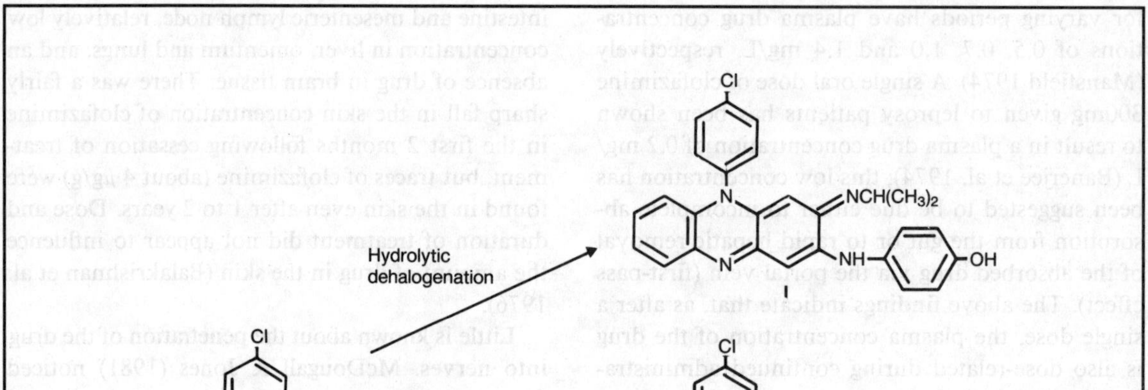

Fig. 4. *In vivo* metabolic pathways of clofazimine in humans. Metabolite I: 3-(*p*-hydroxyanilino)-10-(*p*-chlorophenyl)-2,10-dihydro-2-isopropyliminophenazine; metabolite II: 3-(*p*-chloroanilino)-10-(*p*-chlorophenyl)-4,10-dihydro-4-hydroxy-2-isopropyliminophenazine; metabolite III: 3-(hydroxy)-10-(*p*-chlorophenyl)-2,10-dihydro-2-isopropyl-iminophenazine. Metabolites II and III are excreted in urine after conjugation to D-glucopyranosiduronic acid, while metabolite I is excreted in free form (after Feng et al. 1981, 1982).

is excreted unchanged (Feng et al. 1981, 1982; Levy 1974). The low excretion rate of clofazimine and its metabolites is probably due to the long residence time of the drug in the body. Presumably an equilibrium between intake and output of the drug would eventually be reached, but when this occurs for a given dose of the drug is not certain. The clofazimine metabolites found in urine could also be the products of intestinal bacterial metabolism of the parent drug which is deposited on intestinal walls (Feng et al. 1982). In addition to urinary excretion, a small amount of the drug is also eliminated in the sebum and sweat (Vischer 1969).

The mean terminal half-life has been reported to be 10.6 ± 4.0 days on administration of a single dose of clofazimine 50mg and 8.8 ± 1.0 days after dosing with 50mg daily for 8 days together with food (Lanyi et al. 1987).

Spectral studies have shown binding of clofazimine to deoxyribonucleic acid, non-involvement of an intercalation and involvement of binding to guanine residues as possible events in the mode of action of the drug (Morrison & Morley 1976, 1977). Unidimensional cross-resistance between clofazimine and rifampicin has been reported, suggesting an involvement of clofazimine in transcription (Morrison 1972). Clofazimine resistance appears to be extremely rare and there is only 1 reliable report of such a case (Warndorff-van Diepen 1982).

1.4 Ethionamide and Prothionamide

The thioamides ethionamide and prothionamide are very potent bactericidal antileprosy drugs, surpassed in this respect only by rifampicin. The pharmacokinetics of both the thioamides and their circulatory *S*-oxide metabolites have been studied in detail in rats and armadillos (Peters et al. 1983) as well as human volunteers (Jenner & Ellard 1981; Jenner et al. 1984; Jenner & Smith 1987) using HPLC.

The absorption of prothionamide following oral administration appears to be rapid. Peak concentration is reported to occur whithin 30 minutes of ingestion, making an accurate estimation of its absorption half-life difficult; however, it has been calculated to be 18.5 ± 2.7 minutes. Peak plasma ethionamide concentration is reported to be reached in about 90 minutes. Lack of evidence of significant faecal elimination of the unmetabolised drugs and the systemic availabilities calculated for both these drugs (1.1 and 0.9 for ethionamide and prothionamide, respectively) suggest complete absorption from the gut and an absence of first-pass metabolism (Jenner & Smith 1987). It has been reported in single oral dose studies that the elimination half-life of both drugs is about 2 hours, but the plasma concentrations of prothionamide from 1 hour onwards are only about half those of ethionamide (Jenner et al. 1981). The observed differences in the pharmacokinetics of the 2 drugs have been shown not to be due to greater conversion of prothionamide to its metabolite (Peters et al. 1983).

Following intravenous administration, plasma concentrations of thioamides have been reported to decline biexponentially, with half-lives of 7.2 and 5.8 minutes for the distribution phases of ethionamide and prothionamide, respectively (Jenner &

Table III. Mean (± SD) pharmacokinetic parameters of ethionamide and prothionamide in humans, rats and armadillos

Parameters (units)	Humans (n = 1)[a]				Rats (n = 4)[b]		Armadillos (n = 2)[b]
	ETH[c]	PTH[c]	ETH[d]	PTH[d]	PTH[e]	PTH[f]	PTH[g]
AUC(0→∞) [mg/L · min]	55	48	1215	870	11.6 (32.0)[h]	11.9 (17.4)	5.1
t_{max} (min)			90	30			
$t_{½\alpha}$ (min)	7.2	5.8					
$t_{½\beta}$ (h)	1.77 ± 0.07	2.06 ± 0.12	1.6 ± 0.31	1.49 ± 0.13	0.74 (0.69)	0.43 (0.86)	0.52
$t_{½a}$ (min)			18.5 ± 2.7				
Vd (L)	79	93					
f			1.1	0.9			

a Jenner & Smith (1981).
b Peters et al. (1983).
c 25mg intravenous dose.
d 500mg oral dose.
e 32 mg/kg intravenous dose.
f 32 mg/kg oral dose.
g 16 mg/kg intravenous dose.
h Values in parentheses are those for prothionamide-*S*-oxide.

Abbreviations: ETH = ethionamide; PTH = prothionamide; AUC(0→∞) = area under the concentration-time curve from zero time to infinity; t_{max} = time to reach peak serum drug concentration; $t_{½\alpha}$ = half-life of the distribution phase; $t_{½\beta}$ = elimination half-life; $t_{½a}$ = absorption half-life; Vd = apparent volume of distribution; f = bioavailability.

Smith 1987). The reported pharmacokinetic parameters of both drugs in experimental animals and in humans are given in table III.

The thioamides are converted into *S*-oxides in the body, and this metabolite has been reported to have inhibitory and bactericidal activity against *M. leprae* (Matsuo et al. 1981). Prothionamide has not been shown to induce its own metabolism in studies in rats and armadillos, as indicated by lack of significant differences in serum concentrations of either the parent compound or prothionamide-*S*-oxide after single and multiple doses (Peters et al. 1983).

The cumulative urinary excretion of ethionamide and prothionamide has been reported to be around 0.15% and 0.05%, respectively, of the administered dose (Jenner & Ellard 1981).

1.5 Thiacetazone

Thiacetazone (*p*-acetyl amino benzaldehyde thiosemicarbazone) is still used by some physicians as an antileprosy drug, although it does not feature in the widely used 'standard' multidrug regimens because of its relatively lower antileprosy activity and the evolution of drug-resistant bacilli. The use of this drug in the treatment of leprosy was first described by Lowe (1954). While comparing the activity of thiacetazone and thiambutosine in the chemotherapy of experimental leprosy in mice, Colston & Hilston (1976) found that the MIC of thiacetazone was 0.26 mg/L.

Thiacetazone is well absorbed after a single oral dose. Peak serum concentrations have been reported to occur about 4 to 5 hours after administration of a 150mg dose of the drug. However, peak concentrations are reached much later after higher doses (up to 600mg), possibly because absorption of the larger doses is prolonged owing to its low aqueous solubility. Peak drug concentrations are reported to be proportional to the dosage. The half-life of thiacetazone in humans averages a little under 12 hours (Ellard et al. 1974). Reported serum drug concentrations following oral doses of thiacetazone 150mg in tuberculosis patients are shown in table IV.

Thiacetazone is not extensively deacetylated or cleaved to form its metabolites *p*-acetyl amino benzaldehyde and thiosemicarbazone. On average, about 20% of the administered dose is excreted in urine over a period of 3 days, 15% or more representing unchanged drug (Ellard et al. 1974).

1.6 Isoniazid

Isoniazid is bacteriostatic for *M. leprae* (Shepard 1967) and indications for the use of this drug in leprosy are limited from the bacteriological point of view (Pattyn et al. 1981; Shepard 1967). Nevertheless, multidrug regimens comprising rifampicin, dapsone and isoniazid plus prothionamide ('Isoprodian') have been employed by several workers (Depasquale 1975; Freerksen 1975). There is a report that a combination of dapsone with thiacetazone and isoniazid performed well in leprosy treatment (Molesworth 1975). The pharmacokinetics of isoniazid have been extensively reviewed by Weber and Hein (1979) and need not be covered here since the drug has only limited use in the

Table IV. Mean (± SD) concentrations of thiacetazone in serum (mg/L) [after Ellard et al. 1974]

Dosage	Time after dose (h)					
	0	2	4	6	24	48
150mg once (n = 18)		0.9 ± 0.5[a]	1.2 ± 0.6	0.9 ± 0.7	0.3 ± 0.2	0.0 ± 0.2
150mg daily (n = 21)	0.4 ± 0.4[b]		1.2 ± 0.7			
150mg daily (n = 24)	0.5 ± 0.4[c]	1.4 ± 0.7	1.6 ± 0.9	1.2 ± 0.9	0.6 ± 0.4	

a UV photometry.
b UV photometry, colorimetry and fluorimetry.
c UV photometry and fluorimetry.

Table V. Mean (± SD) pharmacokinetic parameters of isoniazid and pyrazinamide (after Acocella et al. 1985)

Parameter (units)	Isoniazid[a] (n = 4)	Pyrazinamide[b] (n = 4)
Dose[c] (mg/kg)	5.6 ± 0.4	24.6 ± 2.4
C_{max} (mg/L)	9.2 ± 1.2 (1.8 ± 0.4)	30.8 ± 3.6 (5.5 ± 1.4)
AUC (0-12h) (mg/L · h)	49.7 ± 7.8 (16.3 ± 4.0)	224.7 ± 21.5 (38.6 ± 3.6)
t_{max} (h)	2.2 ± 0.5 (5.7 ± 1.3)	1.5 ± 0.3 (3.5 ± 0.3)
$t_{½β}$ (h)	3.6 ± 0.4	7.4 ± 1.0 (11.6 ± 5.5)

a Values in parentheses are for acetyl isoniazid.
b Values in parentheses are for pyrazinoic acid.
c Doses given orally.
Abbreviations: C_{max} = peak serum drug concentration; AUC (0-12h) = area under the concentration-time curve from zero time to 12 hours post-dose; t_{max} = time to reach C_{max}; $t_{½β}$ = terminal half-life.

treatment of leprosy. Recently Acocella et al. (1985) have reported on the pharmacokinetics of isoniazid after a single oral dose in patients with chest disease. The pharmacokinetic parameters described in their work are shown in table V.

1.7 Pyrazinamide

'Persister' bacilli are known to exist in leprosy even after several years of chemotherapy (Ellard 1984). On the basis of experience using pyrazinamide together with other antitubercular bactericidal drugs for effectively eliminating the 'persister' organisms in tuberculosis, it is thought that pyrazinamide could serve as a companion antileprosy drug (Katoch et al. 1988). As drug combinations involving pyrazinamide may be used in the future, the pharmacokinetics of this drug are briefly reviewed here.

Absorption of pyrazinamide from the alimentary tract appears to be extremely rapid. Peak serum drug concentrations are achieved within 2 hours, and are dose-related over the range of pyrazinamide 0.5 to 3g for both the drug and its metabolite, pyrazinoic acid. Non-detection of pyrazinamide in faeces collected after administration of 3g of the drug suggests that there is complete absorption of the drug in the alimentary tract (Ellard 1969).

Recently, Acocella et al. (1985) using HPLC have calculated the pharmacokinetic parameters of pyrazinamide and its pyrazinoic acid metabolite (table V). Serum half-life of pyrazinamide is not related to length of treatment (Ellard 1969).

After absorption from the gut, pyrazinamide is rapidly distributed throughout the whole body water (Ellard 1969). The ready penetration of unchanged pyrazinamide into tissue membranes and sciatic nerves of both dogs and rabbits has been reported (Allen et al. 1975; Yu et al. 1957).

Konno et al. (1967) have suggested that pyrazinamide may exert its antituberculosis activity through *in vivo* pyrazinoic acid. Tuberculosis patients have been shown to excrete about 4% of the dose unchanged and 30% as the metabolite, irrespective of the size of the dose up to 3g. Pyrazinamide filtered by the kidney is reabsorbed while pyrazinoic acid is not (Ellard 1969); the elimination half-life of pyrazinamide is 7.4 ± 1.0 hours (table V).

2. *Side Effects of Antileprosy Drugs*

2.1 Dapsone

The most frequent side effects of dapsone are haematological in nature, and are dose-dependent. Methaemoglobinaemia caused by NOH metabolites of dapsone has been reported to be severe in glucose-6-phosphate dehydrogenase-deficient patients and to cause cyanosis, tiredness, dyspnoea, tachycardia, headache, dizziness, nausea and mild jaundice (Zuidema et al. 1986). Haemolysis is the second most important haematological side effect of dapsone, but is not easy to detect following daily doses of 100mg or less in healthy subjects and 50mg or less in healthy glucose-6-phosphate dehydrogenase-deficient individuals (DeGowin 1967).

2.2 Rifampicin

An uncommon side effect of intermittent administration of rifampicin is hepatitis, while even more rare are thrombocytopenia, psychosis and osteomalacia. Most of the side effects such as 'flu'-syndrome shock, dyspnoea, haemolytic anaemia and renal failure, which are associated with intermittent therapy in tuberculosis, are unlikely in leprosy patients receiving monthly doses of rifampicin on the basis of the WHO recommendation (WHO 1982).

Rifampicin reduces the effectiveness of steroids and oral contraceptives. In leprosy patients with adrenal cortical dysfunction it can be dangerous to administer the drug during erythema nodosum leprosum reactions as, in addition to counteracting the effect of exogenous prednisolone, rifampicin also counteracts endogenous cortisol (Jopling 1983).

2.3 Clofazimine

Jopling (1983) has reviewed the side effects of clofazimine, which may be mild or serious. The mild effects are dose-related and reversible, the commonest effect being a red-brown discoloration of the skin and a much darker brownish-black pigmentation of the leprosy lesions. These changes are naturally less obvious in individuals with dark skins. The less common side effects include gastrointestinal symptoms and general dryness of the skin, which may progress to ichthyosis in limbs. Serious side effects are confined to the small bowel and are dose-related. A 'late syndrome' which is of greater significance occurs after long term administration of high dosages of clofazimine. In this condition, persistent diarrhoea, abdominal pain and weight loss are seen.

2.4 Ethionamide and Prothionamide

Both ethionamide and prothionamide give rise to gastrointestinal side effects, but the latter drug appears to be well tolerated when administered in a daily dosage of 500 to 1000mg as used in tuberculosis patients (Fox et al. 1969). Ethionamide has also been reported to cause peripheral neuropathy in high doses (Leggat 1962). A pellagra-like encephalopathy has been described as an uncommon but serious side effect of ethionamide, and simultaneous administration of isoniazid with ethionamide is likely to enhance the occurrence of this condition. Hypothyroidism, hypoglycaemia, alopecia and gynaecomastia are other side effects which have been reported as rare but serious (Jopling 1983). One case of hepatitis among 102 multibacillary leprosy patients receiving monotherapy with ethionamide 500mg daily has been reported by Rollier & Rollier (1972). An unacceptable incidence of hepatotoxicity (4.5 to 15%) on combining thioamides with rifampicin for leprosy treatment has been reported by many workers (Cartel et al. 1983; Ji et al. 1984; Pattyn et al. 1984).

2.5 Thiacetazone

Mild side effects of thiacetazone include gastrointestinal symptoms, transient rash, dizziness, headache and drowsiness. Serious side effects involve skin, blood, liver and hearing. Because of the risk of hepatotoxicity induced by thiacetazone, it is not advisable to give the drug to patients with liver dysfunction (Jopling 1983; Lowe 1954; Pines 1964; Webb 1973).

The frequency of side effects and acceptability of the drug are influenced by racial and geographical factors and therefore a general statement on these aspects may not be meaningful.

3. Pharmacokinetics in Various Pathophysiological States

Dose recommendations in the literature have only an empirical character. For leprosy patients the use of 50 to 100 mg/day of dapsone has been recommended (Zuidema et al. 1986). A decreased bioavailability of the drug after oral administration has been reported in severely leprotic patients (Kubo et al. 1983). A decrease in skin concentrations of dapsone and an increase in urinary excretion of the parent compound and its metabolites have been observed in lepromatous leprosy patients with severe albuminuria (Venkatesan et al., unpublished data). Although renal function impairment occurs frequently in leprosy (Zuidema et al. 1986), its influence on the renal excretion of dapsone and its metabolites has not been studied.

The dosage of rifampicin used in infants and children varies from 300 to 450mg either as a monthly loading dose or as daily administration during initial intensive therapy (Government of India 1982). The dosage in adult leprosy patients is 450mg for those with bodyweight of less than 35kg and 600mg for those weighing more. Whereas a slight decrease in serum drug concentrations in leprosy patients relative to that in healthy subjects has been suggested by Mehta et al. (1985), these workers did not demonstrate a significant difference in the pharmacokinetics of rifampicin between multi- and paucibacillary leprosy patients.

4. *Implications for the Treatment of Leprosy*

The minimum inhibitory concentration of an antileprosy drug is defined as the serum concentration present in mice fed with the minimum effective dose of the drug for effective inhibition of the growth of *M. leprae* in mouse foot pad. Assuming that MIC for *M. leprae* in humans is similar to that in the mouse, the recommended doses of antileprosy drugs must result in serum concentrations much higher than the estimated MIC in experimental mice (table I). The markedly superior ratios of peak serum concentrations to MIC, therefore, denote therapeutic efficacy of the antileprosy drug. MICs have been defined for dapsone (Levy & Peters 1976), rifampicin (Holmes 1974; Holmes & Hilson 1972), prothionamide and ethionamide (Colston et al. 1978a,b) and thiacetazone (Colston & Hilson 1976). It has not been possible to estimate the MIC for clofazimine owing to its uneven distribution and prolonged retention in the tissues.

It appears likely that the therapeutic effect of dapsone is contributed by the unchanged drug and not by its metabolites such as monoacetyl dapsone or other *N*-substituted sulphones (Bawden & Tute 1981). Daily administration of dapsone 100mg to leprosy patients has been reported to produce a trough plasma drug concentration of 0.5 mg/L at any time during the 24-hour dosing interval once steady-state is reached (Halmekoski et al. 1978; Garg et al. 1988). This is roughly 160 times higher than the MIC for this drug.

A single intramuscular injection of acedapsone is reported to produce a serum concentration of 0.015 to 0.085 mg/L (George & Balakrishnan 1986) which is 5 to 25 times more than the MIC for dapsone, although a steady-state concentration of about 0.5 mg/L seems to be desirable for therapeutic efficiency (Zuidema et al. 1986). Recently, Jagannathan & Mahadevan (1986) have suggested an MIC of 0.028 mg/L using their *in vitro* macrophage assay system.

Simultaneous administration of rifampicin has been reported to decrease the half-life of dapsone by a factor of about 2 and lower its plasma, skin and nerve concentrations considerably (Balakrishnan & Seshadri 1981; Gelber & Rees 1975; Gelber et al. 1975; Peters et al. 1977). These studies also show that the serum concentration of dapsone is still about 300 times higher than the MIC for the drug. A monthly pulse of oral rifampicin 600mg (WHO 1982) with an initial intensive therapy of rifampicin 600mg daily for 14 days (Government of India 1982) is the recommended dosage in multidrug regimens (table VI). The effect of rifampicin on blood concentrations and urinary excretion of dapsone during this period of rifampicin administration has not been found to be significant in terms of MIC (George et al. 1988). The dapsone-lowering effect of rifampicin has also not been found to vary among the various phenotypes of acetylators for dapsone (George et al. 1988; Venkatesan et al. 1980).

As may be seen from table VII, simultaneous administration of either prothionamide or clofazimine has not been shown to exert any effect on plasma concentrations, half-life and urinary excretion of dapsone (George et al. 1988; Mathur et al. 1986; Venkatesan et al. 1986). Serum concentrations of dapsone and urinary excretion of the drug and its conjugated metabolites have not been found to differ between patients on dapsone monother-

Table VI. Multidrug regimens recommended by WHO (1982) and Government of India (1982)

Recommendation	Multibacillary leprosy			Paucibacillary leprosy		
	regimen	dosage	duration	regimen	dosage	duration
WHO (1982)	Rifampicin	600 mg monthly pulse[a]	Minimum 2 years or till smear negativity whichever is longer	Rifampicin	600mg monthly pulse	6 months
	Clofazimine[b]	300mg monthly pulse and 50mg daily				
	Dapsone	100mg daily		Dapsone	100mg daily	
Government of India	Rifampicin	600mg daily for initial 14 days[a] and 600mg monthly	Minimum of two years or till smear negativity	Rifampicin	600mg monthly pulse	Minimum 6 months or till clinical inactivity
	Clofazimine, Dapsone	As in WHO (1982)		Dapsone	100mg daily	

a Monthly doses of clofazimine and rifampicin and daily doses of rifampicin are administered to the patients under supervision.
b Where clofazimine is totally unacceptable owing to the coloration of skin lesions that it causes, replacement by 250 to 375mg self-administered daily doses of ethionamide/prothionamide should be considered.

apy for 1 to 3 years and those on multidrug therapy comprising daily dapsone and clofazimine on alternate days together with monthly pulses of rifampicin for the same time period (Venkatesan et al. 1987). However, there is one report that mobilisation of tissue dapsone occurs, based on the observation of increased urinary excretion in 9 of the 17 patients treated with both clofazimine and dapsone (Grabosz & Wheate 1975).

Probenecid has been shown to cause a significant reduction in the urinary excretion of free and conjugated dapsone together with an increase in dapsone concentrations in blood (Goodwin & Sparell 1969). Pyrimethamine is reported to lower peak serum concentrations of dapsone without altering the half-life of dapsone and monoacetyl dapsone (Ahmad & Rogers 1980b).

A single dose of rifampicin 600mg is estimated to maintain the plasma concentration above its MIC for about 24 hours (WHO 1982). The therapeutic efficacy of rifampicin has been reported to be such that 99.9% of *M. leprae* are killed within 4 days of administration of a single oral dose of 600mg (Levy et al. 1976).

Simultaneous administration of *para*-aminosalicylic acid, isoniazid, pyrazinamide or streptomycin in various combinations has not been shown to exert any significant effect on the absorption, metabolism and excretion of rifampicin in tuberculosis patients (Acocella et al. 1985; Boman 1974). Studies of Venkatesan et al. (1986) and Mathur et al. (1986) have not shown any pharmacokinetic interactions between rifampicin and clofazimine or prothionamide (table VII). On the other hand, Mehta et al. (1985) have reported that clofazimine significantly reduced the absorption of rifampicin, resulting in delayed time to reach peak serum concentrations and increased half-life of the drug. Nevertheless, the bioavailability in terms of AUC and peak serum concentrations was not found to be significantly affected. The pharmacokinetic properties of rifampicin have not been found to vary among multibacillary and paucibacillary leprosy patients as reported by Mehta et al. (1985).

The reduced effectiveness of steroids when given concurrently with rifampicin is a point to be noted. This has been suggested to be due to the latter's ability to induce hepatic microsomal enzymes which increase the metabolic degradation of steroids (Jopling 1983). Since rifampicin is administered as a monthly pulse in the WHO regimen, this effect may not be of consequence while treating reactional erythema nodosum leprosum cases of leprosy with steroids.

Probenecid has been reported to increase the plasma concentrations of rifampicin by competing for hepatic uptake (Kenwright & Levi 1973).

In patients receiving clofazimine 100 to 200mg daily, it is not until treatment has continued for about 50 days that the rate of bacterial killing matches that at the start of therapy with dapsone 50mg in lepromatous leprosy patients (Levy et al. 1972). However, clofazimine also displays an anti-inflammatory effect in high doses, and hence is clinically valuable in controlling erythema nodosum leprosum (Browne 1965).

Neither rifampicin nor dapsone diminished the gastrointestinal absorption of simultaneously administered clofazimine (unpublished data). A lowering of the clofazimine content of the skin of leprosy patients receiving both clofazimine and isoniazid has been reported by Venkatesan et al. (1980). Ramu and Iyer (1976) had earlier observed that the intensity of skin colour in 10 cases treated with isoniazid and clofazimine was much less compared with those on clofazimine alone.

When an oral dose of clofazimine 50mg is given daily, it is only after 30 days that the concentration in plasma will come close to steady-state values and that bioavailability (in terms of AUC_{SS}/AUC_1) will be 4.85 times higher. Lanyi et al. (1987) suggested that slow accumulation towards the steady-state could be avoided by giving higher loading doses at the beginning of the treatment, followed

Table VII. Multiple dose pharmacokinetic parameters (mean ± SD/SE) after the last oral dose of dapsone and rifampicin, before and after addition of clofazimine or prothionamide to dapsone or dapsone plus rifampicin regimen, in leprosy patients

Reference	No. of pts	Drug regimen	Dapsone			Rifampicin		
			$t_{1/2\beta}$ (h)	C (24h) (mg/L)	Ae (mg)	$t_{1/2\beta}$ (h)	AUC (0-12h) (mg/L · h)	Ae (mg)
Mathur et al. (1986)	15[a]	Rifampicin + dapsone	18.0 ± 2.1	0.86 ± 0.10	67.9 ± 13.6	3.20 ± 0.31	58.6 ± 6.3	92.6 ± 21.5
		Rifampicin + dapsone + prothionamide	19.0 ± 2.1	0.89 ± 0.15	70.4 ± 11.5	3.70 ± 0.31	60.3 ± 5.2	106.4 ± 24.4
Venkatesan et al. (1986)	15[b]	Rifampicin + dapsone	18.2 ± 1.8	0.89 ± 0.10	72.1 ± 12.7	3.13 ± 0.46	62.9 ± 7.2	97.1 ± 21.3
		Rifampicin + dapsone + clofazimine	18.4 ± 1.5	0.94 ± 0.10	64.8 ± 9.4	3.31 ± 0.48	64.1 ± 9.5	101.4 ± 24.6
George et al. (1988)	30[c]	Dapsone + clofazimine		1.41 ± 0.14[d] (1.39 ± 0.12)				

a Daily administration of rifampicin 600mg and dapsone 100mg for 7 days, followed by the same drug regimen plus prothionamide 500mg daily for a further 7 days.

b Drug regimen as in (a) but clofazimine 100mg replaced prothionamide.

c Dapsone 100mg and clofazimine 100mg (both daily) for 15 days.

d Mean ± SE on the 8th day after oral dose; plasma concentrations on 15th day are given in parentheses.

Abbreviations: $t_{1/2\beta}$ = terminal half-life; C (24h) = plasma drug concentration 24 hours post-dose; Ae = 24-hour urinary excretion; AUC (0-12h) = area under the concentration-time curve from zero time to 12 hours post-dose.

by daily administration of the maintenance dose. However, the findings of Mathur et al. (1985) and Levy (1974) that increased dosage of clofazimine results in increased faecal excretion should be borne in mind. At present the World Health Organization (WHO 1982) recommends a monthly loading dose of 300mg.

Many clofazimine analogues have been tested for their activity against *M. leprae* in the mouse foot pad system, but none has been shown to be as active as the parent drug itself (Levy 1981). Recently, a few clofazimine analogues have been developed by O'Sullivan et al. (1988) and these are active against a clofazimine-resistant *M. smegmatis* strain. These analogues have also been shown to have growth-inhibitory activity against human-derived *M. leprae* in murine macrophage culture.

The pharmacokinetic properties of ethionamide and prothionamide have been reported to differ only slightly and without clinical significance (Jenner & Smith 1987). Experimental studies have also failed to demonstrate any differences in the inhibitory and bactericidal activities of these 2 agents against *M. leprae* (Colston et al. 1978a), or between their sulphoxide metabolites which also possess substantial antimycobacterial activities (Libermann et al. 1963; Matsuo et al. 1981). Although larger doses of ethionamide, as used in tuberculosis treatment, are less well tolerated than prothionamide (Fox et al. 1969), the regularity of intake of both the thioamides self-administered by leprosy patients has been reported to be similar at daily doses of 250mg of either drug (Stanley et al. 1986). Inclusion of thioamides in treating a leprosy patient will be dictated by therapeutic necessity, cost, availability and tolerance of the drug by the patient, and the past history of treatment with either thiacetazone or thioamides, in view of the reported cross-resistance between ethionamide and either prothionamide or thiacetazone in *M. leprae* (Pattyn & Colston 1978) and a probable cross-resistance between thiacetazone and ethionamide or prothionamide (Ji 1985). It would be advisable not to use multidrug regimens containing prothionamide or ethionamide in therapy for patients who previously had been treated with thiacetazone for more than 2 years.

The effect of companion antileprosy drugs on the pharmacokinetics of these thioamides is not known. Prothionamide has not been shown to induece its own metabolism (Peters et al. 1983). A single dose of prothionamide 500mg results in a serum drug concentration which will be above its MIC for 1 day only, thus necessitating the daily administration of the drug for effective chemotherapeutic activity (WHO 1982).

Acknowledgements

The author wishes to thank Dr H. Srinivasan, Director of the Leprosy Institute, for his critical review of the manuscript; Mr Hari Om and Mr Neeraj Dubey for preparing the figures; and Mr Santosh Masih and Mr S.K. Kulshrestha for typing the manuscript.

References

Acocella G. Clinical pharmacokinetics of rifampicin. Clinical Pharmacokinetics 3: 108-127, 1978

Acocella G, Conti R, Luisetti M, Pozzi E, Grassi C. Pharmacokinetic studies on antituberculosis regimens in humans. 1. Absorption and metabolism of the compounds used in the initial intensive phase of the short course regimens: single administration study. American Review of Respiratory Diseases 132: 510-515, 1985

Acocella G, Pagani V, Marchetti M, Baroni GC, Nicolis FB. Kinetic studies on rifampicin. 1. Serum concentration analysis in subjects treated with different oral doses over a period of two weeks. Chemotherapy (Basel) 16: 356-370, 1971

Ahmad RA, Rogers HJ. Plasma and salivary pharmacokinetics of dapsone estimated by thin layer chromatographic method. European Journal of Clinical Pharmacology 17: 129-133, 1980a

Ahmad RA, Rogers HJ. Pharmacokinetics and protein binding of dapsone and pyrimethamine. British Journal of Clinical Pharmacology 10: 519-524, 1980b

Alexander JO'D, Young E, McFayden T, Fraser NG, Duguid WP, et al. Absorption and excretion of ^{35}S-dapsone in dermatitis herpetiformis. British Journal of Dermatology 83: 620-631, 1970

Allen BW, Ellard GA, Gammon PT, King RC, Rees RJW, et al. The penetration of dapsone, rifampicin, isoniazid and pyrazinamide into peripheral nerves. British Journal of Clinical Pharmacology 55: 151-155, 1975

Balakrishnan S, Desikan KV, Ramu G. Quantitative estimation of clofazimine in tissues. Leprosy in India 48 (Suppl. 4): 732-738, 1976

Balakrishnan S, Ramu G. Blood DDS levels and acetylation rates of sulfadimidine in leprosy patients. Leprosy in India 49: 59-64, 1977

Balakrishnan S, Seshadri PS. Drug interactions: the influence of

rifampicin and clofazimine on the urinary excretion of DDS. Leprosy in India 53: 17-22, 1981
Banerjee DK, Ellard GA, Gammon PT, Waters MFR. Some observations on the pharmacology of clofazimine (B 663). American Journal of Tropical Medicine and Hygiene 23: 1110-1115, 1974
Barry VC, Buggle J, Byrne ML, Conalty ML, Winder F. Factors influencing the anti-tuberculosis activity of the rimino compounds. Bulletin of the International Union against Tuberculosis 29: 582-593, 1959
Barry VC, Buggle J, Byrne ML, Conalty ML, Winder F. Absorption, distribution and retention of riminocompounds in the experimental animals. Irish Journal of Medical Sciences 410: 345-352, 1960
Bawden D, Tute MS. Structure-activity relationships of anti-mycobacterial sulphones: a study using physicochemical constants. European Journal of Medicinal Chemistry 16: 299-300, 1981
Biggs JT, Gordon GR, Peters JH. Disappearance rates and plasma protein-binding of dapsone (DDS) and monoacetyl dapsone (MADDS) in animals and man. Federation Proceedings 30: 629, 1971
Boddingius J, Stolz E. Do anti-leprosy drugs reach *Mycobacterium leprae* in peripheral nerves? Lancet 1: 774-775, 1981
Boman G. Serum concentrations and half-life of rifampicin after simultaneous oral administration of aminosalicylic acid or isoniazid. European Journal of Clinical Pharmacology 7: 217-225, 1974
Boman G, Ringberger V-A. Binding of rifampicin by human plasma proteins. European Journal of Clinical Pharmacology 7: 369-373, 1974
Browne SG. 'B 663'–a possible anti-inflammatory action in lepromatous leprosy. Leprosy Review 36: 9-11, 1965
Browne SG, Harman DJ, Waudby H, McDougall AC. Clofazimine (Lamprene B 663) in the treatment of lepromatous leprosy in the United Kingdom: a 12-year review of 31 cases, 1966-1978. International Journal of Leprosy 49: 167-176, 1981
Byrne J, Conalty ML, Jina A. Laboratory studies on the riminophenazines. Tubercle 50 (Suppl.): 22-28, 1969
Cartel JL, Millan J, Guelpa-Lauras CC, Grosset JH. Hepatitis in leprosy patients treated by a daily combination of dapsone, rifampicin and a thioamide. International Journal of Leprosy 51: 461-465, 1983
Chatterjee KR, Poddar RK. Radioactive tracer studies on uptake of DDS by leprosy patients. Proceedings of the Society for Experimental Biology and Medicine 94: 122-125, 1957
Colston MJ, Ellard GA, Gammon PT. Drugs for combined therapy: experimental studies on the anti-leprosy activity of ethionamide and prothionamide, a general review. Leprosy Review 49: 115-126, 1978a
Colston MJ, Hilson GRF. The activity of thiacetazone, thiambutosine and thiocarlide in the chemotherapy of experimental leprosy. International Journal of Leprosy 44: 123-128, 1976
Colston MJ, Hilson GRF, Bannerjee DK. 'The proportional bactericidal test': a method for assessing the bactericidal activity of drugs against *Mycobacterium leprae* in mice. Leprosy Review 49: 7-15, 1978b
Conalty ML, Jackson RD. Uptake by reticuloendothelial cells of riminophenazine B 663. British Journal of Experimental Pathology 43: 650-654, 1962
DeGowin RL. A review of therapeutic and hemolytic effects of dapsone. Archives of Internal Medicine 120: 242-248, 1967
Depasquale G. Rifampicin and isoprodian in combination in the treatment of leprosy. Leprosy Review 46 (Suppl. 2): 179-180, 1975
Desikan KV, Balakrishnan S. Tissue levels of clofazimine in a case of leprosy. Leprosy Review 47: 107-114,1976
Ellard GA. Absorption, metabolism and excretion of di(p-aminophenyl sulphone (dapsone) and di(p-aminophenyl) sulphoxide in man. British Journal of Pharmacology 26: 212-217, 1966
Ellard GA. Absorption, metabolism and excretion of pyrazinamide in man. Tubercle 50: 144-148, 1969
Ellard GA. Rationale of the multi-drug regimens recommended by a WHO study group on chemotherapy of leprosy for control programmes. International Journal of Leprosy 52: 395-401, 1984
Ellard GA, Dickinson JM, Gammon PT, Mitchison DA. Serum concentrations and antituberculosis activity of thiacetazone. Tubercle 55: 41-54, 1974
Faget GH, Pogge RC, Johansen FA, Dinan JF, Prejean VM, et al. Promin treatment of leprosy. Public Health Reports 58: 1729-1741, 1943
Feng PCC, Fenselau CC, Jacobson RR. Metabolism of clofazimine in leprosy patients. Drug Metabolism and Disposition 9: 521-524, 1981
Feng PCC, Fenselau CC, Jacobson RR. A new urinary metabolite of clofazimine in leprosy patients. Drug Metabolism and Disposition 10: 286-288, 1982
Fox W, Robinson DK, Tall R, Mitchison DA, Kent PW, et al. A study of the intolerance to ethionamide, including a comparison with prothionamide, and the influence of a vitamin B-complex additive in prophylaxis. Tubercle 50: 125-143, 1969
Freerksen E. Preliminary experience with combined therapy using rifampicin and isoprodian (L 73 A). Leprosy Review 46 (Suppl. 2): 316, 1975
Furesz S. Chemical and biological properties of rifampicin. Antibiotica et Chemotherapia (Basle) 16: 316-319, 1970
Garg SK, Kumar B, Bakaya V, Lal R, Shukla VK, et al. Plasma dapsone levels in leprotic patients. International Journal of Clinical Pharmacology, Therapy and Toxicology, 26: 552-554, 1988
Gelber RH, Gooi HC, Rees RJW. The effect of rifampicin on dapsone metabolism. Proceedings of the Western Pharmacological Society 18: 330-334, 1975
Gelber RH, Peters JH, Gordon RG, Glazko AJ, Levy L. The polymorphic acetylation of dapsone in man. Clinical Pharmacology and Therapeutics 12: 225-238, 1971
Gelber RH, Rees RJW. Dapsone metabolism in patients with dapsone-resistant leprosy. American Journal of Tropical Medicine and Hygiene 24: 963-967, 1975
George J, Balakrishnan S. Blood dapsone levels in leprosy patients treated with acedapsone. Indian Journal of Leprosy 58: 401-406, 1986
George J, Balakrishnan S, Bhatia VN. Drug interactions during multidrug regimens for treatment of leprosy. Indian Journal of Medical Research 87: 151-156, 1988
Gidoh M, Tsutsumi S. Determination of three main anti-leprosy drugs and their main metabolites in serum by high performance liquid chromatography. Journal of Chromatography 223: 379-392, 1981
Glazko AJ, Chang T, Baukema J, Chang SF, Savory A, et al. Central role of MADDS in the metabolism of DDS. International Journal of Leprosy 37: 462-463, 1969

Glazko AJ, Dill WA, Baukema J, Thompson PE. Metabolic disposition of repository sulfone drugs. International Journal of Leprosy 36: 511-512, 1968a

Glazko AJ, Dill WA, Montalbo RG, Holmes EL. A new analytical procedure for dapsone. Application to blood level and urinary excretion studies in normal men. American Journal of Tropical Medicine and Hygiene 17: 465-473, 1968b

Goodwin CS, Sparell G. Inhibition of dapsone excretion by probenecid. Lancet 2: 884-885, 1969

Government of India. Report of the Working Group on the Eradication of Leprosy. Ministry of Health and Family Welfare, New Delhi, 1982

Grabosz JAJ, Wheate HW. Effect of clofazimine on the urinary excretion of DDS. International Journal of Leprosy 43: 61-62, 1975

Halmekoski J, Matilla MJ, Mustakallio KK. Metabolism and haemolytic effect of dapsone and its metabolites in man. Medical Biology 56: 216-221, 1978

Hocking DR. Neonatal haemolytic disease due to dapsone. Medical Journal of Australia 1: 1130-1131, 1968

Holmes IB. Minimum inhibitory and bactericidal dosages of rifampicin against *Mycobacterium leprae* in the mouse foot pad: relationships to serum concentrations. International Journal of Leprosy 42: 289-296, 1974

Holmes IB, Hilson GRF. The effect of rifampicin and dapsone on experimental *Mycobacterium leprae* infections: minimum inhibitory concentrations and bactericidal action. Journal of Medical Microbiology 5: 251-261, 1972

Immanuel C, Jayasankar K, Narayana ASL, Sarma GR. Self induction of rifampicin metabolism in man. Indian Journal of Medical Research 82: 381-387, 1985

Jagannathan R, Mahadevan PR. Minimum inhibitory concentration of drugs against *Mycobacterium leprae* as determined by an *in vitro* assay. Journal of Biosciences 10: 137-144, 1986

Jenner PJ, Ellard GA. High performance liquid chromatographic determination of ethionamide and prothionamide in body fluids. Journal of Chromatography 225: 245-251, 1981

Jenner PJ, Ellard GA, Gruer PJK, Aber VR. A comparison of the blood levels and urinary excretion of ethionamide and prothionamide in man. Journal of Antimicrobial Chemotherapy 13: 267-277, 1984

Jenner PJ, Smith SE. Plasma levels of ethionamide and prothionamide in a volunteer following intravenous and oral dosages. Leprosy Review 58: 31-37, 1987

Ji B. Drug resistance in leprosy – a review. Leprosy Review 56: 265-278, 1985

Ji B, Chen J, Wang C, Xia G. Hepatotoxicity of combined therapy with rifampicin and daily prothionamide for leprosy. Leprosy Review 55: 283-289, 1984

Jones CR, Ovenell SM. Determination of plasma concentrations of dapsone, monoacetyl dapsone and pyrimethamine in human subjects dosed with maloprim. Journal of Chromatography 163: 179-185, 1979

Jopling WH. Handbook of leprosy, 2nd ed., William Heinemann Medical Books, London, 1978

Jopling WH. Side effects of anti-leprosy drugs in common use. Leprosy Review 54: 261-270, 1983

Karim AKMB, Elfellah MS, Evans DAP. Human acetylator polymorphism: estimate of allele frequency in Libya and details of global distribution. Journal of Medical Genetics 18: 325-330, 1981

Katoch K, Ramu G. Ramanathan U, Sreevatsa. Pyrazinamide as a part of combination therapy for BL-LL patients – a preliminary report. International Journal of Leprosy 56: 1-9, 1988

Kenny MT, Strates B. Metabolism and pharmacokinetics of the antibiotic rifampicin. Drug Metabolism Reviews 12: 159-218, 1981

Kenwright S, Levi AJ. Impairment of hepatic uptake of rifamycin antibiotics by probenecid and its therapeutic implication. Lancet 2: 1401-1405, 1973

Konno K, Feldmann FM, McDermott W. Pyrazinamide susceptibility and amidase activity of tubercle bacilli. American Review of Respiratory Diseases 95: 461-463, 1967

Kubo E, Fukunishi Y, Matsumoto T. Plasma levels of DDS in leprosy patients admitted in the National Sanatorium Oshima Seisho-en. Japanese Journal of Leprosy 52: 29-34, 1983

Lang PG. Sulfones and sulfonamides in dermatology today. Journal of the American Academy of Dermatology 1: 479-492, 1979

Lammintausta K, Kangas L, Lammintausta R. The pharmacokinetics of dapsone and acetylated dapsone in serum and saliva. International Journal of Clinical Pharmacology and Biopharmacy 17: 159-163, 1979

Lanyi Z, Dieterie W, Dubois JP, Theobald W, Vischer W. Pharmacokinetics of clofazimine in healthy volunteers. International Journal of Leprosy 55: 9-15, 1987

Lanyi Z, Dubois JP. Determination of clofazimine in human plasma by thin layer chromatography. Journal of Chromatography 232: 219-223, 1982

Lecaillon JB, Febvre N, Metayer JP, Souppart C. Quantitative assay of rifampicin and three of its metabolites in human plasma, urine and saliva by high performance liquid chromatography. Journal of Chromatography 145: 319-324, 1978

Lecaillon JB, Schoeller JP, Humbert G, Febvre N, Juge F. Pharmacokinetics of rifampicin and three of its metabolites after single oral doses. In Aiache & Hirtz (Eds) Proceedings of the 1st European Congress on Biopharmaceutics and Pharmacokinetics, Vol. 2, pp. 258, Clermont-Ferrand, Paris, 1981

Leggat PO. Ethionamide neuropathy. Tubercle 43: 95-96, 1962

Levy L. Pharmacologic studies of clofazimine. American Journal of Tropical Medicine and Hygiene 23: 1097-1109, 1974

Levy L. Activity of four clofazimine analogues against *Mycobacterium leprae*. Leprosy Review 52: 23-26, 1981

Levy L, Peters JH. Susceptibility of *Mycobacterium leprae* to dapsone as a determinant of patient response to acedapsone. Antimicrobial Agents and Chemotherapy 9: 102-107, 1976

Levy L, Shepard CC, Fasal P. Clofazimine therapy of lepromatous leprosy caused by dapsone-resistant *Mycobacterium leprae*. American Journal of Tropical Medicine and Hygiene 21: 315-321, 1972

Levy L, Shepard CC, Fasal P. The bactericidal effect of rifampicin on *M. leprae* in man: (a) single doses of 600, 900 and 1200mg; and (b) daily doses of 300mg. International Journal of Leprosy 44: 183-187, 1976

Libermann D, Rist N, Grumbach F. Le S-oxyde de l'α-ethylthionamide isonicotinique. Comptes Rendus Hebdamadaires des Séances de l'Académie des Sciences 257: 307-308, 1963

Lowe J. The treatment of leprosy with TBI/698. A report based on 38 months' experience. Leprosy Review 25: 186-199, 1954

Maggi N, Furesz S, Pallanza R, Pelizza G. Rifampicin desacetylation in the human organism. Arzneimittel-Forschung 19: 651-654, 1969

Mansfield RE. Tissue concentrations of clofazimine (B 663) in

man. American Journal of Tropical Medicine and Hygiene 23: 1116-1119, 1974
Mathur A, Venkatesan K, Bharadwaj VP, Ramu G. Evaluation of effectiveness of clofazimine therapy I. Monitoring of absorption of clofazimine from gastrointestinal tract. Indian Journal of Leprosy 57: 146-148, 1985
Mathur A, Venkatesan K, Girdhar BK, Bharadwaj VP, Girdhar A, et al. A study of drug interactions in leprosy – 1. Effect of simultaneous administration of prothionamide on metabolic disposition of rifampicin and dapsone. Leprosy Review 57: 33-37, 1986
Matsuo Y, Tatsukawa H, Murray JF, Peters JH. Prothionamide and prothionamide S-oxide in experimental leprosy. International Journal of Leprosy 49: 302-306, 1981
McDougall AC, Jones RL. Intra-neural ceroid-like pigment following treatment of lepromatous leprosy with clofazimine (B-663, Lamprene). Journal of Neurology, Neurosurgery and Psychiatry 44: 116-120, 1981
Mehta J, Gandhi IS, Sane SB, Wamburkar MN. Effect of clofazimine and dapsone on rifampicin (Lositril) pharmacokinetics in multibacillary and paucibacillary leprosy cases. Indian Journal of Leprosy 57: 297-310, 1985
Modderman ESM, Mericus FWHM, Zuidema J, Hilbers HW, Warndorff T. Dapsone levels after oral therapy and weekly oily injections in Ethiopian leprosy patients. International Journal of Leprosy 51: 191-196, 1983
Molesworth DB. Discussion on combined therapy. Proceedings of the Second International Leprosy Colloquium held at Forschungs Institut, Borstel. Leprosy Review 46 (Suppl. 2): 239, 1975
Morrison NE. Antimycobacterial activity of phenazine compounds. International Journal of Leprosy 40: 219-220, 1972
Morrison NE, Morley GM. Clofazimine binding studies with deoxyribonucleic acid. International Journal of Leprosy 44: 475-481, 1976
Morrison NE, Morley GM. Comparative DNA binding studies with clofazimine and B 1912. International Journal of Leprosy 45: 188-189, 1977
Murray Jr JF, Gordon GR, Peters JH. A chromatographic-fluorometric procedure for the determination of nanogram quantities of antileprotic sulfones. Journal of Laboratory and Clinical Medicine 78: 464-471, 1971
O' Sullivan JF, Conalty ML, Morrison NE. Clofazimine analogues active against a clofazimine resistant organism. Journal of Medicinal Chemistry 31: 561-572, 1988
Pattyn SR, Colston MJ. Cross-resistance amongst thiambutosine, thiacetazone, ethionamide and prothionamide with *Mycobacterium leprae*. Leprosy Review 49: 324-326, 1978
Pattyn SR, Janssens L, Bourland J, Saylan T, Davies EM, et al. The Collaborative Study Group for the Treatment of Leprosy. Hepatotoxicity of the combination of rifampin-ethionamide in the treatment of multibacillary leprosy. International Journal of Leprosy 52: 1-6, 1984
Pattyn SR, Portaels F, Van Loo G, Van den Breen L. Activity of the combination isoniazid, prothionamide and dapsone against *Mycobacterium leprae* and some other mycobacteria. Arzneimittel-Forschung 31: 2155-2157, 1981
Pawlowska I, Pniewski T. Studies on pharmacokinetics of rifampicin in the body of patients with pulmonary tuberculosis. Arzneimittel-Forschung 29: 1906-1909, 1979
Peters JH, Gordon GR, Ghoul DC, Tolentine JG, Walsh GP, et al. The disposition of anti-leprosy drug (dapsone) DDS in Philippine subjects. American Journal of Tropical Medicine and Hygiene 21: 450-457, 1972
Peters JH, Gordon GR, Karat ABA. Polymorphic acetylation of the antibacterials, sulfmethazine and dapsone, in South Indian subjects. American Journal of Tropical Medicine and Hygiene 24: 641-648, 1975
Peters JH, Gordon GR, Murray Jr JF. Disposition of prothionamide in rats and armadillos. International Journal of Leprosy 51: 54-63, 1983
Peters JH, Gordon GR, Murray Jr JF, Meyers WH. Metabolic disposition of dapsone in African leprosy patients. Leprosy Review 50: 7-19, 1979
Peters JH, Murray Jr JF, Gordon GR, Gelber RH. Dapsone in saliva and plasma of man. Pharmacology 22: 162-171, 1981
Peters JH, Murray Jr JF, Gordon GR, Gelber RH, Laing ABG, et al. Effect of rifampicin on the disposition of dapsone in Malaysian leprosy patients. Federation Proceedings 36: 996, 1977
Peters JH, Murray Jr JF, Gordon GR, Jacobson RR. Metabolic-bacteriologic relationship in the chemotherapy of lepromatous patients with dapsone or dapsone-rifampin. International Journal of Leprosy 46: 115-116, 1978
Peters JH, Shepard CC, Gordon GR, Rojas AV, Elizondo DS. The incidence of dapsone resistance in lepromatous patients in Costa Rica: their metabolic disposition of DDS. International Journal of Leprosy 44: 143-151, 1976
Pettit JHS, Rees RJW. Studies on sulfone resistance in leprosy: 2 treatment with riminophenazine derivative (B 663). International Journal of Leprosy 34: 391-397, 1966
Pieters FAJM, Zuidema J. The absolute oral availability of dapsone in dogs and humans. International Journal of Clinical Pharmacology, Therapy and Toxicology 25: 396-400, 1987
Pilheu JA, Sippel JE. Rifampin concentrations in cerebrospinal fluid of patients with tuberculous meningitis. American Review of Respiratory Diseases 111: 240-243, 1975
Pines A. Thiacetazone toxicity in British patients. Tubercle 45: 188-191, 1964
Ramu G, Iyer CGS. Side effects of clofazimine therapy. Leprosy in India 48 (Suppl. 3): 722-731, 1976
Riess W. The optimum dosage schedule for rimactane. In A symposium on rimactane, Basel, 1968, p. 36, Ciba, Basel, 1969
Rocker I. Rifampicin in early pregnancy. Lancet 2: 48, 1977
Rollier R, Rollier M. Traitement de la lèpre lépromateuse par l'éthionamide. Marocos Medicale 52: 148-166, 1972
Sanders SW, Zone JJ, Foltz RL, Tolman KG, Rollins DE. Hemolytic anaemia induced by dapsone transmitted through breast milk. Annals of Internal Medicine 96: 465-466, 1982
Schulz EJ. Forty-four months' experience in the treatment of leprosy with clofazimine [Lamprene (Geigy)]. Leprosy Review 42: 178-187, 1971
Seydel JK. Physico-chemical studies on rifampicin. Antibiotica et Chemotherapia (Basle) 16: 380-391, 1970
Shepard CC. A kinetic method for the study of activity of drugs against *M. leprae* in mice. International Journal of Leprosy 35: 429-435, 1967
Shepard CC, Chang YT. Activity of anti-tuberculosis drugs against *Mycobacterium leprae*. Studies with experimental infection of mouse foot pads. International Journal of Leprosy 32: 260-271, 1964
Shepard CC. Combinations involving dapsone, rifampicin, clo-

fazimine and ethionamide in the treatment of *M. leprae* infections in mice. International Journal of Leprosy 44: 135-139, 1976

Sielger DI, Bryant M, Burley DM, Citnen KM, Standen SM. Effect of meals on rifampicin absorption. Lancet 2: 197, 1974

Stanley JNA, Pearson JMH, Ellard GA. Ethionamide, prothionamide and thiacetazone self administration – studies of patient compliance using isoniazid-marked formulations. Leprosy Review 57: 9-18, 1986

Swain AF, Ahmad RA, Rogers HJ, Leonard JN, Fry L. Pharmacokinetic observations on dapsone in dermatitis herpetiformis. British Journal of Dermatology 108: 91-98, 1983

Venkatesan K, Bharadwaj VP, Ramu G, Desikan KV. A study on drug interactions in leprosy. Leprosy in India 52: 229-235, 1980

Venkatesan K, Mathur A, Bharadwaj VP, Ramu G. The effect of clofazimine treatment on dapsone metabolism in leprosy patients. International Conference on Clinical Pharmacology and Therapeutics, Bombay (India), November 20-22, 1987. Abstract No. FPS 7/8, 1987

Venkatesan K, Mathur A, Girdhar BK, Bharadwaj VP. The effect of clofazimine on the pharmacokinetics of rifampicin and dapsone. Journal of Antimicrobial Chemotherapy 18: 715-718, 1986

Vischer WA. The experimental properties of G30 320 (B 663) – a new anti-leprotic agent. Leprosy Review 40: 107-110, 1969

Warndorff-van Diepen T. Clofazimine resistant leprosy – a case report. International Journal of Leprosy 50: 139-142, 1982

Waters MFR. G30,320 or B 663, Lampren (Geigy): a working party held in London in September 1968. Leprosy Review 40: 21-47, 1969

Webb AH. A thiacetazone toxicity trial in Sarawak. New Zealand Medical Journal 78: 409-412, 1973

Weber WW, Hein DW. Clinical pharmacokinetics of isoniazid. Clinical Pharmacokinetics 4: 401-422, 1979

WHO. Expert Committee on Leprosy. Fifth report. Technical Report Series 607, 1977

WHO. Chemotherapy for leprosy control programs. Report of a WHO study group. Technical Report Series 675, 1982

Yu T, Berger L, Stone DJ, Wolf J, Gutman AB. Effect of pyrazinamide and pyrazinoic acid on urate clearance and other discrete renal functions. Proceedings of the Society for Experimental Biology and Medicine 96: 264-268, 1957

Zuidema J, Modderman ESM, Merkus FWHM. Clinical pharmacokinetics of dapsone. Clinical Pharmacokinetics 11: 299-315, 1986

Zuidema J, Modderman ESM, Merkus FWHM, Hilbers HW. The intramuscular injection of monoacetyl dapsone. Proceedings of the Second International Congress on Biopharmaceuticals and Pharmacokinetics, pp. 240-249, 1984

Zuidema J, Van Ginneken CAM. Clearance concept in salivary drug excretion. Part I. Theory. Pharmaceutica Acta Helvetiae 58: 88-93, 1983a

Zuidema J, Van Ginneken CAM. Clearance concept in salivary drug excretion. Part II. Experiments. Pharmaceutica Acta Helvetiae 58: 136-143, 1983b

Author's address: Dr. *K. Venkatesan*, Central JALMA Institute for Leprosy (Indian Council of Medical Research), Taj Ganj, Agra 282001 (India).

Original Research Article

Clinical Pharmacokinetics 16: 387-391 (1989)
0312-5963/89/0006-0387/$02.50/0

Single-Dose and Steady-State Pharmacokinetics of Doxazosin Given in Combination with Chlorothiazide to Hypertensive Subjects

E.L. Conway, J.J. McNeil, L. Meng, O.H. Drummer, L.G. Howes, K. Raymond and *W.J. Louis*

University of Melbourne, Clinical Pharmacology and Therapeutics Units, Austin Hospital, Heidelberg, Victoria, Australia

Summary *The pharmacokinetics of doxazosin were determined in hypertensive subjects after a single dose of 1mg, and at steady-state while receiving doses of 1, 2, 4 and 8mg of the drug daily. Chlorothiazide 500mg once daily was administered as additional therapy throughout the study. After a single dose doxazosin was rapidly absorbed, with peak plasma drug concentrations (C_{max}) occurring after 2.1 ± 0.4 hours. The elimination half-life in plasma was 10.7 ± 1.2 hours. These parameters remained essentially unchanged during maintenance administration of doxazosin at each of the dose levels. Calculations of C_{max} and area under the concentration-time curve ($AUC_{0\rightarrow\infty}$) indicated that the pharmacokinetic disposition of the drug remained linear over the dose range 1 to 8mg.*

Doxazosin is one of a number of α_1-adrenoceptor antagonist drugs presently being marketed as antihypertensive agents. These drugs have several properties that make them attractive options for first-line therapy in the treatment of hypertension. They reduce peripheral vascular resistance without significant reflex tachycardia (Lund-Johansen 1975; Lund-Johansen et al. 1986), and are relatively free from CNS side effects and adverse effects on respiratory function (Stokes 1984). Moreover, α_1-adrenoceptor antagonists have favourable effects on plasma lipid profiles (Sachs & Dzau 1986) that may help prevent the progression of atheroma in hypertensive subjects.

Doxazosin appears to be effective and well tolerated during long term treatment with once-daily administration of doses ranging from 1 to 16mg (Cox et al. 1986). Measurement of plasma concentrations of the drug at steady-state in patients on stable treatment have indicated that plasma doxazosin concentrations are proportional to dose (Cox et al. 1986); however, to date there has been no analysis of steady-state pharmacokinetics as a function of dose in the same subjects. The purpose of the present study is to compare the pharmacokinetics of doxazosin in hypertensive subjects after a single dose and during maintenance administration of the drug, and to investigate the relationship between dose and pharmacokinetics. The drug was administered as combination therapy with chlorothiazide.

Patients and Methods

Patients

10 subjects with essential hypertension (5 men, 5 women), with a mean age of 57 years (range 39 to 74 years) and a mean weight of 72kg (range 52

to 94kg), participated in the study. All subjects had normal biochemical and haematological indices. Women of childbearing potential or who were lactating were excluded from the study. The protocol was approved by the Hospital Ethics Committee and informed, written consent was obtained from each participant.

Study Design

The study was conducted as an open trial. In the initial 4-week washout period, and throughout the study, patients received chlorothiazide 500mg once daily. They were reviewed fortnightly while on chlorothiazide therapy alone, and entered into the study if their diastolic blood pressure lay in the range 90 to 115mm Hg. Each subject was then investigated on up to 5 occasions, after administration of doxazosin as follows:

(a) 1mg dose;
(b) 1mg once daily for 2 weeks;
(c) 2mg once daily for 2 weeks;
(d) 4mg once daily for 2 weeks;
(e) 8mg once daily for 2 weeks.

The dose of doxazosin was increased only if there were no severe side effects related to blood pressure reduction, systolic blood pressure did not fall below 120mm Hg and there were no other significant drug-related side effects.

On each pharmacokinetic study day patients attended our outpatient clinic in a fasted state at 8.00 a.m.; baseline samples were collected and haemodynamic variables measured. The dose of doxazosin was then administered with 200ml water. Blood samples for drug estimation were collected at 0.25, 0.5, 1, 1.5, 2, 2.5, 3, 4, 6, 8, 12, 24 and 30 hours after administration. The dose of doxazosin which would normally have been taken 24 hours after the commencement of each pharmacokinetic study day was omitted. Before collection of blood samples, duplicate blood pressure and heart rate measurements were taken in the supine and standing positions using a 'Dinamap' automatic sphygmomanometer. No food was allowed until 4 hours after dosing. Standard meals were provided during the first 12 hours at 12 noon and 6.00 p.m. The patients were not hospitalised overnight. They were assessed by general enquiry for symptoms throughout each kinetic study and after each maintenance dosing period.

Assay Procedure

Freshly drawn blood was collected in heparinised tubes and spun for 10 minutes. The plasma was removed and frozen at −20°C. Doxazosin was stable under these conditions. The assay was performed in disposable polypropylene extraction tubes, to which 1ml of plasma, 5ng of prazosin (acting as internal standard), 50μl of 2 mol/L NaOH and 10ml of distilled diethyl ether were successively added. These tubes were then shaken for 10 minutes on a reciprocating shaker and placed in an alcohol bath at −40°C until the plasma layer was frozen. The ether layer was decanted into another polypropylene tube containing 100μl of 0.1% orthophosphoric acid. The tubes were shaken for 10 minutes on the reciprocating shaker and the ether layer was then aspirated away. Any residual ether was removed by drying the tube down under a gentle stream of air. The phosphoric acid layer (50μl) was then injected into a liquid chromatograph fitted with a Waters Model M45 solvent delivery system, an automatic injector (WISP 710 B) and a fluorometric detector (Kratos FS970). The excitation wavelength was 246nm and the emission wavelength was obtained with a 7-60 filter. The sensitivity was maintained at 0.05μA. The mobile phase consisted of 65% methanol and 35% 10 mmol/L ammonium phosphate at pH 4.6.

The column used was a 'Compression Module Column' (Waters, 10mm × 10mm) packed with a 5μm particle size 'Bondapak C18' phase (Whatman). A 'C18' guard column was used to protect the column. The mobile phase was pumped at 2 ml/min.

Under these conditions a clear separation between the internal standard [prazosin (retention time 2.48 minutes)] and doxazosin (retention time 4 minutes) was obtained. The minimum detectable levels of doxazosin were 1 μg/L, with an intraassay coefficient of variation of < 6% and an inter-assay coefficient of variation of < 12%.

Pharmacokinetic Analysis

The terminal elimination half-life ($t_{1/2\beta}$) of doxazosin was determined for each patient from the terminal exponential of the graphs relating the logarithm of the plasma concentrations to the time elapsed since dosing.

The areas under the individual dosing curves (AUC) for the 48 hours after single-dose administration were obtained by the trapezoidal method; to these values were added estimates of the areas beyond the last measured plasma concentration (C^*) obtained from the expression C^*/β (where β is the slope of the terminal exponential of drug elimination). For the maintenance dose studies AUC was calculated during 1 interdose interval (Wagner 1971).

Statistical Analysis

All data have been expressed as mean ± SE unless otherwise indicated. In the maintenance dosing schedule not all subjects proceeded to the 4 and 8mg steady-state levels due to the incidence of side effects. All 10 subjects completed the 1mg single-dose, 1mg steady-state and 2mg steady-state studies and the differences in pharmacokinetic parameters between 1mg single-dose and 1mg steady-state, and between 1mg steady-state and 2mg steady-state, were analysed using paired t-tests. Analysis of the pharmacokinetic parameters at 1, 2, 4 and 8mg steady-state was confined to the 5 subjects who completed all studies, and was carried out using repeated measures analysis of variance.

Results

Pharmacokinetics

Plasma concentrations of doxazosin after single-dose and maintenance administration of the drug are shown in figure 1. The pharmacokinetic parameters derived from these data are shown in table I.

Following administration of a single dose of doxazosin 1mg the drug was absorbed rapidly, with

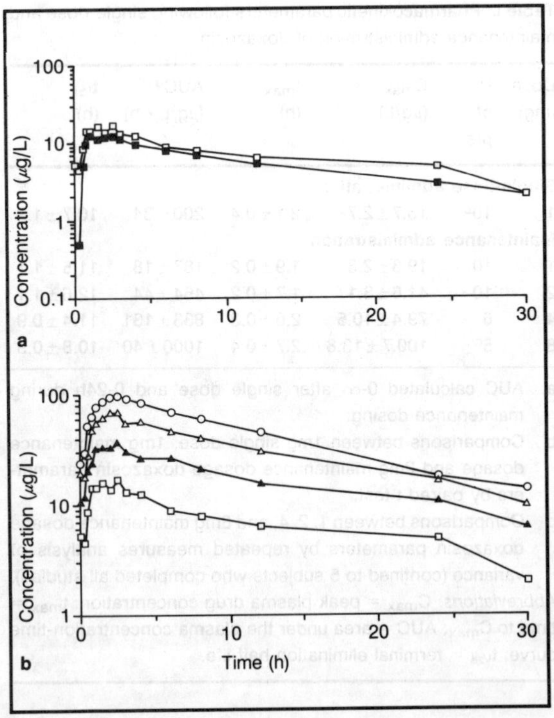

Fig. 1. Plasma concentrations of doxazosin after **(a)** a single dose of 1mg (■) and administration of 1 mg/day for 14 days (□), and **(b)** administration of 1 (□), 2 (▲), 4 (△) and 8 (○) mg/day for 14 days.

peak concentrations (C_{max}) occurring approximately 2 hours after dosing (range 0.75 to 4 hours). The peak concentration achieved varied approximately 6-fold across the 10 subjects, from 6 to 33 μg/L, with a similar 6-fold variability in AUC (65 to 398 μg/L • h). The average $t_{1/2\beta}$ of doxazosin was 10.7 hours (4.2 to 16 hours).

After 14 days' treatment with doxazosin 1mg once daily, the pharmacokinetic disposition of the drug was virtually identical to that following single dose administration. Peak concentrations were again achieved approximately 2 hours after dosing (0.75 to 3 hours). There was a significant increase in C_{max} from 15.7 ± 2.7 to 19.3 ± 2.3 μg/L (paired t-test, p = 0.014), reflecting the residual doxazosin present in the baseline samples collected during maintenance dosing; however, there was no significant difference in AUC. The variability in C_{max}

Table I. Pharmacokinetic parameters following single-dose and maintenance administration of doxazosin

Dose (mg)	No. of pts	C_{max} (μg/L)	t_{max} (h)	AUC[a] (μg/L · h)	$t_{½β}$ (h)
Single-dose administration					
1	10[b]	15.7±2.7	2.1±0.4	200±34	10.7±1.2
Maintenance administration					
1	10	19.3±2.3	1.9±0.2	187±18	11.5±1.1
2	10	41.6±3.1	1.7±0.2	464±44	12.6±1.1
4	6	79.4±10.5	2.0±0.3	833±131	11.4±0.9
8	5[c]	100.7±13.8	2.7±0.4	1000±40	10.8±0.5

a AUC calculated 0-∞ after single dose and 0-24h during maintenance dosing.

b Comparisons between 1mg single dose, 1mg maintenance dosage and 2mg maintenance dosage doxazosin parameters by paired t-test.

c Comparisons between 1, 2, 4, and 8mg maintenance dosage doxazosin parameters by repeated measures analysis of variance (confined to 5 subjects who completed all studies).

Abbreviations: C_{max} = peak plasma drug concentration; t_{max} = time to C_{max}; AUC = area under the plasma concentration-time curve; $t_{½β}$ = terminal elimination half-life.

and AUC across the subjects was less during maintenance administration, with the range from highest to lowest values being 3-fold and 2.5-fold, respectively. The $t_{½β}$ of doxazosin at 1mg steady-state was 11.5 hours, not significantly different from that obtained after the single dose.

Analysis of the pharmacokinetic parameters determined in all 10 patients at 1mg and 2mg steady-state showed there was no significant alteration in time to reach C_{max} (t_{max}) or $t_{½β}$, and that C_{max} and AUC increased linearly with dose. There was a tendency for a lack of proportionality at the highest dose in the increase in AUC and C_{max} in the 5 subjects who completed the studies at all levels (table I), but this was not reflected in the statistical analysis: repeated measures analysis of the kinetic parameters showed no significant changes in t_{max} and $t_{½β}$ but showed that C_{max} and AUC increased linearly with dose ($p = 0.002$ and $p < 0.001$, respectively) across the range 1 to 8mg.

Pharmacodynamics

Both supine and standing blood pressure fell in all subjects following administration of a single dose of doxazosin and during maintenance administration of the drug. The magnitude of the fall averaged 20 to 40mm Hg: however, the study design and lack of placebo control precluded any detailed analysis of the data.

After the first dose of doxazosin 1mg, 5 subjects experienced symptoms of dizziness on standing, and 2 continued to report these symptoms during treatment with doxazosin 1mg once daily (an additional patient who was free of symptoms on the kinetic study day reported dizziness after exercise during maintenance treatment). Only 2 of 10 subjects reported dizziness while receiving doxazosin 2mg, 2 of 6 while receiving a dose of 4mg and 2 of 5 while receiving 8mg of the drug. Other symptoms reported included lethargy, nausea and headache, but these were mild and nonspecific.

Discussion

Doxazosin is a new α_1-adrenoceptor blocking drug chemically related to prazosin. The drugs share similar pharmacological actions; however, the half-life of doxazosin is 9 to 11 hours (Vincent et al. 1983), considerably longer than that of prazosin (2 to 4 hours) [Rubin et al. 1981; McNeil et al. 1988]. Doxazosin has been found to be effective in controlling blood pressure on a once-daily dosing regimen when given either as monotherapy or in combination with thiazide diuretics or β-blockers in the dose range 1 to 6mg (Cox et al. 1986). In the current study the pharmacokinetics of doxazosin (1 to 8mg daily) were determined in hypertensive subjects also receiving chlorothiazide 500mg. The results show that the drug was rapidly absorbed after oral administration, with peak concentrations occurring approximately 2 hours after drug administration and an elimination half-life of approximately 11 hours. These results are similar to those of Vincent et al. (1983, 1986) who determined the pharmacokinetics of doxazosin in healthy volunteers free of any additional drug therapy.

The present results also show that the pharmacokinetics of doxazosin during maintenance administration are similar to those after a single dose, and that the drug obeys approximately linear pharmacokinetics under steady-state conditions over the dose range 1 to 8mg. There was a tendency for a loss of proportionality in AUC at the highest dose, although the significance of this finding is difficult to assess because of the smaller number of subjects who received 8mg. In a recent study patients on different clinically effective doses of doxazosin were assessed, and a linear correlation was found between steady-state plasma concentrations and dose over the range 1 to 16mg (Frick et al. 1986).

Therapeutic Implications

In summary, the present study has demonstrated that the pharmacokinetic disposition of doxazosin in combination therapy with chlorothiazide is not significantly altered during maintenance therapy in hypertensive subjects, and that it remains approximately linear over the dose range 1 to 8mg daily.

Acknowledgements

This work was supported by a programme grant from the National Health and Medical Research Council of Australia, and by Pfizer Pty Ltd.

References

Cox DA, Leader JP, Milson JA, Singleton W. The antihypertensive effects of doxazosin: a clinical overview. British Journal of Clinical Pharmacology 21: 83S-90S, 1986

Frick MH, Halttunen P, Himanen P, Huttunen M, Porsti P, et al. A long-term double-blind comparison of doxazosin and atenolol in patients with mild to moderate essential hypertension. British Journal of Clinical Pharmacology 1: 55S-62S, 1986

Lund-Johansen P. Hemodynamic changes at rest and during exercise in long-term prazosin therapy for essential hypertension. Postgraduate Medical Journal 58 (Suppl.): 45-52, 1975

Lund-Johansen P, Omvik P, Haugland H. Acute and chronic haemodynamic effects of doxazosin in hypertension at rest and during exercise. British Journal of Clinical Pharmacology 21: 45S-54S, 1986

McNeil JJ, Drummer OH, Conway EL, Workman BS, Louis WJ. Effects of age on pharmacokinetics and blood pressure responses to prazosin and terazosin. Journal of Cardiovascular Pharmacology 10: 168-175, 1987

Rubin PC, Scott PJW, Reid JL. Prazosin disposition in young and elderly subjects. British Journal of Clinical Pharmacology 12: 401-404, 1981

Sachs FM, Dzau VJ. Adrenergic effects on plasma lipoprotein metabolism. Speculation on mechanisms of action. American Journal of Medicine 80 (Suppl. 2A): 71-81, 1986

Stokes GS. Prazosin. In Doyle AE (Ed.) Clinical pharmacology of antihypertensive drugs, Handbook of Hypertension, Vol. 5, pp. 350-375, Elsevier, Amsterdam, 1984

Vincent J, Elliot HL, Meredith PA, Reid JL. Doxazosin, an alpha-1-adrenoceptor antagonist: pharmacokinetics and concentration effect relationships in man. British Journal of Clinical Pharmacology 15: 719-725, 1983

Vincent J, Meredith PA, Elliott HL, Reid JL. The pharmacokinetics of doxazosin in elderly normotensives. British Journal of Clinical Pharmacology 21: 521-524, 1986

Wagner JG. Biopharmaceutics and relevant pharmacokinetics. In Drug Intelligence Publications, pp. 242-246, Hamilton Press, Hamilton, Illinois, 1971

Authors' address: Dr. *E.L. Conway*, University of Melbourne, Clinical Pharmacology and Therapeutics Units, Austin Hospital, Heidelberg, Victoria 3084 (Australia).

Clinical Pharmacokinetics

Cumulated Contents, Vol. 16, 1989

Leading Articles

65-73 Protein Binding Drug Displacement Interactions: Fact or Fiction?
MacKichan, J.J.

129-133 Clinical Significance of Differences in Bioavailability of Medroxyprogesterone Acetate Preparations
Stockdale, A.D. and *Rostom, A.Y.*

327-336 Clinical Pharmacokinetics-Pharmacodynamics of Anticancer Drugs
Evans, W.E. and *Relling, M.V.*

Review Articles

Drug Disposition

1-26 Clinical Pharmacokinetics of Non-Opiate Abused Drugs
Busto, U.; *Bendayan, R.* and *Sellers, E.M.*

74-85 Clinical Pharmacokinetics of Clofazimine: A Review
Holdiness, M.R.

193-214 Clinical Pharmacokinetic Properties of the Macrolide Antibiotics: Effects of Age and Various Pathophysiological States (Part I)
Periti, P.; Mazzei, T.; Mini, E. and *Novelli, A.*

215-237 Clinical Pharmacology of 5-Fluorouracil
Diasio, R.B. and *Harris, B.E.*

261-282 Clinical Pharmacokinetic Properties of the Macrolide Antibiotics: Effects of Age and Various Pathophysiological States (Part II)
Periti, P.; Mazzei, T.; Mini, E. and *Novelli, A.*

283-311 Clinical Pharmacokinetics of Epidural and Spinal Anaesthesia
Burm, A.G.L.

337-364 Pharmacokinetics of the Newer Benzodiazepines
Garzone, P.D. and *Kroboth, P.D.*

Clinical Pharmacokinetics and Disease Processes

86-99 Clinical Pharmacokinetics and Therapeutic Use of Hydralazine in Congestive Heart Failure
Mulrow, J.P. and *Crawford, M.H.*

134-161 Clinical Pharmacokinetics in Organ Transplant Patients
Venkataramanan, R.; Habucky, K.; Burckart, G.J. and *Ptachcinski, R.J.*

365-386 Clinical Pharmacokinetic Considerations in the Treatment of Patients with Leprosy
Venkatesan, K.

Pharmacokinetic-Pharmacodynamic Relationships

100-128 Pharmacokinetic-Pharmacodynamic Relationships of Oral Hypoglycaemic Agents: An Update
Marchetti, P. and *Navalesi, R.*

238-253 Clinical Pharmacokinetic Considerations in the Control of Oral Anticoagulant Therapy
Sketty, H.G.M.; Fennerty, A.G. and *Routledge, P.A.*

Pharmacokinetic Drug Interactions

162-179 Food Interactions with Sustained-Release Theophylline Preparations: A Review
Jonkman, J.H.G.

Drug Concentration Monitoring

27-37 Therapeutic Drug Monitoring of Cyclosporin: Practical Applications and Limitations
Rodighiero, V.

Clinical Pharmacokinetic Concepts

38-54 Saturable Pharmacokinetics in the Renal Excretion of Drugs
van Ginneken, C.A.M. and *Russel, F.G.M.*

Original Research Articles

55-64 Influence of Renal Function on the Pharmacokinetics and Cardiovascular Effects of Nisoldipine After Single and Multiple Dosing
van Harten, J.; Burggraaf, J.; van Brummelen, P. and *Breimer, D.D.*

180-185 Lack of Effect of Influenza Vaccine on the Pharmacokinetics of Antipyrine, Alprazolam, Paracetamol (Acetaminophen) and Lorazepam
Scavone, J.M.; Blyden, G.T. and *Greenblatt, D.J.*

186-191 Tianeptine and its Main Metabolite: Pharmacokinetics in Chronic Alcoholism and Cirrhosis
Royer, R.J.; Royer-Morrot, M.J.; Paille, F.; Barrucand, D.; Schmitt, J.; Defrance, R. and *Salvadori, C.*

254-260 Phenytoin Dosage Predictions in Paediatric Patients
Yuen, G.J.; Latimer, P.T.; Littlefield, L.C. and *Mackey, R.W.*

312-316 Clearance of the Antihistamine Doxylamine: Reduced in Elderly Men But Not in Elderly Women
Friedman, H.; Greenblatt, D.J.; Scavone, J.M.; Burstein, E.S.; Ochs, H.R.; Harmatz, J.S. and *Shader, R.I.*

317-325 Co-Trimoxazole (Sulphamethoxazole plus Trimethoprim): Peritoneal Barrier Transfer Pharmacokinetics
Svirbely, J.E.; Pesce, A.J.; Singh, S. and *O'Flaherty, E.J.*

387-391 Single-Dose and Steady-State Pharmacokinetics of Doxazosin Given in Combination with Chlorothiazide to Hypertensive Subjects
Conway, E.L.; McNeil, J.J.; Meng, L.; Drummer, O.H.; Howes, L.G.; Raymond, K. and *Louis, W.J.*

Supplement

1-64 **1.** Quinolone Pharmacokinetics: Focus on Enoxacin
Andriole, V. and *Lode, H.* (Eds)

Clinical Pharmacokinetics
Supplement

Quinolone Pharmacokinetics: Focus on Enoxacin

Guest Editors:
V.T. Andriole
H. Lode

Vol. 16, Supplement 1 (pp. 1-64) 1989
CPKNDH16 (S1) 1-64
ISSN: 0312-5963

USA • UNITED KINGDOM • JAPAN • HONG KONG • AUSTRALIA • NEW ZEALAND

Clinical Pharmacokinetics
Supplement

Supplement Production Team
Manager, Custom Publications: *Maire Neeson*
Senior Project Manager: *Gordon Mallarkey*
Project Managers: *Julia Ralston, Diana Shipp, Sandra U. Wilson*
Associate Project Managers: *Cushla M. Goode, Susan H. Talbot*
Senior Manuscript Editor: *Judith L. Taylor*
Manuscript Editors: *Carol A. d'H. Galvin, Veronica de Lautour*
Production Manager: *Karol Wilczynski*
Production Assistants: *Josie Whitehead, Bruce MacGregor, Gail Waring, Susan Brady*

President and Publisher: Graeme S. Avery
Executive Vice-President, Europe: Peter J. Buckle
Executive Vice-President, USA: Al Sander
Executive Vice-President, Japan: T. Harvey Oakes
Editor-in-Chief: Rennie C. Heel

Editor: George J. Mammen
Senior Managing Editor: Roderick H. Sayce
Senior Editor: Eugene M. Sorkin
Senior Assistant Editor: David R. Britten
Assistant Editor: Scott A. Mataga
Editorial Assistant: Paul C. Jinks

Aim and Scope: The Journal aims to assist in the further development of clinical pharmacokinetics, to promote communication and increased awareness within this specialty area and to further postgraduate education in clinical pharmacology and therapeutics. The Journal places particular emphasis on review articles but also welcomes original research articles. Both types of article consider the pharmacokinetic properties of drugs as related to their actual clinical use. This definition includes bioavailability studies, drug pharmacokinetics, plasma concentration monitoring of pharmacodynamic response, the relationship of drug pharmacokinetics to the therapeutic efficacy or toxicity of drugs etc. – all studied within the context of disease, pregnancy, age or other clinical and pathophysiological determinants of drug response.

USA Postmasters: Send address changes to ADIS Press International Inc., Suite B-30, Oxford Court Business Center, 582 Middletown Blvd, Langhorne, PA 19047. Air freight and mailing in the USA by Publications Expediting Inc., 200 Meacham Avenue, Elmont, NY 11003.

Clinical Pharmacokinetics (ISSN 0312-5963) is published monthly by ADIS Press Limited, 41 Centorian Drive, Private Bag, Mairangi Bay, Auckland 10, New Zealand. Second class postage is paid at Jamaica, NY 11431. Printed in Hong Kong by Caritas Printing Training Centre.

Quinolone Pharmacokinetics: Focus on Enoxacin

Proceedings of a session from the International Congress for Infectious Diseases held in Rio de Janeiro on 20 April 1988

Presented as a service to the medical profession by Parke-Davis Division, Warner-Lambert Company

Guest Editors
V.T. Andriole
H. Lode

Technical Editor
Paul E. Battershill

Clinical Pharmacokinetics is indexed in 'Current Contents', 'Index Medicus' and 'Excerpta Medica'.

Clinical Pharmacokinetics
Supplement

Contents Vol. 16, Supplement 1, 1989

iv **List of Contributors**

v **Foreword**

1-4 Unique Aspects of Quinolone Pharmacokinetics
H. Lode, G. Höffken, K. Borner and *P. Koeppe*

5-24 Pharmacokinetic Disposition of Quinolones in Human Body Fluids and Tissues
F. Sörgel, U. Jaehde, K. Naber and *U. Stephan*

25-31 Clinical Significance of Antibiotic Tissue Penetration
J.J. Schentag

32-37 Tissue Penetration and Clinical Efficacy of Enoxacin in Urinary Tract Infections
S.J. Childs

38-45 Tissue Penetration and Clinical Efficacy of Enoxacin in Respiratory Tract Infections
M.J. Wood

46-51 Review of Tissue Penetration and Clinical Efficacy of Enoxacin in Skin and Skin Structure Infections and in Osteomyelitis
G.A. Pankey

52-58 Enoxacin Absorption and Elimination Characteristics
R.D. Toothaker

59-64 Clinical Overview of Enoxacin
S.H. Zinner

Contributors

Session Chairmen

V.T. Andriole
Infectious Disease Section, Yale University, School of Medicine, Connecticut (USA)

E. Calderón-Jaimes
Instituto Nacional de Perinatologia, Montes Urales, Mexico City (Mexico)

Contributors

S.J. Childs
Department of Surgery, Community Health Sciences, University of Alabama, Tuscaloosa, Alabama (USA)

H. Lode
Medical Department, Klinikum Steglitz, Berlin (Federal Republic of Germany)

G.A. Pankey
Department of Infectious Diseases, Ochsner Clinic, New Orleans, Louisiana (USA)

J.J. Schentag
Clinical Pharmacokinetics Laboratory, Millard Fillmore Hospital, Buffalo, New York (USA)

F. Sörgel
Institute for Biomedical and Pharmaceutical Research, Nürnberg (Federal Republic of Germany)

R.D. Toothaker
Parke Davis Pharmaceutical Research Division, Warner-Lambert Company, Ann Arbor, Michigan (USA)

M.J. Wood
Department of Communicable and Tropical Diseases, East Birmingham Hospital, Birmingham (United Kingdom)

S.H. Zinner
Division of Infectious Diseases, Roger Williams General Hospital, Providence, Rhode Island (USA)

Foreword

In the past 20 years, the sensitivity profiles of many bacteria have changed; this has had a major clinical impact on our antimicrobial use. As a consequence of the increasing resistance of bacteria, we have had to search for agents with more potent antibacterial activity and more useful spectra of activity, as well as more useful pharmacokinetics and fewer side effects. The newer quinolones, including enoxacin, exhibit several of these interesting characteristics.

The purpose of this supplement, a report of the proceedings of a symposium presented at the International Congress for Infectious Diseases in Rio de Janeiro and chaired by Dr Vincent T. Andriole and Dr Ernesto Calderón-Jaimes, is to present a comprehensive review of the pharmacokinetics of enoxacin and to survey clinical experience until now in the context of these pharmacokinetic properties.

Enoxacin pharmacokinetics is an important and timely subject, because the newer quinolone antimicrobials have many characteristics that are especially useful today. Of obvious importance, in this class of agents, is the spectrum of activity, which includes a wide range of clinically important pathogens. Of equal importance, although often less well understood, are the pharmacokinetic characteristics of these agents and their effects on clinical use.

In this publication, Prof. Hartmut Lode provides a review of basic quinolone pharmacokinetics, Prof. Fritz Sörgel reviews the penetration of quinolones into body tissues and fluids, Dr Jerome Schentag provides a comprehensive overview of the antibiotic tissue penetration that places the quinolones in the same context as other classes of antimicrobials, and Dr Roger Toothaker reviews the specific pharmacokinetic data on enoxacin.

The pharmacokinetic data are put into clinical perspective by Dr Stacy Childs, who reviews clinical experience with enoxacin in infections of the urinary tract, Dr Martin Wood, who covers enoxacin treatment of respiratory problems, and Dr George Pankey, who reviews the use of enoxacin in infections of the skin and soft tissues. Stephen Zinner provides a comprehensive overview of published studies of enoxacin in a variety of infections.

Vincent T. Andriole and *Hartmut Lode*

Clinical Pharmacokinetics 16 (Suppl. 1): 1-4 (1989)
0312-5963/89/0001-0001/$2.00/0

Unique Aspects of Quinolone Pharmacokinetics

H. Lode, G. Höffken, K. Borner and *P. Koeppe*

Medical Department of Klinikum Steglitz, Freie Universität, Berlin, Federal Republic of Germany

Summary

Despite some limited differences in pharmacokinetic parameters among the newer quinolones, their pharmacology is characterised by high volumes of distribution, long elimination half-lives, good to excellent bioavailability, low protein binding, limited biotransformation and different elimination pathways (mainly through the kidneys). The unique aspects of quinolones in comparison with β-lactams and aminoglycosides are their higher volumes of distribution, longer elimination half-lives and their intracellular high concentration, especially in phagocytic cells.

Many studies have shown that the pharmacokinetics of the quinolone antimicrobials differ in many respects from the pharmacokinetics of most other groups of antimicrobial agents. Since the older quinolones are characterised by an unfavourable pharmacokinetic profile (low serum concentrations and short half-lives), this paper will focus only on the fluorinated modern quinolones – ciprofloxacin, enoxacin, norfloxacin, ofloxacin and pefloxacin. The introduction of fluorine atoms in the C_6 position and other different side chains in positions C_1 and C_7 resulted in an increased antibacterial activity and favourable pharmacokinetic properties, with high serum concentrations, longer elimination half-lives and excellent bioavailability after oral administration. The results of recent studies of ciprofloxacin and ofloxacin (Borner et al. 1986; Höffken et al. 1985; Lode et al. 1987a) have been incorporated in an analysis of the different pharmacokinetic parameters, which also includes the available data on enoxacin, norfloxacin and pefloxacin.

1. Absorption

The newer quinolones are 80 to 100% bioavailable; exceptions are norfloxacin, which is only 30 to 40% bioavailable after an oral dose, and ciprofloxacin, with a good bioavailability of between 60 and 80%. The rate of absorption from the intestinal tract is rapid, with peak plasma concentrations occurring between 1 and 3 hours after oral administration. The most rapid absorption occurs with ciprofloxacin and ofloxacin and the slowest absorption with enoxacin (Wise et al. 1986). The concomitant ingestion of food alters the peak plasma concentration to a limited degree, but AUC or elimination half-life does not change; the time to reach C_{max} is shorter in the fasting state, and slightly delayed with food with ciprofloxacin (Wingender et al. 1985).

Absorption of the quinolones is reduced by concomitant administration of aluminium and magnesium hydroxide, because of chelate formation (Höffken et al. 1988).

2. Distribution

The newer quinolones are widely distributed throughout the body, with high volumes of distribution exceeding 1.5 to 3.5 L/kg. Volumes range from approximately 100 to more than 300L for adults. The volume of distribution is independent of dose; the clinical consequences of this specific distribution of the quinolones is discussed by Sörgel et al. (this issue pp. 5-24). However, in the literature and in our studies, different volumes of distribution were calculated for the different quinolones. There is a tendency to higher volumes of distribution with ciprofloxacin and lower volumes of distribution with ofloxacin; volumes of distribution with other quinolones range between these 2 extremes (Neuman 1988).

3. Metabolism

The metabolic biotransformation of most fluoroquinolones occurs primarily at the piperazinyl ring in the C_7 position. Some of the metabolites identified to date are common to several of the quinolones. The major metabolites are the oxo-metabolite, the N-desmethyl-metabolite and the desethylene- or the sulfo-metabolite. Some of these metabolites are still active against bacteria; the oxo- and N-formyl-metabolites, in particular, have antimicrobial activity (Borner & Lode 1986).

Biotransformation is extensive with pefloxacin (50 to 85%), medium with ciprofloxacin and enoxacin (15 to 30%), low with norfloxacin (< 15%) and very low with ofloxacin (< 10%).

4. Elimination

The quinolones are excreted by renal, biliary, hepatic and intestinal metabolic pathways. Individual compounds may be eliminated by a combination of routes. The elimination half-lives range from 3 to 5 hours (ciprofloxacin) and 8 to 10 hours (pefloxacin) [Lode et al. 1987b]. Faecal concentrations of the fluoroquinolones are related to the percentage of their gastrointestinal absorption and biliary or intestinal elimination. Biliary concentrations of all the newer quinolones are 2 to 10 times greater than plasma concentrations (Neuman 1988).

Table I. Pharmacokinetic properties of enoxacin (adapted from Wise et al. 1984)

Site, parameter	Enoxacin	
	400mg IV	600mg PO
Serum		
T_{max}(h)		1.9 ± 1.0
C_{max}(mg/L)	5.5 ± 1.8	3.7 ± 0.5
$T_{1/2\beta}$ (h)	5.1 ± 0.4	6.2 ± 1.1
$AUC_{0-\infty}$ (mg/L · h)	17.8 ± 3.5	28.8 ± 4.9
K_a (h^{-1})		2.1 ± 1.1
Blister fluid		
T_{max} (h)	0.5 ± 0.8	3.7 ± 1.0
C_{max} (mg/L)	2.2 ± 0.5	2.9 ± 0.5
$T_{1/2}$ (h)	6.5 ± 0.7	7.2 ± 2.5
$AUC_{0-\infty}$ (mg/L · h)	23.1 ± 2.8	32.8 ± 4.9
Urine		
24-h excretion (% of dose)	46.4 ± 7.7	61.2 ± 7.4

Within the first 24 hours, 30 to 40% of an oral ciprofloxacin dose is excreted in the urine; the total body clearance values for ciprofloxacin reported in the literature range from 15 to 19.5 L/h (Jack et al. 1985) or 18 to 22.8 L/h (Borner et al. 1986). Renal clearance constitutes 56 to 70% of total body clearance (Drusano et al. 1986; Höffken et al. 1985). As these values are about 2 to 3 times greater than normal creatinine clearance, an active tubular secretion mechanism would seem to be involved in the elimination of ciprofloxacin (Höffler et al. 1984). This mechanism also appears to apply to norfloxacin, ofloxacin and enoxacin. Support for this hypothesis also comes from studies involving the administration of probenecid, which inhibits active secretion processes and increases the half-life of ciprofloxacin (Wingender et al. 1984).

The elimination half-life of enoxacin is 5 to 7 hours and appears to increase with the duration of treatment (Wolff et al. 1984). Approximately 60% of an oral dose is excreted by the kidneys within 24 hours (Wise et al. 1984) [table I]. Renal clearance comprises about 30% of the total body clearance of 0.4 to 0.5 L/h/kg after a single dose.

Table II. Comparison of the pharmacokinetic properties of new quinolones

Drug	Oral dose (mg)	Bio-avail-ability (%)	C_{max} (mg/L)	$T_{1/2}$ (h)	Vd (L)	$AUC_{0-\infty}$ (mg/L · h)	Protein binding (%)	Clearance IV/oral (L/h)		Route of elimination (% of dose)		Biotransformation	
								total	renal	renal	faecal	No. of metabolites	% of dose
Cip	500	60-80	1.8-2.8	3.3-5.4	307	7-10	20-40	39.1	21.4	40-60	15	4	6-12
Eno	400	80	2.8-3.6	3.3-5.8	175	16-25	35	21.0	12.0	65-72	18	1	7-15
Nor	400	35-45	1.4-1.8	3.3-5.5	>100	4-5[a]	14	18.0	18.0	30-40	28	5	8
Ofl	400	85-95	3.5-5.3	5.0-7.0	90	28-35	25	12.8	10.4	70-90	4	3	6
Pef	400	90-100	3.8-5.6	7.5-10.0	139	48-58	20-30	8.9	0.4	60		5	50

a AUC_{0-12h}.

Abbreviations: Cip = ciprofloxacin; Eno = enoxacin; Nor = norfloxacin; Ofl = ofloxacin; Pef = pefloxacin.

The elimination half-life of pefloxacin ranges from 8 to 14 hours (Sörgel et al. 1985) and results in accumulation during twice-daily administration. Again, there is an increase in half-life during long term administration.

Some accumulation of ofloxacin occurs during repeated administration because of its half-life of 6 to 8 hours (Humbert et al. 1985). Approximately 80 to 90% is excreted unchanged in the urine within 24 hours (Lode et al. 1987a), which indicates that, in patients with normal renal function, renal elimination probably accounts for less than 20 to 30% of the elimination (table II).

5. Interactions

The reduction of theophylline clearance by those quinolones that are metabolised primarily in the liver (enoxacin and ciprofloxacin) is of clinical relevance (Lode 1988; Schwartz et al. 1988; Wijnands et al. 1984); increased plasma theophylline concentrations were found in patients treated with theophylline and quinolone derivatives.

Furthermore, cimetidine inhibits the hepatic metabolism of pefloxacin and increases its half-life (Sörgel et al. 1988).

6. Unique Aspects of Quinolones

The pharmacokinetics of newer quinolones are characterised by high volumes of distribution, long elimination half-lives, good to excellent bioavailability, low protein binding, limited biotransformation and different elimination pathways, mainly through the kidneys (table III). In comparison with other commonly used antibiotics, such as the β-lactams or aminoglycosides, the longer half-lives of the quinolones, the low (once- or twice-daily) rate of administration and, particularly, the high

Table III. Specific aspects of quinolone pharmacokinetics

After oral administration, moderate to excellent bioavailability
Long biological half-lives
High volumes of distribution
Low protein binding
Mainly renal excretion
Limited biotransformation

volume of distribution provide the basis for successful treatment of intracellular localised infections or other specific localised infections such as osteomyelitis or prostatitis.

References

Borner K, Höffken G, Lode H, Koeppe P, Prinzing C, et al. Pharmacokinetics of ciprofloxacin in healthy volunteers after oral and intravenous administration. European Journal of Clinical Microbiology 5: 179-186, 1986

Borner K, Lode H. Biotransformation von ausgewählten Gyrasehemmern. Infection 14 (Suppl. 1): 54-59, 1986

Drusano GL, Standiford HC, Plaisance K, Forrest A, Leslie J, et al. Absolute oral bioavailability of ciprofloxacin. Antimicrobial Agents and Chemotherapy 30: 444-446, 1986

Höffken G, Lode H, Prinzing C, Borner U, Koeppe P. Pharmacokinetics of ciprofloxacin after oral and parenteral administration. Antimicrobial Agents and Chemotherapy 27: 375-379, 1985

Höffken G, Lode H, Wiley R, Glatzel TD, Sievers D, et al. Pharmacokinetics and bioavailability of ciprofloxacin and ofloxacin: effect of food and antacid intake. Reviews of Infectious Diseases 10 (Suppl. 1): 138-139, 1988

Höffler D, Dalhoff A, Gau W, Beermann D, Michl A. Dose- and sex-independent disposition of ciprofloxacin. European Journal of Clinical Microbiology 3: 363-366, 1984

Humbert G, Brosa R, Couet W, Fourtillan JB, Vincent de Laurier M, et al. Pharmacokinetics of ofloxacin in young healthy subjects (abstract) 14th International Congress of Chemotherapy, Kyoto, 1985

Jack DB, Wilkins MR, Laugher SJ, Kendall MJ, Wise R. A clinical pharmacokinetic study of ciprofloxacin administered chronically as iv bolus doses to young healthy volunteers (abstract S-41-12) 14th International Congress of Chemotherapy, Kyoto, 1985

Lode H, Höffken G, Olschewski P, Sievers B, Borner K, et al. Pharmacokinetics of ofloxacin after oral and parenteral administration. Antimicrobial Agents and Chemotherapy 31: 1338-1342, 1987a

Lode H, Höffken G, Prinzing C, Glatzel P, Wiley R, et al. Comparative pharmacokinetics of new quinolones. Drugs 34 (Suppl. 1): 21-25, 1987b

Neuman N. Clinical pharmacokinetics of 4-quinolones. Clinical Pharmacokinetics 14: 96-121, 1988

Schwartz J, Jauregni L, Lettieri J, Bachmann K. Impact of ciprofloxacin on theophylline clearance and steady-state concentrations in serum. Antimicrobial Agents and Chemotherapy 32: 75-77, 1988

Sörgel F, Brüning I, Stephan U, Lang E. The pharmacokinetics of pefloxacin and its metabolites in healthy volunteers (abstract S-41-10) 14th International Congress of Chemotherapy, Kyoto, 1985

Sörgel F, Mahr G, Koch HU, et al. Effects of cimetidine on the pharmacokinetics of pefloxacin in healthy volunteers. Reviews of Infectious Diseases 10 (Suppl. 1): S137, 1988

Wijnands W, Van Herwaarden C, Vree T. Enoxacin raises plasma theophylline concentrations. Lancet 2: 108-109, 1984

Wingender W, Grade K, Gau W, et al. Pharmacokinetics of ciprofloxacin after oral and IV administration. European Journal of Clinical Microbiology 3: 355-359, 1984

Wingender W, Forster W, Beermann D, Rohweder T. Effect of the gastric emptying time on rat and extent of the systemic availability of ciprofloxacin in humans (abstract) 14th International Congress of Chemotherapy, Kyoto, 1985

Wise R, Lockley R, Dent J, Webberly M. Pharmacokinetics and tissue penetration of enoxacin. Antimicrobial Agents and Chemotherapy 26: 17-19, 1984

Wise R, Lister D, McNully CAM, Griggs D, Andrews JM. The comparative pharmacokinetics of five quinolones. Journal of Antimicrobial Chemotherapy 18 (Suppl. D): 71-81, 1986

Wolff M, Regnier B, Baldoss C, Nkam M, Vachon F. Penetration of pefloxacin into cerebrospinal fluid of patients with meningitis. Antimicrobial Agents and Chemotherapy 26: 289-291, 1984

Author's address: Prof. *Hartmut Lode*, Medical Department, Klinikum Steglitz, Hindenburgdamm 30, D-1000 Berlin 45 (Federal Republic of Germany).

Clinical Pharmacokinetics 16 (Suppl. 1): 5-24 (1989)
0312-5963/89/0001-0005/$10.00/0

Pharmacokinetic Disposition of Quinolones in Human Body Fluids and Tissues

Fritz Sörgel[1], *Ulrich Jaehde*[1], *Kurt Naber*[2] and *Ulrich Stephan*[3]

1 IBMP – Institute for Biomedical and Pharmaceutical Research, Nürnberg, Federal Republic of Germany
2 Department of Urology, Elisabeth-Hospital, Straubing, Federal Republic of Germany
3 Department of Pediatrics, University of Essen, Essen, Federal Republic of Germany

Summary *The unique pharmacokinetic properties as well as the body fluid and tissue penetration of quinolones are discussed.*

Quinolones are well absorbed from the gastrointestinal tract and are eliminated with considerable differences in their terminal half-lives. The major elimination pathways of quinolones are renal excretion and hepatic metabolism. Renally, these drugs undergo the potential excretion mechanisms (glomerular filtration, tubular secretion, reabsorption). In the liver, they are metabolised primarily by oxidation as well as by conjugative pathways. However, the metabolic pattern and extent of metabolism differ significantly between individual agents.

Alterations in the pharmacokinetic disposition of these agents in liver and renal failure as well as in elderly patients are observed as predicted from their excretion pattern. In addition, quinolones can interact with a number of other compounds at hepatic (e.g. with xanthine derivatives), renal (with probenecid) and gastrointestinal (with antacids) sites.

The volume of distribution of quinolones is considerably higher than body volume, which suggests intracellular penetration. Studies on tissue penetration show that concentrations exceeding plasma levels are obtained in most tissues. The highest tissue/plasma concentration ratios are achieved in lung and kidney, whereas concentrations in fat are considerably lower than in plasma.

Body fluid penetration is introduced as a new approach to evaluate distribution kinetics of quinolones. With the exception of those in nasal secretions and ejaculate, body fluid levels of these drugs rarely reach plasma levels. The body fluid penetration model allows for differentiation among individual agents. There is no apparent relationship between differences in body fluid penetration of quinolones and differences in volume of distribution. For the clinical use of these drugs it is important that the concentrations achieved in body fluids and tissues are sufficient to kill most pathogens. A discussion on the relationship between plasma and tissue levels and the MICs of quinolones is, however, beyond the scope of this article.

In the treatment of infections with antibacterial drugs, the concentration at the infection site is an important factor for successful eradication of pathogens. Measurements of β-lactams and aminoglycosides in tissues show that these drugs reach concentrations high enough to kill pathogens, although their volume of distribution is small (Wise 1986). Previous hypotheses based on the determination of the volume of distribution of β-lactams suggested that the volume into which β-lactams distribute is equivalent to the extracellular space (Wise 1986). More recent experience and re-evaluation of that concept, however, support the view that the similarity of the value for volume of distribution of β-lactams and that for the volume of the body's extracellular space is merely numerical rather than of anatomical or physiological meaning. The calculation of the pure pharmacokinetic term 'volume of distribution' from serum or plasma data requires the assumption that the human body can be regarded as a beaker without any diffusion barriers. The volume of distribution simply relates clearance and the elimination rate constant ($CL_{tot} = Vd \times k_e$) and may therefore be of little help when speculating about the concentrations in body fluids or tissues.

Other approaches to predict tissue concentrations were based on plasma concentration versus time curves, protein binding and calculations of volumes of distribution. Even the most sophisticated physiologically based models, however, do not allow the reliable prediction of individual tissue levels. Actual measurement of drug concentrations in tissues and body fluids as reported in this review is, in our opinion, still the most promising approach.

Quinolones differ from β-lactams and most other antibacterials in their high volume of distribution, which exceeds body volume by up to 3-fold. Although it is clear from that finding that the distribution of quinolones cannot be limited to the extracellular space, it is not apparent whether quinolone molecules are bound to the outside of cell membranes or penetrate into the intracellular space. Penetration into host cells is, however, very likely, and is also supported by results on the distribution of these agents in blood cells (Easmon & Crane 1985; Silvain et al. 1987). The shift of drug molecules from extracellular to intracellular space leads to lower quinolone blood levels compared with β-lactams.

In this situation, any additional measurement of drug levels in the extravascular space may help to elucidate the disposition of quinolones in the human body. Numerous investigations of quinolone body fluid and tissue penetration have been performed over the last few years. Recently, our group introduced a new approach to study the penetration of quinolones into secretions of the eye, skin, digestive system, respiratory and genitourinary tracts. Preliminary data previously published by us in abstract form will be presented.

The major aim of this paper is to critically review the data available on basic pharmacokinetic parameters and body fluid and tissue penetration by quinolones. Particular attention will be given to the results generated by our group to ensure identical methods of sampling, sample handling, drug measurement and pharmacokinetic analysis in the studies reported here. Since the pharmacokinetic analysis of body fluid and tissue penetration differs considerably between different authors, we have tried to standardise published data by relating body fluid/tissue and plasma parameters such as C_{max} and AUC values. If authors did not calculate these ratios themselves, we performed the calculations from published data; however, this article does not attempt to include all material published on the issues discussed.

1. Basic Pharmacokinetics

Although there are minor structural differences between quinolones (fig. 1), considerable differences in their pharmacokinetic disposition have been observed. The basic pharmacokinetic parameters for individual quinolones are presented in table I.

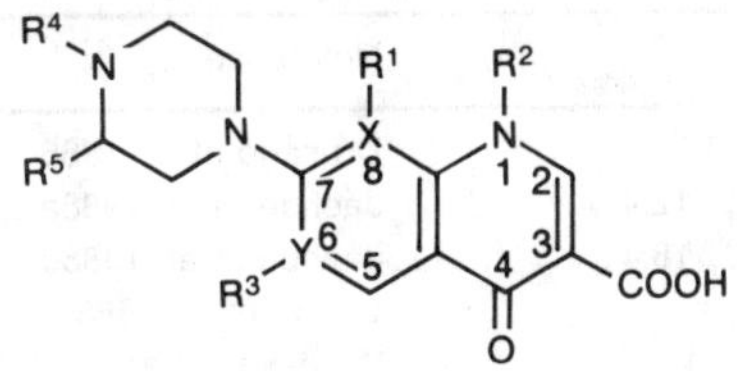

Compound	X	Y	R1	R2	R3	R4	R5
Ciprofloxacin	C	C	H		F	H	H
Difloxacin	C	C	H	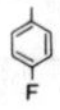	F	CH_3	H
Enoxacin	N	C	-	C_2H_5	F	H	H
Fleroxacin	C	C	F	CH_2-CH_2-F	F	CH_3	H
Lomefloxacin	C	C	F	C_2H_5	F	H	CH_3
Norfloxacin	C	C	H	C_2H_5	F	H	H
Ofloxacin	C	C	-O-CH_2-CH(CH_3)-		F	CH_3	H
Pefloxacin	C	C	H	C_2H_5	F	CH_3	H
Pipemidic acid	N	N	-	C_2H_5	-	H	H
Temafloxacin	C	C	H	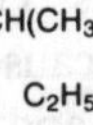	F	H	CH_3

Fig. 1. Chemical structure of quinolones.

1.1 Absorption

The absolute oral bioavailability of quinolones (table II) varies from less than 40% for norfloxacin to virtually complete absorption of fleroxacin, lomefloxacin, ofloxacin and pefloxacin. N-methylation of the piperazine substituent in the 4-position and an additional nitrogen atom located within the nucleus of the quinolone molecule improve the absolute bioavailability of these drugs (Jaehde et al. 1987a; Sörgel et al. 1987a). This is demonstrated by comparisons of norfloxacin with either pefloxacin (N-methylation) or enoxacin (additional N-atom in the 8-position of the quinolone nucleus). The absorption rate constants (k_a) were found to be similar for all quinolones, ranging from 2.1 to 3.2 h^{-1} (Wise et al. 1986) and thus indicating rapid absorption. This is also apparent from the t_{max} values of less than 2 hours observed in many pharmacokinetic studies in which oral quinolone formulations were used.

1.2 Distribution

The penetration of drugs into the extravascular

Table I. Basic pharmacokinetic parameters of quinolones (this table primarily reviews work by our group, since data have been generated by identical analytical and pharmacokinetic methods)

Drug	Dose (mg) [F]	Vd_β (L)	$t_{1/2}$ (h)	CL_{tot} (ml/min)	CL_R (ml/min)	CL_{NR} (ml/min)	Reference
Ciprofloxacin	200 IV	151 ± 28	3.3 ± 0.4	531 ± 56	267 ± 41	264 ± 36	Jaehde et al. 1988a
Difloxacin	400 PO	98 ± 10 (Vd_β/F)	27.1 ± 3.3	41 ± 5.5 (CL_{tot}/F)	4.3 ± 1.4	37[a]	Granneman et al. 1986
Enoxacin	400 IV	211 ± 30	5.1 ± 0.7	479 ± 37	257 ± 15	222 ± 34	Jaehde et al. 1988c
Fleroxacin	400 PO [0.96]	101 ± 22 (Vd_β/F)	10.8 ± 1.6	108 ± 15 (CL_{tot}/F)	68 ± 12	40 ± 15	Sörgel et al. 1988e
Lomefloxacin	400 PO [1][b]	140 ± 46 (Vd_β/F)	6.6 ± 1.1	242 ± 60 (CL_{tot}/F)	172 ± 46	70 ± 22	Metz et al. unpublished data
Norfloxacin	800 PO [0.35]	223 ± 97 (Vd_β/F)	5.0 ± 0.7	506 ± 211 (CL_{tot}/F)	236 ± 56	270[a]	Mahr et al. 1987
Ofloxacin	200 IV	86 ± 10	4.3 ± 0.3	234 ± 28	190 ± 27	44[a]	Lode et al. 1987b
Pefloxacin	400 IV	101 ± 25	10.2 ± 2.6	118 ± 31	11.7 ± 2.3	106 ± 30	Jaehde et al. 1988a
Pipemidic acid	100 IV	116 ± 7	3.1 ± 0.3	428 ± 34	367 ± 41	61[a]	Klinge et al. 1984

a Calculated from mean CL_{tot} and CL_R values.
b Not yet experimentally proven.
Abbreviations: Vd_β = volume of distribution; $t_{1/2}$ = half-life; CL_{tot} = total clearance; CL_R = renal clearance; CL_{NR} = non-renal clearance; F = bioavailability; IV = intravenous; PO = oral.

Table II. Bioavailability (F) of quinolones after oral administration

Drug	Dose (mg)	Formulation	F(%)	Reference
Ciprofloxacin	200	Tablet	69 ± 7	Drusano et al. 1986
	500	Tablet	59.6 ± 12.4	Jaehde et al. 1988a
Enoxacin	400	Tablet	76.5 ± 18.4	Jaehde et al. 1988c
	200	Capsule	87[a]	Chang et al. 1988
Fleroxacin	400	Tablet	99 ± 14	Weidekamm et al. 1987
Norfloxacin	400	Tablet	30-40[a]	MSD Research Laboratories, Rahway, NJ, USA
Ofloxacin	200	Tablet	96[a]	Lode et al. 1987b
Pefloxacin	400	Tablet	98 ± 20	Sörgel et al. 1988c
	600	Tablet	91.0 ± 13.3	Zürcher et al. 1988b
Pipemidic acid	100	Tablet	93.1 ± 11.4	Klinge et al. 1984

a No standard deviation available.

space depends primarily on the following 4 factors:
- protein binding
- lipophilicity
- acid-base properties
- molecular size.

The extent of protein binding determines the amount of drug available for diffusion across capillary membranes. Quinolones exhibit low protein binding, ranging from 14 to 51% (table III). Studies evaluating the high performance liquid chromatography retention behaviour of these agents show that the lipophilicity of quinolones is greatest at a neutral pH (fig. 2), suggesting that a blood pH of 7.4 favours the passage of these compounds through capillary membranes. The pH dependence of lipophilicity may also cause 'ion-trapping' of quinolones in body fluids and tissues with a slightly acid or basic pH (e.g. inflamed tissues), because the quinolone molecule is more ionised in these compartments, which reduces the movement of the molecule back into the plasma. This can lead to higher tissue (body fluid) levels than those in plasma. Although low protein binding, high lipophilicity at blood pH and the relatively small molecular size of quinolones are certainly important factors for an extensive distribution into body fluids and tissues, other factors, such as binding at the outer or inner cell membrane, may be of equal importance.

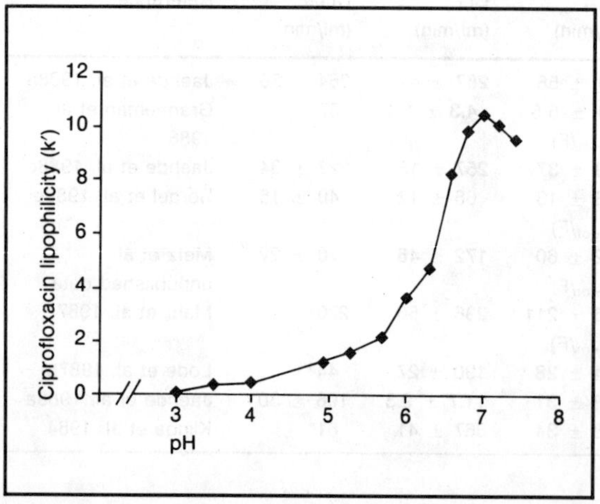

Fig. 2. Lipophilicity (k') of ciprofloxacin as a function of pH (after Gruber et al. 1988) [pH was not elevated beyond 7.4 because of column material decomposition at alkaline pH].

The volume of distribution (Vd_β) of quinolones ranges from 86 to 223L (fig. 3). There is no apparent relationship between the chemical structure of these compounds and the volume of distribution. As with any compilation of literature, data differences appearing between agents may be caused by different methods of pharmacokinetic analysis, i.e. use or non-use of pharmacokinetic models.

Our group has therefore performed several crossover studies with different quinolones. A recent intraindividual crossover comparison of ciprofloxacin and pefloxacin in 12 volunteers resulted in a significantly smaller volume of distribution for pefloxacin (Jaehde et al. 1988a). There-

Table III. Binding of quinolones to plasma proteins

Drug	Protein binding (%)	Reference
Ciprofloxacin	39.6[a]	Höffken et al. 1985
Difloxacin	42[a]	Granneman et al. 1986
Enoxacin	51.2 ± 10.6	Wijnands et al. 1988
Fleroxacin	23.0 ± 1.0	Brandt & Meyer 1985
Norfloxacin	14[a]	MSD Research Laboratories, Rahway, NJ, USA
Ofloxacin	25.0 ± 5.7	Lode et al. 1987b
Pefloxacin	20-30[a]	Montay et al. 1984
Pipemidic acid	15-39[a]	Klinge et al. 1984

a No standard deviation available.

fore, it is believed that distinct differences in the volume of distribution of the individual quinolones do exist; however, the reason for these differences as well as their relevance to tissue penetration are still unclear. Furthermore, the measured volume of distribution cannot be used to predict concentrations of quinolones in body fluids and tissues.

The available literature on body fluid and tissue penetration of quinolones will be reviewed and discussed in sections 3 and 4.

1.3 Elimination

Quinolones are eliminated by renal excretion, hepatic metabolism and probably gastrointestinal secretion. As with most drugs, the dosage regimen is usually based on terminal half-life, which depends on distribution and elimination. According to their half-life, quinolones may be classified into the following 5 groups:

- compounds with a half-life < 4 hours: ciprofloxacin, pipemidic acid
- compounds with a half-life of 4 to 6 hours: enoxacin, norfloxacin, ofloxacin
- compounds with a half-life of 6 to 8 hours: lomefloxacin, temafloxacin
- compounds with a half-life of 9 to 11 hours: fleroxacin, pefloxacin

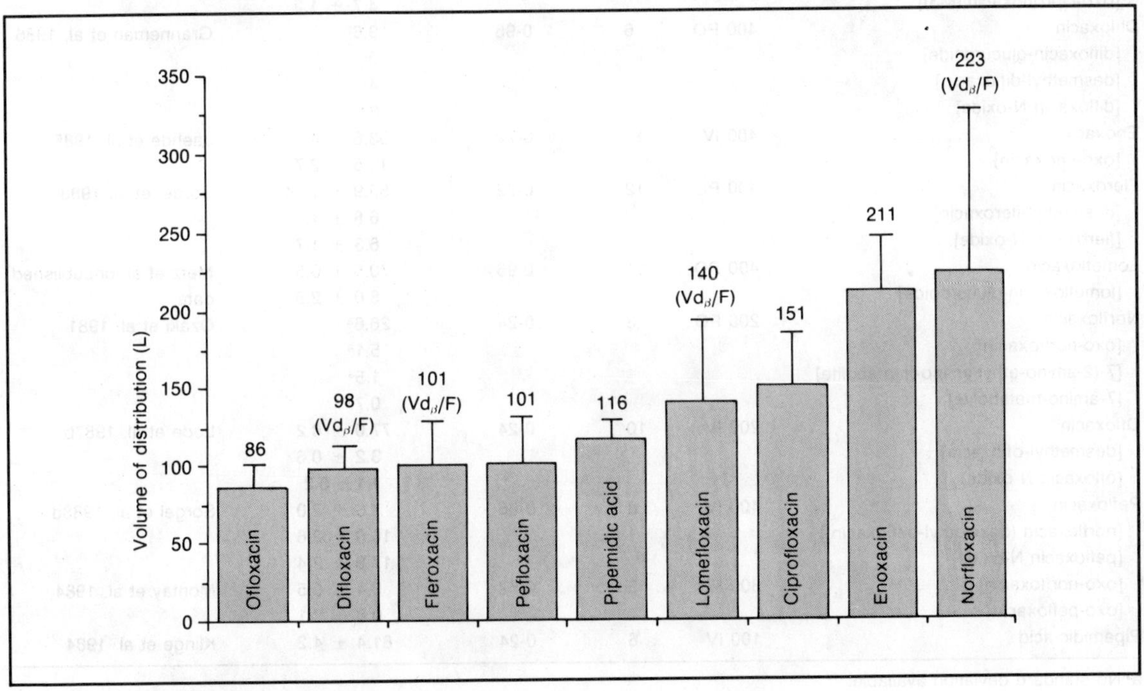

Fig. 3. Volume of distribution (Vd_β) of quinolones (for references see table I).

● compounds with a half-life > 25 hours: difloxacin.

The differences in half-life reflect differences in total clearance and volume of distribution among the individual quinolones (table I).

2. *Handling by Elimination Organs*

2.1 Kidney

Renal excretion is the most important elimination pathway of quinolones and their metabolites. Although ciprofloxacin, enoxacin, fleroxacin, lomefloxacin, norfloxacin, ofloxacin and temafloxacin are primarily excreted unchanged, only 7.6% of parent pefloxacin and 9.6% of parent difloxacin are recovered in urine. Pefloxacin is mostly excreted as metabolites (table IV). Because of their relatively low molecular weight and protein binding, quinolones and their metabolites are excreted largely by glomerular filtration. A renal clearance higher than the glomerular filtration rate (80-120 ml/min in healthy adults) suggests additional tubular secretion, whereas a lower renal clearance suggests tubular reabsorption. As shown in figure 4, ciprofloxacin, enoxacin, norfloxacin, ofloxacin and pipemidic acid are predominantly secreted, while difloxacin and pefloxacin are predominantly reabsorbed. The observed pH dependence of renal

Table IV. Urinary excretion of quinolones and their metabolites in healthy volunteers (this table primarily reviews work by our group, since data have been generated by identical analytical and pharmacokinetic methods)

Parent drug [metabolite]	Dose (mg)	No. of volunteers	Collection time interval (h)	Urinary excretion (% of dose)	Reference
Ciprofloxacin	200 IV	12	0-72	50.4 ± 5.2	Jaehde et al. 1988d
[7-(2-amino-ethyl-amino-)metabolite (M1)]				2.1 ± 0.6	
[sulfonyl-ciprofloxacin (M2)]				3.0 ± 1.8	
[oxo-ciprofloxacin (M3)]				4.7 ± 1.2	
Difloxacin	400 PO	6	0-96	9.6[a]	Granneman et al. 1986
[difloxacin-glucuronide]				10[a]	
[desmethyl-difloxacin]				4[a]	
[difloxacin N-oxide]				3[a]	
Enoxacin	400 IV	11	0-72	53.6 ± 4.1	Jaehde et al. 1988c
[oxo-enoxacin]				12.5 ± 2.7	
Fleroxacin	400 PO	12	0-72	59.9 ± 10.4	Sörgel et al. 1988f
[desmethyl-fleroxacin]				6.8 ± 1.7	
[fleroxacin N-oxide]				6.3 ± 1.7	
Lomefloxacin	400 PO	11	0-96	70.5 ± 5.5	Metz et al. unpublished data
[lomefloxacin-glucuronide]				8.0 ± 2.9	
Norfloxacin	200 PO	3	0-24	26.6[a]	Ozaki et al. 1981
[oxo-norfloxacin]				5.1[a]	
[7-(2-amino-ethyl-amino-)metabolite]				1.5[a]	
[7-amino-metabolite]				0.7[a]	
Ofloxacin	200 IV	10	0-24	77.0 ± 8.2	Lode et al. 1987b
[desmethyl-ofloxacin]				3.2 ± 0.6	
[ofloxacin N-oxide]				1.1 ± 0.2	
Pefloxacin	400 IV	8	0-96	7.6 ± 2.0	Sörgel et al. 1988d
[norfloxacin (desmethyl-pefloxacin)]				16.6 ± 2.6	
[pefloxacin N-oxide]				17.9 ± 2.4	
[oxo-norfloxacin]	800 PO	5	0-72	5.4 ± 0.5	Montay et al. 1984
[oxo-pefloxacin]				0.8 ± 0.1	
Pipemidic acid	100 IV	6	0-24	81.4 ± 4.2	Klinge et al. 1984

a No standard deviation available.

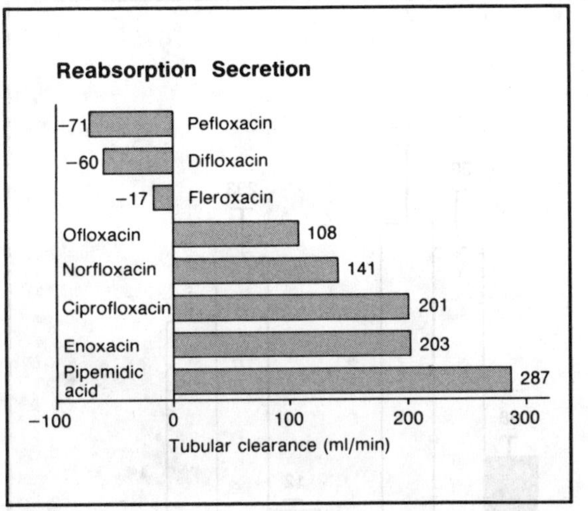

Fig. 4. 'Tubular' clearance (CL_{tub}) of quinolones calculated according to: $CL_{tub} = CL_R - (f_u \times GFR)$, where CL_R = renal clearance; f_u = fraction unbound in plasma; GFR = glomerular filtrate rate (110 ml/min) [for references see tables I and III].

clearance of pefloxacin (fig. 5) supports the hypothesis that pefloxacin undergoes extensive reabsorption in the kidney tubules. The available renal clearance values for the metabolites are higher than those for the respective parent compounds, suggesting that the metabolites undergo a more extensive secretion or less reabsorption in the kidney tubules than the parent compounds (fig. 6).

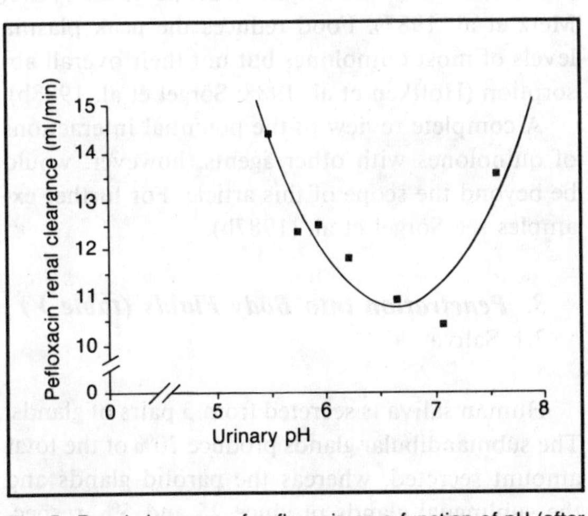

Fig. 5. Renal clearance of pefloxacin as a function of pH (after Jaehde et al. 1987d).

2.2 Liver

All quinolones are metabolised, although the degree of biotransformation varies considerably among agents. The liver is presumably the predominant organ of metabolism for these drugs. Two sites of the molecule have been identified as metabolically unstable: the 3-carboxyl- and, more importantly, the 7-piperazinyl-substituent. The principal metabolic pathways of quinolones at the piperazine ring are shown in figure 7; N-methylated quinolones undergo mainly N-oxidation and N-demethylation, while the non-N-methylated compounds are primarily converted to 3-oxo-metabolites. Other pathways of minor importance are N-acetylation, N-formylation, N-sulphate conjugation, the cleavage of the piperazine ring [formation of 7-(2-aminoethylamino-)metabolites] and the total breakdown of the piperazine ring (formation of 7-amino-metabolites). Although the formation of acylglucuronides in humans has been questioned, studies on difloxacin (Granneman et al. 1986) as well as our recent studies with lomefloxacin (Metz et al. unpublished data) clearly indicate that there is considerable glucuronidation of the 3-carboxyl-group of these 2 agents. Investigations by Mahr et al. (1988) showed that the major metabolites of quinolones are also formed by human liver microsomes. In recent studies with rat liver perfusion, we found (Labisch et al. unpublished data) that the N-oxide-metabolites are reconverted to their respective parent compounds.

2.3 Alterations in the Disease State and in Elderly Patients

The basic pharmacokinetic parameters and the different handling of quinolones by the kidney and liver as described above suggest that renal or liver failure affects the pharmacokinetics of these agents differently. Agents such as difloxacin and pefloxacin are prone to pharmacokinetic changes during impairment of liver function, whereas the pharmacokinetic disposition of ciprofloxacin, enoxacin, fleroxacin, norfloxacin and ofloxacin changes with renal impairment.

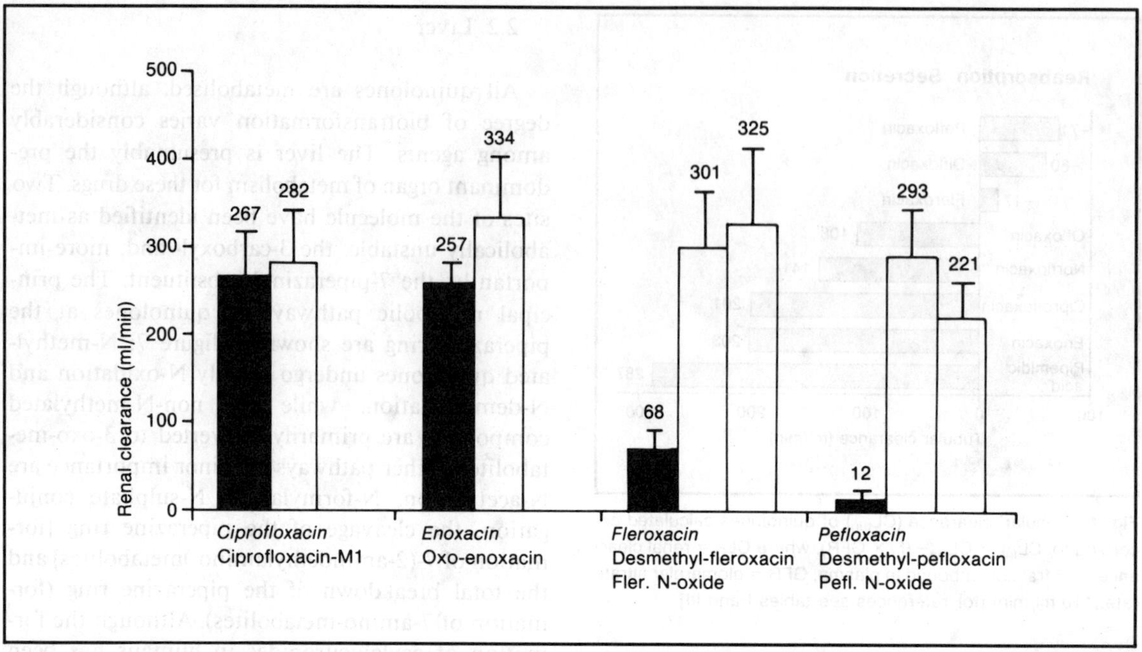

Fig. 6. Renal clearance of quinolones (■) and their metabolites (□) [for references see table I].

Although the age-related changes in liver function are still poorly understood, age-related decreases in kidney function occur and may affect the pharmacokinetics of agents predominantly excreted via the kidneys. In a recent review we analysed the available data, which in general support the hypotheses made from excretory patterns (Sörgel et al. 1987b).

2.4 Pharmacokinetic Interactions with Other Drugs

Quinolones may inhibit the metabolism of other drugs or their metabolism may be inhibited by other agents. The most prominent examples are the inhibition of theophylline, caffeine and antipyrine metabolism by enoxacin (Logemann et al. 1986; Stille et al. 1987; Wijnands et al. 1985) and the inhibition of pefloxacin metabolism by cimetidine (Sörgel et al. 1988a).

Other interactions involving quinolones are the inhibition of tubular secretion by probenecid (Wingender et al. 1985) and a clinically very important inhibition of absorption by antacids containing magnesium and aluminium (Flor et al. 1988; Höffken et al. 1988; Jaehde et al. 1987b; Lode et al. 1987a; Schentag et al. 1987). On the other hand, we found no interaction of pefloxacin with the pharmacokinetics of ceftazidime, metronidazole, piperacillin and tobramycin (Jaehde et al. 1987c; Metz et al. 1987). Food reduces the peak plasma levels of most quinolones but not their overall absorption (Höffken et al. 1988; Sörgel et al. 1988b).

A complete review of the potential interactions of quinolones with other agents, however, would be beyond the scope of this article. For further examples see Sörgel et al. (1987b).

3. Penetration into Body Fluids (table V)

3.1 Saliva

Human saliva is secreted from 3 pairs of glands. The submandibular glands produce 70% of the total amount secreted, whereas the parotid glands and the sublingual glands produce 25 and 5%, respectively. An adult produces approximately 1L of sa-

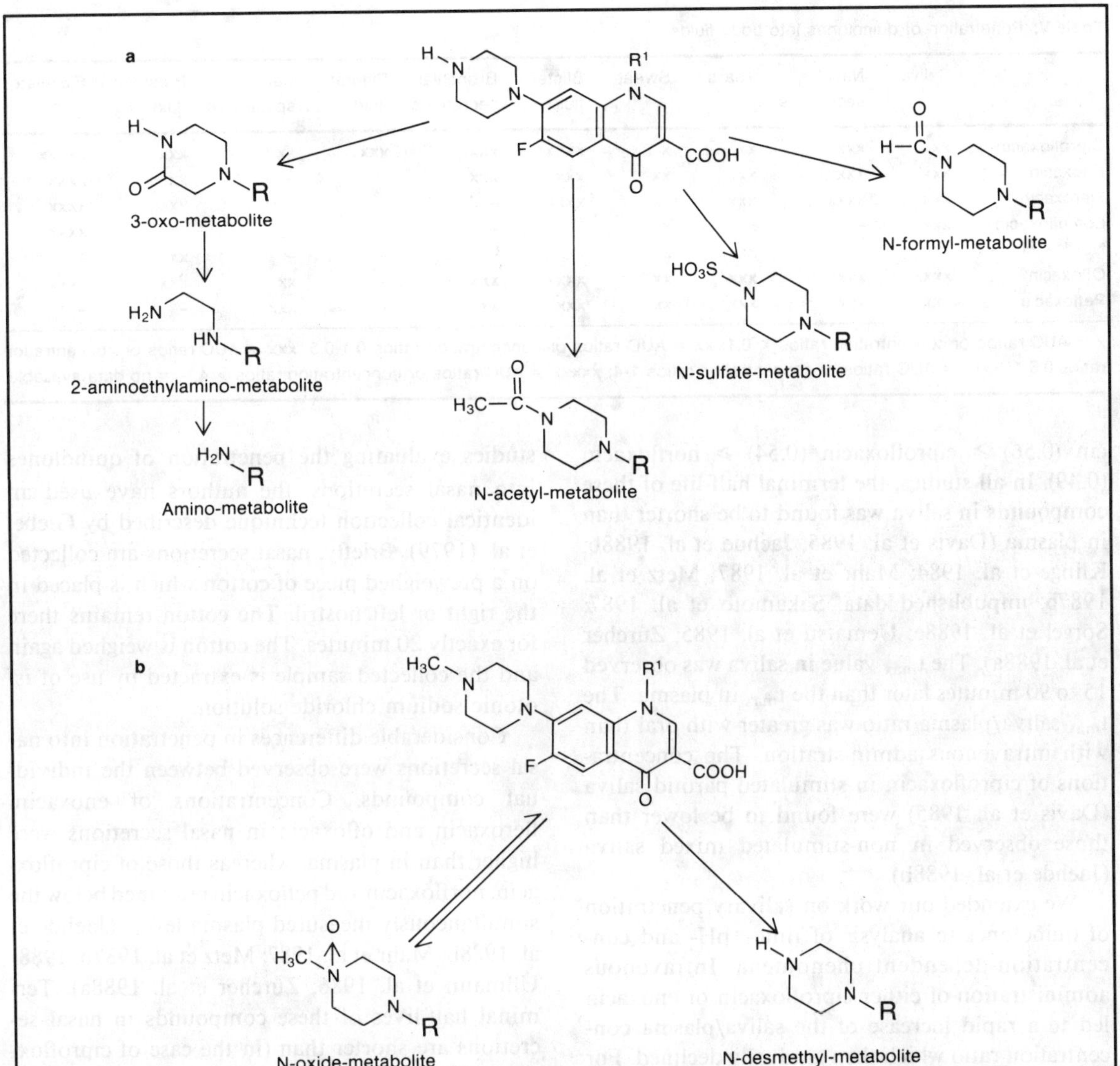

Fig. 7. Principal metabolic pathways of (a) non-N-methylated quinolones and (b) N-methylated quinolones.
Abbreviations: R = nucleus; R[1] = alkyl, fluoroalkyl, fluorophenyl, cyclopropyl.

liva per day. Primary saliva secretion occurs in the acini of the salivary glands, and its composition is modified during its passage through the duct system. Mixed saliva is slightly acid (pH 6.2 to 7.4), and the pH of saliva primarily depends on the concentration of bicarbonate, which tends to increase with increasing flow rate. Therefore, pH analysis of saliva samples must take place immediately after saliva collection to avoid any loss of carbon dioxide.

The AUC ratio between saliva and plasma for mixed, non-stimulated saliva decreases in the following order: ofloxacin (0.89) > enoxacin (0.76) > lomefloxacin (0.72) > fleroxacin (0.66) > pefloxa-

Table V. Penetration of quinolones into body fluids

	Saliva	Nasal secretions	Tears	Sweat	Blister fluid	Bronchial secretions	Pleural fluid	Cerebro-spinal fluid	Prostatic fluid	Ejaculate
Ciprofloxacin	xx	xxx	xx	x	xxxx	xxx	xxx	xx	xxx	xxxxx
Enoxacin	xxx	xxxx	xx	xx	xxxx	xxx	–	–	xx	xxxx
Fleroxacin	xxx	xxxx	xxx	xx	xxxx	–	–	–	xx	xxxx
Lomefloxacin	xxx	–	xx	xx	–	–	–	–	xxx	xxxx
Norfloxacin	xx	xxx	xx	x	xxxx	–	–	–	xx	–
Ofloxacin	xxx	xxxx	xxx	xx	xxxx	xxx	–	xx	xxx	xxxx
Pefloxacin	xxx	xxx	xxx	xx	xxx	xxx	–	xxx	–	–

x = AUC ratios or concentration ratios < 0.1; xx = AUC ratios or concentration ratios 0.1-0.5; xxx = AUC ratios or concentration ratios 0.5-1; xxxx = AUC ratios or concentration ratios 1-4; xxxxx = AUC ratios or concentration ratios > 4; – = no data available.

cin (0.56) ⩾ ciprofloxacin (0.54) ⩾ norfloxacin (0.49). In all studies, the terminal half-life of these compounds in saliva was found to be shorter than in plasma (Davis et al. 1985; Jaehde et al. 1988b; Klinge et al. 1984; Mahr et al. 1987; Metz et al. 1987b, unpublished data; Sakamoto et al. 1987; Sörgel et al. 1988e; Uematsu et al. 1985; Zürcher et al. 1988a). The t_{max} value in saliva was observed 15 to 90 minutes later than the t_{max} in plasma. The t_{max} saliva/plasma ratio was greater with oral than with intravenous administration. The concentrations of ciprofloxacin in stimulated parotid saliva (Davis et al. 1985) were found to be lower than those observed in non-stimulated mixed saliva (Jaehde et al. 1988b).

We extended our work on salivary penetration of quinolones to analysis of time-, pH- and concentration-dependent phenomena. Intravenous administration of either ciprofloxacin or enoxacin led to a rapid increase of the saliva/plasma concentration ratio which then gradually declined. For enoxacin we observed that the saliva/plasma ratio also depends on salivary pH, with higher saliva levels of enoxacin found in the more acidic samples. How these findings may improve an understanding of the physiological mechanisms of salivary gland secretion of quinolones has yet to be determined.

3.2 Nasal Secretions

The nasal glands produce mucous and serous secretions to moisten the nasal epithelium. In all studies evaluating the penetration of quinolones into nasal secretions, the authors have used an identical collection technique described by Giebel et al. (1979). Briefly, nasal secretions are collected on a preweighed piece of cotton which is placed in the right or left nostril. The cotton remains there for exactly 20 minutes. The cotton is weighed again and the collected sample is extracted by use of isotonic sodium chloride solution.

Considerable differences in penetration into nasal secretions were observed between the individual compounds. Concentrations of enoxacin, fleroxacin and ofloxacin in nasal secretions were higher than in plasma, whereas those of ciprofloxacin, norfloxacin and pefloxacin remained below the simultaneously measured plasma levels (Jaehde et al. 1988b; Mahr et al. 1987; Metz et al. 1987b, 1988; Ullmann et al. 1986; Zürcher et al. 1988a). Terminal half-lives of these compounds in nasal secretions are shorter than (in the case of ciprofloxacin and enoxacin) or equal to (in the case of fleroxacin) plasma half-lives.

3.3 Tears

As well as the theoretical understanding of the physiology of drug disposition in tears, penetration of antimicrobials into tears is also of clinical interest for the treatment of keratitis or endophthalmitis (Woo et al. 1985). Tears are produced by the lacrimal system to keep the conjunctiva and the cornea moist and wash away irritating particles. The serous secretory cells of the lacrimal gland resemble those of the parotid gland. After production, tears enter a drainage system which is formed entirely by epithelial cells. Normally, tears replace the loss of water in the eyes caused by evaporation, but with irritation, the rate of tear production is considerably accelerated. To collect tears non-invasively, tear secretion may be stimulated until the nasolacrimal duct cannot remove the fluid fast enough. At this point, the tears run over the cheek and are collected with small capillary tubes. Stimulation by freshly cut onions is a possible way to obtain sufficient tear production and was used in our experiments.

Our results show that concentrations of quinolones in tears remain below the simultaneously determined concentrations in plasma (Jaehde et al. 1988b; Mahr et al. 1987; Metz et al. 1987b, 1988, unpublished data; Sörgel et al. 1988e; Zürcher et al. 1988a). Quinolones can be classified into compounds with a lower penetration into tears (tears/plasma AUC ratio < 0.3: ciprofloxacin, enoxacin, norfloxacin) and those with a higher penetration (tears/plasma AUC ratio > 0.5: fleroxacin, ofloxacin, pefloxacin). The structural feature responsible for this difference may be the methylation of the piperazine ring in the 4-position.

3.4 Sweat

The sweat glands are divided into eccrine and apocrine glands, which differ in morphology and distribution. Apocrine glands occur mainly in the axilla, whereas eccrine glands are distributed over the entire body. In studies designed to measure the penetration of quinolones into sweat, we collected sweat only from the palmar forearm of subjects after pilocarpine iontophoresis. Therefore, only the physiology of eccrine glands will be reviewed.

The eccrine sweat gland consists of a secretory coil and a duct, with the secretory portion of the sweat gland surrounded by a network of capillaries. The fluid secreted is an ultrafiltrate of plasma modified by reabsorption processes during passage through the duct of the sweat gland. Sweat primarily consists of water, sodium chloride, ammonia, urea and uric acid. The pH of sweat is slightly acidic and increases with increasing flow rate towards a neutral pH, indicating that the bicarbonate buffer system plays a major role in regulating this pH (Sato 1977).

All quinolones were found to penetrate into sweat to a lesser degree than into saliva, nasal secretions or tears. The mean AUC ratios range between 0.06 (norfloxacin) and 0.49 (fleroxacin) [Jaehde et al. 1988b; Mahr et al. 1987; Metz et al. 1987b, 1988, unpublished data; Sörgel et al. 1988e; Zürcher et al. 1988a]. As observed for tears, fleroxacin and pefloxacin exhibit the highest penetration into sweat. For enoxacin and fleroxacin, the terminal half-life in sweat was determined and found to be longer than in plasma, suggesting that the penetration rate of quinolones into and from sweat are slower processes than the elimination of these compounds from plasma. In a recent study we showed that sweat/plasma AUC ratios of fleroxacin after multiple dosing did not differ from those after a single dose (Sörgel et al. unpublished data). From these data we conclude that, although drug elimination may be altered with multiple administration (Sörgel et al. 1988g), distribution processes may not be affected.

3.5 Blister Fluid

The measurement of drug concentrations in skin blister fluid can serve as a model for the investigation of the extravascular distribution of pharmacological agents in man. Blisters are artificially produced by cantharides plasters (cantharides-induced blister fluid) or by the application of negative pressure (suction-induced blister fluid).

The fluids produced by these 2 methods differ considerably in their protein content (suction blister 10 to 60% and cantharides blister 70 to 80% of serum protein content) [Bergeron & Brousseau 1986].

Wise et al. (1986, 1987) studied the penetration of 6 quinolones into cantharides-induced blisters. The AUC of ciprofloxacin, enoxacin, norfloxacin and ofloxacin in blister fluid was found to be slightly higher than that in plasma, but it was lower for fleroxacin and pefloxacin. Secondly, the t_{max} was observed considerably later in blister fluid than in plasma, suggesting that quinolones equilibrate slowly in blister fluid. In addition, the terminal half-life of all compounds tested was slightly prolonged in blister fluid compared with plasma. For β-lactam antibiotics, Wise et al. (1980) found a relationship between protein binding and blister fluid penetration. As indicated by a comparison of blister fluid/plasma AUC ratios (Kalager et al. 1985; LeBel et al. 1986; Panneton et al. 1988; Wise et al. 1986, 1987) and available data on protein binding (table III), a similar relationship may not be expected for quinolones.

Using suction-induced blisters, LeBel et al. (1986) and Panneton et al. (1988) found no significant differences in blister fluid penetration when comparing single and multiple dosing of ciprofloxacin and fleroxacin or when the dose of fleroxacin was increased from 400 to 800mg. Whereas penetration of ciprofloxacin into cantharides-induced blisters was higher than that of fleroxacin, the reverse occurred in suction-induced blisters. These differences in blister fluid/plasma AUC ratios between the 2 blister models indicate that the 2 models are not equivalent.

3.6 Bronchial Secretions and Sputum

Although the relationship between antimicrobial concentrations in respiratory secretions and the clinical efficacy of an antimicrobial regimen is still unclear, the penetration of these agents into bronchial secretions and sputum is regarded as an important factor for the treatment of respiratory infections. Bronchial secretions and sputum consist primarily of serous and mucous secretions produced by tubuloalveolar and tracheobronchial glands as well as by the epithelial cells of the bronchial mucosa. Since only small volumes of bronchial secretions are produced by healthy subjects, the penetration of drugs into respiratory secretions is usually investigated in patients with chronic bronchitis or a tracheostomy or in patients undergoing bronchoscopy. Although bronchial secretions are aspirated directly from the trachea or the bronchi, sputum is collected after expectoration and may be contaminated with saliva, leading to alterations of drug levels.

Penetration of quinolones into bronchial secretions and sputum, assessed by the AUC or the concentration ratio between secretions and plasma, does not differ significantly among the individual compounds (Davies et al. 1986; Fong et al. 1987a; Loos et al. 1987, 1988; Metz et al. 1988; Thys et al. 1986). Davies et al. (1986), who studied 4 quinolones, found that penetration of ciprofloxacin (sputum AUC is 53-79% of plasma AUC) was lower than that of enoxacin, ofloxacin and pefloxacin (88-112%). Our work on sputum penetration of pefloxacin in patients with cystic fibrosis shows similar results, and results were also similar for this group of patients with a particularly worsened lung situation (Metz et al. 1988). In general, quinolones exhibit a similar AUC and terminal half-life in respiratory secretions and plasma. No obvious differences between concentrations in bronchial secretions and sputum were observed for these agents.

3.7 Pleural Fluid

The pleura is a membrane consisting of 2 layers, which, by covering the lung, permits the smooth sliding of lungs and chest against each other during respiratory movements. A cavity between the 2 layers contains a thin film of pleural fluid. In some disease states, e.g. infections of the respiratory tract, the volume of pleural fluid increases considerably because of a high permeability of the pleura to water and other substances (Junqueira & Carneiro 1980).

The penetration of ciprofloxacin into pleural fluid varies considerably, with reported mean pleural fluid/plasma ratios ranging from 0.41 to 1.86 (Austgen et al. 1988; Bölcskei et al. 1987; Thys et al. 1986). In all studies, a relatively slow equilibration of ciprofloxacin between plasma and pleural fluid was observed. The terminal half-life in pleural fluid was found to be slightly longer than that in plasma (Thys et al. 1986).

3.8 Cerebrospinal Fluid

The penetrability of the brain capillaries is different from those of other capillaries in the body. Since they exhibit no intercellular gaps, the aqueous flow through the capillaries is strongly reduced. The penetration of drugs into the cerebrospinal fluid (CSF) mainly depends on their degree of ionisation and their lipophilic properties. For many drugs, the rate of diffusion into the CSF was shown to be a function of their lipid to water partition coefficient (Rowland & Tozer 1980). In patients with inflamed meninges, the penetration of drugs into the CSF may be strongly increased because of the abnormal state of the blood-brain barrier membranes (Gibaldi 1984).

The CSF penetration of quinolones was studied by several authors, both in patients with non-inflamed and in patients with inflamed meninges (Bassaris et al. 1986; Dow et al. 1986; Kitzes-Cohen et al. 1986; Stahl et al. 1986; Stübner et al. 1986; Valainis et al. 1986; Wolff et al. 1984). The data suggest that quinolones penetrate faster into the CSF of patients with meningeal infections compared with non-infected patients. When the individual compounds are compared, the concentration ratio between CSF and plasma is considerably higher for ofloxacin and pefloxacin than for ciprofloxacin. Differences in lipophilicity and N-methylation of the piperazine substituent may explain this observation.

3.9 Prostatic Fluid

Quinolones have been successfully used in the treatment of prostatitis (Malinverni & Glauser 1988). This clinical finding correlates well with the concentrations of quinolones found in prostatic tissue and fluid. The pH of prostatic fluid of healthy volunteers is slightly acidic (mean value 6.7), whereas that in patients is slightly basic (mean value 8.1) [Pfau et al. 1978]. The degree of ionisation in plasma and prostatic fluid may play an important role in penetrability of quinolones into prostatic fluid (Madsen et al. 1986).

Nevertheless, penetration of antimicrobials into prostatic fluid is often studied in healthy volunteers, since results in patients with prostatitis vary considerably, probably because of age- and disease-related differences in physiological conditions. The collection of prostatic fluid in healthy volunteers is performed after prostate massage.

Urination between drug administration and prostate massage may lead to contamination of prostatic fluid and hence to falsely high concentrations. We therefore developed a model in which we can estimate contamination of prostatic fluid by urine (Naber et al. 1987a). In the procedure, subjects additionally receive a single intravenous dose of the x-ray contrast agent ioxitalamic acid. This agent is completely excreted by the kidneys and does not penetrate into prostatic fluid. High concentrations of ioxitalamic acid in prostatic fluid indicate contamination by urine. In addition to the measurement of ioxitalamic acid, unusually high metabolite concentrations in prostatic fluid (prostatic fluid/plasma ratios > 5) can also serve to indicate contamination of the samples. In this case, however, the metabolic pattern and the concentrations of metabolites in plasma have to be carefully considered.

There are considerable discrepancies among different investigators regarding the results of quinolone penetration into prostatic fluid (Boerema et al. 1985; Kumon et al. 1985; Naber et al. 1987a,b,c, 1988; Stahl et al. 1986b; Valainis et al. 1986). The wide range of prostatic fluid/plasma ratios reported by Boerema et al. (1985) leads us to speculate that the higher mean prostatic fluid/plasma ratios may be caused by urine-contaminated samples. When our model is used, the data on 4 quinolones show that penetration of these drugs into prostatic fluid increases in the following order: norfloxacin (0.14) < ciprofloxacin (0.27) < fleroxacin (0.30) < enoxacin (0.43). We observed no relationship between the prostatic fluid/plasma ratio of quinolones and the pH of prostatic fluid.

3.10 Ejaculate

Ejaculate, which is a mixture of sperm, prostatic fluid and secretions of the seminal vesicles, the testes and Cowper's glands, has a pH value between 7.2 and 7.6. Prostatic fluid and secretion of the seminal vesicles contribute approximately 20 and 60% of the total ejaculate volume, respectively (Ganong 1981). Ejaculate is usually collected in 2 fractions (split ejaculate) after masturbation: the first fraction contains a higher proportion of prostatic fluid, whereas the second fraction consists mainly of seminal vesicle fluid.

The concentrations of quinolones in ejaculate exceed the plasma concentrations considerably (Mizoguchi et al. 1985; Naber et al. 1988, unpublished data; Schramm 1986). When the 2 ejaculate fractions were compared, there was a tendency for slightly higher concentration ratios in the second fraction. The concentrations of these agents do not seem to depend on pH or volume (Naber et al. unpublished data).

4. Penetration into Tissues (table VI)

4.1 Heart

Sufficient concentrations of quinolones in heart tissues are required in surgical infection prophylaxis and therapy of bacterial endocarditis. Penetration of these agents into cardiac muscle and heart valves was studied in patients undergoing open heart surgery. In the myocardium, pefloxacin and ciprofloxacin levels exceed the respective plasma levels by 2- to 4-fold. The mean concentration ratios between the myocardium and plasma were found to be 2.72 for pefloxacin (Brion et al. 1986) and 2.59 for ciprofloxacin (Schmidt et al. 1988). Brion et al. (1986) observed no time dependence of the myocardium/plasma concentration ratio, suggesting a rapid transfer of pefloxacin into the myocardium and from the myocardium back to the blood. The concentrations of pefloxacin in heart valves were significantly lower than in the myocardium, which might have been caused by a lower blood supply to this area. Mean concentration ratios between valves and plasma were 0.91 (aortic valve) and 1.05 (mitral valve) [Brion et al. 1986].

4.2 Lung

Mean concentration ratios between lung tissue and plasma ranged between 1.96 and 6.50 (Couraud et al. 1985; Lerebours-Pigeonnière et al. 1987; Radtke et al. 1987; Saux et al. 1987; Schlenkhoff et al. 1986; Unertl et al. 1987). Since the results for the individual compounds vary considerably among authors, differences between the compounds cannot be established at present. The lack of time dependence of the lung tissue/plasma ratio suggests that equilibration of quinolones between lung and plasma occurs rapidly. Schlenkhoff et al. (1986) reported that ciprofloxacin reached a lung tissue/plasma ratio of 4.20 within 15 minutes after intravenous injection. This is in accordance with the rich blood supply of the lung.

Table VI. Penetration of quinolones into body tissues

	Heart (myocardium)	Lung	Muscle	Renal	Bone	Skin	Fat
Ciprofloxacin	xxxx	xxxx	xxxx	xxxxx	xx	xxx	xxx
Enoxacin	–	xxxx	xxxx	xxxx	xx	xxx	xx
Ofloxacin	–	xxxx	–	xxxxx	xx	–	–
Norfloxacin	–	–	–	xxxxx	–	–	–
Pefloxacin	xxxx	xxxx	–	–	xx	–	–

x = AUC ratios or concentration ratios < 0.1; xx = AUC ratios or concentration ratios 0.1-0.5; xxx = AUC ratios or concentration ratios 0.5-1; xxxx = AUC ratios or concentration ratios 1-4; xxxxx = AUC ratios or concentration ratios > 4; – = no data available.

4.3 Muscle

The penetration of ciprofloxacin and enoxacin into muscle was studied at different times after administration (Dalhoff et al. 1987; Daschner et al. 1986; Eickenberg & Dalhoff 1985; Malmborg & Rannikko 1988; Schmidt et al. 1988). The muscle/plasma concentration ratio increased during the first 2 hours, with muscle levels exceeding plasma levels 1 hour after administration. This suggests a slower equilibration process compared with the heart and lung. Peak levels in muscle were reached between 1 and 4 hours after administration. There is again a large variability in the muscle/plasma concentration ratios reported by different investigators.

4.4 Fat

Because of its poor blood perfusion, fat equilibrates slowly with blood. The fat/plasma concentration ratio slowly increases with time after drug administration, with fat levels rarely reaching plasma levels (Dalhoff et al. 1987; Daschner et al. 1986; Eickenberg & Dalhoff 1985; Malmborg & Rannikko 1988; Schmidt et al. 1988). Peak levels in fat occur within 2 to 3 hours after administration and decline faster than in plasma. The latter finding is surprising in view of the poor blood supply to fat.

4.5 Skin

The concentrations of quinolones achieved in skin are sufficient to treat skin infections. However, results vary among authors, with skin levels of ciprofloxacin reported to be higher (Dalhoff et al. 1987) and lower (Daschner et al. 1986) than respective plasma levels. Whether these differences are due to different collection techniques or to different groups of patients remains unclear.

4.6 Bone

Penetration of quinolones into bone is of interest for the treatment of osteomyelitis. Bone samples are usually taken during orthopaedic procedures. Their preparation for analysis involves pulverisation and subsequent extraction into phosphate buffer. In detail, however, the sample collection and preparation techniques can vary considerably among different authors. Some authors considered blood contamination and corrected their results by the haemoglobin content and the respective plasma concentration. Others relate the concentration of the antibacterial agent to the inorganic phosphate content of the sample (Adam et al. 1987).

With the exception of data from Braun and Dürig (1986), concentrations of quinolones in bone were found to be lower than in plasma, reaching mean bone/plasma ratios of between 0.27 and 0.55 (Braun & Dürig 1986; Dellamonica et al. 1986; Fong et al. 1986, 1987b; Wittmann & Kotthaus 1986). Braun and Dürig (1986) reported ratios 10 times higher than those reported by other investigators. They also found higher levels of ciprofloxacin in cancellous bone compared with those in cortical bone. Fong et al. (1986) reported a tendency for higher bone/plasma ratios in infected bone samples of patients with osteomyelitis. Wittmann and Kotthaus (1986) measured bone levels of ofloxacin at various times after drug administration and observed that bone levels increased slowly, reaching a peak value 4.5 hours after oral administration. As indicated by a constant bone/plasma ratio during the elimination phase of ofloxacin, the elimination half-life of ofloxacin in bone is similar to that in plasma.

4.7 Renal Tissue

The kidney has a rich blood supply. Renal blood flow, however, differs between the cortex (4-5 ml/min/g of tissue) and the medulla (0.2 ml/min/g in inner medulla, 1.5 ml/min/g in outer medulla) [Sullivan 1974].

As expected from their considerable renal excretion, quinolones reach high concentrations in renal tissue that exceed plasma levels several-fold (Bergeron et al. 1985; Daschner et al. 1986; Malmborg & Rannikko 1988; Noel et al. 1987). Malmborg and Rannikko (1988) investigated the penetration of enoxacin into both the cortex and the medulla of the kidney and found that concentrations of quinolones are higher in the cortex. Daschner et al. (1986) studied the time dependence of the renal tissue/plasma ratio of ciprofloxacin in 25 patients. Tissue/plasma ratio (13.28) peaked 2 to 3 hours after drug administration and then declined rapidly to a nearly constant value of between 6.2 and 7.2.

5. *Conclusions*

In this review the pharmacokinetic basis for a rational clinical use of quinolones has been presented.

Most quinolones are rapidly and completely absorbed from the gastrointestinal tract. Antacids should be given at least 2 hours after oral administration of quinolones to avoid impairment of absorption; however, overall absorption of these agents is not affected by food intake. Terminal half-lives of quinolones are generally longer than those of most β-lactams. In patients with severe renal or hepatic impairment, dose adjustment of quinolones in relation to the excretory pattern of the individual agents is necessary.

The oxidative metabolism of these drugs in the liver is a potential source for interactions with other drugs. Likewise, inhibitors of the cytochrome P-450 system, such as cimetidine, inhibit the metabolism of quinolones. The inhibition of metabolism of xanthine derivatives by some quinolones, particularly enoxacin, is the drug interaction with the highest clinical relevance. Other hepatic interactions may appear as these agents are more widely used in antimicrobial therapy.

Generally, quinolones reach high levels in tissues and exceed the MIC of the most clinically relevant pathogens. To estimate the extent of penetration, we prefer to use the AUC ratio of the respective body fluid and plasma whenever possible. The concentration ratio can be affected by a possible time dependence of the distribution process, which, in the case of quinolones, was observed for some body fluids and tissues. Our new approach to estimate the penetration of drugs into sites outside the plasma includes the measurement of drug levels in saliva, nasal secretions, tears, sweat, prostatic fluid and ejaculate. To reach measurable concentrations in any of these body fluids, it is necessary for the agent to penetrate through epithelial cells and/or intercellular gaps. Thus, results on body fluid penetration also enhance understanding of the cellular uptake of quinolones. The following are advantages of this model over tissue sampling:

- the possibility of frequent sampling of body fluids in the same subject, allowing investigations on the kinetics of drugs outside plasma
- the simultaneous sampling of body fluids in different parts of the body, which makes comparison of several body fluids in 1 individual possible
- study of distribution processes in the normal state without potential interaction with anaesthetics and/or without effect of anaesthetics on organ function, as can be the case when tissue samples are taken during surgery.

Although differences in volume of distribution (Vd_β) among individual quinolones exist, it cannot be concluded that there are also proportional differences in body fluid and tissue levels. In some body fluids, e.g. nasal secretions and tears, compounds with a relatively 'low' volume of distribution such as ofloxacin and fleroxacin reach considerably higher body fluid/plasma ratios than other quinolones.

In clinical practice, differences in distribution between quinolones and other antibiotics have to be considered. Quinolones have a volume of distribution up to 10 times higher than β-lactams. Even though the sensitivity of assays for β-lactams in body fluids is not high enough to detect trace levels, unpublished data from our group suggest that β-lactams do not penetrate significantly into saliva, nasal secretions, tears and sweat. Therefore, we conclude that quinolones, unlike β-lactams, penetrate into cells and from there into body fluids. Without consideration of dose differences, absolute tissue levels of β-lactams are higher than those of quinolones. However, before tissue levels can be related to antimicrobial activity, the MICs, which are clearly lower for quinolones, also need to be considered.

Finally, the application of the unique pharmacokinetic disposition of these agents in clinical practice will help to evaluate the role of this class of agents in antimicrobial therapy.

Acknowledgements

The authors express their gratitude to Andreas Reiter, B.Sc., and Francesca Aweeka, Pharm.D., for their excellent help in the preparation of the manuscript.

Part of the results reported in this article are the fulfilment of the Ph.D. thesis of U. Jaehde at the Freie Universität, Berlin.

References

Adam D, Heilmann HD, Weismeier K. Concentrations of ticarcillin and clavulanic acid in human bone after prophylactic administration of 5.2 g of timentin. Antimicrobial Agents and Chemotherapy 31: 935-939, 1987

Austgen M, Morgenroth A, Seelmann R, Muth P, Sörgel F. Pharmacokinetics and pleural penetration of ciprofloxacin in patients with empyema thoracis. 6th Mediterranean Congress of Chemotherapy, Taormina, May 22-27, 1988. Abstract no. 124, p. 222, 1988

Bassaris HP, Papadakis N, Gogos C, Siamplis D. Penetration of ciprofloxacin into human cerebrospinal fluid. In Neu & Weuta (Eds) Proceedings of the 1st International Ciprofloxacin Workshop, Leverkusen, Nov. 6-8, 1985, pp. 204-205, Excerpta Medica, Amsterdam 1986

Bergeron MG, Brousseau L. Tissue fluid pharmacokinetic models in humans and animals. In Zak O, Sande MA (Eds) Experimental models in antimicrobial chemotherapy, Vol. 1, pp. 71-107, Academic Press, London, 1986

Bergeron MG, Thabet M, Roy R, Lessard C, Foncault P. Norfloxacin penetration into human renal and prostatic tissue after oral administration. Antimicrobial Agents and Chemotherapy 28: 349-350, 1985

Boerema JBJ, Dalhoff A, Debruyne FMY. Ciprofloxacin distribution in prostatic tissue and fluid following oral administration. Chemotherapy 31: 13-18, 1985

Bölcskei P, Burkhardt G, Klatt O, Thoma B, Gill E. Penetration of ciprofloxacin in the pleural fluid. Proceedings of the 5th Mediterranean Congress of Chemotherapy, Cairo, Oct. 26-Nov. 1, 1986, pp. 290-292, 1987

Brandt R, Meyer J. The *in vitro* protein binding of Ro 23-6240 (AM 833) in human, dog and rat plasma. Roche Research Report no. B-104'181, 1985

Braun R, Dürig M. Penetration of ciprofloxacin into human bone tissue. In Neu & Weuta (Eds) Proceedings of the 1st International Ciprofloxacin Workshop, Leverkusen, Nov. 6-8, 1985, pp. 197-200, Excerpta Medica, Amsterdam, 1986

Brion N, Lessana A, Mosset F, Lefevre JJ, Montay G. Penetration of pefloxacin in human heart valves. Journal of Antimicrobial Chemotherapy 17 (Suppl. B): 89-92, 1986

Chang T, Black A, Dunky A, Wolf R, Sedman A, et al. Pharmacokinetics of intravenous and oral enoxacin in healthy volunteers. Journal of Antimicrobial Chemotherapy 21 (Suppl. B): 49-56, 1988

Couraud L, Fourtillan JB, Saux MC, Bryskier A, Vincent du Laurier M. Diffusion of ofloxacin into human lung tissue. Proceedings of the 14th International Congress of Chemotherapy, Kyoto, 1985, pp. 1795-1796, 1985

Dalhoff A, Aigner KR, Eickenberg HU. Penetration activities of ciprofloxacin into muscle, skin and fat following oral administration. Proceedings of the 5th Mediterranean Congress of Chemotherapy, Cairo, Oct 26-Nov 1, 1986, pp. 294-295, 1987

Daschner FD, Westenfelder M, Dalhoff A. Penetration of ciprofloxacin into kidney, fat, muscle and skin tissue. European Journal of Clinical Microbiology 5: 212-213, 1986

Davies BI, Maesen FPV, Teengs JP, Baur C. The quinolones in chronic bronchitis. Pharmaceutisch Weekblad 8: 53-59, 1986

Davis RL, Koup JR, Williams-Warren J, Weber A, Smith AL. Pharmacokinetics of three oral formulations of ciprofloxacin. Antimicrobial Agents and Chemotherapy 28: 74-77, 1985

Dellamonica P, Bernard E, Etesse H, Garraffo R. The diffusion of pefloxacin into bone and the treatment of osteomyelitis. Journal of Antimicrobial Chemotherapy 17 (Suppl. B): 93-102, 1986

Dow J, Chazal J, Frydman AM, Janny P, Woehrle R, et al. Transfer kinetics of pefloxacin into cerebro-spinal fluid after one hour i.v. infusion of 400mg in man. Journal of Antimicrobial Chemotherapy 17 (Suppl. B): 81-87, 1986

Drusano GL, Standiford HC, Plaisance K, Forrest A, Leslie J, et al. Absolute oral bioavailability of ciprofloxacin. Antimicrobial Agents and Chemotherapy 30: 444-446, 1986

Easmon CSF, Crane JP. Uptake of ciprofloxacin by human neutrophils. Journal of Antimicrobial Chemotherapy 16: 67-73, 1985

Eickenberg HU, Dalhoff A. Tissue distribution of ciprofloxacin following oral and intravenous administration. Proceedings of the 14th International Congress of Chemotherapy, Kyoto, 1985, pp. 1612-1613, 1985

Flor S, Guay D, Tack K, Beals B, Weintraub H, et al. Evaluation of the interaction and safety of administration of antacids with ofloxacin. International Congress for Infectious Diseases, Rio de Janeiro, April 17-21, 1988. Abstract no. 706, p. 233, 1988

Fong IW, Ledbetter W, Vandenbroucke A, Simbul W, Rahm V. Penetration of ciprofloxacin after single doses in normal and infected bones. In Neu & Weuta (Eds) Proceedings of the 1st International Ciprofloxacin Workshop, Leverkusen, Nov 6-8, 1985, pp. 201-203, Excerpta Medica, Amsterdam, 1986

Fong IW, Vandenbroucke A, Simbul M. Penetration of enoxacin into bronchial secretions. Antimicrobial Agents and Chemotherapy 31: 748-751, 1987a

Fong IW, Rittenhouse D, Simbul M, Vandenbroucke A. Bone penetration of enoxacin after oral and intravenous dosing. 15th International Congress of Chemotherapy, Istanbul, July 19-24, 1987, abstract no. 1197, p. 325, 1987b

Ganong WF. Review of medical physiology. 10th ed., pp. 344-345, Lange Medical Publications, Los Altos, 1981

Gibaldi M. Biopharmaceutics and clinical pharmacokinetics, 3rd ed., pp. 169-170, Lea & Febiger, Philadelphia, 1984

Giebel W, Schönleber KH, Breuninger H, Ullmann U. Quantitative Bestimmung von Protein, Albumin und Antibiotika im Nasensekret gesunder Probanden. Archives of Oto-Rhino-Laryngology 225: 149-159, 1979

Granneman GR, Snyder KM, Shu VS. Difloxacin metabolism and pharmacokinetics in humans after single oral doses. Antimicrobial Agents and Chemotherapy 30: 689-693, 1986

Gruber G, Jaehde U, Sörgel F, Heiss R, Schunack W. Relationships between the chemical structure and the HPLC capacity factor of gyrase inhibitors and their metabolites in different methanol-water eluents. Fresenius' Zeitschrift für Analytische Chemie 330: 388-389, 1988

Höffken G, Lode H, Prinzing C, Borner K, Koeppe P. Pharmacokinetics of ciprofloxacin after oral and parenteral administration. Antimicrobial Agents and Chemotherapy 27: 375-379, 1985

Höffken G, Lode H, Wiley R, Glatzel TD, Sievers B, et al. Pharmacokinetics and bioavailability of ciprofloxacin and ofloxacin: effect of food and antacid intake. Reviews of Infectious Diseases 10 (Suppl. 1): S138-S139, 1988

Jaehde U, Sörgel F, Schunack W. Influence of lipophilicity on pharmacokinetics of quinolones. 71st Annual Meeting of FASEB, Washington, DC, March 29-April 2, 1987. Abstract no. 3224, 1987a

Jaehde U, Sörgel F, Gottschalk B, Stephan U, Schunack W. Reduced bioavailability of pefloxacin after coadministration with antacids. 1st Biennial Conference on Chemotherapy of Infectious Diseases and Malignancies, Munich, April 26-29, 1987. Abstract no. 280, 1987b

Jaehde U, Sörgel F, Gottschalk B, Stephan U, Schunack W. Pharmacokinetics of pefloxacin and metronidazole after concomitant administration. 1st Biennial Conference on Chemotherapy of Infectious Diseases and Malignancies, Munich, April 26-29, 1987. Abstract no. 278, 1987c

Jaehde U, Malter U, Sörgel F, Gottschalk B, Wiesemann H, et al. Individual factors affecting the pharmacokinetics of pefloxacin. Proceedings of the 15th International Congress of Chemotherapy, Istanbul, July 19-24, 1987. In Berkarda & Kuemmerle (Eds) Progress in antimicrobial and anticancer chemotherapy, Vol. 1, pp. 883-885, Ecomed-Verlag, Landsberg, 1987d

Jaehde U, Zürcher J, Sörgel F, Naber K, Sigl G, et al. Comparative bioavailability and pharmacokinetics of ciprofloxacin and pefloxacin in healthy volunteers. 2nd International Symposium on New Quinolones, Geneva, August 25-27, 1988. Abstract no. 80, 1988a

Jaehde U, Sörgel F, Naber K, Schumacher H, Kraus C, et al. Distribution of ciprofloxacin into various body fluids of healthy volunteers. 6th Mediterranean Congress of Chemotherapy, May 22-27, Taormina, 1988. Abstract no. 340, p. 160, 1988b

Jaehde U, Mahr G, Zürcher J, Naber K, Schunack W, et al. Absolute bioavailability (F), distribution and metabolism of enoxacin in healthy volunteers. 89th Annual Meeting ASCPT, San Diego, March 9-11, 1988. Abstract PII 6-7, Clinical Pharmacology and Therapeutics 43: 157, 1988c

Jaehde U, Zürcher J, Sörgel F, Naber K, Schunack W. Metabolism of ciprofloxacin in man following oral and intravenous administration. 2nd International Symposium on New Quinolones, Geneva, August 25-27, 1988. Abstract no. 145, 1988d

Junqueira LC, Carneiro J. Basic histology, 3rd ed., Lange Medical Publications, Los Altos, 1980

Kalager T, Digranes A, Bergan T, Rolstad T, Ishigam J. Pharmacokinetics of ofloxacin in serum and skin blister. Proceedings of the 14th International Congress of Chemotherapy, Kyoto, 1985, pp. 1765-1766, 1985

Kitzes-Cohen R, Miler A, Gilboa A, Harel D. Penetration of ciprofloxacin into human cerebrospinal fluid: preliminary results. In Neu & Weuta (Eds) Proceedings of the 1st International Ciprofloxacin Workshop, Leverkusen, Nov 6-8, 1985, pp. 206-208, Excerpta Medica, Amsterdam, 1986

Klinge E, Männisto PT, Mäntylä R, Mattila J, Hänninen U. Single- and multiple-dose pharmacokinetics of pipemidic acid in normal human volunteers. Antimicrobial Agents and Chemotherapy 26: 69-73, 1984

Kumon H, Mizuno A, Kishi M, Miyata K, Ohmori H. The concentration of ofloxacin in human prostatic tissue and fluid. Proceedings of the 14th International Congress of Chemotherapy, Kyoto, 1985, pp. 1767-1768, 1985

LeBel M, Vallee F, Bergeron MG. Tissue penetration of ciprofloxacin after single and multiple doses. Antimicrobial Agents and Chemotherapy 29: 501-505, 1986

Lerebours-Pigeonnière G, Gres JJ, Montay G, Bonmarchard G, Dujon A, et al. Diffusion of pefloxacin in lung parenchyma. 15th International Congress of Chemotherapy, Istanbul, July 19-24, 1987. Abstract no. 77, p. 112, 1987

Lode H, Hampel B, Wachter T, Borner K, Koeppe P. Single dose pharmacokinetics of fleroxacin in volunteers, after fasting, a standard breakfast, and antacids. 15th International Congress of Chemotherapy, Istanbul, July 19-24, 1987. Workshop on fleroxacin (Ro 23-6240): a new oral once-a-day quinolone. Abstract, p. 14, 1987a

Lode H, Höffken G, Olschewski P, Sievers B, Kirch A, et al. Pharmacokinetics of ofloxacin after parenteral and oral administration. Antimicrobial Agents and Chemotherapy 31: 1338-1342, 1987b

Logemann C, Ohnhaus EE. Enoxacin, a differential inhibitor of the microsomal liver enzyme system in men. 26th Interscience Conference of Antimicrobial Agents and Chemotherapy, New Orleans, 1986. Abstract no. 481, p. 185, 1986

Loos U, Schwabe HK, Vogel F. Ofloxacin concentrations in human plasma, bronchial secretions, bronchoalveolar lavage and alveolar macrophages. 15th International Congress of Chemotherapy, Istanbul, July 19-24, 1987. Abstract no. 78, p. 112, 1987

Loos U, Marklein G, Scholl H, Hübner U, Kaster H, et al. Bronchopulmonary penetration of ciprofloxacin. 6th Mediterranean Congress of Chemotherapy, Taormina, Italy, May 22-27, 1988. Abstract no. 341, p. 160, 1988

Madsen PO, Dørflinger T, Larsen EH, Gasser TC. Pharmacokinetics of antibacterial agents used for treatment of bacterial prostatitis. In Weidner et al. (Eds) Therapy of prostatitis, pp. 17-20, Zuckschwerdt Verlag, München, 1986

Mahr G, Sörgel F, Naber K. Body fluid penetration and metabolism of norfloxacin in healthy volunteers using a new metabolite specific assay. Proceedings of the 15th International Congress of Chemotherapy, Istanbul, July 19-24, 1987. In Berkarda & Kuemmerle (Eds) Progress in antimicrobial and anticancer chemotherapy, Vol. 1, pp. 883-885, Ecomed-Verlag, Landsberg, 1987

Mahr G, Metz R, Vergin H, Fabian W, Muth P, et al. Metabolism of gyrase inhibitors in perfused rat liver and liver microsomes from different species. 72nd Annual Meeting of FASEB, Las Vegas, May 1-5, 1988. Abstract no. 4414, 1988

Malinverni R, Glauser MP. Comparative studies of fluoroquinolones in the treatment of urinary tract infections. Reviews of Infectious Diseases 10 (Suppl. 1): S153-S163, 1988

Malmborg AS, Rannikko S. Enoxacin distribution in human tissues after multiple oral administration. Journal of Antimicrobial Chemotherapy 21 (Suppl. B): 57-60, 1988

Metz R, Sörgel F, Gottschalk B, Stephan U. Pharmacokinetics of pefloxacin alone and in combination with other antimicrobial agents. 1st Biennial Conference on Chemotherapy of Infectious Diseases and Malignancies, April 26-29, Munich, 1987. Abstract no. 277, 1987a

Metz R, Sörgel F, Naber K. Pharmacokinetics and body fluid penetration of ofloxacin after multiple dosing in healthy volunteers. Proceedings of the 15th International Congress of Chemotherapy, Istanbul, July 19-24, 1987. In Berkarda & Kuemmerle (Eds) Progress in antimicrobial and anticancer chemotherapy, Vol. 2, pp. 1912-1913, Ecomed-Verlag, Landsberg, 1987b

Metz R, Sörgel F, Federspil P, Malter U, Koch HU, et al. Penetration of pefloxacin into saliva, sputum, sweat, tears and nasal secretions. Reviews of Infectious Diseases 10 (Suppl. I): S97, 1988

Mizoguchi H, Maeda Y, Shimizu T. An appraisal of ofloxacin level in semen. Proceedings of the 14th International Congress of Chemotherapy, Kyoto, 1985, pp. 1793-1794, 1985

Montay G, Goueffon Y, Roquet F. Absorption, distribution, metabolic fate, and elimination of pefloxacin mesylate in mice, rats, dogs, monkeys and humans. Antimicrobial Agents and Chemotherapy 25: 436-472, 1984

Naber KG, Sörgel F, Schumacher H, Nausch I, Mahr G. True penetration of quinolones into prostatic fluid of man determined by a new method. 27th Interscience Conference of Antimicrobial Agents and Chemotherapy, October 4-7, New York, 1987. Abstract no. 1270, p. 318, 1987a

Naber KG, Sörgel F, Schumacher H, Metz R. *In vitro* activity of fleroxacin against isolates causing complicated urinary tract infections and concentrations in prostatic fluid in volunteers. 15th International Congress of Chemotherapy, Istanbul, July 19-24, 1987. Workshop on fleroxacin (Ro 23-6240): a new oral once-a-day quinolone. Abstract, p. 13, 1987b

Naber KG, Sörgel F, Kees F, Schumacher H, Metz R, et al. Norfloxacin concentrations in prostatic adenoma tissue (patients) and in prostatic fluid in patients and volunteers. 15th International Congress of Chemotherapy, Istanbul, July 19-24, 1987. In Berkarda & Kuemmerle (Eds) Progress in antimicrobial and anticancer chemotherapy, Vol. 2, p. 352, Ecomed-Verlag, Landsberg, 1987c

Naber KG, Sörgel F, Schumacher H, Sigl G, Zürcher J, et al. Enoxacin concentrations in prostatic and seminal fluid in volunteers. 2nd International Symposium on New Quinolones, Geneva, August 25-27, 1988. Abstract no. 302, 1988

Noel F, Couet W, Lefebvre MA, Akbaraly JP, Mignot A, et al. Diffusion of ofloxacin in human tissues. Proceedings of the 5th Mediterranean Congress of Chemotherapy, Cairo, Oct 26-Nov 1, 1986, pp. 300-301, 1987

Ozaki T, Uchida H, Irikura T. Studies on metabolism of AM-715 in humans by high-performance liquid chromatography. Chemotherapy 29: 128-135, 1981

Panneton AC, Bergeron MG, LeBel M. Tissue penetration of fleroxacin after single and multiple 400 and 800 mg dosage regimens. 5th International Congress for Infectious Diseases, Rio de Janeiro, April 17-21, 1988. Abstract no. 416, p. 26, 1988

Pfau A, Perlberg S, Shapira A. The pH of the prostatic fluid in health and disease: implications of treatment in chronic bacterial prostatitis. Journal of Urology 119: 384-387, 1978

Radtke HJ, Floh W, Böcker R, Hopf G. Distribution of ciprofloxacin in serum, lung and pleural tissue in patients undergoing lung surgery. 15th International Congress of Chemotherapy, Istanbul, July 19-24, 1987. Abstract no. 126, p. 120, 1987

Rowland M, Tozer TN. Clinical pharmacokinetics: concepts and applications, pp. 37-38, Lea & Febiger, Philadelphia, 1980

Sakamoto H, Sasaki J, Uematsu M, Morihana T, Imoto T, et al. Ofloxacin: its blood level, penetration into saliva and distribution in tooth extraction wound. 15th International Congress of Chemotherapy, Istanbul, July 19-24, 1987. Abstract no. 108, p. 117, 1987

Sato K. The physiology, pharmacology and biochemistry of the eccrine sweat gland. Reviews of Physiology, Biochemistry and Pharmacology 79: 51-131, 1977

Saux MC, Grellet J, Couraud L, Leng B, Hazane C. Diffusion of enoxacin into human lung tissue. 15th International Congress of Chemotherapy, Istanbul, July 19-24, 1987. Abstract no. 139, p. 123, 1987

Schentag JJ, Sedman AJ, Wilton JH, Thomas DJ, Schultz RW, et al. Interactions between enoxacin, ranitidine and antacids. 3rd European Congress of Clinical Microbiology, The Hague, 1987. Abstract, 1987

Schlenkhoff D, Knopf J, Dalhoff A. Penetration of ciprofloxacin into human lung tissue. In Neu & Weuta (Eds) Proceedings of the 1st International Ciprofloxacin Workshop, Leverkusen, Nov. 6-8, 1985, pp. 157-159, Excerpta Medica, Amsterdam, 1986

Schmidt W, Eigel P, Zürcher J, Dexling B, Sörgel F. Efficiency of ciprofloxacin prophylaxis in open-heart surgery: examination of its distribution into serum, myocardium, skeletal muscle and mediastinal fat. 2nd International Symposium on New Quinolones, Geneva, August 25-27, 1988. Abstract no. 72, 1988

Schramm P. Ofloxacin: concentration in human ejaculate and influence on sperm motility. Infection 14 (Suppl. 4): 274-275, 1986

Silvain C, Breux JP, Rochard E, Bouquet S, Becq-Giraudon B, et al. Decreased erythrocyte penetration of pefloxacin in cirrhotic patients. Journal of Antimicrobial Chemotherapy 20: 290-292, 1987

Sörgel F, Jaehde U, Naber K, Schunack W. Pharmakokinetik und Analytik von Gyrase-Hemmern. 3. Einfluss der Lipophilie auf die Pharmakokinetik. In Naber et al. (Eds) Gyrase-Hemmer II. FAC 6-10, pp. 1987-1997, Futuramed Verlag, München, 1987a

Sörgel F, Naber KG, Stephan U. Pharmakokinetik und Analytik von Gyrase-Hemmern. 1. Pharmakokinetik – ein Überblick. In Naber et al. (Eds) Gyrase-Hemmer II. FAC 6-10, pp. 1907-1961, Furturamed Verlag, München, 1987b

Sörgel F, Mahr G, Koch HU, Stephan U, Wiesemann HG, et al. Effects of cimetidine on the pharmacokinetics of pefloxacin in healthy volunteers. Reviews of Infectious Diseases 10 (Suppl. 1): S137, 1988a

Sörgel F, Mahr G, Stephan U, Koch HU, Wiesemann HG. Effect of normal and fat-rich food on the absorption of pefloxacin in humans. Reviews of Infectious Diseases 10 (Suppl. 1): S137-S138, 1988b

Sörgel F, Mahr G, Stephan U, Koch HU, Wiesemann HG. Absolute bioavailability and pharmacokinetics of pefloxacin in healthy volunteers. Reviews of Infectious Diseases 10 (Suppl. 1): S93, 1988c

Sörgel F, Koch HU, Malter U, Metz R, Mahr G, et al. Metabolism of pefloxacin in humans. Reviews of Infectious Diseases 10 (Suppl. 1): S95-S96, 1988d

Sörgel F, Metz R, Naber K, Seelmann R, Muth P. Pharmacokinetics of fleroxacin in man. 1. Pharmacokinetics and body fluid penetration of fleroxacin in healthy volunteers. Journal of Antimicrobial Chemotherapy 22 (Suppl. D): 155-167, 1988e

Sörgel F, Seelmann R, Naber K, Metz R, Muth P. Pharmacokinetics of fleroxacin in man. 2. Metabolism of fleroxacin in man. Journal of Antimicrobial Chemotherapy 22 (Suppl. D): 169-178, 1988f

Sörgel F, Jaehde U, Zürcher J, Seelmann R, Muth P, et al. Effect of multiple dosing on nonrenal elimination of quinolones. 28th Interscience Conference of Antimicrobial Agents and Chemotherapy, October 23-26, Los Angeles, 1988. Abstract no. 1443, 1988g

Stahl JP, Croize J, Lefebvre MA, Bru JP, Guyot A, et al. Diffusion of ofloxacin into the cerebrospinal fluid in patients with bacterial meningitis. Infection 14 (Suppl. 4): 254-255, 1986

Stille W, Harder S, Mieke S, Beer C, Shah PM, et al. Decrease of caffeine elimination in man during co-administration of 4-quinolones. Journal of Antimicrobial Chemotherapy 20: 729-734, 1987

Stübner G, Weinrich W, Brands U. Study of the cerebrospinal fluid penetrability of ofloxacin. Infections 14 (Suppl. 4): 250-253, 1986

Sullivan LP. Physiology of the kidney, p. 37, Lea & Febiger, Philadelphia, 1974

Thys JP, Klastersky J, Jacobs F, Berre J, Gangji D, et al. Penetration of ciprofloxacin into bronchial secretions and pleural fluid. In Neu & Weuta (Eds) Proceedings of the 1st International Ciprofloxacin Workshop, Leverkusen, Nov. 6-8, 1985, pp. 153-156, Excerpta Medica, Amsterdam, 1986

Uematsu M, Morihana T, Sekiguchi T, Imoto T, Sasaki J. The pharmacokinetics and saliva penetration of ofloxacin, norfloxacin, enoxacin and pipemidic acid. Proceedings of the 14th International Congress of Chemotherapy, Kyoto, 1985, pp. 1891-1892, 1985

Ullmann U, Giebel W, Dalhoff A, Koeppe P. Single and multiple dose pharmacokinetics of ciprofloxacin. European Journal of Clinical Microbiology 5: 193-196, 1986

Unertl K, Dieterich HJ, Ruckdeschel G, Martin E, Ehret W. Lung tissue and serum concentrations of ciprofloxacin in patients. 15th International Congress of Chemotherapy, Istanbul, July 19-24, 1987. Abstract no. 1195, p. 324, 1987

Valainis G, Thomas D, Pankey G. Penetration of ciprofloxacin into cerebrospinal fluid. European Journal of Clinical Microbiology 5: 75-76, 1986

Weidekamm E, Portmann R, Suter K, Partos C, Dell D, et al. Single- and multiple-dose pharmacokinetics of fleroxacin, a trifluorinated quinolone, in humans. Antimicrobial Agents and Chemotherapy 31: 1909-1914, 1987

Wijnands WJA, Vree TB, Van Herwerden CLA. Enoxacin decreases the clearance of theophylline in man. British Journal of Clinical Pharmacology 20: 583-588, 1985

Wijnands WJA, Vree TB, Baars AM, van Herwaarden CLA. Pharmacokinetics of enoxacin and its penetration into bronchial secretions and lung tissue. Journal of Antimicrobial Chemotherapy 21 (Suppl. B): 67-77, 1988

Wingender W, Beermann D, Föerster D, Graefe KH, Schacht P, et al. Mechanism of renal excretion of ciprofloxacin (Bay o 9867), a new quinolone carboxylic acid derivative, in humans. Proceedings of the 4th Mediterranean Congress of Chemotherapy, Rhodos, 1984. Chemoterapia 4 (Suppl.): 403-404, 1985

Wise R. The clinical relevance of protein binding and tissue concentrations in antimicrobial therapy. Clinical Pharmacokinetics 11: 470-482, 1986

Wise R, Gillett AP, Cadge B, Durham SR, Baker S. The influence of protein binding upon tissue fluid levels of six β-lactam antibiotics. Journal of Infectious Diseases 142: 77-82, 1980

Wise R, Lister D, McNulty CAM, Griggs D, Andrews JM. The comparative pharmacokinetics of five quinolones. Journal of Antimicrobial Chemotherapy 8 (Suppl. D): 71-81, 1986

Wise R, Kirkpatrick B, Ashby J, Griggs DJ. Pharmacokinetics and tissue penetration of Ro 23-6240, a new trifluoroquinolone. 15th International Congress of Chemotherapy, Istanbul, July 19-24, 1987. Workshop on fleroxacin (Ro 23-6240): a new oral once-a-day quinolone. Abstract, p. 15, 1987

Wittmann DH, Kotthaus E. Further methodological improvement in antibiotic bone concentrations measurements: penetration of ofloxacin into bone and cartilage. Infection 14 (Suppl. 4): 270-273, 1986

Wolff M, Regnier B, Daldoss C, Nkam M, Vachon F. Penetration of pefloxacin into cerebrospinal fluid of patients with meningitis. Antimicrobial Agents and Chemotherapy 26: 289-291, 1984

Woo FL, Johnson AP, Imsler MS, George WJ, La Corte WS. Gentamicin, tobramycin, amikacin and netilmicin levels in tears following intravenous administration. Archives of Ophthalmology 103: 216-218, 1985

Zürcher J, Jaehde U, Sörgel F, Naber K, Schumacher H, et al. Distribution of enoxacin and its main metabolite oxo-enoxacin into saliva, nasal secretions, tears and sweat of healthy volunteers. 2nd International Symposium on New Quinolones, August 25-27, Geneva, 1988. Abstract no. 146, 1988a

Zürcher J, Jaehde U, Gottschalk B, Sörgel F, Naber K, et al. Effect of dose on bioavailability, pharmacokinetics and metabolism of pefloxacin following single and multiple dose administration. 2nd International Symposium on New Quinolones, August 25-27, Geneva, 1988. Abstract no. 69, 1988b

Author's address: Dr *Fritz Sörgel*, IBMP – Institut für Biomedizinische und Pharmazeutische Forschung, Harrichstrasse 5, D-8500 Nürnberg 10 (Federal Republic of Germany).

Clinical Pharmacokinetics 16 (Suppl. 1): 25-31 (1989)
0312-5963/89/0001-0025/$3.50/0

Clinical Significance of Antibiotic Tissue Penetration

Jerome J. Schentag

School of Pharmacy, State University of New York at Buffalo and the Clinical Pharmacokinetics Laboratory, Millard Fillmore Hospital, Buffalo, New York, USA

Summary *The concentrations achieved by a particular antibiotic in serum and tissues can be predicted from pharmacokinetic data. These predictions must be evaluated in the broader context of the patient's infection, particularly the MIC of the drug for the infecting organism. What is the relevant measurement – the serum concentration or the tissue to serum ratio? Are the serum and/or tissue concentrations achieved at the site of infection sufficiently in excess of the MIC to eradicate the organism? How long are these levels sustained? How often must the drug be given to keep the concentrations sufficiently in excess of the MIC to eradicate the organisms?*

This presentation will review these questions in the context of the major classes of antibiotics: the β-lactams, aminoglycosides and quinolones.

Tissue penetration is a frequently discussed characteristic of an antibiotic. It is clearly important as regards the effects of the drug and influences both its toxicity and its antibacterial action. To fully illustrate the importance and relevance of antibiotic tissue distribution, this presentation will outline the principles involved in measuring or calculating the tissue to serum ratio. We will also demonstrate why tissue to serum ratios can be misleading when used to predict the antibacterial effects of antibiotics. Finally, differences in tissue distribution among quinolones, β-lactams and aminoglycosides will be considered and related to the potential for class differences in their activity.

The early pharmacokinetic studies determined volume of distribution as the primary mathematical expression of antibiotic distribution. This parameter is estimated from the dosage divided by the serum peak concentration by use of serum profiles such as those shown in figure 1. Volume of distribution expresses distribution as being homogeneous; however, it was quickly appreciated that antibiotics such as aminoglycosides and β-lactams were unevenly distributed in tissues, as their dis-

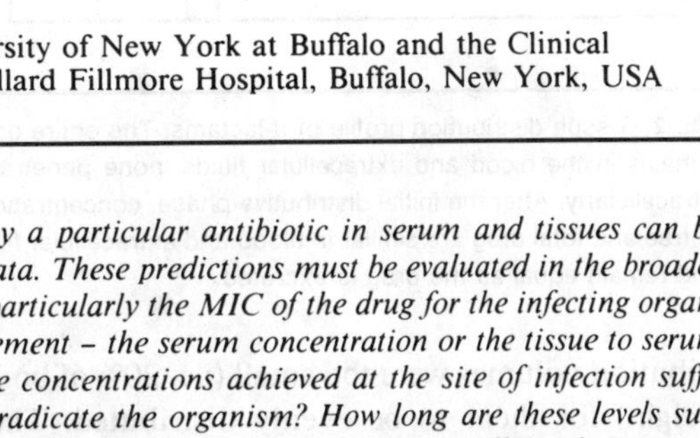

Fig. 1. Serum concentrations *vs* time for representatives of each of the 3 classes of antibiotics – aminoglycosides (▲), quinolones (■) and β-lactams (●) – in patients with normal renal function. Dosages are aminoglycoside 100mg, quinolone 200mg and β-lactam 1000mg.

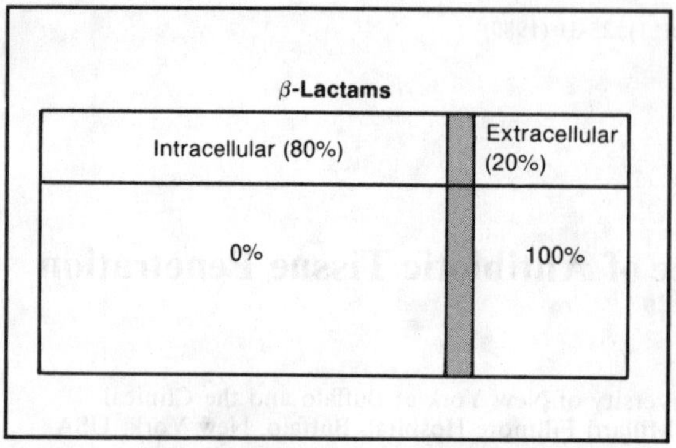

Fig. 2. Tissue distribution profile of β-lactams. The entire dose remains in the blood and extracellular fluids; none penetrates intracellularly. After the initial distributive phase, concentrations of free and total drug are similar in blood and extracellular fluid, and remain equal as the drug is excreted.

tribution volumes were too small (i.e. 20% of bodyweight) for them to be evenly distributed. Their distribution patterns are shown in figures 2 and 3. Measured tissue to serum ratios of these compounds were less than 1 : 1 for most body sites, excluding the excretory organs (Rolinson 1984; Ryan & Cars 1980; Schentag & Gengo 1982; Tsuji et al. 1985). Unfortunately, many investigators focused on the low tissue to serum ratios, and it became a general belief that bacteria involved in tissue infections were exposed to lower antibiotic concentrations than those found simultaneously in blood. Low tissue to serum ratios were used to justify the use of higher dosages to treat tissue infections (Kunin 1981). Further studies which demonstrated poor extravascular penetration (Chisholm et al. 1973; Gerding et al. 1976; Wise et al. 1980) reinforced this viewpoint in the 1980s. Moreover, studies showing that sites such as cerebrospinal fluid (Norrby 1978) and abscess cavities (Barza & Weinstein 1974) had concentrations lower than blood also supported the general view that infection site concentrations were lower than those in blood. Studies of protein binding led some to postulate that protein binding inhibited extravascular penetration (Barza et al. 1974; Drusano et al. 1984; Hoffstedt & Walder 1981; Rolinson 1980) and highly protein-bound antibiotics therefore required higher dosages or were less effective at the same dosage than non-protein-bound antibiotics (Barza et al. 1974; Drusano et al. 1984).

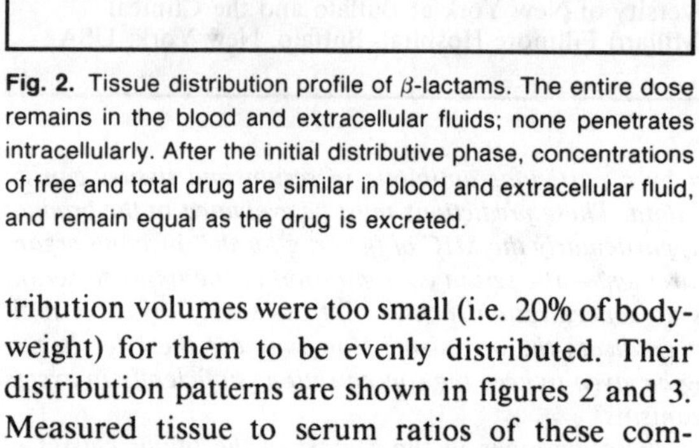

Fig. 3. Tissue distribution profile of aminoglycosides. As with β-lactams, the entire dosage remains in the blood and extracellular fluids. Here, the drug penetrates the cell membrane and binds intracellularly. This active transport mechanism is responsible for very slowly increasing intracellular concentrations and is too slow to be an important determinant of distribution volume. There is, however, a rapid tissue transport pump for these drugs in renal proximal tubular cells, and the higher kidney concentrations are responsible for nephrotoxicity.

Some antibiotics also had the ability to concentrate at body tissue sites. A fundamental observation was the association between the high tissue to serum ratios of aminoglycosides and their nephrotoxicity (Schentag et al. 1977a,b, 1978). Correlations were also observed with efficacy against urinary tract infections such as pyelonephritis (Fabre et al. 1976; Glauser et al. 1979). Kinetic modelling of such uneven tissue distribution required multicompartmental models (Schentag et al. 1977a,b). Logically, this tissue-bound antibiotic displayed little antibacterial action, further complicating the interpretation of tissue concentrations.

In view of these data, most investigators and clinicians readily accepted a lack of correlation between serum and tissue concentrations, and a lack of correlation between serum concentrations and response of the infection (Kunin 1981; Neu 1981). As a consequence, most investigators increased the dosage of β-lactams, partly to offset the perceived defect in tissue penetration. Maximum aminoglycoside dosages were limited by toxicity, and so combination therapy became mandatory.

This 'inadequate tissue penetration' hypothesis

was challenged by studies demonstrating correlations between serum concentrations and efficacy against tissue infections. Studies with aminoglycosides (Moore et al. 1987; Noone et al. 1974), β-lactams (Gengo et al. 1984; Schentag et al. 1984) and quinolones (Michéa-Hamzehpour et al. 1987; Nix et al. 1987) demonstrated correlations between serum concentration and response of infections at extravascular sites. Some of these studies demonstrated good relationships independent of the degree of serum protein binding (Schentag et al. 1984). The primary effects associated with increasing serum protein binding are slowing of excretion (Drusano et al. 1984) and increases in volume of distribution (Reitberg et al. 1984). Clinicians appear equally satisfied with the efficacy of high and low protein-bound antibiotics (Drusano et al. 1984). Evidence is rapidly accumulating in both animal models (Gengo et al. 1984; Michéa-Hamzehpour et al. 1987; Roosendaal et al. 1986; Vogelman et al. 1988) and humans (Drusano 1988; Moore et al. 1987; Nix et al. 1987; Noone et al. 1974; Schentag et al. 1984) that serum concentrations in relation to MIC are the best predictor of response, even for tissue site infections.

The fluoroquinolone antibiotics are a new class of antimicrobial, with markedly different tissue to serum ratios compared with β-lactams and aminoglycosides. Specifically, the quinolone distribution ratios are in excess of 2 : 1 at many tissue sites (Neuman 1988). High tissue penetration would lead to the immediate conclusion that tissue infections would respond at serum concentrations below MIC. Blood levels would not need to exceed MIC, since the drugs concentrate at tissue sites above the serum concentration. Nevertheless, recent studies of concentration versus effect do not validate this viewpoint. Rather, quinolone serum concentrations appear to be better predictors of infection response when related to bacterial MIC (Michéa-Hamzehpour et al. 1987; Nix et al. 1987).

Typical serum concentration versus time curves are shown for these representative antibiotics in figure 1. All 3 classes of antibiotics are likely to have activity against bacteria which can be closely related to their serum concentrations. If this thesis is correct, both the low tissue to serum ratios of aminoglycosides and β-lactams and the high tissue to serum ratios of quinolones are potentially misleading when they are used to describe the response of extracellular Gram-negative bacteria. The remainder of this presentation will attempt to show that serum concentrations predict response better than tissue concentration ratios as long as bacteria are extracellular, and this may also hold true for some intracellular models. This hypothesis applies to all sites which do not have permeability barriers. It may not apply to CNS infections or abscess cavities, which are potential barriers to passive diffusion.

1. Tissue to Serum Ratios

Tissue to serum ratios are measured by administering the dose and then excising tissue at a measured time after the dose. Simultaneously, serum is obtained for comparison with the tissue concentration and for calculation of the ratio. Under ideal conditions, the tissue is excised after the distributive phase has been completed (i.e. after 1 to 2 hours), and the experiment must be performed after a sufficient number of doses have been given to assure steady-state serum and tissue concentrations (Gengo & Schentag 1981, 1982; Van Etta et al. 1983). The excised tissue is blotted to remove excess blood, then weighed and homogenised in a measured volume of buffer. Haemoglobin can be measured if a precise estimate of retained blood is desired (Lowry & Hastings 1942). After homogenisation, the tissue extract is centrifuged, the supernatant removed, its volume recorded, and the supernatant assayed. The concentration in tissue is then determined by use of the following equation:

$$\text{tissue concentration } (\mu g/g) = \frac{\text{concentration in supernatant } (\mu g/ml) \times \text{volume of supernatant (ml)}}{\text{weight of tissue sample (g)}}$$

This tissue concentration in μg/g is then used to determine the tissue to serum ratio by use of the equation below:

$$\text{tissue to serum ratio} = \frac{\text{tissue concentration } (\mu g/g)}{\text{serum concentration } (\mu g/ml)}$$

Clearly, the tissue to serum ratio is based on recovery of a measurable quantity of antibiotic from a homogenised tissue sample. This ratio provides little information on the location of the drug in the piece of excised tissue. However, if bacteria are also distributed evenly in that tissue, the ratio is a useful expression of the exposure to the antibiotic. If bacteria are unevenly distributed, it would be essential to determine whether the distribution of antibiotic is also uneven, and to what extent bacterial distribution coincides with drug distribution.

2. *Bacterial Tissue Distribution*

It is very unlikely that bacteria are evenly distributed throughout infected tissues (Ryan & Cars 1980); thus, the tissue homogenisation method is a potentially misleading index of bacterial exposure to antibiotic. Although some bacteria are trapped in leucocytes (Mandell 1973), bacteria in tissue reside primarily in the extracellular space. It is almost certain that they are excluded from intact cells, since there would be rapid cell death. Furthermore, it is probable that β-lactams and aminoglycosides are also excluded from intact cells (Brown & Percival 1978; Mandell 1973) and are located primarily in blood and extracellular fluids. Therefore, in extracellular infections, bacteria are evenly mixed with the equilibrated antibiotics in extracellular fluids.

The consequence of this perspective is demonstrated for β-lactams in table I and for aminoglycosides in table II. These 2 tables show how virtually all the drug concentrated in blood and extracellular fluid can yield an artificially low tissue to serum ratio. In fact, this ratio is misleading, because the bacteria are exposed to concentrations similar or identical to those in serum. This would explain why serum concentrations predict antibacterial activity. We therefore conclude that low tissue to serum ratios do not reflect the activity of these antibiotics at most sites of infection.

The quinolones present a totally different situation, as shown in figure 4. Here, the tissue to serum ratios exceed 1 : 1 (usually, they exceed 2 : 1). Tissue to serum ratios of this magnitude create excitement, given the belief that these reflect concentrations at the infection site in excess of serum

Table I. Calculation of tissue concentrations and ratios of tissue to serum concentration (non-excretory organs) for β-lactams at a postdistributive serum concentration of 40 μg/ml

Site	Tissue weight (g)	Tissue mass (%)	Concentration (μg/ml)	Amount (μg)
Blood		4	40.0	1.6
Extracellular fluid	1	16	40.0	6.4
Intracellular fluid		80	1.0	0.8
Total				8.8
Tissue to serum ratio: 8.8/40 = 0.22				

Table II. Calculation of tissue concentrations and ratios of tissue to serum concentration (non-excretory organs) for aminoglycosides at a postdistributive serum concentration of 4.0 μg/ml

Site	Tissue weight (g)	Tissue mass (%)	Concentration (μg/ml)	Amount (μg)
Blood		4	4.00	0.16
Extracellular fluid	1	16	4.00	0.64
Intracellular fluid		80	0.01	0.008
Total				0.81
Tissue to serum ratio: 0.81/4.0 = 0.21				

concentrations. A calculation of tissue to serum ratios for a quinolone is shown in table III. These data demonstrate that much of the quinolone in a tissue sample is found inside the cell. Intracellular quinolone concentrations must exceed those in serum by 2- to 3-fold to produce tissue to serum ratios of 2 : 1. This distribution profile is highly useful if the infecting bacteria are intracellular. Quinolones will therefore be the antibiotics of choice, because the aminoglycosides and β-lactams are completely excluded from intracellular infection sites. However, the intracellular penetration of the quinolones may not confer automatic advantages in the treatment of extracellular pathogens, since one consequence of high tissue concentrations is low extracellular concentrations. It is apparent (table IV) that fluid penetration is generally good for all 3 classes of antibiotics, except for impermeable sites such as cerebrospinal fluid. Recent studies in our patients correlate response of extracellular pathogens with quinolone serum concentrations (Nix et al. 1987), indicating that quinolones also conform to the hypothesis of extracellular distribution/extracellular pathogen response developed for aminoglycosides and β-lactams. It is not a disadvantage for these drugs to penetrate cells, but higher systemic dosages are needed for extracellular infections, because doses must compensate for the large fraction of the circulating dosage which is inside cells and therefore not at the extracellular infection site. From a pharmacokinetic perspective, the difference between quinolones and β-lactams is reflected in a quinolone distribution volume in excess of 2 L/kg and perhaps a delay in clearance associated with tissue binding and partitioning. This delay generally yields a longer serum half-life, even in the absence of serum protein binding.

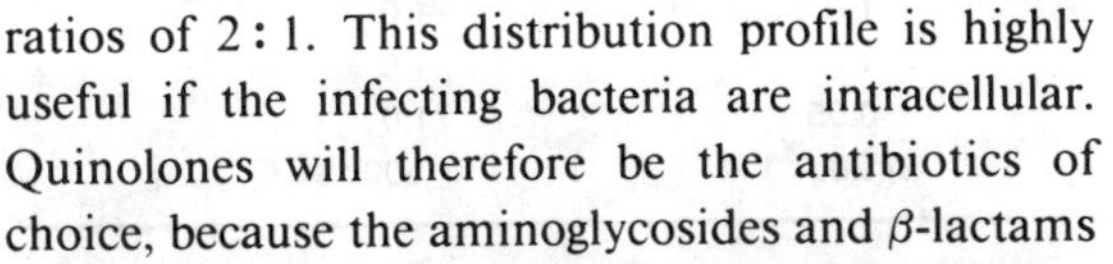

Fig. 4. Tissue distribution profile of the quinolones. These drugs cross the cell membrane readily, and by the end of the distributive phase, they have equilibrated both intracellularly and extracellularly. Concentrations in blood and extracellular fluid are equal, and free concentrations inside the cell are probably similar to blood and extracellular fluid concentrations. Intracellular concentration is unlikely to be greater than 5 : 1, bound to free, to achieve the data shown in table III.

3. *Conclusions*

At non-excreting sites permeable by these drugs, all 3 antibiotic classes show predictable distribution volumes and tissue to serum ratios. However, it will be necessary to measure or estimate the extracellular fluid volume of each organ or tissue site if prediction is to be precise. Values for eliminating

Table III. Calculation of tissue concentrations and ratios of tissue to serum concentration (non-excretory organs) for quinolones at a postdistributive serum concentration of 4.0 μg/ml

Site	Tissue weight (g)	Tissue mass (%)	Concentration (μg/ml)	Amount (μg)
Blood		4	4.0	0.16
Extracellular fluid	1	16	4.0	0.64
Intracellular fluid		66	4.0	2.11
Intracellular organelles		34	21.6	5.89
Total				8.8

Tissue to serum ratio: 8.8/4.0 = 2.2

Table IV. Extracellular fluid distribution ratios for β-lactams, quinolones and aminoglycosides at steady state

Site	Fluid to serum ratios		
	aminoglycosides	β-lactams	quinolones
Cerebrospinal fluid	0.08-0.25	0.1-0.3	0.2-0.4
Pleural fluid	1.0	1.0	1.0
Synovial fluid	0.9	1.0	1.0
Peritoneal fluid	1.0	1.0	1.0
Saliva	0.05	0.05	1.0
Urine	> 500 : 1	> 200 : 1	> 500 : 1

organs such as the liver or kidney will not be predictable if based only on diffusion principles. Knowledge of extracellular fluid volumes, binding characteristics, and transport processes will be needed to accurately describe the concentration ratios of excretory organs.

Of the 3 classes of antibiotics, only the quinolones are potentially useful against intracellular pathogens. This is a predictable consequence of their intracellular penetration and distribution characteristics. Given their approximate 2 : 1 tissue to serum ratio, it is likely that the concentration in intracellular organelles will be as high as 5 times the concentration free in serum or cytoplasm. If this prediction can be verified, the intracellularly active quinolone concentration in cytoplasm will also be quite similar to the serum concentration. Dosages required to inhibit intracellular pathogens would therefore aim for serum concentrations in relation to the bacterial MIC or MBC.

Finally, dosages and dosing intervals for the common extracellular Gram-negative and Gram-positive pathogens should be designed with full consideration of the relationships between antibiotic serum concentrations and the MIC (Schentag et al. 1985). For β-lactams (Schentag et al. 1984) and quinolones (Michéa-Hamzehpour et al. 1987; Nix et al. 1987), trough serum concentrations should invariably be maintained above the MIC and/or MBC. Studies of the phenomenon of early 'breakthrough bacteraemia' strongly reinforce the concept of maintaining antibiotic concentrations above the inhibitory levels for the entire dosing interval (Anderson et al. 1976). For aminoglycosides, troughs may fall below the MIC for a period of time, allowing the advantageous use of the postantibiotic effect (McCormack & Schentag 1987). How long aminoglycoside trough concentrations may be below the MIC remains an unanswered question which is actively being studied.

References

Anderson ET, Young LS, Hewitt WL. Simultaneous antibiotic levels in "breakthrough" gram-negative rod bacteremia. American Journal of Medicine 61: 493-497, 1976

Barza M, Weinstein L. Penetration of antibiotics into fibrin loci *in vivo*. I. Comparison of penetration of ampicillin into fibrin clots, abscesses, and interstitial fluid. Journal of Infectious Diseases 129: 59-65, 1974

Barza M, Samuelsson T, Weinstein L. Penetration of antibiotics into fibrin loci *in vivo*. II. Comparison of nine antibiotics: effect of dose and degree of protein binding. Journal of Infectious Diseases 129: 66-72, 1974

Brown KN, Percival A. Penetration of antimicrobials into tissue culture cells and leukocytes. Scandinavian Journal of Infectious Diseases 14 (Suppl.): 251-260, 1978

Chisholm GD, Waterworth PM, Calnan JS, Garrod LP. Concentration of antibacterial agents in interstitial tissue fluid. British Medical Journal 1: 569-573, 1973

Drusano GL. Role of pharmacokinetics in the outcome of infections. Antimicrobial Agents and Chemotherapy 32: 289-297, 1988

Drusano GL, Ryan PA, Standiford HC, Moody MR, Schimpff SC. Integration of selected pharmacologic and microbiologic properties of 3 new β-lactam antibiotics. A hypothesis for rational comparison. Review of Infectious Diseases 6: 357-363, 1984

Fabre J, Rudhart M, Blanchard P, Reganey C. Persistence of sisomycin and gentamicin in renal cortex and medulla compared with other organs and serum of rats. Kidney International 10: 444-449, 1976

Gengo FM, Schentag JJ. Methicillin distribution in serum and extravascular fluid, and its relevance to normal and damaged heart valves. Antimicrobial Agents and Chemotherapy 19: 836-841, 1981

Gengo FM, Schentag JJ. Rate of methicillin penetration into normal heart valves and experimental endocarditis lesions. Antimicrobial Agents and Chemotherapy 21: 456-459, 1982

Gengo FM, Mannion TW, Nightingale CH, Schentag JJ. Integration of pharmacokinetics and pharmacodynamics of methicillin in the curative treatment of experimental endocarditis. Journal of Antimicrobial Chemotherapy 14: 619-631, 1984

Gerding D, Hall WH, Schierl EA, Marion RE. Cephalosporin and aminoglycoside concentrations in peritoneal capsular fluid in rabbits. Antimicrobial Agents and Chemotherapy 10: 902-911, 1976

Glauser MP, Lyons JM, Braude AI. Prevention of pyelonephritis due to *E. coli* in rats with gentamicin stored in kidney tissue. Journal of Infectious Diseases 139: 172-177, 1979

Hoffstedt B, Walder M. Influence of serum protein binding and mode of administration on penetration of five cephalosporins into subcutaneous tissue fluid in humans. Antimicrobial Agents and Chemotherapy 20: 783-786, 1981

Kunin CM. Dosage schedules of antimicrobial agents: a historical review. Reviews of Infectious Diseases 3: 4-11, 1981

Lowry OH, Hastings AB. Histochemical changes associated with aging I. Methods and calculations. Journal of Biological Chemistry 143: 257-269, 1942

McCormack JP, Schentag JJ. The potential impact of quantitative susceptibility test on the design of aminoglycoside regimens. Drug Intelligence and Clinical Pharmacy 21: 187-191, 1987

Mandell GL. Interaction of intraleukocytic bacteria and antibiotics. Journal of Clinical Investigation 52: 1673-1679, 1973

Michéa-Hamzehpour M, Auckenthaler R, Regamey P, Pechère J-C. Resistance occurring after fluoroquinolone therapy of experimental *Pseudomonas aeruginosa* peritonitis. Antimicrobial Agents and Chemotherapy 31: 1803-1808, 1987

Moore RD, Lietman PS, Smith CR. Clinical response to aminoglycoside therapy: importance of the ratio of peak concentration to MIC. Journal of Infectious Diseases 155: 93-99, 1987

Neu HC. Current practices in antimicrobial dosing. Reviews of Infectious Diseases 3: 12-18, 1981

Neuman H. Clinical pharmacokinetics of the newer antimicrobial 4-quinolones. Clinical Pharmacokinetics 14: 96-121, 1988

Nix DE, Sands MF, Peloquin CA, Vari AJ, Cumbo TJ, et al. Dual individualization of intravenous ciprofloxacin in patients with nosocomial lower respiratory tract infections. American Journal of Medicine 82 (Suppl. 4A): 352-356, 1987

Noone P, Parsons TMC, Pattison JR, Slack RCB, Garfield-Davies D. Experience in monitoring gentamicin therapy during treatment of serious gram-negative sepsis. British Medical Journal 1: 477-481, 1974

Norrby RA. Review of the penetration of antibiotics into CSF, and its clinical significance. Scandinavian Journal of Infectious Diseases 14 (Suppl.): 296-309, 1978

Reitberg DP, Cumbo TJ, Smith IL, Schentag JJ. Effect of protein binding on cefmenoxime steady state kinetics in critical care patients. Clinical Pharmacology and Therapeutics 35: 64-73, 1984

Rolinson GN. The significance of protein binding of antibiotics in antibacterial chemotherapy. Journal of Antimicrobial Chemotherapy 6: 311-317, 1980

Rolinson GN. Tissue penetration of antibiotics. Journal of Antimicrobial Chemotherapy 13: 593-602, 1984

Roosendaal R, Bakker-Woudenberg IAJM, van den Berghe-van Raffe M, Michel MF. Continuous versus intermittent administration of ceftazidime in experimental *Klebsiella pneumoniae* in normal and leukopenic rats. Antimicrobial Agents and Chemotherapy 30: 403-408, 1986

Ryan DM, Cars O. Antibiotic assays in muscle: are conventional tissue levels misleading as indicators of antibacterial activity? Scandinavian Journal of Infectious Diseases 12: 307-309, 1980

Schentag JJ, Gengo FM. Principles of antibiotic tissue penetration and guidelines for pharmacokinetic analysis. Medical Clinics of North America 66: 39-49, 1982

Schentag JJ, Jusko WJ, Vance JW, Cumbo TJ, Abrutyn E, et al. Gentamicin disposition and tissue accumulation on multiple dosing. Journal of Pharmacokinetics and Biopharmaceutics 5: 559-577, 1977a

Schentag JJ, Jusko WJ, Plaut ME, Cumbo TJ, Vance JW, et al. Tissue persistence of gentamicin in man. Journal of the American Medical Association 238: 327-329, 1977b

Schentag JJ, Cumbo TJ, Jusko WJ, Plaut ME. Gentamicin tissue accumulation and nephrotoxic reactions. Journal of the American Medical Association 240: 2067-2069, 1978

Schentag JJ, Smith IL, Swanson DJ, DeAngelis C, Fracasso JE, et al. Role for dual individualization with cefmenoxime. American Journal of Medicine 77 (Suppl. 6A): 43-50, 1984

Schentag JJ, Swanson DJ, Smith IL. Dual individualization – antibiotic dosage calculation forms the integration of *in vitro* pharmacodynamics and *in vivo* pharmacokinetics. Journal of Antimicrobial Chemotherapy 15 (Suppl. A): 47-57, 1985

Tsuji A, Terasaki T, Imaeda N, Nishide K, Nakashima E. Effect of extracellular water volume on the distribution of kinetics of beta lactam antibiotics as a function of age. Journal of Pharmacobio-Dynamics 8: 167-174, 1985

Van Etta L, Fasching CE, Peterson LR, Gerding DN. Comparison study of the kinetics of ceftizoxime penetration into extravascular spaces with known surface area to volume ratios *in vitro* and *in vivo* in rabbits. Antimicrobial Agents and Chemotherapy 23: 49-53, 1983

Vogelman B, Gudmundsson S, Turnidge J, Leggett J, Craig WA. *In vivo* PAE in a thigh infection in neutropenic mice. Journal of Infectious Diseases 157: 287-289, 1988

Wise R, Gillett AP, Codge B, Durham SR, Baker S. The influence of protein binding upon tissue fluid levels of six β-lactam compounds. Journal of Infectious Diseases 142: 79-82, 1980

Author's address: *Jerome J. Schentag*, Clinical Pharmacokinetics Laboratory, Millard Fillmore Hospital, 3 Gates Circle, Buffalo, NY 14209 (USA).

Clinical Pharmacokinetics 16 (Suppl. 1): 32-37 (1989)
0312-5963/89/0001-0032/$3.00/0

Tissue Penetration and Clinical Efficacy of Enoxacin in Urinary Tract Infections

Stacy J. Childs

Department of Surgery, Community Health Sciences, University of Alabama, Tuscaloosa, Alabama, USA

Summary *The fluoroquinolones in general, and particularly enoxacin, show great promise in the treatment of urinary tract infection. Orally administered enoxacin achieves high concentrations in the serum and urine as well as in prostate tissue, kidney and perirenal fat and muscle. These concentrations are generally in excess of the minimum inhibitory concentrations (MIC) for 95% of the common uropathogens, including* Escherichia coli, Pseudomonas aeruginosa, Klebsiella *spp.,* Proteus *spp.,* Enterobacter *spp.,* Serratia marcescens *and* Staphylococcus saprophyticus.

In comparative clinical trials, treatment with oral enoxacin has achieved satisfactory clinical results (symptoms improved or absent) in 67 to 96% of patients and satisfactory bacteriological results (< 10^4 colony count of the original bacteria) in 77 to 98% of patients. Clinical cure or improvement occurred in 94 to 100% of patients in uncontrolled trials, with corresponding satisfactory bacteriological results of 82 to 100%. In a number of studies of patients with difficult-to-treat infections, satisfactory clinical results were achieved in 92 to 100% of patients and satisfactory bacteriological results in 89 to 100% of patients.

Antibiotic treatment of urinary tract infections presents problems, as *in vitro* bacterial susceptibility often correlates poorly with clinical results. Achievement of a bacterial inhibitory concentration of drug at the site of infection is essential for cure and probably more important than the plasma concentration. This is of even greater importance in difficult-to-treat infections such as prostatitis and pyelonephritis, in which bacteria tend to be more 'deeply rooted'. In addition, adequate tissue concentrations in areas such as the prostate and kidneys and in surrounding tissues such as fat and muscle are important in preventing infections associated with urological and renal surgery.

The object of this paper is to review pharmacokinetic and clinical aspects of enoxacin, a new broad spectrum quinolone antibiotic, in the treatment of urinary tract infections. As with other quinolones, enoxacin provides excellent coverage of pathogens most often found in urinary tract infections. In addition, the extensive tissue distribution of enoxacin results in concentrations that exceed MIC levels for most uropathogens.

1. Pharmacokinetics and Tissue Penetration

Wise et al. (1984) studied the pharmacokinetics of a single 600mg oral dose of enoxacin in volunteers. Mean peak serum levels, measured by microbiological assay, were 3.7 μg/ml at a mean of 1.9 hours after administration. In this study, 67% of the dose was recovered in the urine after 24 hours.

Urine levels of enoxacin remained in excess of 0.5 μg/ml for up to 72 hours after a single dose.

The penetration of enoxacin into renal tissues was evaluated by Malmborg and Ranikko (1988) in a study of 6 patients with renal tumours. After oral administration of enoxacin 200mg twice daily for 3 days, concentrations in the renal cortex and renal medulla (measured by microbiological assay) were 9.5 and 8.0 μg/g, respectively, with corresponding tissue : serum ratios of 3.8 and 3.2. Enoxacin also penetrated the surrounding muscle tissue (3.5 μg/g) and fat (0.9 μg/g). The mean (24-hour) urinary excretion was 62.7% of the daily dose.

Bergeron et al. (in press) used a microbiological assay to measure concentrations of a single oral dose of enoxacin 400mg in prostatic tissue obtained during transurethral prostatectomy. The mean concentration in 11 of 13 specimens in which the drug was detectable was 2.1 ± 0.3 μg/g. The ratio of tissue : serum concentration in this group of patients was 1.4 ± 0.2. In another patient, after 3 days of intravenous administration of enoxacin 300mg 3 times daily, the level of drug in the kidney parenchyma was 16.6 μg/ml, and the kidney : serum ratio was 7.7.

Ranikko and Malmborg (1986) administered enoxacin 200mg orally, twice daily for 3 days to 12 patients before transurethral resection. The mean prostatic tissue concentration in these patients, as measured by microbiological assay, was 4.1 ± 1.2 μg/g 3.9 hours after the final dose. The prostate : serum ratio in these patients was 2.1 ± 0.6 and the mean urinary excretion of enoxacin was 241.5 mg/day, or 60.4% of the daily dose.

2. *Activity against Common Urinary Tract Pathogens*

An effective agent for the treatment of urinary tract infections should provide concentrations in tissues and fluids that exceed the MIC_{90} of common uropathogens. The enoxacin MIC_{90} values of pathogens commonly responsible for 95% of urinary tract infections are ≤ 2.0 μg/ml (table I).

Table I. *In vitro* activity of enoxacin against common urinary tract pathogens (after Clarke et al. 1985; Siporin & Towse 1984)

Organism	Enoxacin MIC_{90} (μg/ml)
E. coli	0.5
P. aeruginosa	2.0
Klebsiella spp.	1.0
Proteus spp.	0.5
Enterobacter spp.	0.5
Serratia marcescens	0.5
Staphylococcus saprophyticus	2.0

3. *Therapeutic Trials*

3.1 Uncontrolled Trials

Table II summarises worldwide data from uncontrolled trials of enoxacin in the treatment of uncomplicated and complicated urinary tract infections in nearly 500 patients. Patients in these trials received oral enoxacin 200 or 400mg twice daily for 7 to 14 days. Overall, 305 of 319 evaluable patients (96%) were considered clinically cured or improved, and satisfactory bacteriological results (< 10^4 colony count of the original bacteria) were obtained in 290 of 328 patients (88%). In these studies, a total of only 23 patients were withdrawn because of adverse events, which included headache, nausea and other gastrointestinal symptoms, insomnia and dizziness. Some patients also experienced rashes. Two patients in the multicentre study experienced seizures; these were considered to have no known relationship to treatment.

3.2 Comparative Trials

3.2.1 Comparison with Amoxycillin

Seven-day courses of enoxacin and amoxycillin were compared in a randomised, double-blind, multicentre study in Canada (data on file, Warner-Lambert/Parke Davis; DuBois et al. 1987). 64 patients (1 male, 63 female, mean age 30.2 years) with uncomplicated lower urinary tract infections (predominantly acute cystitis caused by *E. coli*) received 7-day courses of enoxacin 200mg twice daily (n = 30) or amoxycillin 500mg twice daily

Table II. Uncontrolled clinical trials involving enoxacin 200 to 400mg twice daily in genitourinary infections (data on file, Warner-Lambert/Parke Davis; Thomas & Ellis-Pegler 1985)

Principal investigators	No. of patients	Patient characteristics					Outcome (5-9 days post-treatment)					
		age range (mean) [y]	sex (M/F)	urinary tract infection			pyelonephritis (%)	cystitis (%)	prostatitis	other/multi[a] (%)	adverse effects (withdrawals)
				complicated	uncomplicated						
Multicentre (10 countries)	413	14-94 (51.8)	188/233	30	383	Clin[b]	63/66 (95)	129/33 (97)	6/6	39/41 (95)	18
						Bact[c]	57/66 (86)	125/132 (95)	6/6	33/41 (80)	
Claereboudt (Belgium)	20	17-80 (41.4)	12/8	20		Clin	2/3	7/8		3/3	5
						Bact	2/3	10/11		3/3	
Barsotti (Italy)	20	20-65 (48)	4/16	8	12	Clin	10/10	10/10			
						Bact	6/10	10/10			
Ellis-Pegler (New Zealand)	20	17-65 (36)	7/13	5	15	Clin	6/7	12/13			
						Bact	4/7	18/20			
Schmidbauer (Austria)	21	40-89 (66.3)	13/8	8	13	Clin	3/3	13/14	1/1	1/1	
						Bact	2/3	12/14	1/1	1/1	
Total	494		216/278	71	423	Clin	84/89 (94)	171/178 (96)	7/7	43/45 (96)	23
						Bact	71/89 (90)	175/187 (94)	7/7	37/45 (82)	

a Rarer conditions and combinations of these, e.g. ureteritis, urethritis, epididymitis.
b No. of patients with satisfactory clinical outcome/no. of evaluable patients.
c No. of patients with satisfactory bacteriological outcome/no. of evaluable patients.

(n = 34). At the short term follow-up, 86% of enoxacin-treated and 93% of amoxycillin-treated patients were classified as clinically cured or improved, and 90% and 86%, respectively, had satisfactory bacteriological results ($p > 0.05$). 13 enoxacin-treated patients experienced adverse events, 11 of which were definitely or probably related to treatment. Adverse events included headache, nausea and/or vomiting and candidiasis. 18 patients treated with amoxycillin experienced adverse events, 9 of which were definitely or probably related to the study drug. These included diarrhoea, nausea and/or vomiting, mycotic infection and lumbar pain.

Single-dose treatment with enoxacin has been shown to be effective in some patients with uncomplicated urinary tract infection. In a randomised study conducted in Germany (Bischoff 1986), 120 women with acute (n = 55), recurrent (n = 47), or chronic cystitis (n = 18) received single oral doses of enoxacin 400mg (60 patients) or amoxycillin 3g (60 patients). *E. coli* was the most common pathogen, occurring in 57% of the enoxacin group and in 63% of the amoxycillin group. The 7-day follow-up evaluation showed a 96% satisfactory clinical response and a 98% satisfactory bacteriological response for enoxacin, and corresponding values of 85% and 91% for amoxycillin ($p > 0.05$). Adverse events were experienced by 2 patients treated with enoxacin (3.3%) [gastrointestinal disturbances] and 10 who received amoxycillin (16.6%) [allergy and gastrointestinal disturbances].

3.2.2 Comparison with Trimethoprim

A similar study in New Zealand (data on file, Warner-Lambert/Parke Davis) enrolled 53 patients (2 male, 51 female, mean age 27 years) with cystitis. 28 patients received a single oral dose of enoxacin 400mg, and 25 received a single oral dose of trimethoprim 600mg. The predominant organism in both groups was *E. coli.* Of the baseline pathogens susceptible to both agents, enoxacin eradicated 77%, and trimethoprim eradicated 94% ($p > 0.05$). At the 7-day follow-up, 67% of enoxacin-treated patients and 89% of trimethoprim-treated patients were cured or improved. One patient in each group experienced an adverse event (candidiasis).

3.3 Difficult-to-Treat Infections

3.3.1 Complicated Urinary Tract Infections

A number of non-comparative trials have evaluated the efficacy of enoxacin in difficult-to-treat urinary tract infections (table III). One study consisted of 64 patients (30 male, 34 female, median age 58 years) with complicated urinary tract infections caused by pathogens resistant to co-trimoxazole (predominantly *Pseudomonas aeruginosa, E. coli* and *Klebsiella pneumoniae*). These patients received oral enoxacin 400mg twice daily for 14 days. At the short term follow-up evaluation (5 to 9 days after treatment), 59 of 60 evaluable patients (98%) had satisfactory clinical results (cure or improvement), and all patients were classified as bacteriologically cured. Therapy was discontinued in 2 patients because of adverse events (nausea and pruritus) [data on file, Warner-Lambert/Parke Davis].

3.3.2 Paraplegic/Tetraplegic Patients

Two studies of difficult-to-treat urinary tract infections in paraplegic or tetraplegic patients achieved excellent results with twice-daily oral administration of enoxacin (table III). In a multicentre study involving 40 paraplegic or tetraplegic patients with cystitis and/or pyelonephritis, a dosage of enoxacin 400mg twice daily (n = 30) or 200mg twice daily (n = 10) was administered for a mean of 7.7 days. Five to 9 days after the end of treatment, 100% of patients with a single causative pathogen (mainly *E. coli, P. aeruginosa* or *Proteus* spp.) had satisfactory bacteriological results, as did 2 of 4 patients with multiple pathogens. Clinical response was satisfactory in 100% of patients. Therapy had to be discontinued in 5 patients because of adverse events which included nausea and/or vomiting in 4 patients and pruritus in 1 patient (data on file, Warner-Lambert/Parke Davis).

In a similar single-centre study, 20 paraplegic or tetraplegic patients received enoxacin 400mg twice

Table III. Non-comparative studies involving twice-daily enoxacin in difficult-to-treat urinary tract infections (data on file, Warner-Lambert/Parke Davis; Tosolini et al. 1988)

Patient group	No. of patients	Mean study duration (days)	Twice daily dosage (mg)	Results		
				patients with satisfactory clinical outcome (%)	patients with satisfactory bacteriological outcome (%)	no. of patients withdrawn because of adverse effects
Co-trimoxazole-resistant (complicated UTI)	64	14	400	98	100	2
Elderly (mean age 80.4 years)	101	6.5	200 or 400	92	89	3
Paraplegic/tetraplegic	40	7.7	200 or 400	100	91	5
Paraplegic/tetraplegic	20	6.8	400	100	88	

daily for a mean of 6.8 days. The clinical response was 100% satisfactory at the 5- to 9-day follow-up, and the bacteriological response was 88% satisfactory. Three patients reported mild adverse experiences (nausea and/or rash) that were considered to be related to treatment. However, no patient was withdrawn as a result of these (Tosolini et al. 1988).

3.3.3 Elderly Patients

A large group of elderly patients (10 male, 91 female, mean age 80.4 years) with pyelonephritis and/or cystitis received enoxacin 200 or 400mg twice daily for a mean of 6.5 days (table III). 70% of patients had chronic or recurrent infections, most frequently caused by *E. coli, Proteus mirabilis* or *K. pneumoniae.* 92% of these patients were clinically cured or improved. Of the 66 patients eligible for bacteriological evaluation at the 5- to 9-day follow-up, 89% had a satisfactory bacteriological response. This included 93% of *E. coli*, 81% of *P. mirabilis,* and 100% of *K. pneumoniae* infections. A total of 41 adverse events were noted by 29 of 101 patients in this study; 16 adverse events were considered to be definitely or probably related to the drug. Therapy was discontinued in 3 patients because of adverse events; 1 patient had nausea and vomiting and 2 patients had epileptiform seizures, although both of these had a history of cerebrovascular disturbance (data on file, Warner-Lambert/Parke Davis; Huttunen et al. 1988).

3.4 Prophylaxis

The prophylactic use of oral enoxacin in prostate surgery has recently been reported (Desai et al. 1988). In this double-blind study, 32 patients undergoing prostatectomy received 5 doses of enoxacin 200mg (2 preoperative and 3 postoperative doses). Only 2 postoperative urinary tract infections were reported in this group (both in patients with indwelling catheters), compared with 12 infections in a control group of 34 patients who received placebo.

References

Bergeron MG, Roy R, Lessard C, Foucault P. Enoxacin penetration into human renal and prostatic tissues. Antimicrobial Agents and Chemotherapy 32 (9): 1433-1434, 1988

Bischoff W. Vergleichende Untersuchung von Enoxacin mit Amoxicillin bei der akuten unkomplizierten Zystitis der Frau. Infection 14 (Suppl. 3): S209-S210, 1986

Chang T, Black A, Dunky A, Wolf R, Sedman A, et al. Pharmacokinetics of intravenous and oral enoxacin in healthy volunteers. Journal of Antimicrobial Chemotherapy 32 (Suppl. B): 49-56, 1988

Chin N-X, Neu HC. In vitro activity of enoxacin, a quinolone carboxylic acid, compared with those of norfloxacin, new β-lactams, aminoglycosides, and trimethoprim. Antimicrobial Agents and Chemotherapy 24: 754-763, 1983

Clarke AM, Zemcov SJV, Campbell ME. In-vitro activity of pefloxacin compared to enoxacin, norfloxacin, gentamicin, and new β-lactams. Journal of Antimicrobial Chemotherapy 15: 39-44, 1985

Desai K, White LO, Abrams P. Efficacy and pharmacokinetics of enoxacin administered prophylactically for benign prostatic hypertrophy. Reviews of Infectious Diseases 10 (Suppl. 1): S176, 1988

Dubois J, Martel A, Saad WP. Randomized evaluation of enoxacin and amoxicillin in the treatment of urinary tract infec-

tions (abstract 1170). 15th International Congress of Chemotherapy, Istanbul, Turkey, 1987
Huttunen M, Kunnas K, Saloranta P. Enoxacin treatment of urinary tract infections in elderly patients. Journal of Antimicrobial Chemotherapy 21 (Suppl. B): 105-111, 1988
Malmborg A-S, Ranikko S. Enoxacin distribution in human tissue after multiple oral administration. Journal of Antimicrobial Chemotherapy 21 (Suppl. B): 57-60, 1988
Ranikko S, Malmborg A-S. Enoxacin concentration in human prostatic tissue after oral administration. Journal of Antimicrobial Chemotherapy 17: 123, 1986
Siporin C, Towse G. Enoxacin: worldwide in-vitro activity against 22451 clinical isolates. Journal of Antimicrobial Chemotherapy 14 (Suppl. C): 47-55, 1984
Thomas MG, Ellis-Pegler RB. Enoxacin treatment of urinary tract infections. Journal of Antimicrobial Chemotherapy 15: 759-763, 1985
Tosolini FA, Brown DJ, Herbert DB, Geddes A. Enoxacin treatment of urinary tract infections in patients with spinal injuries. Reviews of Infectious Diseases 10 (Suppl. 1): S177-S178, 1988
Wise R, Griggs D, Andrews JR. Pharmacokinetics of the quinolones in volunteers: a proposed dosing schedule. Reviews of Infectious Diseases 10: S83-S89, 1988
Wise R, Lockley R, Dent J, Webberly M. Pharmacokinetics and tissue penetration of enoxacin. Antimicrobial Agents and Chemotherapy 26: 17-19, 1984

Author's address: Dr *Stacy J. Childs*, Alabama Urology Associates, 1006 First Street, Suite 203, Alabaster, Alabama 35007 (USA).

Clinical Pharmacokinetics 16 (Suppl. 1): 38-45 (1989)
0312-5963/89/0001-0038/$4.00/0

Tissue Penetration and Clinical Efficacy of Enoxacin in Respiratory Tract Infections

M.J. Wood

Department of Communicable and Tropical Diseases, East Birmingham Hospital, Birmingham, United Kingdom

Summary

Enoxacin, in common with other new oral 4-quinolones, has a broad spectrum of antimicrobial activity which includes most pulmonary pathogens (with the exception of Streptococcus pneumoniae, *against which its activity is poor); this spectrum has provided the impetus for investigation of its potential in the treatment of respiratory infections.*

Initial pharmacokinetic studies have demonstrated that the drug has a large volume of distribution and achieves concentrations in the secretions of the respiratory tract that are at least as high as those attained in the serum. These concentrations are sufficient to suggest that enoxacin would be effective treatment for most respiratory infections. Furthermore, the concentration of enoxacin that is achieved within the bronchopulmonary tissues is considerably higher than peak serum concentrations and suggests not only that there is an active transport mechanism, but also that the drug could be expected to eradicate organisms in the lungs such as streptococci that are considered moderately sensitive to the drug in vitro.

There are relatively few clinical studies of, and thus limited data on, the efficacy of enoxacin in the treatment of respiratory tract infections. A review of the evidence suggests that enoxacin is as successful as other therapies used in the treatment of acute exacerbations of chronic bronchitis. There have sometimes been failures of eradication of, and occasional superinfections with, pneumococci. Enoxacin is also likely to interact with the metabolism of theophylline and so lead to elevated theophylline plasma concentrations. Hence when these 2 agents are given concurrently, careful monitoring of theophylline concentrations and/or dosage adjustments are recommended. In more chronic infections, particularly those caused by Pseudomonas aeruginosa, *enoxacin seems to be effective, but further comparative studies with more conventional intravenous treatments are required.*

Infections of both the lower and the upper respiratory tract are extremely common and are a frequent indication for antibiotic use in the community and in the hospital. Most community-acquired infections are caused by a relatively small number of predictable pathogens. More unusual pathogens, particularly Gram-negative enteric bacteria and *Pseudomonas aeruginosa*, are implicated in hospital-acquired respiratory infections and in exacerbations of certain types of chronic disease, particularly cystic fibrosis and bronchiectasis. Because of the satisfactory microbiological activity of the new oral 4-quinolones against most of these respiratory pathogens, it is natural that they should be considered for the treatment of respiratory tract infections.

One of the most important factors that determines the efficacy of any drug in the treatment of respiratory tract infections is its penetration to the site of infection in the tissues of the lung or upper respiratory tract at concentrations that exceed the minimum inhibitory concentration (MIC) of the infecting pathogen (Bergogne-Berezin 1981). Indeed, studies have shown that the clinical response depends upon whether the antibiotic concentrations in the sputum are above or below the bacterial MIC (Maesen et al. 1976; May 1965).

The concentration of drug at the site of action depends largely on passive diffusion into the infected tissues (Lambert 1978), which is in turn determined by its degree of ionisation at physiological pH, its lipophilicity and the presence or absence of inflammation (May 1965). Local metabolism of the drug and the clearance of bronchial secretions may also play a major role in determining the drug's clinical effectiveness.

This paper reviews the pharmacokinetic profile of the new quinolone antibiotic, enoxacin, with regard to its ability to penetrate to the site of infection in the respiratory tract and the available evidence of its efficacy in the treatment of respiratory tract infections.

1. Penetration of Enoxacin into Respiratory Tract Tissues

1.1 Absorption and Overall Distribution

The rapidity of absorption of oral enoxacin in volunteers is somewhat variable (Wise et al. 1984) with t_{max} [time required to reach maximum plasma concentrations (C_{max})] ranging from 0.75 to 3 hours, but there is less variability in the maximum serum concentrations attained. After a single oral dose of 600mg the C_{max} is approximately 4.0 mg/L (Wijnands et al. 1988; Wise et al. 1984). In common with the other newer quinolones, enoxacin is widely distributed throughout the body, with a volume of distribution estimated as 113L (Dobbs et al. 1985). Such a high volume of distribution indicates that the tissue levels of enoxacin are often markedly higher than those in serum.

1.2 Sputum Concentrations

Maximum sputum levels of enoxacin are achieved approximately 3 hours after dosing (i.e. approximately 1 hour after peak serum levels) and decline with a half-life of between 4 and 5 hours (Davies et al. 1984; Wijnands et al. 1988) [table I]. In 24 French patients with respiratory tract infections, enoxacin concentrations in expectorated sputum were measured by high performance liquid chromatography (HPLC) at intervals after a 400mg dose on day 3 of treatment (Morel et al. 1987). The ratio of the mean peak sputum to mean peak serum levels was 1.2, with figures ranging from 0.95 to 1.5 for individual patients. The sputum concentrations after 600mg doses of enoxacin have been measured in other studies of patients with respiratory infections (Davies et al. 1984; Wijnands et al. 1988). The Dutch group obtained mean peak sputum concentrations of 6.9 mg/L at steady state after 600mg twice daily for 2 days, a value that equated with a sputum : serum ratio of 0.93 (Wijnands et al. 1988). By contrast, in the study by Davies et al. (1984), somewhat lower peak sputum concentrations (3.7 mg/L) were attained after administration of a single 600mg dose of enoxacin to patients. In this latter study, however, a microbiological assay, as opposed to HPLC, was used; since microbiologically active metabolites are formed from enoxacin, this is a potentially less accurate method of assay.

In all these studies expectorated sputum was assayed; it is possible that this was diluted by saliva, leading to artificially low enoxacin concentrations. To overcome this difficulty of potentially contaminated expectorated sputum, samples can be collected from persons with permanent tracheostomies. In 6 such subjects, administration of enoxacin 400mg twice daily for 7 days resulted in steady-state peak sputum levels ranging from 3.47 to 15.29 mg/L. The ratio of peak sputum concentrations to those in plasma varied from 0.65 to 3.68 and those of the sputum to plasma $AUC_{(0-12)}$ from 0.83 to 3.49, with a mean of 1.61 (Dobbs et al. 1988). These levels are somewhat higher than those obtained after similar doses given to other tracheostomied

Table I. Serum, sputum and lung tissue concentrations of enoxacin obtained after oral administration of 400mg twice daily

Tissue	Peak serum level (mg/L)	Peak tissue level (mg/L)	Tissue : serum ratio	Sputum AUC_{0-12} (mg/L · h)
Sputum/bronchial mucus				
Fong et al. 1987	2.5	2.4	1.0	
Morel et al. 1987	2.4	2.9	1.2	
Dobbs et al. 1988[a]	4.5	7.1	1.7	40.9
Wijnands et al. 1988	4.8	2.7	0.5	
Davies et al. 1984[b]	4.1	3.7	0.9	25.0
Lung tissue				
Newsom & Wells 1987	1.9	7.7	3.9	
Wijnands et al. 1988[c]	2.0	7.0	3.5	
Marlin et al. 1986[d]	3.1	117.0	46.8	

a Healthy subjects.
b Single dose; microbiological assay.
c 600mg single dose.
d Bronchial mucosa.

patients with copious sputum production (Fong et al. 1987) and are comparable with those achieved in expectorated sputum from patients with respiratory infections who were studied on the third day of treatment with enoxacin 600mg twice daily (Wijnands et al. 1988).

1.2.1 Comparison with Other Quinolones

The degree of penetration of enoxacin into purulent sputum determined in these studies compares favourably with that of other newly developed quinolones. A review by Davies et al. (1986) reported the sputum penetration of several quinolones, as judged by the sputum AUC values in relation to the corresponding serum values after a single dose, as enoxacin (400mg) 88.9%, ciprofloxacin (750mg) 76.7%, pefloxacin (400mg) 86.4% and ofloxacin (400mg) 101.2%.

1.3 Lung Tissue Concentrations

Studies in patients undergoing elective pneumonectomy for carcinoma have demonstrated that enoxacin can readily penetrate into lung tissues (Newsom & Wells 1987) [table I]. Administration of a 400mg dose of enoxacin the night before surgery, followed by a second 400mg dose 2 hours preoperatively, resulted in lung tissue concentrations, determined by HPLC, ranging between 1.6 and 12.4 mg/L (mean 7.7 mg/L). These levels were on average 3.9 times higher than levels achieved in plasma. Moreover, drug concentrations from samples that contained predominantly bronchus were not substantially different from the concentrations found in samples that were almost entirely composed of lung parenchyma. Similar results were obtained by Wijnands et al. (1988) after administration of a single 600mg dose of enoxacin given to 15 male patients before thoracotomy for bronchial malignancy. In this study enoxacin concentrations in normal lung tissue peaked at a mean time of 2.8 hours after drug ingestion and were 3.5 times higher than corresponding plasma levels.

Marlin et al. (1986) specifically studied the penetration of enoxacin into the bronchial mucosa. Samples were obtained from patients undergoing fibreoptic bronchoscopy who had been given enoxacin 400mg twice daily for 4 days. The mean tissue concentration of enoxacin, measured 3 to 5 hours after the last dose, was 117 mg/L, but there was a high degree of variation between subjects, with values ranging from 50.7 to 195.8 mg/L. These concentrations were approximately 50 times higher than those in the plasma, and there were no significant differences in the bronchial mucosa to plasma concentration ratios at the different times of sampling. The authors suggested that this remarkable degree of penetration might be explained by either an active transport mechanism (enoxacin apparently exists as a zwitterion at physiological pH) or by enoxacin avidly binding to tissue macromolecules. These results do not correspond to the findings reported by Newsom and Wells (1987) and clearly require further validation, but, if substantiated, they would provide evidence to suggest that enoxacin is concentrated in the mucosa before secretion into sputum.

1.4 Concentrations in Upper Respiratory Tract Secretions

Limited pharmacokinetic data are available for enoxacin in upper respiratory tract infections, but 1 study has reported fluid or tissue to serum ratios of 5 : 1 for middle ear pus, 3 : 1 for sinus mucosa and 2 : 1 for interstitial fluid/lymph (Federspil et al. 1986).

1.5 Effect of Inflammation

In the study of Marlin et al. (1986) there were only 2 patients with active pulmonary infection at the time of bronchial biopsy; therefore, more data are required before it can be determined whether inflammation influences the transport of enoxacin into bronchial tissue. Some suggestion that this might be the case comes from the results of Wijnands et al. (1988). They showed that there was a fall in the ratio of peak sputum to peak plasma concentrations after a single dose from 0.75 (400mg doses) and 1.0 (600mg doses) to 0.56 and 0.9, respectively, when steady state was achieved on the third day of treatment, and that this fall was accompanied by a concomitant reduction in sputum purulence.

2. *Activity of Enoxacin against Respiratory Tract Pathogens*

The rapid and complete penetration of enoxacin into sputum, bronchial mucus and lung tissue results in local concentrations of the drug which exceed the MICs for most respiratory tract pathogens (table II). Enoxacin has excellent activity against the majority of bacteria that are responsible for upper and lower respiratory tract infections. Enterobacteriaceae, *Haemophilus influenzae* and *Legionella* spp. are particularly susceptible to enoxacin *in vitro*, with MIC_{90} values of < 1 mg/L (Chin & Neu 1983; Fallon & Brown 1985; Siporin & Towse 1984). The susceptibilities of *Branhamella* spp. (Davies et al. 1986), *P. aeruginosa* and *Staphylococcus aureus* also fall within the range of achievable tissue concentrations (Chin & Neu 1983; Siporin & Towse 1984), but many strains of *Streptococcus pneumoniae* (Chin & Neu 1983; Siporin & Towse 1984), and *Mycoplasma pneumoniae* (Fallon & Brown 1985) are less susceptible to enoxacin, and their MICs fall outside the concentrations of enoxacin attained in sputum or lung tissue (but not necessarily outside the concentrations reported in bronchial mucosa).

Table II. Mean MIC_{90} of enoxacin against common respiratory pathogens (from Chin & Neu 1983; Davies et al. 1986; Fallon & Brown 1985; Siporin & Towse 1984)

Organism	Mean MIC_{90} (mg/L)
Enterobacteriaceae	< 1.0
Haemophilus influenzae	0.125
Legionella spp.	< 0.5
Branhamella spp.	2.0
Staphylococcus aureus	2.0
Pseudomonas aeruginosa	4.0
Mycoplasma pneumoniae	5.0
Streptococcus pneumoniae	8.0-16.0

3. *Enoxacin in the Treatment of Respiratory Tract Infections*

The pharmacokinetic profile of enoxacin, coupled with its microbiological activity, thus appears to make the drug suitable for the treatment of respiratory tract infections, especially those caused by Gram-negative pathogens. Recent clinical experience largely supports this optimism.

3.1 Efficacy in Lower Respiratory Tract Infections

3.1.1 Open Label Studies

Excellent clinical and bacteriological efficacy has been obtained with enoxacin in the treatment of lower respiratory tract infections (table III). The majority of cases treated have been acute exacerbations of chronic bronchitis and bronchopneumonia or bronchiectasis caused by *H. influenzae, P. aeruginosa* or *S. pneumoniae.* A multicentre, non-comparative, open study of oral enoxacin in the treatment of serious lower respiratory tract infections included 121 evaluable patients given either 400mg (107 patients) or 600mg (14 patients) twice daily (data on file, Warner Lambert International). Although the clinical response was uniformly good, the bacteriological results varied according to the pathogen involved. A high success rate was achieved against infections caused by *H. influenzae* (100% eradicated) and Enterobacteriaceae (92%), but the results were somewhat less satisfactory against *S. pneumoniae* (76%) and *P. aeruginosa* (61%).

These observations have been substantiated by Wijnands et al. (1986), who evaluated the efficacy of enoxacin against 43 respiratory tract infections in 39 patients. Most patients had chronic obstructive pulmonary disease, and patients with *P. aeruginosa* infections were particularly selected; 23 of the 43 courses were given to patients with proven bronchiectasis who were chronically colonised with *P. aeruginosa.* These patients were treated with enoxacin 600mg twice daily, whereas other infections were treated with enoxacin 400mg twice daily. Although the clinical response was satisfactory in the patients with *P. aeruginosa* infections, only 6 of the cases (26%) responded fully to treatment, as defined by the complete eradication of the pathogen. In a further 12 cases (52%), however, there was a clear reduction in sputum purulence and *Pseudomonas* growth. Furthermore, it was noted that 2- to 4-fold rises in MICs compared with pretreatment values were observed for most of the *P. aeruginosa* strains that persisted in the sputum, and that these strains with increased MICs remained in the patients' sputum for several months. In 20 non-pseudomonal infections in the same study, a much higher bacteriological response rate (90%) was achieved, and only 1 strain of *S. aureus* persisted in the sputum.

Davies et al. (1984) treated 15 elderly patients with acute exacerbations of chronic obstructive airways disease with enoxacin 600mg twice daily. After 3 days of treatment most strains of *S. pneumoniae* had not been eradicated from the sputum; however, further assessment was not possible, since, in the majority of the patients, treatment had to be

Table III. Enoxacin in the treatment of lower respiratory tract infections

Study	No. of infections	Clinical response rate (%)	Bacteriological response rate (%)
Open label studies			
International (data on file, Warner Lambert)	121	91	82
Wijnands et al. 1986	43	91	56[a]
Philip-Joet et al. 1988	20	85	83
Versus amoxycillin (Prigogine et al. 1988)			
enoxacin	23	83	88
amoxycillin	14	93	71
Versus co-trimoxazole (Maasilta et al. 1988)			
enoxacin	24	88	
co-trimoxazole	26	96	

a Bacteriological response rate 90% for non-pseudomonal infections.

discontinued because of severe adverse reactions involving the gastrointestinal or nervous systems. A further group of 20 hospitalised patients with chronic obstructive lung disease complicated by pneumonia (8 patients) or other infective exacerbations were treated in Marseilles by Philip-Joet et al. (1988). The predominant pathogens, again *H. influenzae, S. pneumoniae* and *P. aeruginosa,* were treated with enoxacin 400mg twice daily for 7 to 10 days. Three patients failed to respond clinically (including 1 patient with legionnaires' disease), and in 2 cases, the responsible pathogen (1 strain each of *S. aureus* and *S. pneumoniae*) was not eradicated.

3.1.2 Comparison with Other Agents

There have been 2 published comparative studies of enoxacin and other antibiotics in lower respiratory tract infections. In 1, the efficacy of enoxacin (400mg 12-hourly) in Gram-negative lower respiratory tract infections was compared with that of amoxycillin (1g 8-hourly) in 43 hospitalised patients with exacerbations of chronic bronchitis or bronchiectasis (Prigogine et al. 1988). Although the study was initially randomised, the treatment was changed to enoxacin if, in the amoxycillin group, the pathogen isolated was subsequently found to be resistant to amoxycillin. 37 of the 43 cases were evaluable (23 enoxacin and 14 amoxycillin). The overall clinical and bacteriological results showed no significant difference between the 2 groups (table III), although the small numbers treated make this conclusion of little worth. In the enoxacin group, 2 pathogens persisted at the end of therapy (both *P. aeruginosa*), 1 infection with *H. influenzae* relapsed and in 3 cases superinfections with *S. pneumoniae* occurred. In the amoxycillin group there were 4 relapses of *H. influenzae.*

The efficacy of enoxacin (400mg twice daily) was also found to be comparable with that of co-trimoxazole, when studied in 50 evaluable patients with serious lower respiratory tract infections (Maasilta et al. 1988). This study included 4 patients with pneumonia, but the protocol specifically excluded patients with pneumococcal infections. Overall, there was little toxicity noted, but at the end of treatment 13 patients had *Candida albicans* isolated from sputum cultures. It is not clear which group 4 of these patients were in, but 3 of the remaining 9 had received enoxacin and 6 co-trimoxazole.

3.1.3 Comparison with Other Quinolones

Enoxacin also compares favourably with other newly developed quinolones in the treatment of acute exacerbations of chronic bronchitis. In a recent review, good to excellent results were obtained at follow-up 7 days after the end of therapy in the following percentage of patients: enoxacin (400mg twice daily) 64%, ciprofloxacin (750mg twice daily) 58%, pefloxacin (400mg twice daily) 68% and ofloxacin (400mg twice daily) 67% (Davies et al. 1986).

3.2 Efficacy in Upper Respiratory Tract Infections

There have been few studies of enoxacin in the treatment of upper respiratory tract infections (URTI) [table IV].

3.2.1 Open Studies

The results from an open, multicentre study of patients with otitis media, sinusitis, tonsillitis and other URTI indicated excellent clinical responses, but the bacteriological response rate was influenced by the large number of infections caused by *P. aeruginosa* that were included (data on file, Warner Lambert International). The patients studied in the brief report by Federspil et al. (1986) also included many with chronic, often pseudomonal, infections of the upper airways. No bacteriological results were included in this paper.

3.2.2 Comparative Study

The only published comparative study of enoxacin in URTI is against amoxycillin in the treatment of chronic suppurative otitis media (Krajewski et al. 1988). The patient population in this study consisted of 40 black South African patients with severe and long-standing disease. After 10 days of treatment with enoxacin (400mg twice daily), the

Table IV. Enoxacin in the treatment of upper respiratory tract infections

Study	No. of infections	Clinical response rate (%)	Bacteriological response rate (%)
Open label studies			
International (data on file, Warner Lambert)	109	89	71
Federspil et al. 1986	60	82	
Versus amoxycillin (Krajewski 1988)			
enoxacin	21	53	50
amoxycillin	19	32	56

clinical and bacteriological response rates were comparable with those achieved with amoxycillin (table IV). Moreover, audiological assessments indicated that there was a tendency for bone conduction to be improved only in those patients who had received enoxacin, and, using a measurement of 'overall effectiveness', enoxacin appeared significantly superior ($p < 0.05$).

4. *Safety Profile*

Enoxacin has proved to be generally well tolerated in these studies. Occasional rashes have been reported (Philip-Joet et al. 1988), and, in common with other quinolones, enoxacin may produce gastric pain or nausea in a small proportion of patients (Federspil et al. 1986; Maasilta et al. 1988).

4.1 Interaction with Theophylline

The study of Davies et al. (1984) documented a high incidence of side effects when enoxacin was given in combination with theophylline; this led to discontinuation of enoxacin therapy in 9 of their 15 patients. Subsequent studies have provided evidence that the metabolism of enoxacin to 4-oxo-enoxacin uses the enzyme that metabolises theophylline, thus leading to reduced clearance and hence elevated plasma concentrations of the latter drug (Wijnands et al. 1985). This is not always a clinical problem: in the study of Philip-Joet et al. (1988), for example, the plasma concentration of theophylline was found to rise from 12.5 to 25 mg/L in 1 of 2 patients monitored, but none of the 9 patients receiving concurrent theophylline-enoxacin therapy developed any signs of toxicity. Careful monitoring of theophylline concentrations and/or dosage adjustments is, however, recommended whenever the 2 agents are given concurrently (Wijnands et al. 1985).

5. *Conclusion*

The results of these clinical studies suggest that enoxacin, in common with the other quinolones, can be used for acute purulent respiratory infections. However, some reservations about the use of enoxacin in these infections must be expressed. Of paramount concern is the relatively poor *in vitro* activity against pneumococci; although in many instances therapy of such infections has been successful, the overall bacteriological efficacy of enoxacin against this pathogen in lower respiratory tract infections is only 78% (data on file, Warner Lambert International). The overgrowth of *S. pneumoniae* reported in some studies (Prigogine et al. 1988; Wijnands et al. 1986) has been noted with other quinolones, notably ciprofloxacin, used to treat exacerbations of chronic bronchitis (Davies et al. 1986) and is a further argument against the empirical use of these agents in chronic chest disease.

Limited clinical experience has been gained with enoxacin in the treatment of *P. aeruginosa* infections, but the results obtained by Wijnands et al. (1986) suggest that rises in the MIC of enoxacin against this organism are likely to occur during treatment of infections. Similar findings have been obtained for ciprofloxacin (Roberts et al. 1985), but the clinical significance of this phenomenon for the use of the quinolones in patients with chronic pseudomonal infections and cystic fibrosis has yet to be clarified.

References

Bergogne-Berezin E. Penetration of antibiotics into the respiratory tree. Journal of Antimicrobial Chemotherapy 8: 171-174, 1981

Chin N-X, Neu HC. *In vitro* activity of enoxacin, a quinolone carboxylic acid, compared with those of norfloxacin, new beta-lactams, aminoglycosides, and trimethoprim. Antimicrobial Agents and Chemotherapy 24: 754-763, 1983

Davies BI, Maesen FPV, Teengs JP. Serum and sputum concentrations of enoxacin after single oral dosing in a clinical and bacteriological study. Journal of Antimicrobial Chemotherapy 14 (Suppl. C): 83-89, 1984

Davies BI, Maesen FPV, Teengs JP, Baur C. Neue orale Chinolon-Verbindungen bei chronischer Bronchitis. Infection 14 (Suppl. 1): S73-S78, 1986

Dobbs BR, Grazeley LR, Stewart IA, Edwards IR. Pharmacokinetics and penetration of enoxacin into sputum. In Ishigami (Ed.) Recent advances in chemotherapy 1985, pp. 1735-1736, Tokyo University Press, Tokyo, 1985

Dobbs BR, Gazeley LR, Stewart IA, Edwards IR. Pharmacokinetics and sputum penetration of enoxacin after twice daily oral dosing for seven days. Journal of Antimicrobial Chemotherapy 21 (Suppl. B): 61-66, 1988

Fallon RJ, Brown WM. Sensitivity of Legionellaceae, meningococci and mycoplasmas to the quinolones ciprofloxacin and enoxacin. Chemioterapia 4 (Suppl.): 466-467, 1985

Federspil PJ, Lind A, Tiesler E, Schmidt B. Clinical and pharmacokinetic studies on enoxacin in ear, nose and throat infections. Infection 14 (Suppl. 3): S211-S212, 1986

Fong IW, Vandenbroucke A, Simbul M. Penetration of enoxacin into bronchial secretions. Antimicrobial Agents and Chemotherapy 31: 748-751, 1987

Krajewski MJ. Effectiveness of enoxacin in the treatment of chronic suppurative otitis media. Reviews of Infectious Diseases 10 (Suppl. 1): S248, 1988

Lambert HP. Clinical significance of tissue penetration of antibiotics in the respiratory tract. Scandinavian Journal of Infectious Diseases 14 (Suppl.): 262-266, 1978

Maasilta P, Mattson K, Leionen M, Nissinen A, Renkonen O-V. Enoxacin compared with trimethoprim-sulfamethoxazole in the treatment of lower respiratory tract infections in patients with chronic obstructive pulmonary disease. Reviews of Infectious Diseases 10 (Suppl. 1): S221-S222, 1988

Maesen FPV, Beeuweks H, Davies BI, Bujtendijk HJ, Brombacher PJ, et al. Bacampicillin in acute exacerbations of chronic bronchitis – a dose-range study. Journal of Antimicrobial Chemotherapy 2: 279-285, 1976

Marlin GE, Braud PD, Whelan AJ, Somogyi AA. Penetration of enoxacin into human bronchial mucosa. American Review of Respiratory Diseases 134: 1209-1210, 1986

May JR. The bacteriology and chemotherapy of chronic bronchitis. British Journal of Diseases of the Chest 59: 57-65, 1965

Morel C, Vergnaud M, Malbruny B, Bernard Y. Diffusion dans le mucus bronchique de l'énoxacine administrée par voie orale chez l'homme. Pathologie Biologie (Paris) 35: 781-784, 1987

Newsom SWB, Wells FC. Penetration of enoxacin into lung tissue. 15th International Congress of Chemotherapy, Istanbul, 1987

Philip-Joet F, Nourrit J, Frances Y, Arnaud A. Enoxacin in the treatment of lower respiratory tract infections. Journal of Antimicrobial Chemotherapy 21 (Suppl. B): 125-129, 1988

Prigogine P, Glupczynski Y, Carpiaux JP, Blogie M, Yourassowsky E, et al. Enoxacin in acute exacerbations of chronic bronchitis: a comparison with amoxycillin. Journal of Antimicrobial Chemotherapy 21 (Suppl. B): 131-136, 1988

Roberts CM, Batten J, Hodson ME. Ciprofloxacin-resistant *Pseudomonas.* Lancet 1: 1442, 1985

Siporin C, Towse G. Enoxacin: worldwide *in vitro* activity against 22451 clinical isolates. Journal of Antimicrobial Chemotherapy 14 (Suppl. C): 47-55, 1984

Wijnands WJA, Vree TB, van Herwaarden CLA. Enoxacin decreases the clearance of theophylline in man. British Journal of Clinical Pharmacology 20: 583-588, 1985

Wijnands WJA, Van Griethuysen AJA, Vree TB, Van Klinkeren B, van Herwaarden CLA. Enoxacin in lower respiratory tract infections. Journal of Antimicrobial Chemotherapy 18: 719-727, 1986

Wijnands WJA, Vree TB, Baars AM, van Herwaarden CLA. Pharmacokinetics of enoxacin and its penetration into bronchial secretions and lung tissue. Journal of Antimicrobial Chemotherapy 21 (Suppl. B): 67-77, 1988

Wise R, Lockley R, Webberly M, Adhami ZN. The pharmacokinetics and tissue penetration of enoxacin and norfloxacin. Journal of Antimicrobial Chemotherapy 14 (Suppl. C): 75-81, 1984

Author's address: *M.J. Wood,* Department of Communicable Diseases, East Birmingham Hospital, Birmingham, B9 5ST (United Kingdom).

Clinical Pharmacokinetics 16 (Suppl. 1): 46-51 (1989)
0312-5963/89/0001-0046/$3.00/0

Review of Tissue Penetration and Clinical Efficacy of Enoxacin in Skin and Skin Structure Infections and in Osteomyelitis

George A. Pankey

Department of Infectious Diseases, Ochsner Clinic and Ochsner Foundation Hospital, New Orleans, Louisiana, USA

Summary *Enoxacin achieves a high penetration into skin tissue and blister fluid, reaching a maximum serum concentration (C_{max}) of 3.7 mg/L at a time to reach maximum concentration (t_{max}) of 1.9 hours and a blister-fluid C_{max} of 2.9 mg/L at a t_{max} of 3.7 hours after an oral dose of 600mg. The half-life of enoxacin is 6.2 hours in serum and 7.2 hours in blister fluid.*

In a multicentre, open, non-comparative trial, clinical cure or improvement in skin or skin structure infections was achieved after oral administration of enoxacin 200 to 600mg twice daily in 88% of 196 evaluable patients. Overall satisfactory bacteriological response was obtained in 76% of patients. In a multicentre, randomised, double-blind trial comparing oral enoxacin 400mg twice daily with cephalexin 500mg twice daily, satisfactory clinical outcome was achieved in 92% of 73 evaluable patients receiving enoxacin and in 99% of 72 evaluable patients receiving cephalexin. Furthermore, there was no statistically significant difference between the bacteriological efficacy of the 2 agents. In 3 single-centre trials, satisfactory clinical results were achieved in 75 to 100% of patients, and satisfactory bacteriological results occurred in 47 to 76% of patients after administration of oral enoxacin 400mg twice daily for 7 to 14 days.

In vitro *uptake of enoxacin in bone leads to a concentration of 300 μg/g, with 83% being retained by bone after 3 washings with saline at pH 7.2. Clinical trials involving oral enoxacin in osteomyelitis are currently under way.*

Enoxacin is a third generation, 4-quinolone bactericidal antimicrobial agent. It is of clinical value in the treatment of a variety of infections, including uncomplicated and complicated urinary tract infections, respiratory tract infections, enteric infections, sexually transmitted diseases, osteomyelitis, and infections of the skin and skin structures (Kietzmann 1986; Neuman 1988; Shah & Frech 1986; Wijnands 1986; Williams 1986).

The clinical efficacy of enoxacin depends to a major degree on the agent's pharmacokinetic properties. This article summarises the pharmacokinetic properties that relate particularly to infections of the skin and skin structures. The results of the major clinical trials of enoxacin in the treatment of these infections are presented. Pharmacokinetic data which relate to the clinical value of enoxacin in infections of bone are also reviewed.

Table I. Pharmacokinetic parameters measured in serum and blister fluid after oral administration of enoxacin 600mg (after Wise et al. 1986)

Parameter	Serum	Blister fluid
C_{max} (mg/L)	3.7 ± 0.5	2.9 ± 0.5
t_{max} (h)	1.9 ± 1.0	3.7 ± 1.0
$t_{1/2}$ (h)	6.2 ± 1.1	7.2 ± 2.5

1. Pharmacokinetics

1.1 Tissue Penetration

Enoxacin has pharmacokinetic properties very appropriate for use in the oral therapy of infections of the skin and skin structures (table I). It is well absorbed from the gastrointestinal tract and has an oral bioavailability (capsule formulation) of 89% (Chang et al. 1988). A biological plate diffusion technique was used to detect levels of enoxacin in serum: *Escherichia coli* SCH 12655 was used as the indicator organism, and antibiotic medium No. 1 (CM 327 Oxoid), pH 6.6, was used for growth. Standards were prepared in human serum. Assay plates were incubated overnight in air at 37°C. The lower limit of sensitivity was 0.01 mg/L for enoxacin. High serum concentrations are achieved: oral enoxacin in a dose of 600mg resulted in a maximum serum concentration (C_{max}) of 3.7 ± 0.5 mg/L at a mean time to reach maximum concentration (t_{max}) of 1.9 ± 1.0 hours after administration (Wise et al. 1986). Furthermore, a C_{max} of 2.9 ± 0.5 mg/L was achieved in cantharides-induced blister fluid within 3.7 ± 1.0 hours after administration, with the drug remaining in the blister fluid for at least 12 hours at a concentration greater than that in serum (Wise et al. 1986). These concentrations are above the minimum inhibitory concentrations (MICs) of enoxacin for many pathogenic organisms involved in these infections (Parish & Witkowski 1986). For example, the ranges of MIC_{90} for *Proteus mirabilis, Pseudomonas aeruginosa,* methicillin-sensitive *Staphylococcus aureus* and *Staphylococcus epidermidis* are 0.25 to 1, 0.5 to 4, 2 to 8 and 1 to 8 mg/L, respectively (Parish & Witkowski 1986). However, streptococci do not fall within the therapeutic spectrum of enoxacin.

1.2 Half-Life

The half-life ($t_{1/2}$) of enoxacin is 6.2 ± 1.1 hours in serum and is even longer, 7.2 ± 2.5 hours, in blister fluid (Wise et al. 1986). These half-lives of enoxacin allow twice-daily dosing; a great convenience for patients and a supporter of patient compliance. Enoxacin thus arrives in dermal tissues and tissue fluid (as indicated by its concentration in experimentally induced blister fluid), where it achieves effective maximal concentration within 3 to 5 hours. Its half-life enables the maintenance of bactericidally effective concentrations with dosing every 12 hours.

1.3 Burn Transudate Concentration

Van der Auwera et al. (1986) studied the pharmacokinetics and toxicity of oral enoxacin in 13 severely burned patients (mean 3° burned body surface area, 29.7%). Enoxacin was given in a dose of 400mg, twice daily for 7 doses. Mean creatinine levels were less than 1 mg/dl. No toxicity was observed and the tolerability of the drug was noted to be excellent. Serum C_{max} was 1.06 mg/L and t_{max} was 0.5 to 1.0 hours after the first dose, and they were 1.17 mg/L and 2 hours, respectively, after the seventh dose. C_{max} and t_{max} in burn transudate were 0.25 mg/L and 4 hours, respectively, after the first dose and 0.29 mg/L and 4 hours after the seventh dose.

These pharmacokinetic considerations serve as an important basis for the results of clinical trials of enoxacin in the treatment of skin and soft tissue infections.

2. Multicentre Trials

2.1 Non-Comparative Open Trial

A multicentre, non-comparative, open trial of oral enoxacin 200 to 600mg twice daily in the treatment of skin and skin structure infections was carried out by 15 investigators in 5 countries and similar protocols were used. The following data are a composite of those from all study centres (personal communication, Warner-Lambert Company); individual studies have been reported elsewhere (Mensing 1985, 1986; Petri & Tronnier 1986).

The mean age of the 292 patients entered into the study (166 men, 126 women) was 51.3 years (range 12 to 94 years). Therapy was completed by 263 patients (90%), and the mean duration of treatment was 9.3 days (range 1 to 87 days). Adverse experiences resulted in the withdrawal of 23 patients (8%), and 6 patients (2%) withdrew from the study for other reasons, including resistant baseline pathogens in 3 cases. A major reason for elimination of patients from evaluation was failure to isolate a baseline pathogen. Of the 196 patients (74%) who were evaluable at the end of the trial, 4 patients had cellulitis, 25 had impetigo, 22 had folliculitis, 29 had superficial wound infections, 46 had leg ulcers, 7 had chancroid, 26 had multiple infections and 37 had other types of skin or skin structure infections, including abscesses, pyodermas, acne and infected sebaceous cysts.

Of the 196 evaluable patients, 88% had a satisfactory clinical outcome, i.e. there was either clinical cure (complete disappearance of all signs and symptoms of infection, including fever) or improvement (satisfactory, but not complete, remission of signs and symptoms of infection). The highest failure rate (28%) was seen with leg ulcers, which are notoriously difficult to clear of infection and cure because of underlying vascular disease.

Overall, there was a 76% satisfactory bacteriological response rate. Eradication of the baseline pathogen was considered a satisfactory bacteriological response, even if the baseline pathogen was replaced by another pathogen. *S. aureus* was the most frequently encountered pathogen; it was present as a single pathogen in 29% of cases and was alone or 1 of multiple pathogens in 40% of patients eligible for analysis of bacteriological efficacy.

Satisfactory bacteriological response rates were 71% for *S. aureus* (35 of 49 patients) 100%, for *S. epidermidis* (10 of 10), 82% for *P. aeruginosa* (8 of 9) and 81% for *P. mirabilis* (13 of 16). When 2 pathogens were identified at baseline, there was a 77% satisfactory response.

Thus, in this multicentre study, overall satisfactory clinical response was obtained in 88% of patients, and overall satisfactory bacteriological response was obtained in 76% of patients.

2.2 Double-Blind Comparison with Cephalexin

In another pivotal multicentre study, enoxacin was compared with cephalexin in the treatment of patients with skin and skin structure infections. Six different investigators in the United States carried out identical randomised double-blind protocols which involved the administration of either 400mg of enoxacin or 500mg of cephalexin every 12 hours for 7 days.

Enoxacin was given to 121 patients and cephalexin to 114 patients. No patient had a history of prior treatment failure with cephalexin. Patients were enrolled only if they had superficial skin or skin structure infections, including conditions such as folliculitis, impetigo, infected eczema, cellulitis or ulcers, infected surgical sites or infected cysts. Clinical response was evaluated at the end of therapy on day 7; bacteriological response was evaluated on day 7 and at a follow-up evaluation on day 14. The following data are combined for all study centres (personal communication, Warner-Lambert Company); reports from individual study centres have appeared elsewhere (King & Vire 1985; Parish & Witkowski 1986).

Of 121 patients receiving enoxacin, 102 were evaluable, and of 114 patients receiving cephalexin, 99 were evaluable. After excluding patients whose baseline pathogens were not susceptible to the antimicrobial agents and those in whom no baseline pathogen was identified, there remained 73 enoxacin patients and 72 cephalexin patients available for analyses of clinical efficacy. 52 patients in the enoxacin treatment group and 56 patients in the cephalexin group were available for analyses of bacteriological efficacy at the end of treatment.

A satisfactory clinical outcome, i.e. cure or improvement, was achieved in 92% of patients receiving enoxacin and 99% of those receiving cephalexin ($p = 0.04$). It may be relevant that a greater percentage of patients in the enoxacin group than in the cephalexin group (31% versus 18%) had infections for 4 weeks or longer before the institution of the study medications. Four of the 6 clinical failures in the enoxacin group occurred in patients who had had long-standing infections. Moreover, 4 of these clinical failures had *S. aureus* as a pathogen and 2 had other species of *Staphylococcus*. The single failure in the cephalexin group had both a non-aureus staphylococcus and a diphtheroid at baseline.

There was no statistically significant difference between the 2 groups regarding satisfactory bacteriological response, either at the end of therapy (enoxacin 67% satisfactory, versus cephalexin 71%) or at the short term follow-up (enoxacin 76% satisfactory, versus cephalexin 77%).

This study demonstrated that both enoxacin and cephalexin were clinically and bacteriologically effective in the treatment of skin and skin structure infections. Both treatments were well tolerated. Of a total of 114 patients in the cephalexin group, 1 was withdrawn because of moderate CNS effects. Seven of 121 patients treated with enoxacin were withdrawn because of adverse events, which consisted of abdominal cramping, bloating and diarrhoea (1 patient), mild nausea (4 patients), mild rash (1 patient) and mild anxiety and dizziness (1 patient).

3. *Single-Centre Studies*

3.1 Non-Comparative Open Trials

Kietzmann (1986) conducted an independent clinical study of enoxacin in the treatment of bacterial skin diseases. It was an open non-comparative study involving 20 men between the ages of 25 and 80 years. They were given oral enoxacin 400mg twice daily for 7 to 14 days.

Clinical cure or improvement was seen in 88% of the 18 patients who completed the study. In addition, pathogens were eradicated in 11 of the 18 patients (61%), and there were no recurrences. The only adverse effect ascribed to enoxacin was nausea in 1 patient.

Ten patients had infected vascular ulcers, conditions in which bacterial cure is rarely achieved, even though results are satisfactory from a clinical viewpoint. This may partly explain the difference between the 88% clinical success rate and the 61% bacterial success rate in the study.

In a similar open study, Quintero-Perez et al. (1986) administered oral enoxacin 400mg twice daily for a mean duration of 10 days. Of the 21 patients included in the study, 8 had abscesses, 5 cellulitis, 5 infected ulcers and 3 infected wounds. Most lesions were on the lower extremities and were acute, severe, and present in patients with non-insulin-dependent diabetes mellitus. 16 of the 21 patients (76%) had complete clinical and bacteriological resolution. Enoxacin was well tolerated, and no side effects were noticed. Therapy resulted in the elimination of 9 of 9 (100%) Gram-positive pathogens, 15 of 18 (83%) Enterobacteriaceae, and 1 of 2 (50%) *P. aeruginosa*.

3.2 Comparison with Cephalexin

Fraki et al. (1986) compared enoxacin with cephalexin in the treatment of moderate to severe skin infections (mainly impetigo and infected superficial wounds). 61 patients were randomised to treatment with either oral enoxacin 400mg twice daily or oral cephalexin 500mg 3 times daily for 7 to 14 days.

Satisfactory clinical response (cure or improvement) was 100% for the enoxacin group and 91% for the cephalexin group. Satisfactory bacteriological outcome (eradication of initial pathogen or eradication plus reinfection) was 67% in the enoxacin group and 84% in the cephalexin group. The differences in clinical and bacteriological outcome between the treatment groups were not statistically significant. No severe side effects or laboratory abnormalities due to therapy were noted with either agent. However, 9 enoxacin-treated patients and 5 cephalexin-treated patients experienced adverse effects (nausea, vomiting and diarrhoea) that were considered to be related to treatment. Enoxacin was regarded as a good treatment modality for skin infections, especially those due to Gram-negative bacteria.

4. Bone Infections

The newer quinolones are able to penetrate into inorganic bone in significant concentrations (Bauernfeind et al. 1985), thus contributing to their promise as oral therapy for osteomyelitis. Most cases of osteomyelitis are caused by *S. aureus* or *P. aeruginosa* (Bauernfeind et al. 1985); no oral antibacterial agents other than the quinolones have both of these organisms within their spectrum of activity.

Bauernfeind et al. (1985) have found, as a result of *in vitro* studies of 5 quinolones (ciprofloxacin, norfloxacin, ofloxacin, pefloxacin, enoxacin), that these agents are taken up in high concentrations by inorganic bone. There is no major difference in their uptake in bone or their elution from bone by washing with saline at pH 7.2. Enoxacin achieves a concentration of 300 μg/g in inorganic bone, with 83% of this concentration remaining after 3 washings with saline. Antibacterial activity in pieces of bone previously exposed to ciprofloxacin, ofloxacin, pefloxacin and enoxacin was demonstrated by rapid killing of *S. aureus.*

Studies are now under way to evaluate the clinical efficacy of enoxacin in osteomyelitis. An individual case has been reported of a patient with osteomyelitis of the spine who was cured by oral enoxacin. Osteomyelitis in this instance was due to 2 strains of *P. aeruginosa* (Bailey & Newman 1985). These strains were resistant to tobramycin, amikacin, third generation cephalosporins and semi-synthetic penicillins.

5. Therapeutic Implications

Enoxacin is well absorbed from the gastrointestinal tract, penetrates well into skin and blister fluid and achieves concentrations above MICs for most skin pathogens. In addition, it has a half-life that allows twice-daily dosing. These beneficial pharmacokinetic properties of enoxacin, combined with its clinical and bacteriological efficacy, safety and excellent patient acceptance, as demonstrated in clinical trials, make it a valuable oral agent for the treatment of infections of the skin and skin structures.

The potential for curing osteomyelitis (a condition that has usually required protracted courses of parenteral antibiotics) with an oral antibacterial agent such as enoxacin suggests the possibility of great cost savings and convenience to patients.

References

Bailey RR, Newman E. Oral enoxacin used to cure spinal osteomyelitis due to aminoglycoside-resistant Pseudomonas aeruginosa. New Zealand Medical Journal 98: 508, 1985

Bauernfeind A, Wittmann DH, Holl M, Petermuller C. Uptake of 4-quinolones into inorganic bone and antibacterial activity in the bone. Chemioterapia 4 (Suppl.): 487-488, 1985

Chang T, Black A, Dunky A, Wolf R, Sedman A, et al. Pharmacokinetics of intravenous and oral enoxacin in healthy volunteers. Journal of Antimicrobial Chemotherapy 32 (Suppl. B): 49-56, 1988

Fräki JE, Väätäinen N, Hollmen A. Comparison of enoxacin versus cephalexin in treatment of skin infections. International Symposium on New Quinolones, Geneva, July 17-19, p. 132, 1986

Kietzmann H. Enoxacin treatment of bacterial skin infections and sexually transmitted disease. In Percival A (Ed.) Quinolones – their future in clinical practice, International Congress and Symposium Series, No. 104, pp. 59-64, Royal Society of Medicine Services, London, 1986

King Jr LE, Vire CG. A comparison of enoxacin and cephalexin in the treatment of patients with skin and skin structure infections. In Ishigami J (Ed.) Recent advances in chemotherapy, antimicrobial Section 2, Proceedings of the 14th International Congress of Chemotherapy, pp. 1751-1752, University of Tokyo Press, Kyoto, 1985

Mensing H. Enoxacin in bacterial skin infection: a bacteriologically controlled clinical study. In Ishigami J (Ed.) Recent advances in chemotherapy, antimicrobial Section 2, Proceedings of the 14th International Congress of Chemotherapy, pp. 1753-1754, University of Tokyo Press, Kyoto 1985

Mensing H. Ergebnisse der Behandlung bakterieller Entzündungen der Haut mit Enoxacin. Infection 14 (Suppl. 3): S217-S218, 1986

Neuman M. Clinical pharmacokinetics of the newer antibacterial 4-quinolones. Clinical Pharmacokinetics 14: 96-121, 1988

Parish LC, Witkowski JA. The quinolones and dermatologic practice. International Journal of Dermatology 25: 351-356, 1986

Petri H, Tronnier H. Efficacy of enoxacin in the treatment of bacterial infections of the skin with regard to photosensitization. Infection 14 (Suppl. 3): S213-S216, 1986

Quintero-Perez NP, Perez-Ruvalcaba JA, Morales-Reyes JJ, Huitron-Ramirez JA, Rodreguez-Chagollan JJ, et al. Enoxacin (Enox) in the treatment of skin and skin structure infections (SSI). International Symposium on New Quinolones, Geneva, July 17-19, p. 129, 1986

Shah PM, Frech K. Overview of clinical experience with the quinolones. In Percival A (Ed.) Quinolones – their future in clinical practice, International Congress and Symposium Series No. 104, pp. 29-43, Royal Society of Medicine Services, London, 1986

Van der Auwera P, Martin A, Arnould JP, VanderKelen A, Kets E. Pharmacology of enoxacin given orally in severely burned patients (abstract, p.96) International Symposium on New Quinolones, Geneva, July 17-19, 1986

Wijnands WJA. The use of enoxacin in respiratory tract infection.

In Percival A (Ed.) Quinolones – their future in clinical practice, International Congress and Symposium Series, No. 104, pp. 51-57, Royal Society of Medicine Services, London 1986

Williams G. The use of enoxacin in urinary tract infections. In Percival A (Ed.) Quinolones – their future in clinical practice, International Congress and Symposium Series No. 104, pp. 45-50, Royal Society of Medicine Services, London, 1986

Wise R, Lister D, McNulty CAM, Griggs D, Andrews JM. The comparative pharmacokinetics of five quinolones. Journal of Antimicrobial Chemotherapy 18 (Suppl. D): 71-81, 1986

Author's address: Dr *George A. Pankey*, Department of Infectious Diseases, Ochsner Clinic, 1514 Jefferson Highway, New Orleans, LA 70121 (USA).

Clinical Pharmacokinetics 16 (Suppl. 1): 52-58 (1989)
0312-5963/89/0001-0052/$3.50/0

Enoxacin Absorption and Elimination Characteristics

Roger D. Toothaker

Parke Davis Pharmaceutical Research Division, Warner-Lambert Company, Ann Arbor, Michigan, USA

Summary

Enoxacin, a new fluoroquinolone antibiotic, is rapidly and extensively absorbed after oral administration and has a bioavailability independent of dose and only slightly delayed by concurrent food. Plasma concentrations are similar for both intravenous and oral administration. The $t_{1/2}$ for enoxacin ranges from 4 to 6 hours, which allows effective twice-daily administration without significant accumulation. Plasma enoxacin concentrations may be slightly higher in elderly subjects, but this change does not necessitate dosage adjustment in older patients with adequate renal function. Enoxacin and ciprofloxacin decrease the clearance of coadministered theophylline, whereas ofloxacin does not appear to greatly alter methylxanthine clearance. Maalox® (a magnesium-aluminium hydroxide antacid) significantly decreases the oral bioavailability of ciprofloxacin, ofloxacin and enoxacin, and use of these agents with antacids should be avoided. Enoxacin is a highly effective oral anti-infective agent with excellent bioavailability characteristics, a relatively slow rate of elimination and simple, well-defined requirements for dosage modification in patients with renal dysfunction.

Recent synthetic modifications of the early quinolone anti-infectives, such as nalidixic acid and oxolinic acid, have improved the antibacterial activity and pharmacokinetic characteristics of these agents and resulted in a new class of highly potent, orally absorbed anti-infectives called the fluoroquinolones. Enoxacin, one of the first of these new agents to reach the international market, represents a major advance in the ability to treat successfully a wide range of bacterial infections. The present discussion will focus on the absorption and elimination characteristics of enoxacin which are pertinent to the practical use of the drug.

1. Route of Administration

The absence of oral antibiotics with sufficient antibacterial activity and coverage had previously forced physicians to resort to parenteral therapy for the treatment of serious bacterial infections.

1.1 Oral Bioavailability

The availability of enoxacin as an oral product provides the physician with an alternative to intravenous administration. Enoxacin is rapidly absorbed after oral administration, with maximum plasma concentration (C_{max}) values reached within 0.5 to 3 hours after administration (Somogyi et al. 1987). Enoxacin has been reported to have an oral bioavailability of 89% from capsules (Chang et al. 1988), resulting in maximum plasma drug concentrations sufficient to inhibit susceptible pathogens. The low hepatic extraction of enoxacin limits the effect of first-pass metabolism, a factor which may actually contribute to the lower bioavailability seen for ciprofloxacin (Höffken et al. 1988). This high oral bioavailability for enoxacin is independent of the dose size administered (Chang et al. 1988), which means that a change in the dose size will result in a proportional change in plasma drug concentrations. In contrast, some studies have shown that the bioavailabilities of ciprofloxacin and norfloxacin are less at higher therapeutic dose levels (Borner et al. 1986; Swanson et al. 1983).

1.2 Effect of Food

Co-ingested food has been shown to alter the rate and extent of absorption of many different drugs and can even change the rate at which the body eliminates a drug. The type and extent of such effects depend on many factors, including the type of food ingested (Toothaker & Welling 1980). The influence of food on the oral absorption of enoxacin was studied in 15 healthy subjects (Somogyi et al. 1987). Enoxacin 400mg was given orally after an overnight fast, with a standard carbohydrate breakfast, or with a high fat breakfast. Mean plasma enoxacin concentrations for the 3 treatment regimens are shown in figure 1. The amount of enoxacin absorbed was not changed by the ingestion of food, and food also did not alter the rate of enoxacin elimination. Although the high fat meal did

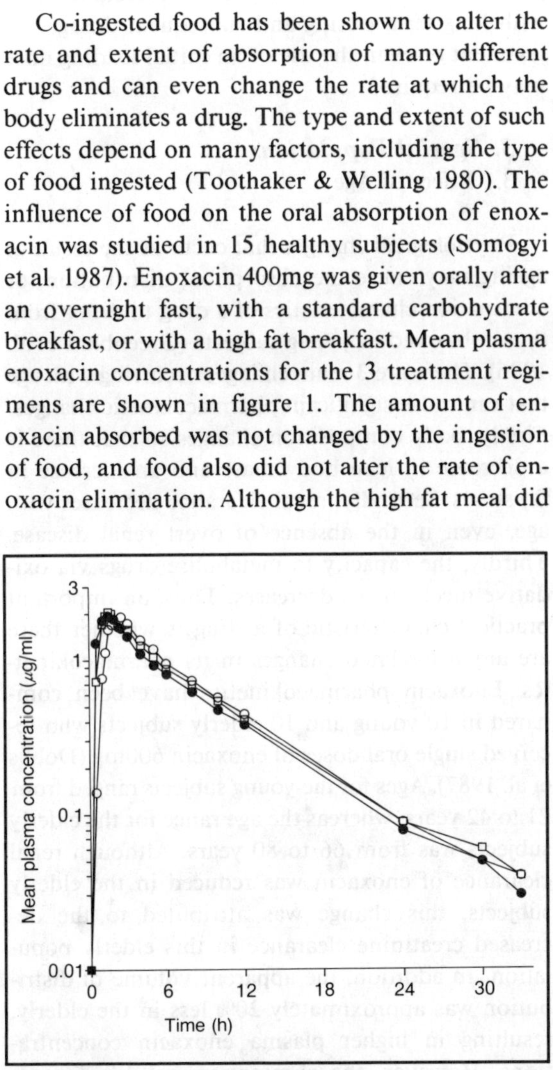

Fig. 1. Effect of a standard carbohydrate (○) or high fat (□) meal compared with an overnight fast (●) on the plasma concentrations of a single oral dose of enoxacin 400mg in 15 healthy subjects (adapted with permission from Somogyi et al. 1987).

not alter the rate of drug absorption, time to reach maximum plasma concentrations (t_{max}) was lengthened by the carbohydrate meal to 2.3 hours compared with 1.4 hours in the fasting subjects. This small shift in t_{max} is not expected to be clinically important, since the peak and trough concentrations of enoxacin were not altered. Thus, patients can take enoxacin whether or not they have eaten. Similar effects of food on drug absorption rates have been observed with ciprofloxacin (Ledergerber et al. 1985), ofloxacin (Kalager et al. 1986) and pefloxacin (Mahr et al. 1988). However, a recent report has suggested that the concurrent administration of food may also slightly decrease ciprofloxacin bioavailability (Gonzalez et al. 1988).

1.3 Comparison with Intravenous Administration

The rapid and extensive oral absorption of enoxacin results in plasma drug concentrations which are similar to those observed after intravenous administration. Concurrent development of an intravenous form of enoxacin will give the physician the option of treating by either route. Figure 2 compares plasma enoxacin concentrations observed after administration of 200mg either orally or as a 1-hour intravenous infusion (Chang et al. 1988). Absolute concentrations and the overall concentration profiles were similar for both routes of administration. Thus, either route should give similar therapeutic effect. Treatment of serious infections which are susceptible to these agents should no longer require parenteral therapy and thus hospitalisation, although patients unable to take oral medication can still benefit from the intravenous formulation of enoxacin.

2. *Elimination*

2.1 Metabolism

Metabolic clearance accounts for about half of the clearance of enoxacin (Chang et al. 1988). Other quinolones such as ofloxacin are mainly eliminated unchanged by the kidneys (Lockley et al. 1984; Wong et al. 1988). These differences in the

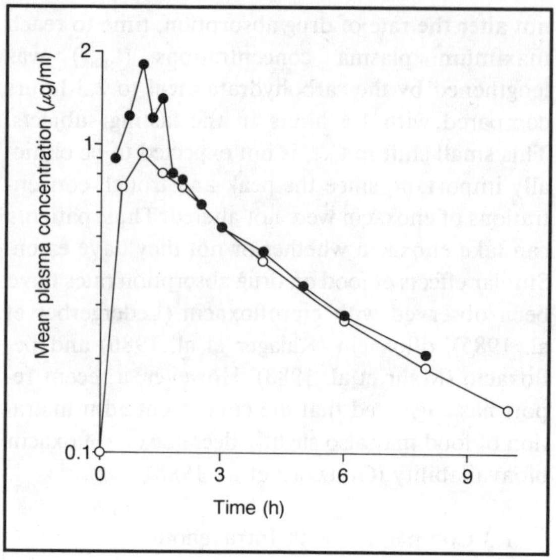

Fig. 2. Mean plasma enoxacin concentration-time profiles for enoxacin 200mg given orally (○) or as a 1-hour intravenous infusion (●) in 8 healthy subjects (adapted with permission from Chang et al. 1988).

renal and hepatic clearances of the quinolones contribute to differences in the effects of renal dysfunction on the pharmacokinetics of the compounds. The metabolites of enoxacin have much less antibacterial activity than the parent drug and achieve much lower concentrations in plasma and urine than seen for the parent drug (Van der Auwera et al. 1985; Vree et al. 1985), which simplifies the therapeutic monitoring of drug concentrations of enoxacin. In contrast, pefloxacin is almost completely demethylated to form the active component norfloxacin, as well as other non-active metabolites (Barre et al. 1984; Sörgel et al. 1988a).

2.2 Rate of Elimination

Even though enoxacin is partially eliminated by metabolism, high concentrations of active unchanged drug are achieved in the urine (Chang et al. 1988). The elimination half-life for enoxacin ($t_{1/2}$) generally ranges from 4 to 6 hours (Wolf et al. 1984), allowing effective twice-daily administration without significant accumulation. In contrast, $t_{1/2}$ values of 0.5 to 2 hours for many β-lactam antibiotics require that these drugs be given 3 to 4 times daily (Barza & Weinstein 1976). Other quinolones exhibit $t_{1/2}$ values of from 10 hours for pefloxacin and fleroxacin (Griggs et al. 1988; Weidekamm et al. 1987) to as long as 28 hours for difloxacin (Granneman et al. 1986), which may make once-daily administration possible for some of these compounds. However, quinolones with $t_{1/2}$ values greater than enoxacin may exhibit accumulation with long term dosing and subsequent dosage adjustment or even the use of an initial loading dose may be required.

3. *Special Populations*

3.1 Effect of Age

Physiological changes that occur as the result of ageing may cause the absorption, distribution, or elimination characteristics of a drug to differ from those observed in young subjects (Greenblatt et al. 1986). There are 3 main changes occurring with age that can cause significant pharmacokinetic changes. Firstly, body composition changes so that there is a decrease in lean body mass and an increase in fat stores. Secondly, renal clearance decreases with age, even in the absence of overt renal disease. Thirdly, the capacity to metabolise drugs via oxidative mechanisms decreases. Thus, an important practical characteristic of a drug is whether there are any age-related changes in its pharmacokinetics. Enoxacin pharmacokinetics have been compared in 10 young and 10 elderly subjects who received single oral doses of enoxacin 600mg (Dobbs et al. 1987). Ages for the young subjects ranged from 21 to 42 years, whereas the age range for the elderly subjects was from 66 to 80 years. Although renal clearance of enoxacin was reduced in the elderly subjects, this change was attributed to the decreased creatinine clearance in this elderly population. In addition, the apparent volume of distribution was approximately 20% less in the elderly, resulting in higher plasma enoxacin concentrations. However, the elimination half-life for enoxacin was similar for both groups of subjects, apparently because of the similar decreases in both clearance and volume of distribution in the elderly.

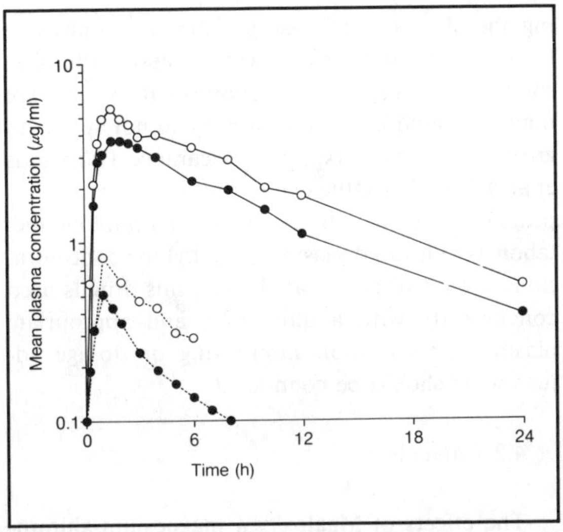

Fig. 3. Mean plasma concentrations for single oral doses of enoxacin 400mg in 10 young (●—●) and 10 elderly (○—○) subjects or ciprofloxacin 100mg in 6 young (●···●) and 9 elderly (○···○) subjects (adapted with permission from Dobbs et al. 1987 and Ball et al. 1986).

Thus, plasma enoxacin concentrations may be slightly higher in elderly subjects because of a decrease in the apparent volume of distribution, but this change does not necessitate a dosage adjustment. Furthermore, the elimination characteristics of the drug should not be altered in older patients with adequate renal function. As shown in figure 3, similar results have been observed for ciprofloxacin (Ball et al. 1986) but maximum plasma concentrations and the area under the plasma concentration-time curve for ciprofloxacin in elderly subjects were more than twice those for young subjects. In elderly subjects receiving ofloxacin 200mg orally every 12 hours, the elimination half-life increased from about 6 hours on day 1 to almost 18 hours on day 7 (Graber et al. 1988). This change in ofloxacin half-life in the elderly was accompanied by significant drug accumulation, which was not observed in young subjects given the same drug regimen. In contrast, when enoxacin 200mg was given orally twice daily to elderly patients with urinary tract infections (Wise et al. 1987), steady-state plasma concentrations were reached within 3 days and enoxacin elimination half-lives were similar to those seen in young subjects. The investigators concluded that enoxacin dosage adjustment was not necessary.

3.2 Effect of Renal Dysfunction

Decreased drug elimination rates in the elderly have been correlated with observed decreases in renal or hepatic function. The effects of such types of dysfunction differ between drugs, depending on the percentage of dose eliminated by each of the 2 elimination processes. Enoxacin is less affected by renal dysfunction than ofloxacin, as shown in the plot (fig. 4) of the 2 drugs in patients with creatinine clearances (Cl_{cr}) of 15 to 30 ml/min (Fillastre et al. 1987; Nix et al. 1988). Consequently, enoxacin can be used without dosage adjustment in patients with certain degrees of renal dysfunction, and the dosage adjustment for severe dysfunction is less than that necessary for ofloxacin (table I). The dosage interval should be doubled (or the dose halved) when creatinine clearance falls below 20 to 30 ml/min for norfloxacin, ciprofloxacin and en-

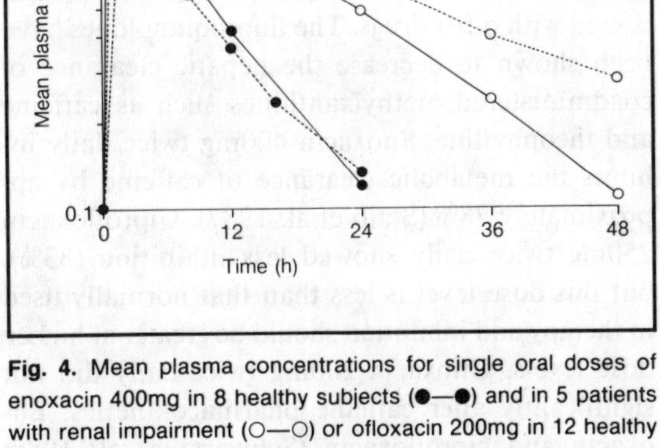

Fig. 4. Mean plasma concentrations for single oral doses of enoxacin 400mg in 8 healthy subjects (●—●) and in 5 patients with renal impairment (○—○) or ofloxacin 200mg in 12 healthy subjects (●···●) and in 7 patients with renal impairment (○···○) [creatinine clearances < 30 ml/min] (adapted with permission from Nix et al. 1988 and Fillastre et al. 1987).

Table I. Recommended dosage interval modifications for the fluoroquinolones in patients with renal dysfunction

	Renal function		References
	< 50 ml/min	< 20 ml/min	
Cip	NC	2×	Boelart et al. 1985
Eno	NC	2×	Nix et al. 1988
Nor	NC	2×	Fillastre et al. 1984
Ofl	2×	4×	Fillastre et al. 1987

Abbreviations: Cip = ciprofloxacin; Eno = enoxacin; Nor = norfloxacin; Ofl = ofloxacin; NC = no change.

oxacin (Boelaert et al. 1985; Fillastre et al. 1984; Nix et al. 1988). The same adjustment is necessary for ofloxacin at Cl_{cr} values less than 50 ml/min, with a 4-fold adjustment necessary at Cl_{cr} values less than 20 ml/min (Fillastre et al. 1987; Mignot et al. 1988). Studies with enoxacin, norfloxacin, ciprofloxacin and ofloxacin have shown that haemodialysis is not an efficient way of clearing quinolones from patients with renal dysfunction (Boelaert et al. 1985; Dorfler et al. 1987; Fillastre et al. 1984; Nix et al. 1988).

4. Drug Interactions

4.1 Methylxanthines

Although these new agents promise to provide excellent activity after oral administration, several important pharmacokinetic interactions have been observed when the fluoroquinolones are coadministered with other drugs. The fluoroquinolones have been shown to decrease the hepatic clearance of coadministered methylxanthines such as caffeine and theophylline. Enoxacin 400mg twice daily inhibits the metabolic clearance of caffeine by approximately 78% (Staib et al. 1987). Ciprofloxacin 250mg twice daily showed less inhibition (33%), but this dose level is less than that normally used in therapy and inhibition should be greater at higher dose levels. Ofloxacin 200mg twice daily did not significantly alter caffeine pharmacokinetics. Enoxacin and ciprofloxacin (Schwartz et al. 1988; Wijnands et al. 1986) also show significant interactions with theophylline, with enoxacin decreasing the clearance of coadministered theophylline by 50 to 60% and a 30% decrease reported for ciprofloxacin. Drugs such as ofloxacin which are mainly cleared by renal processes do not appear to greatly alter methylxanthine clearance (Wijnands et al. 1986). Thus, the extent of this interaction appears to correlate with the extent of quinolone metabolism. Elevated plasma theophylline concentrations should be anticipated when this drug is used concurrently with a quinolone, and appropriate plasma concentration monitoring or dosage adjustments should be conducted.

4.2 Antacids

The effects of Maalox®, a magnesium-aluminium hydroxide antacid, on the oral bioavailability of ciprofloxacin and ofloxacin were examined in 10 healthy subjects (Höffken et al. 1988). Maalox® decreased the oral bioavailability of ciprofloxacin by 91%, and the bioavailability of ofloxacin was decreased by 73%. The effect of antacids on enoxacin bioavailability is similar to that seen with ofloxacin, with bioavailability decreased by 50 or 73% with Maalox® given, respectively, 2 hours or 30 minutes before enoxacin (Schentag et al. 1987). Because of these large decreases in bioavailability when given with antacids, coadministration of all fluoroquinolones with aluminium-magnesium type antacids should be avoided if possible.

4.3 Histamine H_2-Receptor Blocking Agents

The effects of the histamine H_2-receptor blockers ranitidine and cimetidine on quinolone pharmacokinetics have been studied. Ciprofloxacin and ofloxacin are not affected by concurrent ranitidine therapy (Höffken et al. 1988), whereas ranitidine slightly decreases enoxacin bioavailability (Schentag et al. 1987). Although cimetidine decreases the plasma clearance of coadministered pefloxacin by about 26% (Sörgel et al. 1988b), it would be expected to have a smaller effect on other quinolones because they depend less on metabolic clearance than pefloxacin (section 2.1).

4.4 Warfarin

The potential for a pharmacokinetic interaction between warfarin and enoxacin has been studied (Toon et al. 1987). Enoxacin 400mg twice daily for 8 days decreased the clearance of the R-isomer of warfarin, but did not affect the pharmacokinetics of the more pharmacologically active S-isomer. No effect of enoxacin was observed on prothrombin times or Factor VII clotting times. Thus, although clotting times should be monitored when warfarin and enoxacin are coadministered, a clinically significant interaction is not anticipated. Information on the influence of other quinolones on warfarin pharmacokinetics is still awaited.

4.5 Other Agents

Interaction studies between the fluoroquinolones and other agents such as phenytoin (Thomas et al. 1986) and chlorpropamide (Logemann & Ohnhaus 1986) have been reported, but most observed interactions have been relatively minor in nature or are not expected to alter therapeutic efficacy. However, enoxacin appears to decrease the oral bioavailability of glibenclamide (Logemann & Ohnhaus 1986) and coadministration of these 2 drugs should be done with caution.

5. Conclusion

Enoxacin is a highly effective oral anti-infective agent that possesses an excellent bioavailability and slow rate of elimination relative to β-lactam antibiotics. These characteristics, coupled with the relative lack of influence of food on its absorption, make oral enoxacin an easy and convenient drug to administer. Dosage modification in renal dysfunction is simple and well defined. Several of the fluoroquinolone antibacterials exhibit significant interactions with antacids and methylxanthines such as theophylline and caffeine. These interactions, although sufficiently important to require dosage adjustment or even contraindication, are well documented and should not extensively compromise the utility of these agents.

References

Ball AP, Fox C, Ball ME, Brown IRF, Willis JV. Pharmacokinetics of oral ciprofloxacin, 100 mg single dose, in volunteers and elderly patients. Journal of Antimicrobial Chemotherapy 17: 629-635, 1986

Barre J, Houin G, Tillement JP. Dose-dependent pharmacokinetic study of pefloxacin, a new antibacterial agent in humans. Journal of Pharmaceutical Sciences 73: 1379-1382, 1984

Barza M, Weinstein L. Pharmacokinetics of the penicillins in man. Clinical Pharmacokinetics 1: 297-308, 1976

Boelaert J, Valcke Y, Schurgers M, Daneels R, Rousseneu M, et al. The pharmacokinetics of ciprofloxacin in patients with impaired renal function. Journal of Antimicrobial Chemotherapy 16: 87-93, 1985

Borner K, Höffken G, Lode H, Koeppe P, Prinzing C, et al. Pharmacokinetics of ciprofloxacin in healthy volunteers after oral and intravenous administration. European Journal of Clinical Microbiology 5: 179-186, 1986

Chang T, Black A, Dunky A, Wolf R, Sedman A, et al. Pharmacokinetics of intravenous and oral enoxacin in healthy volunteers. Journal of Antimicrobial Chemotherapy 32 (Suppl. B): 49-56, 1988

Dobbs BR, Gazeley LR, Campbell AJ, Edwards IR. The effect of age on the pharmacokinetics of enoxacin. European Journal of Clinical Pharmacology 33: 101-104, 1987

Dorfler A, Shulz W, Burkhardt F, Zichner M. Pharmacokinetics of ofloxacin in patients on haemodialysis treatment. Drugs 34 (Suppl. 1): 62-70, 1987

Fillastre JP, Hannedouche T, Leroy A, Humbert G. Pharmacokinetics of norfloxacin in renal failure. Journal of Antimicrobial Chemotherapy 14: 439, 1984

Fillastre J, Leroy A, Humbert G. Ofloxacin pharmacokinetics in renal failure. Antimicrobial Agents and Chemotherapy 31: 156-160, 1987

Gonzalez M, Magana J, Heyd A, Lettieri J, Krol G, et al. The effect of food on the bioavailability of ciprofloxacin. Pharmaceutical Research 4: S94, 1988

Graber H, Ludwig E, Arr M, Lanyi P. Pharmacokinetics of ofloxacin in young and elderly patients. Reviews of Infectious Diseases 10: S106, 1988

Granneman GR, Kim MS, Shu VS. Difloxacin metabolism and pharmacokinetics in humans after single oral doses. Antimicrobial Agents and Chemotherapy 30: 689-693, 1986

Greenblatt DJ, Abernethy DR, Shader RI. Pharmacokinetic aspects of drug therapy in the elderly. Therapeutic Drug Monitoring 8: 249-255, 1986

Griggs D, Lister D, Andrews J, Wise R. Pharmacokinetics and inflammatory-fluid penetration of pefloxacin. Reviews of Infectious Diseases 10 (Suppl. 1): S98, 1988

Höffken G, Lode G, Wiley R, Glatzel TD, Sievers D, et al. Pharmacokinetics and bioavailability of ciprofloxacin and ofloxacin: effect of food and antacid intake. Reviews of Infectious Diseases 10: S138-S139, 1988

Kalager T, Digranes A, Bergan T, Rebstad T. Ofloxacin: serum and skin blister fluid pharmacokinetics in the fasting and nonfasting state. Journal of Antimicrobial Chemotherapy 17: 795-800, 1986

Ledergerber B, Bettex JD, Joos B, Flepp M, Luthy R. Effect of standard breakfast on drug absorption and multiple-dose pharmacokinetics of ciprofloxacin. Antimicrobial Agents and Chemotherapy 27: 350-352, 1985

Lockley MR, Wise R, Dent J. The pharmacokinetics and tissue penetration of ofloxacin. Journal of Antimicrobial Chemotherapy 14: 647-652, 1984

Logemann C, Ohnhaus E. Enoxacin, a differential inhibitor of the microsomal liver enzyme system in man. International Symposium on New Quinolones, Geneva, Switzerland, 139, 1986

Mahr G, Stephan U, Koch HU, Wiesemann HG. Effect of normal and fat-rich food on the absorption of pefloxacin in humans. Reviews of Infectious Diseases 10: S137-S138, 1988

Mignot A, Couet W, Lefebvre MA, Fourtillan JB, Fillastre JP, et al. Pharmacokinetics of ofloxacin in patients with renal failure. Reviews of Infectious Diseases 10 (Suppl. 1): S108, 1988

Nix DE, Schultz RW, Frost RW, Sedman AJ, Thomas DJ, et al. The effect of renal impairment and haemodialysis on single dose pharmacokinetics of oral enoxacin. Journal of Antimicrobial Chemotherapy 21 (Suppl. B): 87-95, 1988

Schentag JJ, Sedman AJ, Wilton JH, Thomas DJ, Schultz RW, et al. Interactions between enoxacin, ranitidine and antacids. 3rd European Congress of Clinical Microbiology, The Hague, Netherlands, Abstract no. 256, 1987

Schwartz J, Jauregui L, Lettieri J, Bachmann K. Impact of ciprofloxacin on theophylline clearance and steady-state concentrations in serum. Antimicrobial Agents and Chemotherapy 32: 75-77, 1988

Somogyi AA, Bochner F, Keal JA, Rolan PE, Smith M. Effect of food on enoxacin absorption. Antimicrobial Agents and Chemotherapy 31: 638-639, 1987

Sörgel F, Koch H, Malter U, Metz R, Mahr G, et al. Metabolism of pefloxacin in humans. Reviews of Infectious Diseases 10 (Suppl. 1): S95, 1988a

Sörgel F, Mahr G, Koch H, Stephan U, Wiesemann H, et al. Effects of cimetidine on the pharmacokinetics of pefloxacin in healthy volunteers. Reviews of Infectious Diseases 10 (Suppl. 1): S137, 1988b

Staib AH, Harder S, Mieke S, Beer C, Stille W, et al. Gyrase-inhibitors impair caffeine elimination in man. Methods and Findings in Experimental and Clinical Pharmacology 9: 193-198, 1987

Swanson BN, Boppana VK, Vlasses PH, Rotmensch HH, Ferguson RK. Norfloxacin disposition after sequentially increasing oral doses. Antimicrobial Agents and Chemotherapy 23: 284-288, 1983

Thomas D, Humphrey G, Kinkel A, Sedman A, Rowland M, et al. A study to evaluate the potential pharmacokinetic interaction between oral enoxacin and oral phenytoin. Pharmaceutical Research 3: 99S, 1986

Toon S, Hopkins K, Garstang F, Aarons L, Sedman A, et al. Enoxacin-warfarin interaction: pharmacokinetic and stereochemical aspects. Clinical Pharmacology and Therapeutics 42: 33-41, 1987

Toothaker RD, Welling PG. The effect of food on drug bioavailability. Annual Reviews of Pharmacology and Toxicology 20: 173-199, 1980

Van der Auwera P. A profile of *in vitro* studies of the gyrase inhibitor, enoxacin. Journal of International Biomedical Information and Data 6 (Suppl. 1): 19-32, 1985

Vree TB, Baars AM, Wijnands WJA. High-performance liquid chromatography and preliminary pharmacokinetics of enoxacin and its 4-oxo metabolite in human plasma, urine, and saliva. Journal of Chromatography 343: 449-454, 1985

Weidekamm E, Portmann R, Suter K, Partos C, Dell D, et al. Single and multiple-dose pharmacokinetics of fleroxacin, a trifluorinated quinolone, in humans. Antimicrobial Agents and Chemotherapy 31: 1909-1914, 1987

Wijnands WJA, Vree TB, Van Herwaarden CLA. The influence of quinolone derivatives on theophylline clearance. British Journal of Clinical Pharmacology 22: 677-683, 1986

Wise R, Baker S, Misra M, Griggs D. The pharmacokinetics of enoxacin in elderly patients. Journal of Antimicrobial Chemotherapy 19: 343-350, 1987

Wolf R, Eberl R, Dunky A, Mertz N, Chang T, et al. The clinical pharmacokinetics and tolerance of enoxacin in healthy volunteers. Journal of Antimicrobial Chemotherapy 14 (Suppl. C): 63-69, 1984

Wong F, Flor S, Huang SM, Tran-Phan H, Weintraub H. Metabolism of 14C-ofloxacin in healthy male subjects after single dose administration. Pharmaceutical Research 4: S-101, 1988

Author's address: Dr *Roger D. Toothaker*, Parke-Davis Pharmaceutical Research Division, Warner-Lambert Company, 2800 Plymouth Road, Ann Arbor, MI 48105 (USA).

Clinical Pharmacokinetics 16 (Suppl. 1): 59-64 (1989)
0312-5963/89/0001-0059/$3.00/0

Clinical Overview of Enoxacin

Stephen H. Zinner
Department of Medicine, Roger Williams General Hospital, Brown University, Providence, Rhode Island, USA

Summary *Enoxacin is a new fluoroquinolone that will be available as oral and intravenous preparations. This drug is bactericidal for a wide range of organisms, including* Staphylococcus aureus, S. epidermidis, *Enterobacteriaceae and* Pseudomonas aeruginosa. *In addition,* Neisseria gonorrhoeae *is exquisitely susceptible, as is* Branhamella catarrhalis. *The evaluation of the clinical activity of enoxacin is still relatively new, but published studies reveal a good deal of potential in the treatment of infections caused by susceptible bacteria in the urinary tract, upper and lower respiratory tracts, bones and joints, and the gastrointestinal tract. The general use of this drug has been associated with few adverse reactions. Further published data, as well as the results of comparative trials now in progress, will permit a thorough clinical evaluation of this useful drug.*

Enoxacin (1-ethyl-6-fluoro-1, 4-hydro-4-oxl-7-piperazin-1-yl-1,8-naphthyridine-3-carboxylic acid) is a synthetic antibacterial drug of the fluoroquinolone class. The fluoroquinolones, derivatives of nalidixic acid, have been introduced in the past few years with the promise of broad spectrum antibacterial activity, widespread distribution into tissues and body fluids, favourable pharmacokinetics and excellent absorption after oral administration. Like other fluoroquinolones, enoxacin is rapidly bactericidal against a broad spectrum of bacteria. Enoxacin shows rapid concentration-dependent bacterial killing (similar to that of the aminoglycosides), with a long postantibiotic effect and activity against organisms in their stationary phase. The mechanism of action of enoxacin is the inhibition of the A-subunit of bacterial DNA gyrase, the enzyme responsible for the negative supercoiling of bacterial DNA.

The antibacterial spectrum of enoxacin [defined as including organisms with a minimum inhibitory concentration (MIC) ≤ 2.0 mg/L] includes Enterobacteriaceae such as *Escherichia coli* (MIC_{90} = 0.25 mg/L), *Salmonella* and *Shigella* species (MIC_{90} = 0.25 mg/L), *Klebsiella* and *Enterobacter* species (MIC_{90} = 1 mg/L), *Proteus* species (MIC_{90} = 0.5 mg/L), *Serratia marcescens* (MIC_{90} = 1 mg/L), etc.; *Pseudomonas aeruginosa* (MIC_{90} = 2 mg/L), *Yersinia* species (MIC_{90} = 0.25 mg/L), *Neisseria gonorrhoeae* (MIC_{90} = 0.015 mg/L), *N. meningitidis* (MIC_{90} = 0.06 mg/L), *Haemophilus influenzae* (MIC_{90} = 0.12 mg/L); *Legionella* species (MIC_{90} = 0.25 mg/L), *Branhamella catarrhalis* (MIC_{90} = 0.25 mg/L), methicillin-susceptible *Staphylococcus aureus* (MIC_{90} = 1 mg/L), methicillin-resistant *S. aureus* (MIC_{90} = 2 mg/L) and *S. epidermidis* (MIC_{90} = 1 mg/L). Other Gram-positive cocci including *Streptococcus pneumoniae, S. pyogenes* and *Enterococcus faecalis (S. faecalis),* as well as *Listeria monocytogenes, Bacteroides fragilis* and other anaerobic Gram-negative rods, are less susceptible or resistant to enoxacin. *In vitro* activity has been demonstrated against *Chlamydia trachomatis,* but the genital mycoplasma (*Ureaplasma urealyticum*) is resistant (Chin & Neu, 1983; Heifetz et al. 1988).

Enoxacin is formulated for oral and intravenous administration and achieves peak serum concentrations of 3.7 mg/L after administration of a 600mg oral dose. Enoxacin is minimally bound to serum proteins and has a large volume of distribution; it has a serum elimination half-life of approximately 5 hours, justifying the usual 12-hourly dosage intervals (Chang et al. 1988; Wise et al. 1984).

1. Clinical Uses of Enoxacin

1.1 Respiratory Tract Infections

Enoxacin and other quinolones are likely to prove useful for the treatment of infections in the upper and lower respiratory tract caused by susceptible organisms.

With respect to otitis media and sinusitis in adults, enoxacin may prove effective in the treatment of infections caused by *S. aureus, B. catarrhalis* and *H. influenzae. S. pneumoniae* and other streptococci are likely to be non-responsive to enoxacin because of the higher MICs for these bacteria. In several small studies, enoxacin has proven to be an effective antibacterial for the treatment of lower respiratory tract infections caused by susceptible species of Gram-negative rods, including *E. coli, Klebsiella* species, and *P. aeruginosa,* as well as *H. influenzae, B. catarrhalis* and *S. aureus.* Wijnands et al. (1985a) have reported sputum enoxacin concentrations of 2.5 mg/L and 5.2 mg/L after single oral doses of 400mg and 600mg, respectively; mean tissue concentrations after an oral dose of 600mg were much higher at 8.2 mg/L, suggesting considerable accumulation in lung tissue. The authors reported eradication or reduction in growth of *P. aeruginosa* from patients with lower respiratory tract infections treated with 600mg of enoxacin twice daily; 11 of 14 patients showed clinical improvement or cure. In the same study, all 12 patients with chronic obstructive pulmonary disease, bronchiectasis or other lower respiratory tract infections caused by organisms other than *P. aeruginosa* showed cure or improvement, although 2 of the 12 patients had bacteriological evidence of pneumococci present at the end of the therapy.

Wijnands et al. (1986) extended these data to include a total of 45 patients with lower respiratory tract infections who were treated with enoxacin in an open non-comparative trial. *Pseudomonas* species were eradicated from the sputum of 6 of 23 patients from whom they had been cultured before treatment, and the number of organisms were reduced in another 12 of these 23 patients. Clinical improvements occurred in 20 of 23 patients infected with *Pseudomonas* strains and in 19 of 20 patients infected with other organisms. *S. aureus* was not eradicated from the sputum of 2 patients infected with this species. However, pneumococci were eradicated from 3 patients, despite the high MICs reported for the latter species, suggesting that some patients with pneumococcal pneumonia might be successfully treated with enoxacin or other fluoroquinolones, possibly because of accumulation of the drug in lung tissue.

Unfortunately, the eradication of *S. pneumoniae* was not consistently reported. For example, Wijnands et al. (1986), as well as other reports, showed a 2- to 4-fold increase in the MIC for strains of this species remaining in the sputum during therapy. Davies et al. (1984) treated patients with oral enoxacin 600mg twice daily; within 3 days of treatment, *B. catarrhalis, H. influenzae* and *P. aeruginosa* were eradicated from most patients infected with these species, but in 4 of 6 patients infected with *S. pneumoniae,* sputa continued to culture this organism.

In another study in respiratory tract infections, Philip-Joet et al. (1988) reported cure or improvement with a dosage of enoxacin 400mg twice daily in 6 of 8 patients with pneumonia, in 9 of 10 patients with bronchitis and in both patients with bronchiectasis and infection. Bacteriologically, enoxacin resulted in the eradication of *H. influenzae* from all 4 patients, *S. pneumoniae* from 2 of 3 patients, *P. aeruginosa* from all 3 patients and *Legionella pneumophila* from a single infected patient.

Prigogine et al. (1988) compared enoxacin 400mg twice daily with amoxycillin in the treatment of acute exacerbations of chronic bronchitis caused by Gram-negative bacilli. Clinical responses occurred in 83% of enoxacin-treated patients and 93% of amoxycillin-treated patients, with 76% of the presumed pathogens eradicated by enoxacin and 71% by amoxycillin. Enoxacin did not eradicate *P. aeruginosa* from the 2 patients so infected.

Patients with cystic fibrosis infected with *P. aeruginosa* have also been treated with enoxacin, and fair to good clinical improvement has been reported, although the organism usually persists in puta and the MIC may increase (Miller et al. 1985).

Some strains of *Mycobacterium tuberculosis* and *. avium intracellulare* may be susceptible *in vitro* enoxacin and other fluoroquinolones, but clinical ults are limited. Similarly, although the MIC for *pneumophila* is in the susceptible range, clinical erience in the treatment of legionnaires' disease enoxacin has been limited.

hus, although the number of published cases all, enoxacin shows promise as an effective in the oral treatment of respiratory tract ins caused by susceptible organisms.

Urinary Tract Infections

acin, as well as other fluoroquinolones, is ective in the treatment of infections at all of the urinary tract. Approximately 61% of oxacin is excreted unchanged in the urine and another 15% is excreted as an active metabolite. Urinary concentrations after a 600mg oral dose of enoxacin were in excess of 250 mg/L (Wise et al. 1984). In addition, prostatic concentrations after doses of 200mg twice daily for 3 days were in excess of 4 μg/g 4 hours after the last dose (Ranniko & Malmborg 1986). Tissue concentrations in the renal cortex were greater than 9.9 mg/kg after a single 600mg oral dose (Bates & Elder 1988).

Several new trials of enoxacin for the treatment of urinary tract infections have been reported, but not all of them will be reviewed here. As examples, Thomas and Ellis-Pegler (1985) reported cures in 12 of 13 patients with covert bacteriuria or cystitis and in 4 of 7 patients with pyelonephritis treated with 200 or 400mg 12-hourly for 7 to 14 days. Successfully eradicated organisms included *E. coli, S. epidermidis, S. saprophyticus* and *P. mirabilis*. Few patients either failed or were reinfected with *E. faecalis*.

In another study of complicated urinary tract infections, including those in patients with renal transplants, neurogenic bladders, ileal loops and obstructive uropathy with or without indwelling bladder catheters, enoxacin 400mg twice daily orally resulted in clinical cure in 24 of 25 evaluable patients. The infecting organisms (which included *P. aeruginosa, E. coli, Morganella morganii, E. aerogenes, E. faecalis* and some combinations thereof) were all eradicated at the end of therapy. However, 48% of patients had relapsed or were reinfected by 4 to 6 weeks after therapy (Foot et al. 1988).

Huttunen et al. (1988) evaluated 67 elderly patients with urinary infections (53 with pyelonephritis, 17 with indwelling catheters) and reported 100% eradication of the infecting organism at the end of treatment with enoxacin 200 or 400mg twice daily for 4 to 14 days. These organisms included *E. coli, Proteus* species, *Klebsiella* species, *Pseudomonas* species and Gram-positive cocci. However, 30% of these patients were reinfected or had relapsed by 4 to 6 weeks of follow-up.

In a comparative trial of enoxacin with co-trimoxazole in the treatment of patients with complicated urinary tract infections (urethral stricture or stenosis, urinary calculi, neurogenic bladder, prostatitis or prostatic obstruction), Cox (1988) reported clinical cures in all patients in both groups. Microbiological eradication was reported for 87% of the 23 enoxacin-treated patients and for all of the 23 patients treated with co-trimoxazole (not statistically different). Organisms isolated in this trial included *E. coli, K. pneumoniae, P. mirabilis, Enterobacter* species and *S. marcescens*. Although clinical studies are very limited, enoxacin is likely to be effective in the treatment of bacterial prostatitis because of its high concentration in this organ. Additional studies of patients with proven bacterial aetiologies are needed to fully establish a role for enoxacin and other quinolones in these infections.

1.3 Sexually Transmitted Diseases

N. gonorrhoeae is exquisitely susceptible to enoxacin, and enoxacin has been found to be effective in the treatment of infections caused by this organism. For example, Tegelberg-Stassen et al. (1986) treated 123 women with uncomplicated urogenital gonorrhoea with enoxacin 200mg or 400mg as single-dose therapy. Bacteriological cure rates for the 86 evaluable patients were 98.7% in those treated with 200mg and 100% for those who received enoxacin 400mg. Similarly, van der Willigen et al. (1987) treated 155 men with uncomplicated urethral gonorrhoea with enoxacin 200mg or 400mg as a single oral dose. 90% of 77 evaluable patients receiving enoxacin 200mg were culture negative 7 to 14 days after treatment, and 92% of 78 patients who received 400mg had no evidence of *N. gonorrhoeae* at follow-up. Single dose enoxacin was not effective in eradicating *C. trachomatis* from patients in either of these 2 studies. In contrast, in a study reported only in abstract form, enoxacin was effective in removing *C. trachomatis* from the urinary tract of over 80% of the patients (Siboulet et al. 1986). Nonetheless, it is unlikely that single-dose enoxacin therapy will be universally effective in the treatment of *Chlamydia* infections.

In additional studies in gonorrhoea, Siboulet et al. (1988) used 200, 400 and 600mg single doses, as well as 400mg administered twice, in the treatment of 200 patients with uncomplicated urethral or endocervical gonorrhoea. Eradication rates were in excess of 90% with all regimens and were 100% for the 600mg single dose and the 400mg dose administered twice. Various reports in abstract form only have been presented that suggest that single-dose enoxacin therapy is also effective in anorectal and pharyngeal gonococcal infections (Samarasinghe et al. 1986).

A single 1200mg dose of enoxacin compared favourably with trimethoprim 3200mg plus sulfametrole 640mg in the treatment of chancroid (Siboulet et al. 1988).

1.4 Gastrointestinal Infections

The pronounced *in vitro* activity of the quinolones against Enterobacteriaceae makes it likely that enoxacin will be active in the treatment of bacterial diarrhoea caused by susceptible organisms. For example, DeMol et al. (1987) reported the successful eradication of *Shigella* species (many isolates of which were resistant to ampicillin, chloramphenicol and co-trimoxazole) and *Campylobacter jejuni* from 21 patients with bacillary dysentery.

1.5 Use in Immunologically Compromised Patients

Enoxacin and other quinolones are likely
prove useful in the prophylaxis of Gram-negati
rod bacteraemia in neutropenic patients by me
of the eradication of colonic microflora. In
study, Edlund et al. (1987) treated normal vo
teers with enoxacin 400mg twice daily for 7
and showed the suppression or elimination o
ceptible Enterobacteriaceae. There were no
titative increases in numbers of yeasts or
positive cocci during the trial, and no signi
changes in the colony counts of anaerobic
isms were reported.

Two studies have been published in whic
rofloxacin or norfloxacin were used in the prop
laxis of Gram-negative rod bacteraemia in neutropenic patients (Dekker et al. 1987; Karp et al. 1987). Both these trials were associated with a dramatic decrease in the number of episodes of Gram-negative rod bacteraemia, but bacteraemia did occur because of Gram-positive cocci, including *S. pneumoniae* and *E. faecalis*. There are limited published data describing the role of enoxacin as a prophylactic agent.

Enoxacin has not been studied extensively in patients with profound neutropenia and bacteraemia, but it is likely that it might play an important role administered either alone or in combination with other agents in the treatment of these patients. Further studies are needed.

1.6 Supporting Structure Infections

Fluoroquinolones are likely to prove effective in the treatment of osteomyelitis caused by susceptible strains of staphylococci and Gram-negative bacteria. However, published data for enoxacin are not available at this time, although several studies are in progress.

1.7 Other Infections

Although human data pertaining to the use of enoxacin are unavailable at present, experimental animal data reveal the successful treatment of endocarditis and meningitis caused by susceptible strains of bacteria. In addition, good results have been obtained in animal models of intra-abdominal infections. Further studies and published reports are needed to fully evaluate the clinical role of enoxacin, administered intravenously and orally, in the treatment of these and other infections.

2. *Adverse Effects*

Many reports have reviewed the adverse effects of the quinolone antibacterials, and these appear to be shared in large part by all members of this class (Smith 1987). In some studies, certain side effects have been reported in 5 to 25% of patients receiving these drugs, although side effects requiring discontinuation of therapy are less frequent, occurring in 1 to 3% of patients.

Anorexia, nausea, vomiting, diarrhoea and metallic taste are occasionally reported. Rash, pruritus and photosensitivity have also been reported. Crystalluria may occur with each of these drugs, especially at large doses. Adequate fluid intake will minimise this effect.

Various central nervous system effects have been reported with enoxacin and other quinolones; these include tremulousness, anxiety, insomnia, seizures, etc. Patients who are concomitantly treated with theophylline derivatives may be at increased risk of central nervous system toxicity, because the clearance of these compounds is reduced by some quinolones, notably enoxacin (Wijnands et al. 1985b). However, therapeutic monitoring of theophylline or decreasing the theophylline dose by approximately one-half or one-third will usually permit cotreatment with the fluoroquinolones without an increased risk of side effects.

References

Bates SA, Elder MG. An evaluation of pelvic tissue concentrations after oral administration of enoxacin. Journal of Antimicrobial Chemotherapy 21 (Suppl. B): 79-85, 1988

Chang T, Black A, Dunky A, Wolf R, Sedman A, et al. Pharmacokinetics of intravenous and oral enoxacin in healthy volunteers. Journal of Antimicrobial Chemotherapy 21 (Suppl. B): 49-56, 1988

Chin NX, Neu HC. *In vitro* activity of enoxacin, a quinolone carboxylic acid, compared with those of norfloxacin, new beta-lactams, aminoglycosides and trimethoprim. Antimicrobial Agents and Chemotherapy 24: 754-763, 1963

Davies BI, Maesen FPV, Teengs JP. Serum and sputum concentrations of enoxacin after single oral dosing in a clinical and bacteriological study. Journal of Antimicrobial Chemotherapy 14 (Suppl. C): 83-89, 1984

Dekker AW, Rozenberg-Arska M, Verhoef J. Infection prophylaxis in acute leukemia: a comparison of ciprofloxacin with trimethoprim-sulfamethoxazole and colistin. Annals of Internal Medicine 106: 7-12, 1987

De Mol P, Mets T, Lagasse R, Vandepitte J, Mutwewingabo A, et al. Treatment of bacillary dysentery: a comparison between enoxacin and nalidixic acid. Journal of Antimicrobial Chemotherapy 19: 695-698, 1987

Edlund C, Lidbeck A, Kager L, Nord CE. Effect of enoxacin on colonic microflora of healthy volunteers. European Journal of Clinical Microbiology 6: 298-300, 1987

Foot M, Williams G, Want S, Roe M, Quaghebeur G, et al. An open study of the safety and efficacy of enoxacin in complicated urinary tract infections. Journal of Antimicrobial Chemotherapy 21 (Suppl. B): 97-103, 1988

Heifetz CL, Bien PA, Cohen MA, Dombrowski ME, Griffin TJ, et al. Enoxacin: *in-vitro* and animal evaluation as a parenteral and oral agent against hospital bacterial isolates. Journal of Antimicrobial Chemotherapy 21 (Suppl. B): 29-42, 1988

Huttunen M, Kunnas K, Saloranta P. Enoxacin treatment of urinary tract infections in elderly patients. Journal of Antimicrobial Chemotherapy 21 (Suppl. B): 105-111, 1988

Karp, JE, Merz WG, Hendricksen C, Laughon B, Redden T, et al. Oral norfloxacin for prevention of Gram-negative bacterial infections in patients with acute leukemia and granulocytopenia. Annals of Internal Medicine 106, 1-7, 1987

Miller MG, Ghoneim AT, Littlewood JM. Use of enoxacin in a patient with cystic fibrosis. Lancet 1: 646, 1985

Philip-Joet F, Nourrit J, Frances Y, Arnaud A. Enoxacin in the treatment of lower respiratory tract infections. Journal of Antimicrobial Chemotherapy 21 (Suppl. B): 125-129, 1988

Prigogine T, Glupczynski Y, Carpiaux JP, Blogie M, Yourassowsky E, et al. Enoxacin in acute exacerbations of chronic bronchitis: a comparison with amoxycillin. Journal of Antimicrobial Chemotherapy 21 (Suppl. B): 131-136, 1988

Ranniko S, Malmborg A-S. Enoxacin concentration in human prostatic tissue after oral administration. Journal of Antimicrobial Chemotherapy 17: 123, 1986

Samarasinghe PL, Bakhtiar M, Sonex C. The use of enoxacin as single-dose oral treatment of anal and pharyngeal gonorrhea. Second World Congress on Sexually Transmitted Diseases, Paris, June 1986, Abstract C-37-03, 1986

Siboulet A, Bohbot JM, Catalan F. Enoxacine dans le traitement des infections urétro-génitales, à *Neisseria gonorrhoeae* et à *Chlamydia trachomatis*. Second World Congress on Sexually Transmitted Diseases, Paris, June 1986, Abstract C-37-06, 1986

Siboulet A, Bohbot JM, Catalan F. Enoxacin in the treatment of sexually transmitted diseases. Journal of Antimicrobial Chemotherapy 21 (Suppl. B): 119-124, 1988

Smith CR. The adverse effects of fluoroquinolones. Journal of Antimicrobial Chemotherapy 19: 709-711, 1987

Tegelberg-Stassen MJ, van der Willigen AH, van der Hoek JC, Wagenvoort JH, van Vliet HJ, et al. Treatment of uncomplicated urogenital gonorrhoea in women with a single dose of enoxacin. European Journal of Clinical Microbiology 5: 395-398, 1986

Thomas MG, Ellis-Pegler RB. Enoxacin treatment of urinary tract infections. Journal of Antimicrobial Chemotherapy 15: 759-763, 1985

van der Willigen AG, van der Hoek JCS, Wagenvoort JHT, van Vliet HJA, van Klingeren B, et al. Comparative double-blind study of 200- and 400-mg enoxacin given orally in the treatment of acute uncomplicated urethral gonorrhea in males. Antimicrobial Agents and Chemotherapy 31: 535-538, 1987

Wijnands WJA, Van Herwaarden CLA, Van Griethuysen AJA, Vree TB. The effect and safety of enoxacin in lower respiratory tract infections Chemioterapia 4 (Suppl.): 504-506, 1985a

Wijnands WJA, Vree TB, Van Herwaarden A. Enoxacin decreases the clearance of theophylline in man. British Journal of Clinical Pharmacology 20: 583-588, 1985b

Wijnands WJA, van Griethuysen AJA, Vree TB, Van Klingeren B, van Herwaarden CLA. Enoxacin in lower respiratory tract infections. Journal of Antimicrobial Chemotherapy 18: 719-727, 1986

Wise R, Lockley R, Webberly M, Adhami N. The pharmacokinetics and tissue penetration of enoxacin and norfloxacin. Journal of Antimicrobial Chemotherapy 14 (Suppl. C): 75-81, 1984

Author's address: Dr *Stephen H. Zinner*, Head, Division of Infectious Diseases, Brown University, Roger Williams General Hospital, 825 Chalkstone Avenue, Providence, RI 02908 (USA).

t
re
L.
ex
wi

is s
age
fect

1.

Er
very
levels
en